Simulations and Applications of Augmented and Virtual Reality

Simulations and Applications of Augmented and Virtual Reality

Topic Editors

Radu Comes

Dorin-Mircea Popovici

Calin Gheorghe Dan Neamtu

Jing-Jing Fang

MDPI

Basel • Beijing • Wuhan • Barcelona • Belgrade • Novi Sad • Cluj • Manchester

Topic Editors

Radu Comes
Design Engineering and Robotics
Technical University of Cluj-Napoca
Cluj-Napoca
Romania

Dorin-Mircea Popovici
Mathematics and Computer Science
Ovidius University of Constanta
Constanta
Romania

Calin Gheorghe Dan Neamtu
Design Engineering and Robotics
Technical University of Cluj-Napoca
Cluj-Napoca
Romania

Jing-Jing Fang
Department of Mechanical Engineering
National Cheng Kung University
Tainan
Taiwan

Editorial Office
MDPI AG
Grosspeteranlage 5
4052 Basel, Switzerland

This is a reprint of the Topic, published open access by the journals *Applied Sciences* (ISSN 2076-3417), *Computers* (ISSN 2073-431X), *Sensors* (ISSN 1424-8220) and *Virtual Worlds* (ISSN 2813-2084), freely accessible at: https://www.mdpi.com/topics/136V6RM67T.

For citation purposes, cite each article independently as indicated on the article page online and as indicated below:

Lastname, A.A.; Lastname, B.B. Article Title. *Journal Name* **Year**, *Volume Number*, Page Range.

ISBN 978-3-7258-4139-4 (Hbk)
ISBN 978-3-7258-4140-0 (PDF)
https://doi.org/10.3390/books978-3-7258-4140-0

Cover image courtesy of Radu Comes

Contents

virtual worlds

MDPI

Article

Cybersickness in Virtual Reality Questionnaire (CSQ-VR): A Validation and Comparison against SSQ and VRSQ

Panagiotis Kourtesis [1,2,*], Josie Linnell [2], Rayaan Amir [2], Ferran Argelaguet [3,4] and Sarah E. MacPherson [2]

1 Department of Psychology, National and Kapodistrian University of Athens, 15772 Athens, Greece
2 Department of Psychology, University of Edinburgh, Edinburgh EH8 9YL, UK
3 Institut National de Recherche en Sciences et Technologies du Numérique (Inria), de l'Université de Rennes, 35042 Rennes, France
4 Institut de Recherche en Informatique et Systèmes Aléatoires (IRISA), de Centre National de la Recherche Scientifique (CNRS), 35042 Rennes, France
* Correspondence: pkourtesis@psych.uoa.gr

Citation: Kourtesis, P.; Linnell, J.; Amir, R.; Argelaguet, F.; MacPherson, S.E. Cybersickness in Virtual Reality Questionnaire (CSQ-VR): A Validation and Comparison against SSQ and VRSQ. *Virtual Worlds* **2023**, 2, 16–35. https://doi.org/10.3390/virtualworlds2010002

Academic Editors: Radu Comes, Dorin-Mircea Popovici, Calin Gheorghe Dan Neamtu and Jing-Jing Fang

Received: 19 December 2022
Revised: 9 January 2023
Accepted: 17 January 2023
Published: 29 January 2023

Correction Statement: This article has been republished with a minor change. The change does not affect the scientific content of the article and further details are available within the backmatter of the website version of this article.

Abstract: Cybersickness is a drawback of virtual reality (VR), which also affects the cognitive and motor skills of users. The Simulator Sickness Questionnaire (SSQ) and its variant, the Virtual Reality Sickness Questionnaire (VRSQ), are two tools that measure cybersickness. However, both tools suffer from important limitations which raise concerns about their suitability. Two versions of the Cybersickness in VR Questionnaire (CSQ-VR), a paper-and-pencil and a 3D–VR version, were developed. The validation of the CSQ-VR and a comparison against the SSQ and the VRSQ were performed. Thirty-nine participants were exposed to three rides with linear and angular accelerations in VR. Assessments of cognitive and psychomotor skills were performed at baseline and after each ride. The validity of both versions of the CSQ-VR was confirmed. Notably, CSQ-VR demonstrated substantially better internal consistency than both SSQ and VRSQ. Additionally, CSQ-VR scores had significantly better psychometric properties in detecting a temporary decline in performance due to cybersickness. Pupil size was a significant predictor of cybersickness intensity. In conclusion, the CSQ-VR is a valid assessment of cybersickness with superior psychometric properties to SSQ and VRSQ. The CSQ-VR enables the assessment of cybersickness during VR exposure, and it benefits from examining pupil size, a biomarker of cybersickness.

Keywords: cybersickness; virtual reality; SSQ; VRSQ; sensitivity; cognition; reaction time; motor skills; eye tracking; pupil size

1. Introduction

Virtual reality (VR) is a promising form of technology that facilitates applications in many areas, such as education [1], professional training [2], cognitive assessment [3], mental health therapy [4], and entertainment [5]. Nevertheless, beyond the advantages that VR brings to these fields, a limitation of VR is the presence of cybersickness that affects a percentage of users [6]. Cybersickness symptomatology includes nausea, disorientation, and oculomotor symptoms. Although there are similarities between cybersickness and simulator sickness, cybersickness differs from simulator sickness in terms of the frequency and severity of the types of symptoms [7]. Specifically, users experiencing cybersickness report increased general discomfort due to nausea and disorientation-related symptoms [7]. Cybersickness also differs from motion sickness as cybersickness is triggered by visual stimulation, while motion sickness is triggered by actual movement [8].

Although there is not a comprehensive theoretical framework for cybersickness, the most frequent and predominant one is the sensory conflict theory [6,8,9]. This theoretical framework suggests that cybersickness symptomatology stems from a sensorial conflict between the vestibular (inner ear) and the visual system [6,9]. In simple terms, the perception of postural balance relies on a combination of visual, vestibular, and proprioceptive input. Conflicting motion perception cues of the visual, proprioception, and vestibular systems postulate to cause cybersickness. The technological reason for this conflict is vection, an illusory sense of motion that occurs in VR. Vection is one of the main reasons for experiencing cybersickness in VR [10,11]. Specifically, motions such as linear and angular accelerations appear to induce cybersickness in the user.

1.1. Cybersickness, Cognition, and Motor Skills

Beyond the obvious decrease in user experience in VR, cybersickness may also negatively affect the cognitive and/or motor performance of the user. Given that VR is used for applications that require intact cognitive and motor abilities (e.g., educational, research, clinical, and training applications), the presence of cybersickness has serious consequences for the implementation of VR in these applications. Recent systematic reviews of the literature suggest that cybersickness may substantially, yet temporarily, decrease the cognitive and/or motor performance of the user in immersive VR studies [12–14]. Dahlman et al. [15] postulated that motion sickness significantly decreases users' verbal working memory. Comparably, in immersive VR, Varmaghani et al. [16] conducted a study (N = 47) in which the participants formed two groups: a VR group (N = 25) and a control group (N = 22; playing a board game). The results indicated that the VR group did not show an increase in visuospatial processing ability, while the control group did. Thus, this outcome postulated that cybersickness affects visuospatial processing and/or learning ability.

In another study, Mittelstaedt et al. [17] examined cybersickness and cognition (reaction time, spatial processing, visuospatial working memory, and visual attention processing) in pre- and post-sessions in VR. The findings showed that cybersickness modulated a slower reaction speed and prevented an expected improvement in visual processing speed [17]. These results suggest that cybersickness has a negative effect on attentional processing and reaction times, while spatial abilities and visuospatial memory remain intact. In the same vein, the studies of Nalivaiko et al. [18] (N = 26) and Nesbitt et al. [10] (N = 24) examined the effect of cybersickness on reaction times. In both studies, reaction speed substantially slowed. Interestingly, slower reaction times were significantly correlated with an increase in the intensity of cybersickness [10,18], indicating that cybersickness intensity may be associated with temporary cognitive and/or motor decline. However, no study has examined whether cybersickness intensity predicts cognitive or motor decline. Finally, while the above studies support the notion that cybersickness may decrease cognitive and/or motor skills, they all evaluated cybersickness after VR exposure. No study has assessed cybersickness during exposure.

1.2. Cybersickness Questionnaires

The Simulator Sickness Questionnaire (SSQ) is a 4-point Likert scale that was designed to assess simulator sickness in aviators [19]. The SSQ is the tool that has been used most frequently to measure cybersickness due to exposure to VR [13]. However, simulator sickness differs from cybersickness symptomatology. In the latter, disorientation and nausea symptoms are more frequent and intense [7]. Thus, despite its use in VR studies, the SSQ is not specific to cybersickness symptoms that a user may experience in VR. Indeed, a recent study showed that the SSQ does not have adequate psychometric properties to evaluate cybersickness in VR [20]. However, there is a variant of the SSQ, namely the VR sickness questionnaire (VRSQ), that was recently developed [21] using items directly derived from the SSQ. In the development and validation study of the VRSQ, researchers attempted to isolate the items of the SSQ that are pertinent to cybersickness [21]. Nevertheless, this development and validation study suffered from serious limitations. Firstly, the sample size was small (i.e., 24 participants), and the stimuli diversity was limited. Notably, the factor analyses accepted only items pertinent to oculomotor and disorientation symptoms, while they rejected all items pertinent to nausea (i.e., 7 items) [21]. The latter is very problematic because it is well-established that nausea is the second (after disorientation) most frequent type of symptom of cybersickness [7,22–24]. Furthermore, both the SSQ and the VRSQ examine symptoms after VR exposure (not during) and produce scores that cannot be easily interpreted. Finally, when developing the SSQ and the VRSQ, the available guidelines for designing and developing a Likert scale tool were not considered.

There is scientific consensus regarding the design of Likert scale questionnaires. The literature suggests that a 7-point Likert scale is substantially better than a 5-point (or less) one [25–28]. The 7-point design offers a greater variety of responses, which better captures the diversity of the individuals' views or experiences. Furthermore, combining numbers (e.g., 6) with corresponding text (e.g., strongly disagree) facilitates a better understanding of the differentiation between the available responses [25–28]. These suggestions have been considered and adopted in the development of the VR Neuroscience Questionnaire (VRNQ) and the Cybersickness in VR Questionnaire (CSQ-VR) [29]. The CSQ-VR is derived from the VR Induced Symptoms and Effects (VRISE) section of the VR Neuroscience Questionnaire (VRNQ), which has been found to have very good structural and construct validity [29]. Additionally, the VRISE section of the VRNQ has been validated against the SSQ and the Fast Motion Sickness Scale [30]. The advantages of the VRISE over the SSQ pertain to its short administration (only 5 items/questions) and its production of easily comprehensible outcomes [30]. However, the scoring of the VRISE is inverse (i.e., higher scores indicate milder symptom intensity). In addition, oculomotor symptoms were assessed by only one question in the VRISE.

The CSQ-VR was designed in line with the aforementioned guidelines (i.e., using a 7-point scale and combining text with numbers), while also addressing the previous shortcomings (i.e., inverse scoring and one oculomotor question) of the VRISE section of the VRNQ. The CSQ-VR assesses the whole range of cybersickness symptoms, including nausea, disorientation, and oculomotor symptoms. There are two questions for each type of symptom. Each question is presented on a 7-item Likert Scale and the responses are offered in the form of combined text and numbers, ranging from "1-absent feeling" to "7-extreme feeling". The CSQ-VR produces a total score and three sub-scores: nausea, disorientation, and oculomotor. Each sub-score corresponds to a type of symptom and is calculated by adding the two corresponding responses. The total score is the sum of the three sub-scores. The design of the CSQ-VR yielded the maintenance of the advantages associated with the VRISE of the VRNQ (i.e., very short administration, easy and interpretable scoring, comprehensible questions and responses, and an examination of all types of cybersickness symptoms) and the improvement of the weaker aspects (i.e., the addition of one more oculomotor question and positive scoring, where larger numbers indicate stronger symptoms). Finally, the CSQ-VR was not only developed in a paper-and-pencil form, but also in a 3D form that can be used in any virtual environment to examine cybersickness while the user is in VR. This VR version of the CSQ-VR also benefits from eye tracking to measure gaze fixations and pupil size (i.e., pupillometry). Because pupil size is associated with negative emotions [31], pupillometry may offer a physiological metric of cybersickness intensity.

1.3. Research Aims

This study aims to examine the validity of the paper-and-pencil version and the VR version of the CSQ-VR in detecting and evaluating cybersickness symptoms. The validity is examined against that of the SSQ and the VRSQ, which are considered valid tools to measure cybersickness. Furthermore, as there is an association between cybersickness and cognitive and motor performance, this study offers a comparison between the CSQ-VR (both versions), the SSQ, and the VRSQ in detecting temporary cognitive and/or motor decline due to cybersickness. The VR version of the CSQ-VR is expected to facilitate an ongoing examination of cybersickness while the user is immersed. Finally, the utility of pupillometry in predicting cybersickness intensity is also be explored.

2. Materials and Methods

2.1. Virtual Environment Development

The virtual environment was developed using the Unity3D game engine. The interactions with the environment were developed using SteamVR SDK. Because gaming experience may modulate task performance [3], the virtual hands/gloves of SteamVR SDK were used to ensure an ergonomic and effortless interaction. Notably, none of the interactions required button presses. Instead, interactions were facilitated by simply touching the object (initial selection) and continuously touching the object (to confirm the selection). In addition, SteamVR virtual hands/gloves do not represent any gender or race, so their utilization prevents confounding effects from these variables [32].

To ensure an understanding and the seamless completion of the tasks, users received instructions in video, audio, and written form. For each task's instructions, audio clips with neutral naturalistic voices were produced using Amazon Polly. The audio feedback was spatialized using the SteamAudio plugin. SRapinal SDK was used for eye tracking and facilitating pupillometry. Finally, randomization of the experimental blocks within and between participants and the extraction of the data into a CSV file, as well as the facilitation of the experimental design and control, were achieved using bmlTUX SDK [33].

Linear and Angular Accelerations in VR

Based on the relevant literature, linear and angular accelerations are efficient in inducing significant cybersickness symptoms in users in a relatively short time (e.g., 5–10 min) [10,12,13,18,24,29,34]. Correspondingly, a ride of 5 min was developed. Because the ride had to be repeated three times (i.e., a total 15 min ride) for each participant, a 5 min duration was preferred. The ride was designed as an animation of the platform that the user was standing on (see Figure 1). The direction of motion was always forward (except in the last stage; see reversed *z*-axis). The movements of the platform were similar to those of a roller coaster. The ride included the following accelerations in this specific order: (1) linear (*z*-axis); (2) angular (*z*- and *y*-axes); (3) angular (*z*-, *x*-, and *y*-axes); (4) angular (roll axis); (5) extreme linear (*z*-axis); (6) angular (yaw axis); and (7) extreme linear (*y*-axis followed by reversed *z*-axis). The environment had simple black-and-white surroundings (see Figure 1). This background was used to ensure that the symptoms were strictly induced by vection and not due to other reasons, such as intense colors. Additionally, having the squared/tiled design offered cues for the participants to perceive vection and altitude changes.

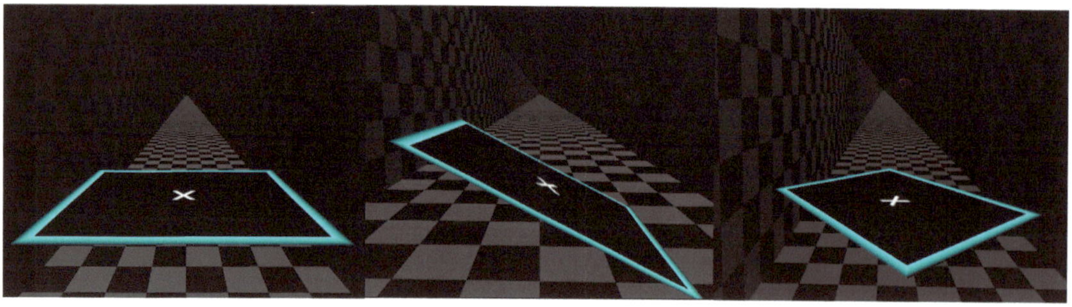

Figure 1. Examples of Linear (**Left**) and Angular (**Centre** and **Right**) Accelerations during the Ride.

2.2. Cognitive and Psychomotor Skills' Assessment

The aims of this study required the examination of cybersickness, cognition, and motor skills to be repeated while the user was immersed in VR. For these reasons, immersive VR versions of well-established tests were developed. For the development of these VR cognitive and psychomotor tasks, the specific design and development guidelines and recommendations for cognitive assessments in immersive VR were followed [35].

2.2.1. Verbal Working Memory

A VR version of the Backward Digit Span Task (BDST; [36]) was developed and used. The VR BDST requires participants to listen to a series of digits and remember and recall them in the reverse order of their presentation. For example, when the digits were 2, 4, and 3, then participants had to respond in the reverse order (i.e., 3, 4, and 2). Therefore, the first step involved listening to the digits. After this step, a keypad appeared in front of the participants. Using the keypad, users had to provide the digits in the reverse order. To indicate a number, participants had to touch the white box button displaying the equivalent number (see Figure 2). Continuous touch of the button for one second confirmed the response. After confirmation, if the response was correct, the button turned green and made a positive sound. In contrast, if the response was incorrect, then the button turned orange and made a negative sound. When a mistake was made or all the digits were provided correctly, the trial ended. In every second successful trial, the length of the digit sequence increased. When the participant made two subsequent mistakes within the same digit sequence length (e.g., 3 digits), or when they finished the last trial (i.e., second trial with a sequence length of 7 digits), then the task ended. The total score of the VR BDST was determined by adding together the total number of correct trials and the highest digit sequence length that was performed in at least one trial. A video displaying the task and its procedures can be found here: https://www.youtube.com/watch?v=1H8cqci-lFs (accessed on 16 January 2023).

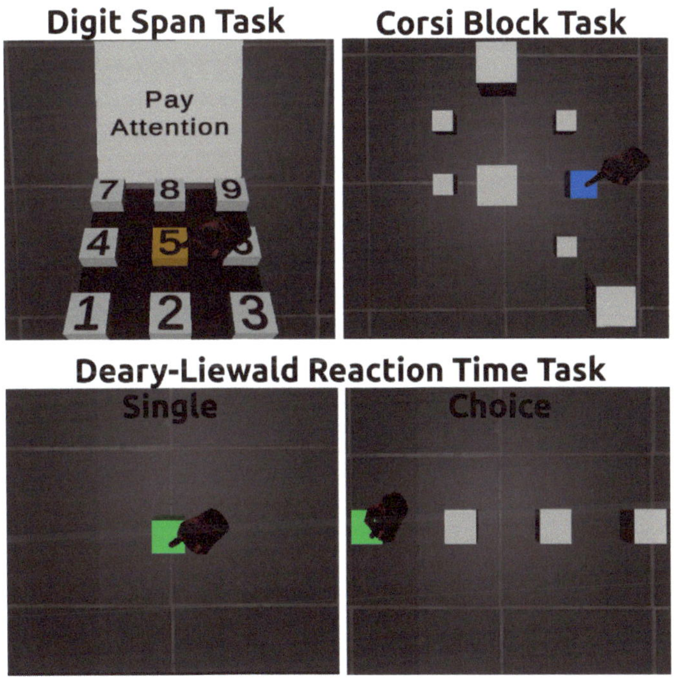

Figure 2. Digit Span Task (**Upper Left**), Corsi Block Task (**Upper Right**), and Deary–Liewald Reaction Time Tasks (**Bottom**).

2.2.2. Visuospatial Working Memory

Visuospatial working memory was assessed using the Backward Corsi Block Test (BCBT) [37]. A VR version of the BCBT was developed. This task consists of 27 white boxes where each one is placed in a different position based on the *x*-, *y*-, and *z*-axes. Nevertheless, only 9 boxes out of the 27 possible boxes were shown to the participants at one time (see

Figure 2). The 9 boxes were presented at the beginning of each trial. Then, a number of these boxes (depending on the current sequence length) were randomly presented (turning blue and making a bell sound) in sequential order, with each box presented for one second. After the presentation of the sequence, participants had to select the boxes in reverse order. Participants had to touch a cube (the cube turned blue on touch) and keep touching it for one second to select the cube. When a cube was selected, it either turned green and made a positive sound (i.e., correct response), or it turned orange and made a negative sound (i.e., an error). The trial ended when the participants either made a mistake or they correctly selected all the targets in their reverse order. The sequence lengths were initially two boxes, with two trials for each length. The number of boxes in the sequence was increased by one box when at least one of the two trials of the same length/span was correct. When the participant incorrectly recalled two sequences of the same length, the task ended. Equally, when the second trial of the last length/span (i.e., 7 cubes) was performed, the task ended. The sequence lengths increased by up to seven cubes. The total score is the sum of the span (the longest correct sequence length) and the total number of correct sequences. A video displaying the task and its procedures can be found here: https://www.youtube.com/watch?v=MLilvkyMt-g (accessed on 16 January 2023).

2.2.3. Psychomotor Skills

To assess reaction times, a VR version of the Deary–Liewald Reaction Time (DLRT) task [38] was developed and used. The DLRT encompasses two tasks. One task assesses simple reaction time (SRT), and the other task examines choice reaction time (CRT). For the SRT task, participants had to observe a white box and touch it as soon as the box changes color to blue (see Figure 2). There are 20 trials/repetitions in the SRT task. In the CRT task, there are four boxes, which are aligned horizontally (see Figure 2). Randomly, one of the four boxes changes its color to blue. When the box turns blue, participants are required to touch the box as fast as possible (see Figure 2). The CRT task includes 40 trials/repetitions. For both the SRT and CRT, the participants were instructed to touch the boxes as fast as possible using the most convenient hand. There was a practice session at the start of both the SRT and the CRT to ensure that the instructions were understood by the participants. A video displaying the task and its procedures can be found here: https://www.youtube.com/watch?v=wXdrt0PjNsk (accessed on 16 January 2023).

As in the original version, the SRT produces a score that is the average reaction time across the 20 trials. Similarly, the CRT produces a score that is the average reaction time across the 40 trials, for the correct responses only. However, in addition, given that the VR version of the CRT is enhanced by eye tracking, the time required to attend to the target was also measured (attentional time, i.e., the time from the appearance of the target until the gaze of the user falls on it). Additionally, eye tracking facilitated the calculation of the time required to touch the target once it had been attended to (motor time). Finally, similarly to the original version, the overall time between the target's presentation and its selection (reaction time) was also calculated. Thus, the VR version of the CRT produces three scores:

(1) the reaction time (RT) to indicate overall psychomotor speed,
(2) the attentional time (AT) to indicate attentional processing speed,
(3) the motor time (MT) to indicate movement speed.

2.3. Cybersickness Questionnaires

The Motion Sickness Susceptibility Questionnaire (MSSQ) [39] was completed prior to enrolment to reduce the likelihood of a participant experiencing severe symptoms of cybersickness. The MSSQ is a 3-point Likert scale with 18 items/questions examining the experience of motion sickness using diverse means of transport. Nine items refer to the experience of motion sickness as a child, and the other nine items refer to such experiences as an adult. The nine questions are hence repeated in both sections. The MSSQ produces three scores: a child score; an adult score; and a total score, which is the addition of the previous two scores.

The SSQ and the VRSQ were administered pre- and post-exposure to VR to assess the intensity of cybersickness symptoms. Both the SSQ and VRSQ are 4-point Likert scales. The SSQ was developed for individuals that are trained using simulators (e.g., aviators) [19]. The SSQ has 16 questions, which are grouped under three categories: nausea; disorientation; and oculomotor. Four scores are produced, including one for each category and a total score. The calculation of the scores is made by a formula offered by the developers of the SSQ [19]. The maximum score is 100 for each category, and 300 for the total score. On the other hand, the VRSQ is derived from the SSQ, and it contains 9 items (i.e., approximately half of the SSQ items), which are grouped under two categories: disorientation and oculomotor (i.e., the nausea items are excluded) [21]. The VRSQ produces three scores, including one for each category and a total score, which is the sum of the two sub-scores divided by two. The maximum score for each sub-score is 100. As discussed above (see Section 1.2), while both the SSQ and VRSQ appear to be valid tools, they suffer from certain limitations:

- The SSQ is not specific to cybersickness, and the frequency and intensity of symptoms substantially differ between simulator sickness and cybersickness.
- The VRSQ does not consider nausea symptoms, and nausea symptoms are the second most frequent type of symptoms in cybersickness.
- VRSQ validation was performed in a study with a small sample size and a limited diversity of stimuli.
- Both the SSQ and VRSQ, being 4-point Likert scales, were not designed in line with the design guidelines for Likert scale questionnaires.

Cybersickness in VR Questionnaire

The CSQ-VR is an improved version of the VRISE section of the VRNQ. The VRISE section has been found to have very good structural validity in a study where participants were exposed to three diverse kinds of VR software and environments [29]. Additionally, the VRISE section of the VRNQ was previously validated and compared against the SSQ [30]. The VRISE of the VRNQ appeared superior to the SSQ due to its shorter administration time (i.e., 5 items instead of 16 items) and the enhanced interpretability of the scores (i.e., scores calculated by a simple addition, instead of a complex formula). However, the VRISE section of the VRNQ had only one item for oculomotor symptoms and the score was inversed (i.e., a higher score indicated a weaker intensity of that symptom). To address these limitations, the CSQ-VR was developed based on the VRISE section of the VRNQ. Comparably to the VRNQ, the CSQ-VR was designed and developed by following the design guidelines for Likert scales, i.e., a 7-point Likert scale, and combining text with numbers in the responses (see [25–28]). The CSQ-VR is a 7-point Likert scale that includes six questions for the assessment of the three types of symptoms of cybersickness, which form the following respective sub-scores: nausea; vestibular; and oculomotor. Each category includes two questions. The total score is the sum of the three scores, which a maximum score of 42 (14 for each sub-score). The paper-and-pencil version of the CSQ-VR can be found in the Supplementary Materials.

Moreover, a 3D version of the CSQ-VR has also been developed to assess cybersickness while the user is immersed in VR. A user interface (UI) for the VR version of the CSQ-VR was designed and developed. In the UI, the question appears in the upper area and the response (in red letters) appears in the middle area. The users change their response by touching the corresponding number or sliding along the slider (see Figure 3). Furthermore, based on the established link between pupil size and affective/emotional state [31], eye tracking was integrated to facilitate ophthalmometry and pupillometry. To measure fixation duration, invisible eye-tracking targets were placed in front of the text, while their height and width were always matched to the displayed text per line (see Figure 3). Moreover, the measurement of pupil size was continuous while the user responded to the CSQ-VR questions. Pupillometry yields measurements of average pupil size (right and left), which can be used as a physiological metric of negative emotion. Finally, a video showing the procedures of a questionnaire in VR can be found here: Link to the Video (accessed on 16 January 2023).

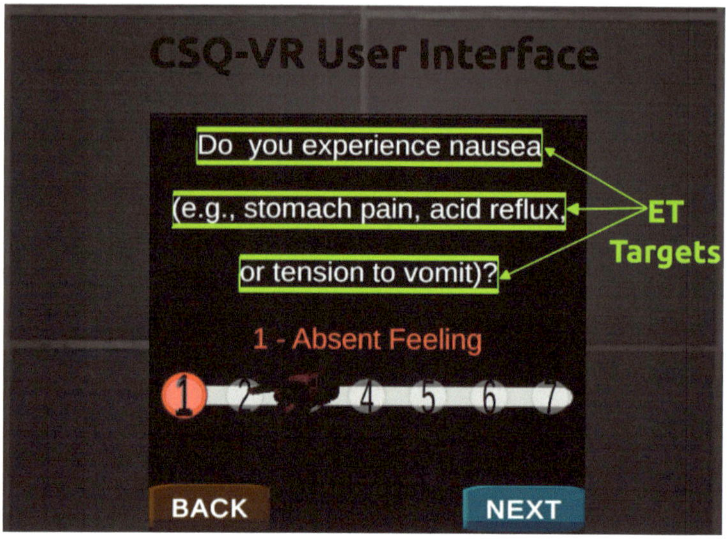

Figure 3. User Interface and Eye-Tracking (ET) Targets of the VR version of CSQ-VR. Note: Eye-tracking targets were not visible to the user.

2.4. Participants and Procedures

Thirty-nine participants (22 females, 17 males) were recruited with a mean age of 25.28 years [*SD* = *3.25, Range* = *22–36*] and a mean education of 17.23 years [*SD* = *1.60, Range* = *13–20*]. The recruitment was performed via opportunity sampling using the University of Edinburgh's internal mailing lists, alongside advertisements on social media. The study was approved by the School of Philosophy, Psychology, and Language Sciences (PPLS) Ethics Committee of the University of Edinburgh. Informed and written consent was obtained from all participants prior to their participation. Participants were compensated with 20 GBP each for their time and effort.

The MSSQ was completed before enrolment to reduce the likelihood of severe symptoms following VR exposure. In line with the MSSQ author's suggestions [39], the 75th percentile was used as a parsimonious cut-off score for inclusion in the study. This allowed us to exclude individuals who are susceptible to experiencing strong cybersickness symptomatology (i.e., the upper 25th percentile of the population). The included participants were then invited to attend the experiment. Upon arrival, participants were informed of the study's aims and procedures, and the adverse effects that they may experience. The participants then provided informed consent in written form.

Firstly, an induction on how to wear the headset and use and hold the controllers was offered to every participant. An HTC Vive Pro Eye was used, which embeds an eye-tracker with a 120 Hz refresh rate and a tracking accuracy of 0.5–1.1°. Secondly, the participants provided the following demographic data by responding to a questionnaire: age; sex; gender; education; dominant eye; VR experience; computing experience; and gaming experience. The dominant eye was determined using the Miles test [40]. Note that VR/computing/gaming experiences were calculated by adding the scores from two questions (6-item Likert scale) for each one. The first question was pertinent to the participant's ability (e.g., 5: highly skilled) to operate a VR/computer/game, and the second one was pertinent to the frequency of operating them (e.g., 4: once a week).

Before VR exposure, participants responded to the CSQ-VR (paper version), SSQ, and VRSQ. Participants were then immersed in VR. Note that for the assessments and rides, participants were always in a standing position in the middle of the VR area (see the X mark in Figure 1). The first part included the tutorials, during which a video tutorial for each task was offered, alongside the corresponding verbal and written instructions. After each tutorial, the participant performed the corresponding task. This part formed the baseline assessment of each participant. The baseline assessment included the following: the VR version of CSQ-VR (Cybersickness); the verbal working memory task (BDST); the visuospatial working memory task (BCBT); and the reaction time task (DLRT; see Figure 2). After the baseline assessment, the first ride started. After each ride, the participants performed an assessment identical to the baseline (i.e., CSQ-VR, BDST, BCBT, DLRT). On top of the baseline assessment, the participants were exposed to three rides and three respective assessments. The whole procedure in VR lasted approximately 100 min for each participant. After the VR session, participants responded to the CSQ-VR (paper version), SSQ, and VRSQ. Then, refreshments rich in electrolytes were offered to the participants. Moreover, the participants rested for 10–15 min before leaving the premises. The participants were instructed to avoid driving and using heavy machinery for the rest of the day.

2.5. Statistical Analyses

Descriptive statistical analyses were performed to provide an overview of the sample. Reliability analyses were conducted to examine the internal consistency of the CSQ-VR. The recommended thresholds for Cronbach's α were used to interpret the internal consistency (i.e., adequate = 0.6–0.7, good = 0.7–0.8, and very good = 0.8–0.95) [41]. Pearson's correlational analyses were performed to examine the validity of the CSQ-VR versions against the SSQ and the VRS post-exposure (i.e., after the VR session). Because the SSQ is considered the gold standard and it has a structure (i.e., three sub-scores: nausea; oculomotor; and disorientation) similar to the CSQ-VR, the convergent validity (i.e., correlations) of the CSQ-VR was assessed against the SSQ. Receiver operating characteristic (ROC) and area under the curve (AUC) analyses were performed to appraise the psychometric properties of the CSQ-VR, SSQ, and VRSQ in detecting temporary cognitive and motor decline due to cybersickness. The thresholds of AUC > 0.7 and metric score > 1.5 were used in line with the respective recommendations for determining the suitability of the tool [42,43]. The temporary decline was based on the performance on the assessment after each ride. In agreement with the consensus of the American Academy of Clinical Neuropsychology for determining a substantial decrease in performance, two standard deviations from the mean were used [44]. Thus, when the performance (i.e., score) on the assessment after the respective ride was 2 standard deviations from the mean of the baseline assessment, the performance was defined as abnormal (i.e., temporary decline). Note that the two standard deviations had to indicate a worse performance and thus be greater for reaction and motor times (i.e., slower reaction or motor speed) and smaller for the verbal and visuospatial working memory (i.e., poorer performance). Finally, the predictive ability of pupil size was examined by performing a mixed model regression analysis. The analysis was performed using *Jamovi* statistical software (descriptive statistics, reliability, ROC, and AUC analyses) [45], as well as *R* (transforming the data, plots design, and correlation and regressions analyses) [46]. As the variables violated the normality assumption, we used the *bestNormalize* R package [47] to transform and centralize the data. The distribution of the data was then normal. The transformed data were used for parametric analyses (i.e., correlations and mixed regression analysis). Furthermore, the psych (correlational analyses) [48], the *ggplot2* (plots) [49], and the *lme4* (regression analyses) [50] R packages were used to perform the respective analyses.

3. Results

The descriptive statistics of the sample are displayed in Table 1. Concerning the intensity of cybersickness symptoms, it can be observed that the participants predominantly experienced moderate symptoms. There were no dropouts during the experiment. The descriptive statistics for the VR version of the CSQ-VR, per experimental stage, are presented in Table 2.

Table 1. Descriptive Statistics.

	Mean (SD)	Range	Max. Score
Sex (22F/17M)	-	-	-
Age	25.28 (3.22)	22–36	-
Years of Education	15.14 (5.18)	13–20	-
VR Experience	2.67 (0.92)	2–6	14
Computing Experience	10.36 (0.80)	9–12	14
Gaming Experience	5.54 (2.97)	2–12	14
MSSQ Child Score	4.69 (3.34)	0–13.50	27
MSSQ Adult Score	3.91 (3.20)	0–11.25	27
MSSQ Total Score	8.60 (5.23)	0–20.13	54
Pupil Size (mm)	5.37 (0.90)	3.70–8.32	-
CSQ-VR (VR) Total Score *	10.63 (4.97)	6–28	42
CSQ-VR (VR) Nausea Score *	3.18 (1.56)	2–9	14
CSQ-VR (VR) Vestibular Score *	3.66 (2.43)	2–13	14
CSQ-VR (VR) Oculomotor Score *	3.79 (1.70)	2–9	14
CSQ-VR Total Score	12.23 (4.96)	6–27	42
CSQ-VR Nausea Score	3.51 (1.68)	2–9	14
CSQ-VR Vestibular Score	3.97 (2.41)	2–10	14
CSQ- VR Oculomotor Score	4.74 (1.81)	2–10	14
SSQ-Total Score	67.24 (48.09)	0–223.66	300
SSQ-Nausea Score	24.22 (22.09)	0–95.40	100
SSQ-Disorientation Score	9.40 (9.98)	0–44.88	100
SSQ-Oculomotor Score	33.62 (21.84)	0–83.38	100
VRSQ-Total Score	19.17 (13.27)	0–59.17	100
VRSQ-Disorientation Score	11.62 (13.27)	0–60.00	100
VRSQ-Oculomotor Score	26.71 (15.63)	0–58.33	100

* (VR) = VR version; Pupil Size measured while responding to the VR version of CSQ-VR.

Table 2. Descriptive Statistics of the VR version of CSQ-VR per Experimental Stage.

Experimental Stage	CSQ-VR Scores *	Mean (SD)	Range	Max. Score
Baseline	Total Score	7.59 (2.09)	6–16	42
	Nausea Score	2.23 (0.54)	2–4	14
	Vestibular Score	2.38 (0.85)	2–6	14
	Oculomotor Score	2.79 (1.11)	2–6	14
Ride 1	Total Score	10.79 (4.35)	6–24	42
	Nausea Score	3.41 (1.37)	2–8	14
	Vestibular Score	3.97 (2.47)	2–12	14
	Oculomotor Score	3.41 (1.41)	2–8	14
Ride 2	Total Score	11.87 (5.03)	6–23	42
	Nausea Score	3.54 (1.57)	2–8	14
	Vestibular Score	4.13 (2.56)	2–12	14
	Oculomotor Score	4.21 (1.73)	2–9	14
Ride 3	Total Score	12.26 (6.19)	6–28	42
	Nausea Score	3.54 (2.02)	2–9	14
	Vestibular Score	4.15 (2.91)	2–13	14
	Oculomotor Score	4.56 (2.00)	2–9	14

* Scores of the VR version of CSQ-VR during the exposure to VR.

3.1. Reliability and Validity

Interpretation of the outcomes was based on the recommendations offered by Ursachi et al. [41]. Based on them, Cronbach's α of 0.6–0.7 is an acceptable score, 0.7–0.8 is a good score, and 0.8–0.95 is a very good score. The overall internal consistency of the questionnaire (i.e., the total score's reliability) was evaluated by considering each questionnaire's sub-scores. The internal consistency of the sub-categories (i.e., the reliability of the sub-score) was examined by considering the respective items/questions. The reliability analyses revealed that all sub-scores of the CSQ-VR had good internal consistency (see Table 3). Specifically, the total score and the vestibular sub-score showed very good internal consistency, while the nausea and oculomotor sub-scores revealed good internal consistency. However, Cronbach's α of the oculomotor sub-score was at the margins between good and adequate internal consistency.

Table 3. Reliability (Internal Consistency) of CSQ-VR, SSQ, and VRSQ.

Questionnaire	Scores	Cronbach's α
CSQ-VR	Total Score	0.865
	Nausea	0.792
	Vestibular	0.934
	Oculomotor	0.704
SSQ	Total Score	0.810
	Nausea	0.676
	Disorientation	0.809
	Oculomotor	0.744
VRSQ	Total Score	0.806
	Disorientation	0.718
	Oculomotor	0.654

The internal consistency was based on the sub-scores of the total score, and the sub-scores were based on their respective items. Based on [41], Cronbach's α of 0.6–0.7 is acceptable, 0.7–0.8 is good, and 0.8–0.95 is very good.

Both the SSQ and VRSQ total scores showed good internal consistency; however, both were substantially lower than the internal consistency of the CSQ-VR total score (see Table 3). The nausea score of the SSQ showed an acceptable internal consistency, which was significantly lower than the almost very good internal consistency of the nausea score of the CSQ-VR. The disorientation score of the SSQ revealed marginally very good internal consistency, while the disorientation score of the VRSQ indicated marginally good internal consistency. Both disorientation scores (SSQ and VRSQ) were significantly lower than the almost excellent internal consistency of the CSQ-VR. Finally, the oculomotor score of the SSQ showed good internal consistency that was higher than the marginally good internal consistency of the oculomotor score of the CSQ-VR. On the other hand, the oculomotor score of the VRSQ revealed adequate internal consistency. The oculomotor score of the VRSQ and the nausea score of the SSQ were the two scores that were below the parsimonious threshold of 0.7. Overall, the CSQ-VR appeared to have superior internal consistency compared to the SSQ and the VRSQ.

The scores of the CSQ-VR (both versions) were significantly correlated with the corresponding scores of the SSQ. Overall, the analyses revealed moderate to strong correlations between the scores. The paper-and-pencil version of the CSQ-VR was strongly associated with the SSQ (see Figure 4). Their total scores especially, as well as their oculomotor scores, revealed a very strong correlation between them. Although the correlations for the nausea and vestibular scores were weaker than those observed above, they were still strong correlations (see Figure 4). Similarly, the VR version of the CSQ-VR was strongly associated with the SSQ (see Figure 5). In particular, their total scores indicated a strong correlation between them. While the correlations for their sub-scores were weaker than those between the total score, they were still moderate to strong correlations (see Figure 5). These results postulate the convergent validity of both versions of the CSQ-VR. Additionally, given that all sub-scores were substantially associated, the construct validity of the CSQ-VR is strongly supported.

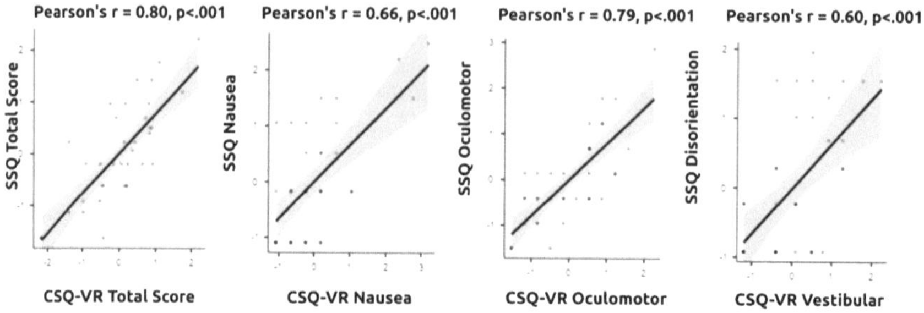

Figure 4. Correlations between the scores of the CSQ-VR (paper-and-pencil version) and the SSQ.

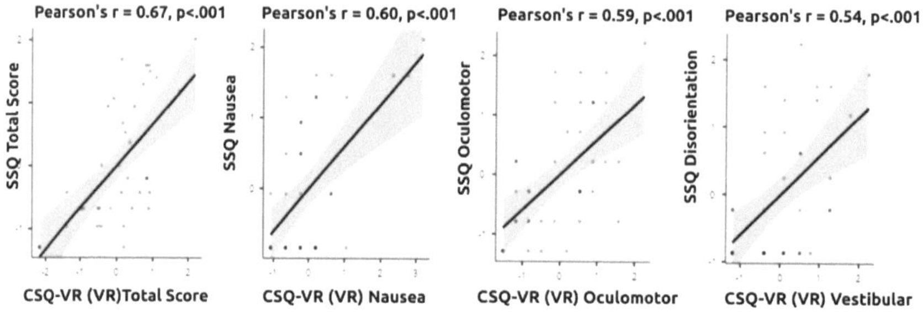

Figure 5. Correlations between the scores of the CSQ-VR (VR version) and the SSQ.

Furthermore, the scores for both versions of the CSQ-VR were strongly associated with the VRSQ scores (see Table 4). The total scores of the CSQ-VR versions showed the strongest correlations with the total score of the VRSQ. The oculomotor scores of the CSQ-VR and VRSQ equally revealed robust associations between them. Although the vestibular scores indicated weaker correlations compared to the other scores, the correlations were moderate (see Table 4). These outcomes further support the convergent and construct validity of both versions of the CSQ-VR.

Table 4. Correlations between the scores of CSQ-VR (both versions) and the VRSQ.

Correlation Pair		Pearson's r	*p*-Value
CSQ-VR–Total Score	VRSQ–Total Score	0.77	<0.001
CSQ-VR–Oculomotor	VRSQ–Oculomotor	0.75	<0.001
CSQ-VR–Vestibular	VRSQ–Disorientation	0.55	<0.001
CSQ-VR (VR)–Total Score	VRSQ–Total Score	0.65	<0.001
CSQ-VR (VR)–Oculomotor	VRSQ–Oculomotor	0.62	<0.001
CSQ-VR (VR)–Vestibular	VRSQ–Disorientation	0.52	<0.001

(VR) = VR version.

3.2. *Detection of Temporary Decline due to Cybersickness*

As mentioned above, the temporary decline was defined by two standard deviations from the mean of the baseline assessment. This definition is in line with the guidelines of the American Academy of Clinical Neuropsychology for determining whether performance is abnormal [44]. Eleven observations were detected which met the criterion for temporary cognitive/motor decline. Six of these were pertinent to reaction speed (i.e., longer reaction times) and five of them were applicable to motor speed (i.e., slower). Thus, all temporary declines were found for the DLRT task. A trend was also observed where, when motor speed was substantially slower (i.e., a decline), reaction speed also substantially declined. Finally, these declines were all found in three participants. Thus, only three participants experienced a temporary decline in their psychomotor skills. These results indicate that susceptibility to experiencing a temporary decline due to cybersickness may be attributed to individual differences.

The ROC–AUC analyses provide cut-off scores for each questionnaire where the optimal sensitivity (i.e., the detection of true positives) and specificity (i.e., the exclusion of true negatives) are achieved. Following the recommendations for ROC–AUC analyses and psychometrics [42,43] to determine the suitability of a questionnaire to detect temporary decline, two criteria were set as follows: (1) AUC > 70% and (2) metric score > 1.5, both of which had to be met. The ROC–AUC analyses for declines in reaction time (i.e., slower reaction times) showed that only the total scores for both versions of the CSQ-VR met the criteria (see Table 5). Similarly, the ROC–AUC analyses for motor speed decline indicated that only the total scores for both versions of the CSQ-VR met the criteria. Furthermore, the two versions of the CSQ-VR showed the best sensitivity and specificity in detecting a temporary decline in reaction time and motor speed, while the VRSQ and SSQ showed significantly smaller psychometric properties (see Tables 5 and 6 and Figure 6). These results postulate that the total scores for both versions of the CSQ-VR have superior psychometric properties to the total scores of the SSQ and VRSQ. Additionally, only the CSQ-VR total scores are suitable for detecting a temporary decline in reaction speed and/or motor speed.

Table 5. Psychometric Properties of the CSQ-VR, SSQ, and VRSQ in detecting Reaction Speed Decline.

Cybersickness Score	Cut-Off	Sensitivity (%)	Specificity (%)	PPV (%)	NPV (%)	AUC (%)	Metric Score
CSQ-VR–Total Score	10	100%	75%	15.15%	100%	87%	1.75
CSQ-VR (VR)–Total Score	9	100%	75%	15.15%	100%	86.5%	1.75
SSQ–Total Score	83.36	80%	68.75%	10.26%	98.72%	66.1%	1.49
VRSQ–Total Score	20	100%	53.57%	8.77%	100%	66.6%	1.54

(VR) = VR version. Based on [42] and [43], the following thresholds were set and had to be met: AUC > 70% and metric score > 1.5.; PPV = positive predictive value (i.e., the ratio of true positives); NPV = negative predictive value (i.e., the ratio of true negatives).

Table 6. Psychometric Properties of the CSQ-VR, SSQ, and VRSQ in detecting Motor Speed Decline.

Cybersickness Score	Cut-off	Sensitivity (%)	Specificity (%)	PPV (%)	NPV (%)	AUC (%)	Metric Score
CSQ-VR–Total Score	10	100%	75.68%	18.18%	100%	86.9%	1.76
CSQ-VR (VR)–Total Score	9	100%	75.68%	18.18%	100%	88%	1.76
SSQ–Total Score	83.36	83.33%	69.37%	12.82%	98.72%	68%	1.53
VRSQ–Total Score	20	100%	54.05%	10.53%	100%	67.53%	1.54

(VR) = VR version. Based on [42] and [43], the following thresholds were set and had to be met: AUC > 70% and metric score > 1.5; PPV = positive predictive value (i.e., the ratio of true positives); NPV = negative predictive value (i.e., the ratio of true negatives).

The psychometric properties of the sub-scores of each questionnaire were also examined. In detecting a temporary decline in reaction speed or motor speed, only the vestibular/disorientation scores of the questionnaires met the criteria of suitable psychometric properties (see Tables 7 and 8). However, the nausea score of the VR version of the CSQ-VR also met the criteria for detecting both. The best sensitivity and specificity in detecting a temporary decline in either reaction or motor speed was observed for the vestibular score of the paper-and-pencil version of the CSQ-VR, closely followed by the same score for the VR version of the CSQ-VR (see Tables 7 and 8 and Figure 7). The sensitivity and specificity of the disorientation scores of the SSQ and VRSQ were substantially lower compared to the CSQ-VR. However, the sensitivity and specificity of the disorientation score of the SSQ were significantly higher than the ones for the disorientation score of the VRSQ.

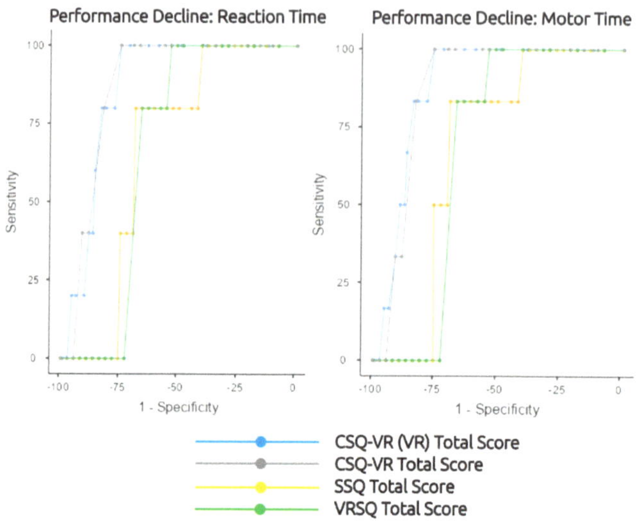

Figure 6. Sensitivity and Specificity of the CSQ-VR, SSQ, and VRSQ Total Scores in detecting Reaction Time (**Left**) and Motor Speed (**Right**) Decline. Note: (VR) = VR version.

Table 7. Psychometric Properties of the CSQ-VR, SSQ, and VRSQ Vestibular/Disorientation Scores in detecting Reaction Speed Decline.

Cybersickness Score	Cut-Off	Sensitivity (%)	Specificity (%)	PPV (%)	NPV (%)	AUC (%)	Metric Score
CSQ-VR–Nausea	3	60%	67.86%	7.69%	97.44%	65.3%	1.28
CSQ-VR–Vestibular	***5***	***100%***	***77.68%***	***16.67%***	***100%***	***92.6%***	***1.78***
CSQ-VR–Oculomotor	7	40%	93.75%	22.22%	97.22%	65.8%	1.34
CSQ-VR(VR)–Nausea	***3***	***100%***	***66.96%***	***11.09%***	***100%***	***83.6%***	***1.67***
CSQ-VR(VR)–Vestibular	***4***	***100%***	***70.54%***	***13.16%***	***100%***	***86.7%***	***1.71***
CSQ-VR (VR)–Oculomotor	6	40%	90.18%	15.38%	97.12%	61.2%	1.30
SSQ–Nausea	47.7	40%	88.39%	13.33%	97.06%	60.04%	1.28
SSQ–Disorientation	***11.22***	***100%***	***64.29%***	***11.11%***	***100%***	***70.1%***	***1.64***
SSQ–Oculomotor	45.48	80%	58.04%	7.84%	98.48%	67.9%	1.38
VRSQ–Disorientation	***20***	***80%***	***74.01%***	***12.12%***	***98.81%***	***73.06%***	***1.54***
VRSQ–Oculomotor	33.33	100%	53.57%	8.77%	100%	63.4%	1.54

(VR) = VR version. Based on [42] and [43], the following thresholds were set and had to be met: AUC > 70% and metric score > 1.5; PPV = positive predictive value (i.e., the ratio of true positives); NPV = negative predictive value (i.e., the ratio of true negatives).

Table 8. Psychometric Properties of the CSQ-VR, SSQ, and VRSQ Vestibular/Disorientation Scores in detecting Motor Speed Decline.

Cybersickness Score	Cut-Off	Sensitivity (%)	Specificity (%)	PPV (%)	NPV (%)	AUC (%)	Metric Score
CSQ-VR–Nausea	2	100%	32.43%	7.41%	100%	62.6%	1.32
CSQ-VR–Vestibular	***5***	***100%***	***78.38%***	***20%***	***100%***	***94.4%***	***1.78***
CSQ-VR–Oculomotor	7	33.33%	93.69%	22.22%	96.3%	61%	1.27
CSQ-VR(VR)–Nausea	***3***	***100%***	***67.57%***	***14.29%***	***100%***	***85.1%***	***1.68***
CSQ-VR(VR)–Vestibular	***4***	***100%***	***71.17%***	***15.79%***	***100%***	***89.3%***	***1.71***
CSQ-VR (VR)–Oculomotor	6	33.33%	90.09%	15.38%	96.15%	56.5%	1.23
SSQ–Nausea	47.7	50%	89.19%	20%	97.06%	65.08%	1.39
SSQ–Disorientation	***11.22***	***100%***	***64.86%***	***13.33%***	***100%***	***70.3%***	***1.65***
SSQ–Oculomotor	45.48	83.33%	58.56%	9.8%	98.48%	67.8%	1.42
VRSQ–Disorientation	***20***	***82.3%***	***74.77%***	***15.15%***	***98.81%***	***75%***	***1.58***
VRSQ–Oculomotor	33.33	100%	54.05%	10.53%	100%	63.5%	1.54

(VR) = VR version. Based on [42] and [43], the following thresholds were set and had to be met: AUC > 70% and metric score > 1.5; PPV = positive predictive value (i.e., the ratio of true positives); NPV = negative predictive value (i.e., the ratio of true negatives).

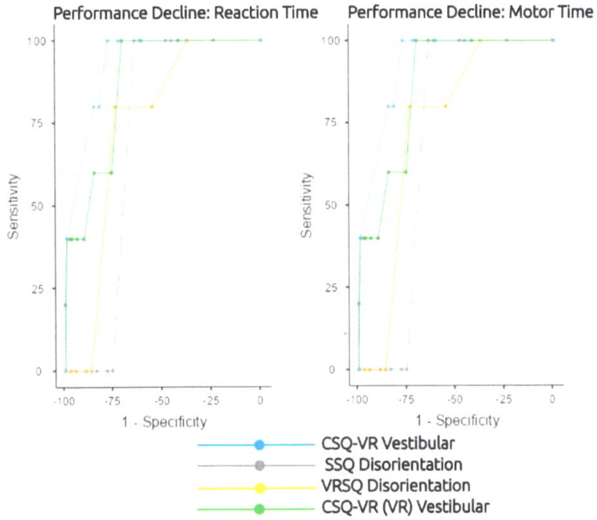

Figure 7. Sensitivity and Specificity of the CSQ-VR, SSQ, and VRSQ Vestibular/Disorientation Scores in detecting Reaction Time (**Left**) and Motor Speed (**Right**) Decline. Note: (VR) = VR version.

3.3. Mixed Model Regression Analysis

A mixed model regression analysis was conducted to determine whether pupil size can be a biomarker/predictor of cybersickness. The analysis indicated that the model with pupil size as a predictor of the total score on the VR version of the CSQ-VR was significant. Pupil size also revealed a relatively high beta (negative) coefficient, postulating that cybersickness intensity substantially increases as pupil size decreases (see Figure 8). Furthermore, the fixed effects of pupil size, alongside the random effects of the participants, appear to explain 50% of the variance in the intensity of cybersickness. These outcomes postulate that pupil size is a significant predictor of the intensity of cybersickness, and it can therefore be considered as a biomarker of cybersickness.

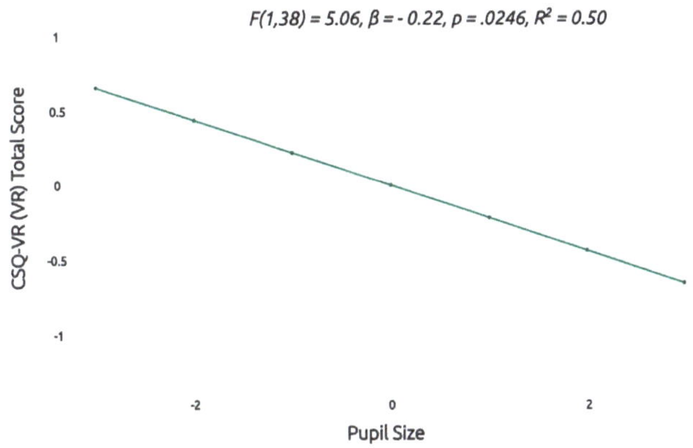

Figure 8. Mixed Regression Model of Pupil Size Predicting Cybersickness Intensity.

4. Discussion

The CSQ-VR is an adapted and enhanced version of the VRISE section and sub-score of the VNRQ. Based on the recommendations by Ursachi et al. [41] for Cronbach's α, the CSQ-VR displayed good to very good internal consistency. This finding is aligned with the high structural validity and internal consistency of the VRNQ and its VRISE sub-score, which have previously been observed [29]. Additionally, the total scores and sub-scores of both versions of the CSQ-VR showed robust correlations with their respective sub-scores and total scores of the SSQ and VRSQ. This finding supports the findings of Somrak et al. [30] in which the VRISE sub-score of the VRNQ was significantly correlated with the SSQ total score. Nevertheless, the current study meticulously examined the reliability and validity of the total scores and the sub-scores of both versions of the CSQ-VR. Beyond their convergent validity, the associations between the sub-scores of the CSQ-VR (both versions) (i.e., nausea, vestibular, and oculomotor) and the equivalent sub-scores of the SSQ support the construct validity of both versions of the CSQ-VR in examining the whole range of cybersickness symptomatology. Therefore, both the paper-and-pencil and the VR versions of the CSQ-VR are highly reliable and are valid tools for measuring the presence and intensity of cybersickness symptoms in VR.

4.1. Comparison of CSQ-VR, SSQ, and VRSQ

Several studies have reported that the SSQ does not have adequate psychometric properties for measuring cybersickness in VR [20,51,52]. The findings of this current study are aligned with the previous literature. The inadequacy and inappropriateness of the SSQ for measuring cybersickness in VR have also been confirmed. Specifically, the overall and sub-scores for the SSQ and the VRSQ displayed internal consistency which was substantially inferior to the respective internal consistency of the CSQ-VR total score and sub-scores. Moreover, the nausea item of the SSQ revealed internal consistency that was below the parsimonious threshold of 0.7 for Cronbach's α, which is required for a tool to be used in research and professional settings [53]. Likewise, the oculomotor sub-score of the VRSQ was well below this threshold. Given that the VRSQ has only two sub-scores (i.e., disorientation and oculomotor), half of the test was found to be unreliable. This finding agrees with the serious limitations reported in VRSQ development and validation, which was conducted using smartphone VR (i.e., Samsung Gear VR) and not PC or standalone VR, a very simplistic task (i.e., target selection) and stimuli (i.e., small and large buttons), which were not efficient in inducing adequate levels of cybersickness in a relatively small sample [21]. As a result, all the items pertinent to nausea, which is the second most frequent symptom of cybersickness in VR [7,22–24,51], were dropped. Thus, it comes as no surprise that both the SSQ and VRSQ displayed problematic consistencies in certain sub-scores and overall inferior reliability for the total and sub-scores of the CSQ-VR.

Furthermore, the SSQ has received criticism for its highly complex structure and scoring [30,51]. The CSQ-VR has previously been strongly preferred over the SSQ because of its easily calculated and interpretable scores [30]. The VRSQ, derived from the SSQ, has predominantly maintained the SSQ structure and scoring system, although the VRSQ scoring system requires somewhat simpler calculations. Nevertheless, as was also seen in this study, both the SSQ and VRSQ suffer in terms of structure. Additionally, given that the design of the questions and available responses use a Likert scale that is essential for collecting reliable and informative data [25–28], the CSQ-VR has an advantage over the SSQ and VRSQ. Both the SSQ and VRSQ use a 4-point Likert scale, while the relevant literature suggests that a 7-point Likert scale, especially when combining a number with textual information (e.g., "*6–Very Intense Feeling*") like in the CSQ-VR, are substantially more efficient in providing useful and representative self-reports [25–28]. The design of the general instructions (i.e., "*Please, from 1 to 7, circle the response that better corresponds to the presence and intensity of the symptom.*") and questions (e.g., "*Nausea A: Do you experience nausea (e.g., stomach pain, acid reflux, or tension to vomit)?*") are also more explicit in the CSQ-VR than the equivalent design in the SSQ and VRSQ (i.e., general instruction: "*Circle how much each symptom below is affecting you now.*"; question: "*Nausea*"). Finally, the SSQ has 16 questions measuring the whole range of symptoms. The VRSQ has nine questions, but it measures only the vestibular and oculomotor-related symptoms, while the CSQ-VR is shorter, measuring the whole range of cybersickness with only six questions. Therefore, the

CSQ-VR is a shorter questionnaire with an overall superior design to the SSQ and VRSQ, which was also reflected in the psychometric properties examined in this study.

The previous literature has shown that cybersickness, particularly when symptoms are strong, may affect the cognitive and/or motor skills of the user [12–14], especially their reaction speed [10,17,18]. It is thus assumed that a questionnaire designed to measure cybersickness would also be effective in detecting relevant declines in performance. The total score for both versions of the CSQ-VR showed high sensitivity and specificity in detecting these temporary declines in performance due to cybersickness, while the psychometric properties of the total scores of the SSQ and VRSQ were substantially lower and inadequate. Furthermore, two sub-scores (nausea and vestibular) of the CSQ-VR were also highly sensitive and specific in the detection of temporary declines, while the equivalent scores of the SSQ and VRSQ (which does not include a nausea score) were either significantly inferior or inadequate. Thus, the CSQ-VR is the only questionnaire that is effective in detecting these temporary declines in performance modulated by cybersickness. Given that VR is implemented in education [1], professional training [2], neuropsychological assessments [54], and therapy [4], where cognitive and motor skills should be reliable, it is essential that a tool should be able to provide information that these skills may have been compromised by cybersickness symptomatology. Finally, beyond these applications, VR is gradually becoming established as a research tool in scientific fields, such as human–computer interactions [55] and psychological sciences [3], where cybersickness may compromise the reliability of the scientific findings [12]. Thus, the detection of a participant whose performance has been compromised by cybersickness enables the exclusion of this participant or observation from the analyses and assures the data's reliability.

Nevertheless, as was also observed in this study, a participant's performance may not be affected throughout the experiment. In previous studies, changes in the intensity of cybersickness during exposure can occur in terms of an increase due to aggravation [22] or a decrease due to cultivated tolerance [56]. Therefore, the continuous or repetitive assessment of cybersickness is required while the participant/user is immersed. Instead of excluding all of a participant's observations, the CSQ-VR allows a researcher to drop only those particular observations where a participant's performance was affected by cybersickness. Considering that the VR version of the CSQ-VR has shown comparable (and sometimes superior) psychometric properties to its paper-and-pencil version, it can detect specific compromised observations/performance and suggest its exclusion from analyses. Nevertheless, beyond self-reports, there are other neuro and biomarkers that have been used to detect and measure cybersickness [8]. Specifically, researchers have efficiently implemented electroencephalography [57,58] and eye tracking [59,60] to detect and appraise the occurrence and intensity of cybersickness. The VR version of the CSQ-VR also benefits from eye-tracking metrics. In this study, pupil size was found to be a significant predictor of cybersickness. A decrease in pupil size indicated higher intensity cybersickness and vice versa, a pattern that has been previously observed between pupil size and negative emotions [31]. Previously, pupil size has been included in a deep fusion model for predicting cybersickness [60]; however, its relationship, predictive ability and contribution to this model were not evaluated, preventing a conclusion of whether pupil size is a biomarker of cybersickness. This study provides evidence postulating that pupil size is indeed a biomarker of cybersickness, as well as its intensity. The VR version of the CSQ-VR thus has an additional advantage of incorporating pupillometry.

4.2. Limitations and Future Studies

The current study also has limitations that should be considered. The sample consisted of young adults, which prevented the examination of cybersickness in a more age-diverse population. Future studies should attempt to examine cybersickness in a sample with a greater age spectrum to enable the study of age differences in tolerance and/or susceptibility towards cybersickness. Additionally, this study implemented a parsimonious inclusion criterion based on the MSSQ scores (i.e., excluding individuals who scored higher than the 75th percentile and could experience substantially more frequent and stronger cybersickness symptomatology). Given that the intensity and prevalence of cybersickness substantially differ across individuals, future studies should explore the effects of cybersickness on cognitive and motor skills in a sample that may experience stronger symptoms. Finally, the assessment included only working memory and psychomotor tests. Future studies should strive to examine more complex cognitive functions (e.g., episodic memory or decision making) and motor skills (e.g., tasks that require fine motor skills and accuracy).

5. Conclusions

The CSQ-VR is a short, valid and reliable tool of cybersickness, which has superior psychometric properties to the SSQ and VRSQ. Additionally, the paper-and-pencil and the VR versions of the CSQ-VR were highly sensitive and specific in detecting temporary performance declines that were modulated by cybersickness. The VR version of the CSQ-VR provides further advantages by facilitating an assessment of cybersickness in the virtual environment while the participant/user is immersed. Finally, the VR version of the CSQ-VR benefits from pupillometry (i.e., measurement of pupil diameter), which was found to predict the presence and intensity of cybersickness. Pupillometry may thus be applied in VR as a biomarker of positive (e.g., amusement) and negative (e.g., frustration) emotions.

Supplementary Materials: The Cybersickness in Virtual Reality Questionnaire (CSQ-VR) can be downloaded at: https://osf.io/4w9cs.

Author Contributions: Conceptualization, P.K., F.A. and S.E.M.; methodology, P.K., F.A. and S.E.M.; software, P.K.; validation, P.K., F.A. and S.E.M.; formal analysis, P.K.; investigation, J.L. and R.A.; resources, P.K.; data curation, J.L. and R.A.; writing—original draft preparation, P.K., J.L. and R.A.; writing—review and editing, P.K., F.A. and S.E.M.; visualization, P.K.; supervision, P.K. and S.M; project administration, P.K. and S.E.M.; funding acquisition, J.L. and R.A. All authors have read and agreed to the published version of the manuscript.

Funding: This research received no external funding.

Institutional Review Board Statement: The study was conducted in accordance with the Declaration of Helsinki, and approved by the Philosophy, Psychology and Language Sciences Research Ethics Committee of the University of Edinburgh (269-2122/4; 14 June 2022).

Informed Consent Statement: Informed consent was obtained from all subjects involved in the study.

Data Availability Statement: The data presented in this study are available on request from the corresponding author. The data are not publicly available due to the ethical approval requirements.

Acknowledgments: This work was funded by the School of Philosophy, Psychology and Language Sciences of the University of Edinburgh. The authors would like to thank the uCreate Studio of the University of Edinburgh for providing them with the VR equipment and tech support.

Conflicts of Interest: The authors declare no conflict of interest.

References

1. Radianti, J.; Majchrzak, T.A.; Fromm, J.; Wohlgenannt, I. A systematic review of immersive virtual reality applications for higher education: Design elements, lessons learned, and research agenda. *Comput. Educ.* **2019**, *147*, 103778. [CrossRef]
2. Xie, B.; Liu, H.; Alghofaili, R.; Zhang, Y.; Jiang, Y.; Lobo, F.D.; Li, C.; Li, W.; Huang, H.; Akdere, M.; et al. A Review on Virtual Reality Skill Training Applications. *Front. Virtual Real.* **2021**, *2*, 645153. [CrossRef]
3. Kourtesis, P.; MacPherson, S.E. How immersive virtual reality methods may meet the criteria of the National Academy of Neuropsychology and American Academy of Clinical Neuropsychology: A software review of the Virtual Reality Everyday Assessment Lab (VR-EAL). *Comput. Hum. Behav. Rep.* **2021**, *4*, 100151. [CrossRef]
4. Emmelkamp, P.M.; Meyerbröker, K. Virtual Reality Therapy in Mental Health. *Annu. Rev. Clin. Psychol.* **2021**, *17*, 495–519. [CrossRef] [PubMed]
5. Cruz-Neira, C.; Fernández, M.; Portalés, C. Virtual Reality and Games. *Multimodal Technol. Interact.* **2018**, *2*, 8. [CrossRef]
6. Rebenitsch, L.; Owen, C. Estimating cybersickness from virtual reality applications. *Virtual Real.* **2020**, *25*, 165–174. [CrossRef]
7. Stanney, K.M.; Kennedy, R.S.; Drexler, J.M. Cybersickness is Not Simulator Sickness. In Proceedings of the Human Factors and Ergonomics Society Annual Meeting; SAGE Publications: New York, NY, USA, 1997; Volume 41, pp. 1138–1142.

8. Davis, S.; Nesbitt, K.; Nalivaiko, E. A Systematic Review of Cybersickness. In Proceedings of the 2014 Conference on Interactive Entertainment, Newcastle, Australia, 2 December 2014; Blackmore, K., Nesbitt, K., Smith, S.P., Eds.; ACM: New York, NY, USA, 2014. [CrossRef]
9. LaViola, J.J. A discussion of cybersickness in virtual environments. *ACM SIGCHI Bull.* **2000**, *32*, 47–56. [CrossRef]
10. Nesbitt, K.; Davis, S.; Blackmore, K.; Nalivaiko, E. Correlating reaction time and nausea measures with traditional measures of cybersickness. *Displays* **2017**, *48*, 1–8. [CrossRef]
11. Kim, J.; Palmisano, S.; Luu, W.; Iwasaki, S. Effects of Linear Visual-Vestibular Conflict on Presence, Perceived Scene Stability and Cybersickness in the Oculus Go and Oculus Quest. *Front. Virtual Real.* **2021**, *2*, 582156. [CrossRef]
12. Kourtesis, P.; Collina, S.; Doumas, L.A.A.; MacPherson, S.E. Technological Competence Is a Pre-condition for Effective Implementation of Virtual Reality Head Mounted Displays in Human Neuroscience: A Technological Review and Meta-Analysis. *Front. Hum. Neurosci.* **2019**, *13*, 342. [CrossRef]
13. Saredakis, D.; Szpak, A.; Birckhead, B.; Keage, H.A.D.; Rizzo, A.; Loetscher, T. Factors Associated with Virtual Reality Sickness in Head-Mounted Displays: A Systematic Review and Meta-Analysis. *Front. Hum. Neurosci.* **2020**, *14*, 96. [CrossRef] [PubMed]
14. Conner, N.O.; Freeman, H.R.; Jones, J.A.; Luczak, T.; Carruth, D.; Knight, A.C.; Chander, H. Virtual Reality Induced Symptoms and Effects: Concerns, Causes, Assessment & Mitigation. *Virtual Worlds* **2022**, *1*, 130–146. [CrossRef]
15. Dahlman, J.; Sjörs, A.; Lindström, J.; Ledin, T.; Falkmer, T. Performance and Autonomic Responses during Motion Sickness. *Hum. Factors: J. Hum. Factors Ergon. Soc.* **2009**, *51*, 56–66. [CrossRef]
16. Varmaghani, S.; Abbasi, Z.; Weech, S.; Rasti, J. Spatial and attentional after effects of virtual reality and relations to cybersickness. *Virtual Real.* **2021**, *26*, 659–668. [CrossRef]
17. Mittelstaedt, J.M.; Wacker, J.; Stelling, D. VR aftereffect and the relation of cybersickness and cognitive performance. *Virtual Real.* **2018**, *23*, 143–154. [CrossRef]
18. Nalivaiko, E.; Davis, S.L.; Blackmore, K.; Vakulin, A.; Nesbitt, K. Cybersickness provoked by head-mounted display affects cutaneous vascular tone, heart rate and reaction time. *Physiol. Behav.* **2015**, *151*, 583–590. [CrossRef]
19. Kennedy, R.S.; Lane, N.E.; Berbaum, K.; Lilienthal, M.G. Simulator Sickness Questionnaire: An Enhanced Method for Quantifying Simulator Sickness. *Int. J. Aviat. Psychol.* **1993**, *3*, 203–220. [CrossRef]
20. Sevinc, V.; Berkman, M.I. Psychometric evaluation of Simulator Sickness Questionnaire and its variants as a measure of cybersickness in consumer virtual environments. *Appl. Ergon.* **2019**, *82*, 102958. [CrossRef] [PubMed]
21. Kim, H.K.; Park, J.; Choi, Y.; Choe, M. Virtual reality sickness questionnaire (VRSQ): Motion sickness measurement index in a virtual reality environment. *Appl. Ergon.* **2018**, *69*, 66–73. [CrossRef]
22. Sharples, S.; Cobb, S.; Moody, A.; Wilson, J.R. Virtual reality induced symptoms and effects (VRISE): Comparison of head mounted display (HMD), desktop and projection display systems. *Displays* **2008**, *29*, 58–69. [CrossRef]
23. Bohil, C.; Alicea, B.; Biocca, F.A. Virtual reality in neuroscience research and therapy. *Nat. Rev. Neurosci.* **2011**, *12*, 752–762. [CrossRef]
24. Palmisano, S.; Mursic, R.; Kim, J. Vection and cybersickness generated by head-and-display motion in the Oculus Rift. *Displays* **2017**, *46*, 1–8. [CrossRef]
25. Dawes, J. Do Data Characteristics Change According to the Number of Scale Points Used? An Experiment Using 5-Point, 7-Point and 10-Point Scales. *Int. J. Mark. Res.* **2008**, *50*, 61–104. [CrossRef]
26. Joshi, A.; Kale, S.; Chandel, S.; Pal, D.K. Likert Scale: Explored and Explained. *Br. J. Appl. Sci. Technol.* **2015**, *7*, 396–403. [CrossRef]
27. Taherdoost, H. What is the best response scale for survey and questionnaire design; review of different lengths of rating scale/attitude scale/Likert scale. *Int. J. Acad. Res. Manag.* **2019**, *8*, 1–10.
28. Wakita, T.; Ueshima, N.; Noguchi, H. Psychological Distance between Categories in the Likert Scale. *Educ. Psychol. Meas.* **2012**, *72*, 533–546. [CrossRef]
29. Kourtesis, P.; Collina, S.; Doumas, L.A.A.; MacPherson, S.E. Validation of the Virtual Reality Neuroscience Questionnaire: Maximum Duration of Immersive Virtual Reality Sessions without the Presence of Pertinent Adverse Symptomatology. *Front. Hum. Neurosci.* **2019**, *13*, 417. [CrossRef]
30. Somrak, A.; Pogačnik, M.; Guna, J. Suitability and Comparison of Questionnaires Assessing Virtual Reality-Induced Symptoms and Effects and User Experience in Virtual Environments. *Sensors* **2021**, *21*, 1185. [CrossRef]
31. Partala, T.; Surakka, V. Pupil size variation as an indication of affective processing. *Int. J. Hum.-Comput. Stud.* **2003**, *59*, 185–198. [CrossRef]
32. Schwind, V.; Knierim, P.; Tasci, C.; Franczak, P.; Haas, N.; Henze, N. "These Are Not My Hands!": Effect of Gender on the Perception of Avatar Hands in Virtual Reality. In Proceedings of the 2017 CHI Conference on Human Factors in Computing Systems, New York, NY, USA, 6–11 May 2017; pp. 1577–1582. [CrossRef]
33. Bebko, A.O.; Troje, N.F. bmlTUX: Design and Control of Experiments in Virtual Reality and Beyond. *I-Perception* **2020**, *11*. [CrossRef]
34. Bonato, F.; Bubka, A.; Palmisano, S. Combined Pitch and Roll and Cybersickness in a Virtual Environment. *Aviat. Space Environ. Med.* **2009**, *80*, 941–945. [CrossRef] [PubMed]
35. Kourtesis, P.; Korre, D.; Collina, S.; Doumas, L.A.A.; MacPherson, S.E. Guidelines for the Development of Immersive Virtual Reality Software for Cognitive Neuroscience and Neuropsychology: The Development of Virtual Reality Everyday Assessment Lab (VR-EAL), a Neuropsychological Test Battery in Immersive Virtual Reality. *Front. Comput. Sci.* **2020**, *1*. [CrossRef]

36. Wechsler, D. *Wechsler Bellevue Adult Intelligence Scale*; Williams & Wilkins: Baltimore, MD, USA, 1939.
37. Corsi, P.M. Human memory and the medial temporal region of the brain. *Diss. Abstr. Int.* **1972**, *34*, 891.
38. Deary, I.J.; Liewald, D.; Nissan, J. A free, easy-to-use, computer-based simple and four-choice reaction time programme: The Deary-Liewald reaction time task. *Behav. Res. Methods* **2010**, *43*, 258–268. [CrossRef] [PubMed]
39. Golding, J.F. Predicting individual differences in motion sickness susceptibility by questionnaire. *Pers. Individ. Differ.* **2006**, *41*, 237–248. [CrossRef]
40. Roth, H.L.; Lora, A.N.; Heilman, K.M. Effects of monocular viewing and eye dominance on spatial attention. *Brain* **2002**, *125*, 2023–2035. [CrossRef]
41. Ursachi, G.; Horodnic, I.A.; Zait, A. How Reliable Are Measurement Scales? External Factors with Indirect Influence on Reliability Estimators. *Procedia Econ. Financ.* **2015**, *20*, 679–686. [CrossRef]
42. Power, M.; Fell, G.; Wright, M. Principles for high-quality, high-value testing. *Evid.-Base. Med.* **2013**, *18*, 5–10. [CrossRef]
43. Streiner, D.L.; Cairney, J. What's under the ROC? An Introduction to Receiver Operating Characteristics Curves. *Can. J. Psychiatry* **2007**, *52*, 121–128. [CrossRef]
44. Guilmette, T.J.; Sweet, J.J.; Hebben, N.; Koltai, D.; Mahone, E.M.; Spiegler, B.J.; Stucky, K.; Westerveld, M.; Participants, C. American Academy of Clinical Neuropsychology consensus conference statement on uniform labeling of performance test scores. *Clin. Neuropsychol.* **2020**, *34*, 437–453. [CrossRef]
45. The Jamovi Project [Computer Software]. Available online: http://www.jamovi.org (accessed on 1 January 2020).
46. R Core Team. *A Language and Environment for Statistical Computing*; R Foundation for Statistical Computing: Vienna, Austria, 2022. Available online: https://www.R-project.org/ (accessed on 12 December 2022).
47. Peterson, R.A.; Cavanaugh, J.E. Ordered quantile normalization: A semiparametric transformation built for the cross-validation era. *J. Appl. Stat.* **2019**, *47*, 2312–2327. [CrossRef] [PubMed]
48. Revelle, W. *psych: Procedures for Psychological, Psychometric, and Personality Research*; Northwestern University: Evanston, IL, USA, 2018. Available online: https://CRAN.R-project.org/package=psych (accessed on 12 December 2022).
49. Wickham, H. *ggplot2: Elegant Graphics for Data Analysis*; Springer-Verlag: New York, NY, USA, 2016. Available online: https://ggplot2.tidyverse.org (accessed on 12 December 2022)ISBN 978-3-319-24277-4.
50. Bates, D.; Mächler, M.; Bolker, B.; Walker, S. Fitting Linear Mixed-Effects Models Using lme4. *J. Stat. Softw.* **2015**, *67*, 48. [CrossRef]
51. Bouchard, S.; Berthiaume, M.; Robillard, G.; Forget, H.; Daudelin-Peltier, C.; Renaud, P.; Blais, C.; Fiset, D. Arguing in Favor of Revising the Simulator Sickness Questionnaire Factor Structure When Assessing Side Effects Induced by Immersions in Virtual Reality. *Front. Psychiatry* **2021**, *12*, 739742. [CrossRef] [PubMed]
52. Iii, W.B.S. Psychometric Evaluation of the Simulator Sickness Questionnaire as a Measure of Cybersickness. Ph.D. Thesis, Iowa State University, Ames, IA, USA, 2017. [CrossRef]
53. Nunnally, J.C. Psychometric Theory—25 Years Ago and Now. *Educ. Res.* **1975**, *4*, 7–21. [CrossRef]
54. Kourtesis, P.; Collina, S.; Doumas, L.A.; MacPherson, S.E. Validation of the Virtual Reality Everyday Assessment Lab (VR-EAL): An Immersive Virtual Reality Neuropsychological Battery with Enhanced Ecological Validity. *J. Int. Neuropsychol. Soc.* **2020**, *27*, 181–196. [CrossRef]
55. Karray, F.; Alemzadeh, M.; Abou Saleh, J.; Arab, M.N. Human-Computer Interaction: Overview on State of the Art. *Int. J. Smart Sens. Intell. Syst.* **2008**, *1*, 137–159. [CrossRef]
56. Stanney, K.; Lawson, B.D.; Rokers, B.; Dennison, M.; Fidopiastis, C.; Stoffregen, T.; Weech, S.; Fulvio, J.M. Identifying Causes of and Solutions for Cybersickness in Immersive Technology: Reformulation of a Research and Development Agenda. *Int. J. Hum.–Comput. Interact.* **2020**, *36*, 1783–1803. [CrossRef]
57. Jeong, D.; Yoo, S.; Yun, J. Cybersickness Analysis with EEG Using Deep Learning Algorithms. In Proceedings of the 2019 IEEE Conference on Virtual Reality and 3D User Interfaces (VR), Osaka, Japan, 23–27 March 2019; pp. 827–835. [CrossRef]
58. Krokos, E.; Varshney, A. Quantifying VR cybersickness using EEG. *Virtual Real.* **2021**, *26*, 77–89. [CrossRef]
59. Lopes, P.; Tian, N.; Boulic, R. Eye Thought You Were Sick! Exploring Eye Behaviors for Cybersickness Detection in VR. In Proceedings of the 13th ACM SIGGRAPH Conference on Motion, Interaction and Games, New York, NY, USA, 16–18 October 2020. [CrossRef]
60. Islam, R.; Desai, K.; Quarles, J. Cybersickness Prediction from Integrated HMD's Sensors: A Multimodal Deep Fusion Approach using Eye-tracking and Head-tracking Data. In Proceedings of the 2021 IEEE International Symposium on Mixed and Augmented Reality (ISMAR), Bari, Italy, 4–8 October 2021; pp. 31–40. [CrossRef]

virtual worlds MDPI

Communication

Current Perspective of Metaverse Application in Medical Education, Research and Patient Care

Irene Suh [1], Tess McKinney [2] and Ka-Chun Siu [1,*]

[1] Department of Health & Rehabilitation Sciences, University of Nebraska Medical Center, Omaha, NE 68198, USA
[2] Global Center for Health Security, University of Nebraska Medical Center, Omaha, NE 68198, USA
* Correspondence: kcsiu@unmc.edu; Tel.: +1-(402)-559-8464

Abstract: As virtual and augmented reality simulation technologies advance, the use of such technologies in medicine is widespread. The advanced virtual and augmented systems coupled with a complex interactive, immersive environment create a metaverse. The metaverse enables us to connect with others in a virtual world free of spatial restrictions and time constraints. In the educational aspect, it allows collaboration among peers and educators in an immersive 3D environment that can imitate the actual classroom setting with learning tools. Metaverse technology enables visualization of virtual 3D structures, facilitates collaboration and small group activities, improves mentor–mentee interactions, provides opportunities for self-directed learning experiences, and helps develop teamwork skills. The metaverse will be adapted rapidly in healthcare, boost digitalization, and grow in use in surgical procedures and medical education. The potential advantages of using the metaverse in diagnosing and treating patients are tremendous. This perspective paper provides the current state of technology in the medical field and proposes potential research directions to harness the benefits of the metaverse in medical education, research, and patient care. It aims to spark interest and discussion in the application of metaverse technology in healthcare and inspire further research in this area.

Keywords: virtual reality; augmented reality; mixed reality; health professions education

Citation: Suh, I.; McKinney, T.; Siu, K.-C. Current Perspective of Metaverse Application in Medical Education, Research and Patient Care. *Virtual Worlds* **2023**, *2*, 115–128. https://doi.org/10.3390/virtualworlds2020007

Academic Editors: Radu Comes, Dorin-Mircea Popovici, Calin Gheorghe Dan Neamtu and Jing-Jing Fang

Received: 1 March 2023
Revised: 18 March 2023
Accepted: 21 March 2023
Published: 18 April 2023

1. Introduction

The use of augmented reality (AR) and virtual reality (VR) in healthcare has been on the rise, leading to an expansion in the market size for these technologies. The market size for AR and VR in healthcare was US 2.0 billion in 2020, and it is expected to continue growing at a compound annual growth rate of 27% until 2028 [1]. This suggests that there is a growing demand for AR and VR in healthcare and a potential for these technologies to transform the way healthcare services are delivered. Furthermore, the COVID-19 pandemic era boosted the adaptation of the metaverse to use the benefit of virtual and real-world space [2]. Experiences of the metaverse need to be expanded, so that the healthcare providers and educators can understand the necessity of its use [3]. Meta-education and metaverse-powered online distance education have been introduced and accelerated in development that can emerge as rich, hybrid formal and informal learning experiences in online 3D virtual environments [4]. The concept of the metaverse satisfies all the concerns of interactions between humans and computers and the integration between the virtual and real worlds [5].

Immersive learning environments involve using virtual and augmented reality technologies to create more engaging and effective learning experiences [6]. These technologies can help simulate real-world scenarios, provide interactive feedback, and personalize learning, based on the needs and preferences of individual learners. Immersive learning environments can be created using various tools and technologies, such as 3D modeling software, game engines, and specialized hardware like head-mounted displays or haptic feedback devices. These tools can be used to simulate real-world environments, such as a hospital room, a factory floor, or a natural ecosystem, which can help learners develop skills and knowledge in a safe and controlled setting [7].

Web-based data processing innovations have been used to assess performance improvement and satisfaction levels in medical education and clinical care since 2006 [7]. Computer-based or computerized virtual patients simulating real-life clinical scenarios-based learning consistently showed higher learning outcomes [8]. As learning with computerized intervention gained popularity, trainees and students were allowed to perform anamnesis and physical exams, make diagnoses, and finalize therapeutic decisions in a safe environment; as a result, trainees could refine their clinical skills [9]. The metaverse could promote experiential learning through integrating effective educational approaches, such as problem-solving-based learning, game-based learning, and scenario-based learning [9]. These interventions have now become more realistically developed.

Surgical training simulators have been revolutionized by AR and VR, and they have coupled with machine learning tools. These revolutionized surgical simulators could provide trainees with life-like training, hyper-realistic simulations, and instant feedback [8]. Development of VR and AR simulation technologies in healthcare systems could be applied to not only surgeries, but also diagnostics, rehabilitation, training, and education [1].

Metaverse

The metaverse is an internet-based application that needs to be supported by AR, VR, and artificial intelligence [10]. Kye et al. [11] proposed a model for the metaverse that includes four primary pillars: AR, lifelogging, mirror world, and virtual worlds. It is a universal platform that supports innovation, communication, and shared knowledge. The four pillars are complementary to each other and form an interconnected roadmap to maximize the use of virtual technology for educational applications. Augmented reality expends real-world information to enhance knowledge, while lifelogging captures, stores, and shares experiences with others. The mirror world reflects the real world and provides external information, and the virtual world builds a simulated environment with digital information.

The metaverse is a unique and different concept from existing virtual technologies. It is envisioned as a fully interconnected virtual space where users can move seamlessly between different environments. Unlike existing virtual technologies, typically standalone applications, or platforms, the metaverse is designed to be a network of connected virtual spaces, allowing for more extensive and diverse experiences [12,13]. The metaverse is also designed to be a persistent space, meaning that a user's digital identity and avatar can exist across different platforms and applications, allowing for continuity of interaction and experience (Figure 1). This differs from existing virtual technologies, where users' experiences are often isolated within a particular platform or application [13,14].

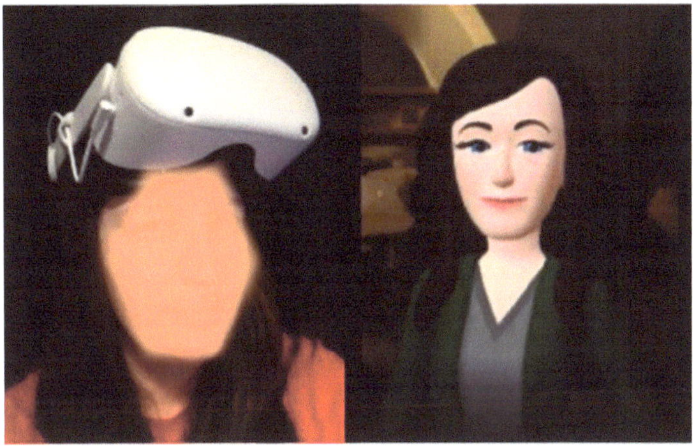

Figure 1. Metaverse avatar creation: Tess McKinney is pictured here (**left**) with her avatar (**right**) that she uses in the metaverse on the Horizon World platform and EngageVR platform.

Another key difference is that the metaverse is designed to be a space where users can create and share their content, interact with other users, and build communities around shared interests (Figure 2). This differs from existing virtual technologies, where users are often limited to pre-existing content or experiences [13]. Furthermore, the metaverse is designed to be an immersive environment, providing users with a sense of presence and embodiment within the virtual space. This differs from existing virtual technologies, which often rely on more limited forms of immersion, such as 2D displays or simple controllers [13,14]. The metaverse represents a significant step forward in virtual technology, offering a more extensive, interconnected, and immersive space for users to interact and create. While the technology to fully realize the metaverse is still developing, it can potentially transform how we interact with each other and the world around us [13,14]. The utilization of the metaverse for education is full of possibilities and unlimited. The metaverse creates a new dimension for students to learn new knowledge in 3D space and immersive environments. Such utilization has expanded substantially during and after the recent COVID-19 pandemic. More applications beyond science, technology, and engineering education are developing, such as medical training, research, and patient care. The following sections highlight those health-related potentials of using the metaverse.

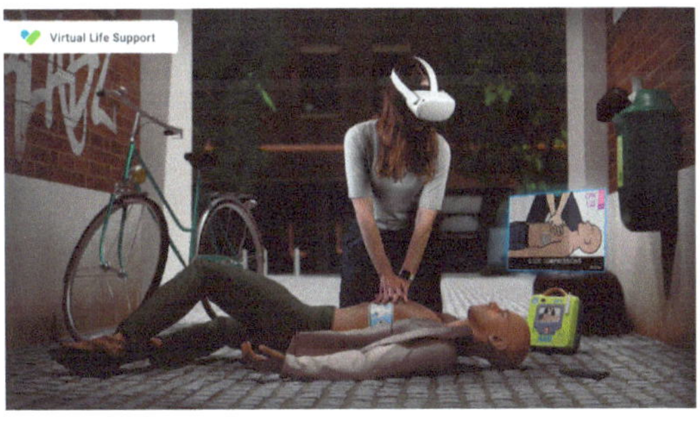

(**a**)

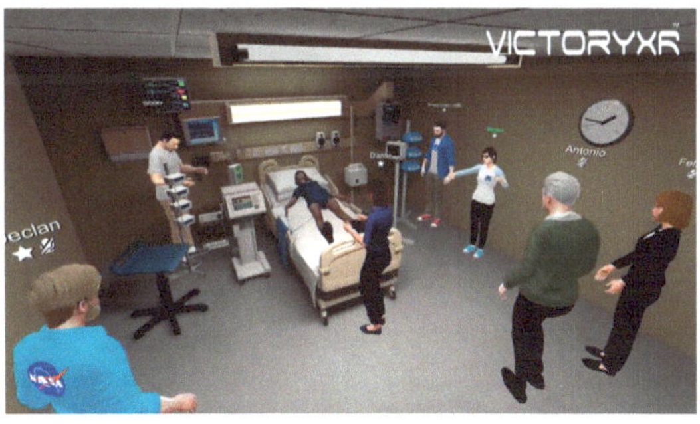

(**b**)

Figure 2. *Cont.*

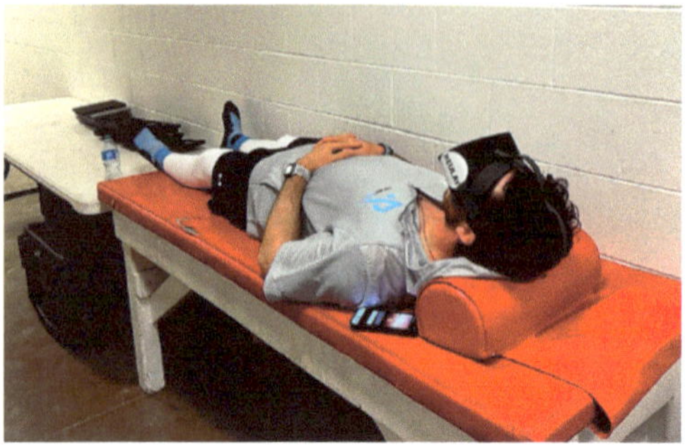

(c)

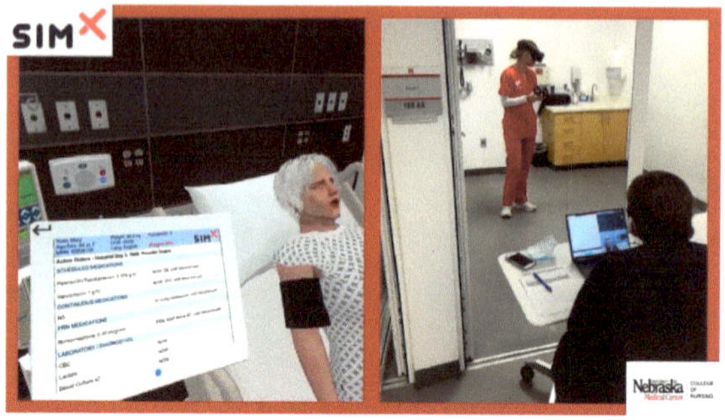

(d)

Figure 2. (**a**) Virtual Life Support utilizing passthrough VR with AR with an Oculus Quest 2 created by VR Lab. CPR and AED Training [15]. (**b**) Reulay, a mental health company, leverages virtual reality for mental wellbeing: decreasing stress and increasing focus [16]. (**c**) Class being held to learn about patients in a Metaversity using VictoryXR multiplayer IVR software [17]. (**d**) UNMC College of Nursing student working with faculty to go through a scenario on Sepsis. Faculty are involved in this simulation by becoming the patient voice or extras within the simulation to help the student practice real-world simulations. This simulation is multiplayer and contains a laptop moderator and an Immersive Virtual Reality headset [18].

2. Significance of the Metaverse in Healthcare Systems

The process to adopt the metaverse in healthcare has grown rapidly. The urgent need for digital transformation within healthcare settings was accelerated since the outbreak of the coronavirus in 2019 [19]. Furthermore, telehealth care services have gained significant attention and acceptance due to the evolving COVID-19 pandemic [20]. Before the COVID-19 pandemic, only 43% of healthcare facilities could provide services remotely [21,22]. Now, the usage of telemedicine has grown to 95% [23]. With the increased needs of digitalization of telemedicine services, the metaverse was highlighted and boosted research interests in supporting the importance of immersive VR technology [20].

The combination of augmented and mixed reality with the metaverse offers a novel approach to visualizing images and pinpointing targets in image-guided procedures [24]. The application of the metaverse can provide realistic consultations through personalized avatars that are interconnected [7]. The advent of the metaverse made it possible to interconnect online with the synergistic combination of augmented, virtual, and mixed reality. It happened to present a new era of immersive and real-time experiences to enhance human-to-human social interaction and connection [25]. The avatar is the digital representation of the player character in the metaverse [26]. The metaverse concept is increasingly used in healthcare to create personalized patient avatars. These avatars can represent a patient's unique physical, mental, and emotional characteristics and provide a more personalized approach to healthcare [26].

One potential application of personalized avatars is in patient education. By creating a virtual patient representation, healthcare providers can help patients better understand their medical conditions and treatment options. For example, a patient with a heart condition could be shown a virtual representation of their heart and how it functions, helping them to better understand their condition and how it can be managed. Personalized avatars can also simulate medical procedures and treatments, allowing healthcare providers to test different approaches before performing them on real patients. This can help reduce the risk of complications and improve outcomes. Another potential use of personalized avatars is in telemedicine. By creating a virtual patient representation, healthcare providers can conduct virtual visits and consultations, providing more personalized care even when patients are not physically present in the same location. The use of personalized avatars in healthcare is an exciting development that has the potential to improve patient outcomes and provide more personalized and effective care. The metaverse provides a powerful platform for creating and utilizing these avatars, and it will likely play an increasingly important role in future healthcare [27].

A review study in pain management by Chan et al. [28] found that VR interventions were effective in reducing pain intensity and providing pain relief, both during and after the intervention. The VR interventions were particularly effective in managing procedural pain, such as during medical procedures like wound dressing changes or dental procedures. Additionally, the studies showed that VR interventions improved patient satisfaction, decreased anxiety and stress, and enhanced the overall healthcare experience. This review suggests that VR may be a promising tool in pain management and can be used as an adjunct to pharmacological and non-pharmacological interventions [28]. Another study by Ahmadpour et al. [29] has shown that use of computer-generated images and sounds to create a simulated environment can be a tool to distract patients from pain sensations or to provide relaxation and mindfulness exercises. In acute pain management, VR interventions have been used to provide distraction during painful medical procedures such as burn wound care, dental procedures, and injections. The immersive environment can reduce the patient's focus on the pain, providing a sense of control and reducing anxiety. In chronic pain management, VR interventions have been used to provide relaxation exercises and cognitive-behavioral therapy techniques. Patients can enter calming virtual environments and practice mindfulness exercises or guided imagery, which can reduce pain intensity and distress. There is growing evidence of the effectiveness of VR interventions for acute and chronic pain management, and it has been shown to be safe and well-tolerated by patients. The VR interventions offer a non-pharmacological approach to pain management, which can be particularly beneficial for patients who cannot tolerate or do not want to take pain medication [29].

2.1. Applications in Education for Healthcare

As the metaverse came into daily life, its applications have been applied in educational settings [11]. The metaverse can be used to create virtual classrooms and training environments, which can be particularly useful for fields that require hands-on learning or simulations, such as medicine [11,26]. One of the key benefits of using the metaverse is to provide learners with immediate and personalized feedback [30]. For example, a medical student practicing a surgical procedure in a VR environment can receive real-time feedback on their technique and performance. This feedback can help learners identify areas to improve and adjust their approach accordingly [8], as shown in Figure 2d.

Chen et al. [30] suggest that using an immersive, blended pedagogy that combines traditional classroom instruction with immersive learning experiences in the metaverse can enhance student engagement and improve learning outcomes, particularly in the areas of patient care and scientific inquiry during the COVID-19 pandemic. They noted that the pandemic has disrupted traditional classroom instruction, making it difficult for educators to provide students with the hands-on experiences and interactions with patients that are essential for learning in healthcare fields. They found that the active learning strategies implemented in the metaverse promoted engagement and scientific inquiry, providing a safe and immersive environment for students to practice and develop their skills. This approach may be beneficial for educators facing pandemic-related disruptions to traditional classroom instruction, as it provides hands-on experiences and interactions with patients that may not be possible in a physical classroom [30]. Immersive learning technology in the metaverse is an exciting and rapidly evolving field that has the potential to transform the way we learn and teach. By leveraging the latest technologies and pedagogical approaches, the metaverse can provide learners with engaging, effective, and personalized learning experiences that help them develop the knowledge and skills they need to succeed [8].

Like virtual anatomy classes, medical students can learn about human anatomy through interactive virtual lessons, including the ability to manipulate and explore virtual cadavers (Figure 3). Virtual medical education simulations can also be used for medical students to practice diagnosing and treating patients, practice procedures, and practice decision-making in a safe, controlled environment. Furthermore, the full-scale scenario-based simulator training can be developed to help the learner acquire interpersonal communication skills, teamwork, leadership, decision-making, the ability to prioritize tasks under pressure, and stress management [31]. With the full-scale scenario-based simulator, medical students can engage in virtual patient encounters to practice their clinical skills, including taking medical histories, performing physical exams, and communicating with patients [32]. Remote collaboration, training, and learning can be near with metaverse technology to connect with one another and receive training from experts, even if they are located in different parts of the world. Virtual conferences and workshops can remotely continue their education and keep them up to date with the latest developments in their fields [32]. These are just a few examples of how metaverse technology can be used in education for healthcare.

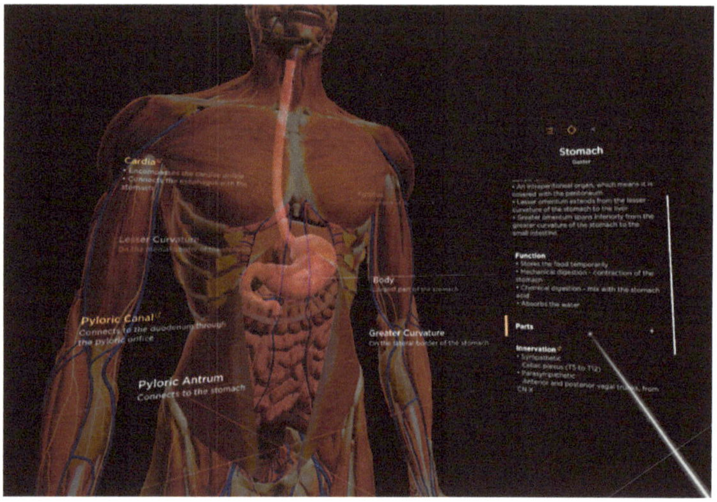

Figure 3. Dissection of human anatomy using 3D/VR/AR/and computer-based simulation application [33].

The metaverse can play a useful role in enhancing the performance of the medical trainees [34]. The metaverse has the great potential to transform medical education by providing students with realistic and engaging learning experiences. It can help to improve their skills, reduce medical errors, and prepare them for the challenges of real-world medical practice [27]. Active learning strategies can be effectively used in the metaverse to improve student engagement in a blended learning environment [30]. The authors discussed how immersive technologies can provide students with opportunities to engage in experiential learning, which can be challenging in traditional classroom settings. By integrating virtual patient scenarios and scientific inquiry into the metaverse, students can develop critical thinking skills and gain practical experience in patient care. The authors suggest that using active learning strategies in the metaverse can lead to better student outcomes, including increased student motivation, improved retention rates, and higher levels of engagement [26]. The possibilities are endless, and technology continues to evolve, so the use cases for the metaverse in education for healthcare will likely expand in the coming years.

2.2. Applications in Research

The metaverse is a concept that refers to a shared, immersive virtual space where people can interact and communicate with one another. It is an emerging technology with many potential applications in research. With the metaverse, researchers can conduct experiments in a controlled, immersive environment. According to Bhugaonkar et al. [35], psychologists could use the metaverse to study social interactions or communication, while economists could use it to study decision-making under different conditions [35]. The authors also noted that these technologies have the potential to improve healthcare outcomes by providing more immersive and interactive training experiences, enhancing patient engagement and motivation, and enabling remote monitoring and care delivery [35].

Psychologists Krijn et al. [36] used VR to study the effectiveness of exposure therapy for social anxiety disorder. Virtual reality exposure therapy (VRET) is a type of therapy that uses VR technology to simulate anxiety-provoking situations in a safe and controlled environment. VRET is typically used to treat anxiety disorders like phobias, social anxiety disorder, and post-traumatic stress disorder. The researchers found that VRET was more effective than traditional exposure therapy in reducing social anxiety symptoms [36]. VRET has the advantage of being more flexible and accessible since it can be done remotely and at the patient's own pace [36]. In a neuroscience study by Spiers and Maguire [37], the researchers used VR to investigate the neural mechanisms underlying spatial memory. They were able to identify the brain regions that are selectively activated during spatial memory tasks and determine their role in memory consolidation. The researchers found that the hippocampus, a brain region associated with memory, was more active when participants navigated through a virtual environment than when they viewed static images [37]. This research provided insights into the neural processes underlying spatial memory and highlighted the potential of VR technology for investigating brain function in real-world contexts [37].

The advantage of using the metaverse is that it enables collaborative research. The metaverse can facilitate collaboration among researchers who are physically separated, allowing them to work together in a virtual space as if they were in the same room [38]. The state-of-the-art human–computer interaction (HCI) in the metaverse is an area of active research and development. HCI in the metaverse involves designing intuitive and natural ways for users to interact with virtual objects and other users, as well as creating immersive and engaging user experiences [38].

According to Zhao et al. [39], the metaverse can be used to create interactive 3D visualizations of data, which can be helpful for understanding complex information or communicating research findings to a wider audience. The metaverse has the potential to transform many aspects of our lives, but it also requires significant advancements in technology and conceptual design [39]. Overall, the metaverse has the potential to revolutionize the way that research is conducted and communicated, and it is an exciting area of study with many potential applications.

2.3. Applications in Patient Care

As of now, the metaverse in healthcare is still in its early stages of development and has not been widely implemented. However, there have been some initial experiences and experiments with using VR and AR technologies to enhance healthcare [40,41]. VR and AR can be used to improve patient education and engagement. Patients can use VR and AR technologies to better understand their medical conditions and treatments, which can improve adherence to treatment plans and ultimately lead to better health outcomes [40]. Virtual healthcare platforms are being developed that aim to provide a more immersive and personalized healthcare experience. These platforms use a combination of virtual and physical components to provide remote medical consultations and diagnosis [41]. In summary, while there are some initial experiences and experiments with using the metaverse in healthcare, the concept is still in its early stages of development, and it will likely be some time before we see widespread implementation of this technology in healthcare [40,41]. More potential applications of the metaverse in patient care are in Table A1 (Appendix A).

3. Limitations and Challenges

One of the main limitations of the metaverse is data management, security, and privacy of the patient's information [42]. Since it requires higher ethical standards to protect patients' information, the rules and regulations need to be cautiously reviewed and formulated [40]. The metaverse needs to provide various tools and techniques to users, so that they can preserve privacy. As metaverse technologies evolve, data management science should develop together. Furthermore, healthcare providers and medical training programs may include additional courses that can cover data ethics and cybersecurity.

Despite considerable research relating to metaverse technologies, little attention has been paid to the standardization of medical education programs. Educational research is needed to assess whether the metaverse improves the learning experience of medical students, which will help academic research departments compare and evaluate the effectiveness of different programs [8]. More educationalists, social scientists, and learning technologists need to be involved since developing and maintaining a virtual environment for medical education can be technically challenging and requires significant resources [7,11,43].

Additional limitations would be the computer capacity and internet bandwidth for image streaming, especially in rural areas with lack of internet connectivity [10]. Both students and educators also need smartphones or computers with enough processing capacity and internet bandwidth for virtual and augmented reality [1]. The hardware for virtual and augmented reality, such as visors or glasses, are required for a truly immersive experience, but these items are costly [9]. Technical and equipment supports would be required for the underprivileged areas and underserved students.

Some users may experience discomfort or other negative effects using virtual and augmented systems, such as dizziness, headaches, or nausea [12]. These factors can significantly impact their willingness to use the technology and affect their overall experience with the metaverse. While these technologies have the potential to revolutionize various aspects of our lives, it is critical to ensure that they are accessible and enjoyable for all users. Designers and developers should consider these factors and work to minimize potential side effects through improvements in hardware, software, and user interface development [12].

The use of metaverse technology in education for healthcare is a promising development with potential benefits, but it must be approached with careful consideration and ongoing evaluation to ensure its effectiveness and safety.

4. Future Direction and Recommendation

The metaverse is coming to us. As technology advances, it will bring us new immersive and imaginary worlds [10]. An immersive 3D environment could provide a better perception of the surrounding environment. It could be applied in diverse medical fields such as neuroscience, psychology, dentistry, and other interventions that allow immersive places [33]. The synergy effect of collaboration across multiple disciplines remains a crucial opportunity for educational research in the metaverse. The future of the metaverse in education for healthcare is promising and can potentially enhance medical education and training [9–11]. If integrated with artificial intelligence and machine learning, advances can enhance the interactivity and realism of metaverse environments, providing a more immersive and practical learning experience.

The metaverse's diverse applications are evolving daily, and developers' perception is changing as they create new metaverses [42]. The developers may create a more sustainable and economic metaverse platform that can be easily applied to medical education and healthcare providers. Healthcare professionals would be needed to educate medical trainees and prepare them to advance to meet new opportunities [9–11], and medical educators need to pinpoint the incorporation of these applications. The metaverse is revolutionizing medical education, patient care, treatment, surgical training, and research [9–11,44]. It could enhance the overall quality of patient care and improve the quality of medical procedures, diagnosis, and treatment.

5. Summary

The metaverse cannot take the place of clinical practice. Interactions with patients are essential skills that healthcare professionals acquire [42]. However, the metaverse in education in healthcare has great potential to be an interactive and immersive application that can be modified for each person [21]. It can support educators to implement interactions with patients as well as trainees that can be more caring in many ways.

The metaverse can be included to enhance the quality of education, research, and patient care. It could bring new possibilities to facilitate healthcare professionals having a positive experience within a risk-free environment [33]. The metaverse is a fully immersive virtual world that integrates human life's social, economic, and cultural aspects. The metaverse extends virtual worlds, aiming to provide users with a more comprehensive and engaging experience [14,45]. Revolutionized technologies and the metaverse can be used in diverse medical fields, and the application can benefit patients, healthcare providers, and trainees. The use of metaverse technology in education for healthcare is a promising development with potential benefits. However, it must be carefully considered and evaluated to ensure its effectiveness and safety. Collaboration with multiple disciplinary areas would be anticipated to evaluate the long-term effects of the metaverse for medical education in the future.

Author Contributions: Conceptualization, I.S. and K.-C.S.; oginal draft preparation, I.S. and T.M.; writing—review and editing, I.S., T.M. and K.-C.S.; visualization, T.M.; supervision, K.-C.S.; project administration, I.S. and K.-C.S.; funding acquisition, K.-C.S. All authors have read and agreed to the published version of the manuscript.

Funding: This project is supported by the National Institute of Biomedical Imaging and Bioengineering of the National Institutes of Health under award number (1R56EB030053-01A1).

Institutional Review Board Statement: Not Applicable.

Informed Consent Statement: Not Applicable.

Data Availability Statement: Not Applicable.

Conflicts of Interest: The authors declare no conflict of interest.

Appendix A

Table A1. Application in Patient Care.

Types	Pros	Cons
Virtual reality (VR) therapy [44] VR can be used as a therapeutic tool to help patients with a range of conditions, including anxiety, phobias, post-traumatic stress disorder (PTSD), and pain management.	i. Controlled Environment: VR allows therapists to create a controlled and safe environment in which patients can confront their fears and anxieties. ii. Customizable: VR experiences can be customized to suit individual needs, making the therapy more effective. iii. Being Immersed: VR creates an immersive experience that can be more effective than traditional therapy methods in treating conditions such as phobias and PTSD. iv. Accessibility: VR therapy is more accessible to patients who may not be able to participate in traditional exposure therapy due to physical limitations or fears of leaving the house.	i. Cost: VR equipment can be expensive, making it less accessible to some patients. ii. Limited Research: The use of VR for treating anxiety, phobias, and PTSD is still in the early stages of development and there is limited research on its long-term effects. iii. Unrealistic: Some patients may not respond well to VR therapy because they perceive the experience as unrealistic or too artificial.

Table A1. *Cont.*

Types	Pros	Cons
Virtual consultations [35] The metaverse can be used to facilitate virtual consultations between patients and healthcare providers, allowing patients to access care from anywhere. This can be particularly useful for patients in remote or underserved areas, or for those who have mobility issues.	i. Accessibility: Virtual consultations can increase access to healthcare for patients who may have difficulty traveling to see a healthcare provider in person, such as those with mobility issues or who live in rural areas. ii. Convenience: Virtual consultations can be more convenient for both patients and healthcare providers as they can be done from the comfort of one's own home or office. iii. Timesaving: Virtual consultations can save time compared to traditional in-person consultations as they eliminate the need for traveling. iv. Reduced costs: Virtual consultations can potentially reduce costs associated with travel and parking.	i. Technical issues: Virtual consultations can be disrupted by technical issues such as poor internet connectivity or equipment malfunctions. ii. Reduced personal interaction: Virtual consultations may lack the personal interaction and human touch that can be important in building a therapeutic relationship between a healthcare provider and patient. iii. Limited examination: Virtual consultations may limit the examination that can be performed compared to an in-person consultation, as the healthcare provider may not be able to physically touch or observe the patient. iv. Data security: Virtual consultations may raise concerns about the security of personal and medical information, as it is transmitted electronically.
Telerehabilitation [46] The metaverse can be used to deliver rehabilitation services to patients remotely, enabling them to complete therapy exercises at home or in other locations.	i. Increased access to rehabilitation services: Telerehabilitation with the metaverse can increase access to rehabilitation services for patients who may not have access to traditional rehabilitation facilities due to geographic or mobility limitations. ii. Improved outcomes: The systematic review by de Araújo et al. found that VR rehabilitation was effective in improving outcomes such as motor function, balance, and activities of daily living in individuals with spinal cord injuries. iii. Customized and immersive rehabilitation experience: The metaverse allows healthcare providers to create customized virtual environments that simulate real-world scenarios, providing a more engaging and motivating rehabilitation experience for patients. iv. Increased safety: VR rehabilitation provides a controlled and safe setting for patients to practice and improve their skills, minimizing the risk of further injury.	i. Access to technology: Not all patients may have access to the necessary technology and equipment for telerehabilitation with the metaverse, such as VR headsets. ii. Cost: The cost of technology and equipment for telerehabilitation with the metaverse can be a barrier for some patients and healthcare providers. iii. Technical difficulties: Technical difficulties or malfunctions of the equipment can disrupt the rehabilitation experience and may require additional support. iv. Limited ability to assess physical performance: The virtual environment may not fully replicate real-world scenarios, making it difficult for healthcare providers to accurately assess physical performance.

Table A1. *Cont.*

Types	Pros	Cons
Telemedicine [35] The metaverse could be used to provide remote medical consultations, allowing patients to see a doctor or specialist in a virtual environment. This could be especially useful for people living in remote or underserved areas.	i. Convenient for patients: Telemedicine enables patients to access healthcare services from the comfort of their homes, saving them time and effort in traveling to see a doctor. ii. Improved access to care: Telemedicine can provide healthcare services to patients in remote and underserved areas, improving access to care. iii. Increased efficiency: Telemedicine can reduce wait times for appointments and improve the efficiency of the healthcare system. iv. Cost-effective: Telemedicine can be a more cost-effective solution compared to traditional in-person visits. v. Better continuity of care: Telemedicine can improve the continuity of care for patients, as they can easily communicate with their healthcare provider between appointments.	i. Technical challenges: Telemedicine can be limited by technology and may require patients to have access to reliable internet, a computer or smartphone, and other necessary equipment. ii. Quality of care concerns: The quality of care provided through telemedicine may not be as high as in-person visits, as certain physical exams and procedures cannot be performed remotely. iii. Limited patient-provider interaction: Telemedicine may not provide the same level of patient–provider interaction as in-person visits, as patients may feel less connected to their healthcare provider. iv. Privacy and security risks: Telemedicine can also pose privacy and security risks, as personal health information may be vulnerable to hacking and cyberattacks. v. Reimbursement issues: Telemedicine may also face reimbursement issues, as insurance companies may not cover all telemedicine services.
Patient education [47] The metaverse can be used to provide interactive, immersive patient education experiences, which can be more engaging and effective than traditional methods.	i. Improving rehabilitation outcomes: The study focuses on the use of VR as a rehabilitation tool after knee surgery. By incorporating VR exercises into the rehabilitation process, patients can improve their physical performance, balance, and gait, resulting in a faster recovery and better outcomes. ii. Increased patient satisfaction: Patients in the study reported a high level of satisfaction with VR-based rehabilitation compared to traditional physical therapy. iii. Personalized rehabilitation: The study found that the level of difficulty of the VR exercises had a significant impact on patient outcomes. By tailoring the exercises to the patient's specific abilities and progress, the rehabilitation program can be personalized to meet each patient's unique needs.	i. Potential for technological limitations: The use of VR technology for rehabilitation may be limited by the availability and accessibility of the equipment, as well as the technical skills required to operate it. Patients may also experience discomfort or motion sickness while using VR, which could limit the feasibility of this approach for some patients.

Table A1. *Cont.*

Types	Pros	Cons
Social support [44] The metaverse can be used to connect patients with similar conditions and provide a sense of community and social support.	i. Greater control: Virtual reality exposure therapy (VRET) provides the therapist with greater control over the patient's exposure to anxiety-provoking stimuli, allowing them to carefully tailor the treatment to the patient's specific needs and progress at a pace that they can handle. ii. Increased engagement and motivation: VRET provides a highly immersive and engaging experience, which can increase patient motivation to participate in therapy and adhere to treatment plans. iii. Safe and controlled environment: VRET allows patients to confront anxiety-provoking stimuli in a safe and controlled environment, without the risks associated with exposure in real-life situations. iv. Efficacy: VRET has been found to be effective in reducing symptoms of anxiety disorders, with some studies reporting results that are comparable to traditional in vivo exposure therapy.	i. Limited generalizability: VRET may not always generalize to real-life situations, as the stimuli presented in VR may differ from those encountered in the real world. This can limit the effectiveness of the therapy in some cases. ii. Technical limitations: The quality of the VR experience can be impacted by technical limitations, such as the quality of the graphics or the performance of the hardware. This can potentially detract from the effectiveness of the therapy. iii. Cost: VRET can be expensive to implement, as it requires specialized equipment and software. This can limit its accessibility to some patients who may not have access to the necessary resources.
Medical Visualization [39] The metaverse could be used to create interactive 3D visualizations of medical data, such as CT scans, MRI images, and microscopic samples. This could make it easier for doctors and researchers to understand and analyze medical data and could also be used to create VR experiences that help patients understand their diagnosis and treatment.	i. Improved understanding of medical data: By creating interactive 3D visualizations of medical data, doctors and researchers can better understand and analyze complex medical data. This can lead to more accurate diagnoses and better treatment decisions. ii. Enhanced patient education: Using VR experiences, patients can better understand their diagnosis and treatment, which can improve their engagement in the treatment process and their overall outcomes. iii. Greater efficiency: Medical visualization can help doctors and researchers process complex medical data more efficiently, leading to faster diagnoses and treatment decisions. iv. Reduced risk: Using VR to visualize medical data can reduce the need for invasive procedures or surgeries, which can reduce the risk of complications and speed up recovery times.	i. Cost: Developing high-quality, interactive VR visualizations can be expensive, which may limit their availability to certain institutions or patients. ii. Technical challenges: Creating 3D visualizations of medical data requires specialized technical expertise and resources, which may be a barrier to adoption. iii. Limited accessibility: VR technology may not be accessible to all patients, particularly those with certain disabilities or conditions that make it difficult to use. iv. Ethical concerns: There may be ethical concerns around the use of VR to visualize sensitive medical data, particularly if there are privacy or confidentiality risks.

Table A1. *Cont.*

Types	Pros	Cons
Mental Health treatment [44] This could be used for providing virtual therapy sessions, creating virtual support groups, and providing VR exposure therapy for people suffering from anxiety and post-traumatic stress disorder (PTSD).	i. Increased access to care: Virtual therapy sessions and virtual support groups can be more accessible and convenient for people who may have difficulty accessing in-person mental health services due to geographical, financial, or other barriers. ii. Greater anonymity: Virtual therapy and support groups can provide a greater sense of anonymity and privacy, which may make it easier for people to share about their mental health struggles. iii. More engaging and immersive therapy: VR exposure therapy can create a more immersive and realistic experience for people receiving treatment for anxiety and PTSD, which may lead to more effective therapy outcomes. iv. Customizable experiences: Virtual technology can be used to create personalized and customizable therapy experiences, such as virtual environments that are tailored to a person's specific fears or triggers.	i. Technical issues: Virtual technology may be subject to technical issues that could disrupt therapy sessions, such as internet connectivity problems, hardware failures, or software glitches. ii. Lack of personal connection: Virtual therapy and support groups may lack the personal connection and face-to-face interactions that some people may prefer in traditional therapy settings. iii. Potential for distractions: Virtual therapy sessions may be more susceptible to distractions from the person's environment, such as notifications from their phone or other digital devices. iv. Ethical and legal concerns: Virtual therapy may raise ethical and legal concerns related to privacy, security, and informed consent. For example, ensuring that personal health information is kept confidential and secure may be more challenging in a virtual environment.

References

1. Flavián, C.; Ibáñez-Sánchez, S.; Orús, C. The impact of virtual, augmented and mixed reality technologies on the customer experience. *J. Bus. Res.* **2019**, *100*, 547–560. [CrossRef]
2. Ramesh, P.V.; Joshua, T.; Ray, P.; Devadas, A.K.; Raj, P.M.; Ramesh, S.V.; Ramesh, M.K.; Rajasekaran, R. Holographic elysium of a 4D ophthalmic anatomical and pathological metaverse with extended reality/mixed reality. *Indian J. Ophthalmol.* **2022**, *70*, 3116–3121. [CrossRef] [PubMed]
3. Iwanaga, J.; Muo, E.C.; Tabira, Y.; Watanabe, K.; Tubbs, S.J.; D'Antoni, A.V.; Rajaram-Gilkes, M.; Loukas, M.; Khalil, M.K.; Tubbs, R.S. Who really needs a Metaverse in anatomy education? A review with preliminary survey results. *Clin. Anat.* **2023**, *36*, 77–82. [CrossRef] [PubMed]
4. Mystakidis, S. Metaverse. *Encyclopedia* **2022**, *2*, 486–497. [CrossRef]
5. Qiu, C.S.; Majeed, A.; Khan, S.; Watson, M. Transforming health through the metaverse. *J. R. Soc. Med.* **2022**, *115*, 484–486. [CrossRef] [PubMed]
6. Morgado, L.; Allison, C.; Beck, D.; Penicheiro, F. Immersive Learning Research. *J. Univers. Comput. Sci.* **2018**, *24*, 70–71. [CrossRef]
7. Hilty, D.M.; Alverson, D.C.; Alpert, J.E.; Tong, L.; Sagduyu, K.; Boland, R.J.; Mostaghimi, A.; Leamon, M.L.; Fidler, D.; Yellowlees, P.M. Virtual reality, telemedicine, web and data processing innovations in medical and psychiatric education and clinical care. *Acad. Psychiatry* **2006**, *30*, 528–533. [CrossRef]
8. Cook, A.; Erwin, P.J.; Triola, M.M. Computerized Virtual Patients in Health Professions Education: A Systematic Review and Meta-Analysis. *Acad. Med.* **2019**, *85*, 1589–1602. [CrossRef]
9. Sandrone, S. Medical education in the metaverse. *Nat. Med.* **2022**, *28*, 2456–2457. [CrossRef]
10. A Whole New World: Education Meets the Metaverse. Available online: https://www.brookings.edu/research/a-whole-new-world-education-meets-the-metaverse/ (accessed on 20 February 2023).
11. Kye, B.; Han, N.; Kim, E.; Park, Y.; Jo, S. Educational applications of metaverse: Possibilities and limitations. *J. Educ. Eval. Health Prof.* **2020**, *18*, 32. [CrossRef]
12. Chang, E.; Kim, H.T.; Yoo, B. Virtual Reality Sickness: A Review of Causes and Measurements. *Int. J. Hum.-Comput. Interact.* **2020**, *36*, 1658–1682. [CrossRef]
13. Lombardi, J.; Lombardi, M. Opening the Metaverse. In *Online Worlds: Convergence of the Real and the Virtual*; Human-Computer Interaction Series; Bainbridge, W., Ed. Springer: London, UK, 2010; pp. 111–122. [CrossRef]
14. Nevelsteen, K.J. Virtual world defined from a technological perspective and applied to video games mixed reality and the metaverse. *Comput. Animat. Virtual Worlds* **2018**, *29*, e1752. [CrossRef]
15. Virtual Life Support™, Created by VR Lab. Available online: virtuallifesupport.eu (accessed on 15 March 2023).
16. Reulay, Inc. Available online: www.reulay.com (accessed on 15 March 2023).
17. VictoryXR. Available online: www.victoryxr.com (accessed on 16 March 2023).

18. University of Nebraska Medical Center- Lincoln College of Nursing and SimX. Available online: www.simxvr.com (accessed on 23 March 2023).
19. Center for Systems Science and Engineering (CSSE) at Johns Hopkins University. COVID-19 Dashboard. Available online: https://coronavirus.jhu.edu/map.html (accessed on 20 January 2023).
20. Wong, M.Y.Z.; Gunasekeran, D.V.; Nusinovici, S.; Sabanayagam, C.; Yeo, K.K.; Cheng, C.Y.; Tham, Y.C. Telehealth demand trends during the COVID-19 pandemic in the top 50 most affected countries: Infodemiological evaluation. *JMIR Public Health Surveill.* **2021**, *7*, e24445. [CrossRef] [PubMed]
21. Kala, N. Revolutionizing Medical Education with Metaverse. *Int. J. Sci. Res. Comput. Sci. Eng. Inf. Technol.* **2022**, *8*, 26–32. [CrossRef]
22. Metaverse: The Next Frontier for Health 4.0. Available online: https://www.netscribes.com/metaverse-in-healthcare/ (accessed on 22 January 2023).
23. Jnr, A.B. Integrating telemedicine to support digital health care for the management of COVID-19 pandemic. *Int. J. Healthc. Manag.* **2021**, *14*, 280–289. [CrossRef]
24. Vergara, D.; Rubio, M.P.; Lorenzo, M. On the design of virtual reality learning environments in engineering. *Multimodal. Technol. Interact.* **2017**, *1*, 11. [CrossRef]
25. Rahaman, T. Into the Metaverse—Perspectives on a New Reality. *Med. Ref. Serv. Q.* **2022**, *41*, 330–337. [CrossRef]
26. Zhang, X.; Chen, Y.; Hu, L.; Wang, Y. The metaverse in education: Definition, framework, features, potential applications, challenges, and future research topics. *Front. Psychol.* **2022**, *13*, 1016300. [CrossRef]
27. Bansal, G.; Rajgopal, K.; Chamola, V.; Xiong, Z.; Niyato, D. Healthcare in Metaverse: A Survey on Current Metaverse Applications in Healthcare. *IEEE Access* **2022**, *10*, 119914–119946. [CrossRef]
28. Chan, E.; Foster, S.; Sambell, R.; Leong, P. Clinical efficacy of virtual reality for acute procedural pain management: A systematic review and meta-analysis. *PLoS ONE* **2018**, *27*, 13. [CrossRef]
29. Ahmadpour, N.; Randall, H.; Choksi, H.; Gao, A.; Vaughan, C.; Poronnik, P. Virtual Reality interventions for acute and chronic pain management. *Int. J. Biochem. Cell Biol.* **2019**, *114*, 105568. [CrossRef] [PubMed]
30. Chen, Y.; Lin, W.; Zheng, Y.; Xue, T.; Chen, C.; Chen, G. Application of Active Learning Strategies in Metaverse to Improve Student Engagement: An Immersive Blended Pedagogy Bridging Patient Care and Scientific Inquiry in Pandemic. *SSRN Electron. J.* **2022**. [CrossRef]
31. Al-Elq, A.H. Simulation-based medical teaching and learning. *J. Fam. Community Med.* **2010**, *17*, 35–40. [CrossRef] [PubMed]
32. Thomason, J. MetaHealth—How will the Metaverse Change Health Care? *J. Metaverse* **2021**, *1*, 13–16.
33. [33]Medical Augmented Intelligence (MAI) Is a Pioneer in the Field of Medical VR Innovations Creating the Google Maps of the Human Body. Available online: www.mai.ai/bodymap/ (accessed on 16 March 2023).
34. Javaid, M.; Haleem, A. Virtual reality applications toward medical field. *Clin. Epidemiol. Glob. Health* **2020**, *8*, 600–605. [CrossRef]
35. Bhugaonkar, K.; Bhugaonkar, R.; Masne, N. The Trend of Metaverse and Augmented & Virtual Reality Extending to the Healthcare System. *Cureus* **2022**, *12*, e29071. [CrossRef]
36. Krijn, M.; Emmelkamp, P.M.G.; Olafsson, R.P.; Biemond, R. Virtual reality exposure therapy of anxiety disorders: A review. *Clin. Psychol. Rev.* **2004**, *24*, 259–281. [CrossRef]
37. Spiers, H.J.; Maguire, E.A. Neural substrates of driving behaviour. *NeuroImage* **2007**, *36*, 245–255. [CrossRef]
38. State-of-the-Art Human-Computer-Interaction in Metaverse. Available online: https://think.taylorandfrancis.com/special_issues/international-journal-human-computer-interaction-metaverse/ (accessed on 21 January 2023).
39. Zhao, Y.; Jiang, J.; Chen, Y.; Liu, R.; Yang, Y.; Xue, X.; Chen, S. Metaverse: Perspectives from graphics, interactions and visualization. *Vis. Inform.* **2022**, *6*, 56–67. [CrossRef]
40. Chengoden, R.; Victor, N.; Huynh-The, T.; Yenduri, G.; Jhaveri, R.H.; Alazab, M.; Gadekallu, T.R. Metaverse for Healthcare: A Survey on Potential Applications, Challenges and Future Directions. *IEEE Access* **2023**, *11*, 12765–12795. [CrossRef]
41. Halbig, A.; Babu, S.K.; Gatter, S.; Latoschik, M.E.; Brukamp, K.; von Mammen, S. Opportunities and challenges of virtual reality in healthcare–a domain experts' inquiry. *Front. Virtual Real.* **2022**, *3*, 837616. [CrossRef]
42. Petrigna, L.; Musumeci, G. The Metaverse: A New Challenge for the Healthcare System: A Scoping Review. *J. Funct. Morphol. Kinesiol.* **2022**, *7*, 63. [CrossRef] [PubMed]
43. Sandrone, S.; Carlson, C.E. Future of Neurology & Technology: Virtual and Augmented Reality in Neurology and Neuroscience Education Applications and Curricular Strategies. *Neurology* **2021**, *97*, 740–744. [CrossRef]
44. Carl, E.; Stein, A.T.; Levihn-Coon, A.; Pogue, J.R.; Rothbaum, B.; Emmelkamp, P.; Powers, M.B. Virtual reality exposure therapy for anxiety and related disorders: A meta-analysis of randomized controlled trials. *J. Anxiety Disord.* **2019**, *61*, 27–36. [CrossRef]
45. Metaverse Continuum. Available online: https://www.accenture.com/us-en/services/metaverse-index?c=acn (accessed on 14 March 2023).
46. de Araújo, A.V.L.; Neiva, J.F.O.; Monteiro, C.B.M.; Magalhães, F.H. Efficacy of Virtual Reality Rehabilitation after Spinal Cord Injury: A Systematic Review. *Biomed. Res. Int.* **2019**, *13*, 7106951. [CrossRef]
47. Lee, M.; Suh, D.; Son, J.; Kim, J.; Eun, S.D.; Yoon, B. Patient perspectives on virtual reality-based rehabilitation after knee surgery: Importance of level of difficulty. *J. Rehabil. Res. Dev.* **2016**, *53*, 239–252. [CrossRef]

applied sciences

MDPI

Article

Understanding VR-Based Construction Safety Training Effectiveness: The Role of Telepresence, Risk Perception, and Training Satisfaction

Joon Woo Yoo, Jun Sung Park and Hee Jun Park *

Department of Industrial Engineering, Yonsei University, Seoul 03722, Republic of Korea
* Correspondence: h.park@yonsei.ac.kr

Abstract: The use of virtual reality as a safety training technology is gaining attention in the construction industry. While current studies focus mainly on the development of VR-based safety training programs, studies focusing on improving its effectiveness is still lacking. Thus, this study aims to understand the psychological process of training transfer and determine the factors that affect VR safety training effectiveness. The study analysed survey data from 248 construction workers who finished construction safety training using VR using PLS-SEM. The results show that the telepresence experienced through the VR and the risk perception of the trainees regarding occupational accidents significantly affect their satisfaction with VR safety training, which affected its effectiveness. Considering that the use of VR in the construction safety training context is still in its early stages, the results of our study, which comprehensively analyses both the technological and psychological aspects of VR safety training, could provide meaningful implications to VR training content developers. Furthermore, the theoretical approach of our study could be implemented in future studies focusing on the topic of training effectiveness.

Keywords: virtual reality; telepresence; training transfer; training satisfaction; safety training

Citation: Yoo, J.W.; Park, J.S.; Park, H.J. Understanding VR-Based Construction Safety Training Effectiveness: The Role of Telepresence, Risk Perception, and Training Satisfaction. *Appl. Sci.* **2023**, *13*, 1135. https://doi.org/10.3390/app13021135

Academic Editors: Radu Comes, Dorin-Mircea Popovici, Calin Gheorghe Dan Neamtu and Jing-Jing Fang

Received: 6 December 2022
Revised: 9 January 2023
Accepted: 13 January 2023
Published: 14 January 2023

1. Introduction

The construction industry often requires several workers to perform hands-on tasks to produce a final product. This makes construction workers especially vulnerable to occupational accidents, such as falling or electrocution [1]. According to a report from the Korean Ministry of Employment and Labor (MoEL), the construction industry recorded 9.41 accidents per 1000 workers in 2018, while the average rate for all industries was only 5.36 [2]. Furthermore, according to Zhao and Lucas [3], 80% of the occupational accidents in the construction industry are caused by human error, with at least 49% being due to unawareness or misjudgment, meaning that they are preventable.

Over the years, various efforts to improve the safety of construction workers have been made, one of them being the implementation of mandatory safety training. Since 2012, construction workers in South Korea have been obligated to complete a four-hour basic safety and health training. The training focuses mainly on introducing various hazards in a construction site and ways to prevent accidents from happening therein. The workers must also complete additional training every time they change workplaces or when they operate special equipment, such as excavators.

However, despite these training sessions and their content, the current safety training has not resulted in an improvement in accident rates in the construction industry. According to the Korean MoEL, the construction industry exhibited an increase in the number of accidents per 1000 workers from 7.48 in 2015 to 9.41 in 2018, in contrast with the downward trend of accident rates in other industries [2]. The increase in accident rate implies that the knowledge and skills garnered from the safety training are not being transferred to the workplace.

To enhance the effectiveness of safety training and promote safe working practices of construction workers, different training methods and technologies are being employed and tested with the current safety training. For example, advances in the IT sector have promoted the use of e-learning as a tool for safety training. Compared with the traditional training method, the use of e-learning has reduced training costs dramatically while the quality of the training has improved [4].

Recently, the e-learning trend has further advanced with the adoption of virtual reality (VR) technology. VR safety training allows construction workers to interact in a virtual environment using a head-mounted display and a controller [3,5]. This allows them to experience various workplace hazards and practice safe working procedures in a safe, controlled environment [6,7]. In addition, a systematic review of literature on VR/AR use in the educational context found that the use of VR/AR technology enhances interactivity, encourages collaborative learning, and increases learner satisfaction [8]. Furthermore, owing to the COVID-19 pandemic, the use of VR as a training tool is gaining attention because it can be conducted with minimal human contact [9].

Although the adoption of VR safety training in the construction industry is rapidly increasing, studies on understanding the factors that increase VR safety training effectiveness are still lacking. Some studies have focused on developing a VR training system and comparing its effectiveness to that of other training methods using ANOVA or a paired sample *t*-test as analysis methods; nevertheless, simply demonstrating that the VR method is more effective fails to explain the reason for its effectiveness. For example, Sacks et al. [10] found that trainees who completed VR safety training showed higher test scores for certain construction tasks compared with those who received traditional classroom training; however, the researchers failed to explain the reason for the effectiveness of the VR-trained group in selective tasks. This type of methodological approach to understanding effectiveness has led researchers to assert that research on training effectiveness lacks a theoretical basis [11].

Therefore, this study aims to employ a more theoretical approach to explain VR construction safety training effectiveness. Specifically, we utilize the technology acceptance model (TAM) to determine the specific features of VR safety training and risk perception toward occupational accidents that affect the workers' perception toward VR safety training and finally, training transfer. Consequently, we aim to provide timely implications for improving the effectiveness of construction safety training using VR.

2. Theoretical Background

2.1. Training Transfer

Training transfer is defined as the implementation of knowledge or skill obtained from the training to the actual workplace and is one of the primary criteria for evaluating its effectiveness [12]. Because the training of human resources requires investing a significant amount of both time and money, improving the transfer of training has been a persistent issue for both researchers and practitioners. More specifically, according to Baldwin and Ford [13], only 10% of the total investment in human resource training and development leads to the successful transfer of the training content. Increasing the overall transfer is particularly important, because the accident and fatality rate of construction workers remains high despite the government-mandated training.

According to prior studies, factors affecting training transfer can be broadly divided into two categories: individual factors and organizational factors. Individual factors are related to the trainees' characteristics or the characteristics of the training content. For example, job function, job position, or training satisfaction are some widely used individual factors that affect training transfer [14]. In contrast, organizational factors, such as transfer climate or organizational support, are related to the characteristics of the organization to which the trainee belongs [14,15].

However, because this study focuses mainly on identifying the characteristics of VR training that affect effectiveness, organizational factors are not of interest. Therefore, this study develops a research model that focuses on identifying the individual factors and technological characteristics of the VR construction safety training that affect its effectiveness.

2.2. Modified Technology Acceptance Model

The TAM was developed by Davis in order to explain the effect of a user's beliefs on their attitude and behaviour regarding a new technology [16]. Specifically, the TAM explains that a user's perceived usefulness and ease of use of a new technology affects their attitude toward its use, which then affects their behavioural intention and actual usage behaviour.

TAM is one of the most powerful and commonly used theoretical models for explaining the adoption of new technologies. It has been utilized to explain and predict the adoption behaviour of e-commerce, ride-sharing services, and mobile-learning [17–19]. It has also been revised and extended in follow-up studies, leading to the development of modified models such as TAM2 and TAM3, which are intended to explain technology acceptance more effectively by adding factors such as subjective norm and self-efficacy [20,21]. Despite these moderations, perceived usefulness, perceived ease of use, behavioural intention, and acceptance/use behaviour remain the key constructs.

TAM itself, however, fails to consider the distinctive features of specific technologies and contexts. To overcome this shortcoming, researchers have extended the TAM by adding technological or usage-specific factors that affect the user's belief. For example, to study the acceptance of VR in aeronautical assembly tasks, Sagnier et al. [22] analysed the effect of technology-specific factors, such as pragmatic quality and hedonic quality stimulation. Similarly, to explain the use of ICT among senior citizens, Guner and Acarturk [23] utilized social influence, anxiety, and self-satisfaction as external variables affecting the user's perceived usefulness and perceived ease of use. Therefore, in the current study, we consider both technology-specific and usage-specific external variables that reflect the distinctive features of VR construction safety training.

Another shortcoming of the TAM is that in cases where technology usage is mandatory, such as a system mandated by company policy, predicting acceptance through usage intention is rather inadequate. In such cases where users were mandated to adopt a certain system, satisfaction was found to be an effective predictor of user acceptance or performance [24]. Therefore, because the adoption VR construction safety training is mandatory, we adopted training satisfaction as a predictor of user acceptance.

2.3. VR and Telepresence

Telepresence, defined as the feeling of being present in an environment constructed through certain communication media, is one of the key features that characterize VR [25,26]. In fact, Steuer [25] defined VR as "a real or simulated environment where the user experiences telepresence."

Furthermore, Steuer [25] introduced two dimensions that influence telepresence within the VR environment: vividness and interactivity. Vividness, also known as realness, is defined as the richness of the mediated virtual environment. The higher the number of senses the medium stimulates and the better the medium replicates the human sensory experience, the higher the vividness of the VR [27]. Interactivity is defined as the degree to which users of the medium can manipulate the mediated environment in real time. The faster the medium responds to the user's commands, the wider the range of manipulation. The more similar the response of the virtual environment is to that expected in the real world, the higher the interactivity [26]. That is, if users feel that they have control over their actions in the virtual environment, they experience a higher level of interactivity.

A number of studies have employed telepresence, vividness, and interactivity as key concepts for studying VR adoption. For example, Kim and Ko [28] studied the influence of the use of VR on flow experience and satisfaction. Their study found that users of VR showed a significantly higher level of vividness and interactivity compared with those of traditional 2D media, which led to a higher level of telepresence. They also found that telepresence significantly impacted the users' flow experience, which affected their overall satisfaction. Other studies such as Jang and Park [29] and Wu et al. [30] found that display quality and interactivity positively affected the presence felt by the user, which affected their continued intention to use VR games and credibility of VR news.

In the construction safety training context, studies have not yet focused specifically on telepresence. Instead, most studies have focused on comparing the effectiveness of VR safety training and traditional training. For example, Sacks et al. [10] tested the effectiveness of a VR safety training system compared with that of the traditional training method. The results showed that while VR safety training showed higher test results for some tasks, such as stone cladding work, it had no observable advantages in overall safety training. Other studies, such as that by Zhao and Lucas [3], focused on developing and testing a VR training program for construction workers.

Because telepresence is a crucial factor that distinguishes VR training from the traditional classroom training method, understanding how it affects training effectiveness provides a key implication for our study. Hence, the two dimensions of telepresence are utilized as external variables of the TAM that affect the trainee's beliefs regarding VR safety training.

3. Research Model and Hypotheses

Prior studies on VR safety training have focused mainly on comparing the effectiveness of the VR training method with that of traditional methods. However, simply comparing the performance between different training groups fails to explain the reason for the effectiveness of one training method over another. This has been a major issue in studies related to measuring training effectiveness. Clark et al. [31] specifically mentioned that "without a theoretical basis for studying the techniques ... researchers are often at a loss either to explain why they are effective or to predict their effectiveness in other settings".

Therefore, this study aims to provide an explanation for the effectiveness of the use of VR as a safety training tool. Specifically, by applying the TAM, we explain the effect of the characteristics of VR construction safety training on trainees' beliefs regarding VR safety training, which affect the trainee's satisfaction and the training effectiveness. Our research model is presented in Figure 1.

3.1. Modified TAM

The TAM posits that an individual's belief, specifically their perceived usefulness and perceived ease of use concerning a certain technology, affects their attitude, usage intention, and acceptance of the technology. The two cognitive beliefs presented in TAM are perceived usefulness and perceived ease of use, which are each defined, respectively, as "the degree to which a user believes that the use of a certain system would enhance their performance" and "the degree to which a user believes that using a certain system would be free of effort [16]".

Prior studies have confirmed the effectiveness of TAM when explaining and predicting acceptance of a newly emerging technology [32,33]. In a training or education context, TAM has been utilized to study an individual's intention to use e-learning or other newly introduced training tools. For example, Chang et al. [34] adopted the TAM to study the factors affecting students' intention to use e-learning. They found that although perceived ease of use had no significant effect on perceived usefulness, both perceived usefulness and perceived ease of use positively affected students' intention to use e-learning. Additionally, Wu and Vu [35] confirmed the positive effect of perceived usefulness and perceived ease of use on an aviation student's intention to use an augmented reality maintenance training system.

Additionally, in cases where technology adoption is mandatory, satisfaction was found to be an effective indicator of user acceptance. For example, to study the acceptance of web-based training among construction professionals, Park et al. [24] utilized user satisfaction as a variable replacing usage intention in the TAM model. Similarly, Nah et al. [36] applied 'symbolic adoption' as an alternative to usage intention regarding the acceptance of an enterprise system, and measured the construct through items such as 'I am excited about using the SAP system in my workplace'.

Therefore, based on prior studies, we defined perceived usefulness as the degree to which a trainee believed that the VR safety training would enhance their performance, and perceived ease of use as the degree to which a trainee believed that the VR safety training would be free of effort. Furthermore, based on studies employing the TAM as a theoretical basis for studying the acceptance of technologies in a mandatory setting, we present the following hypotheses:

H1. *Perceived usefulness has a positive effect on training satisfaction.*

H2. *Perceived ease of use has a positive effect on training satisfaction.*

H3. *Perceived ease of use has a positive effect on perceived usefulness.*

3.2. External Variables of TAM

3.2.1. Telepresence in VR

Telepresence is a multi-dimensional concept consisting of vividness and interactivity [25]. While vividness is determined by the sensory breadth and depth perceived by the user, interactivity is determined by the response speed, range, and mapping of the VR technology. In summary, higher levels of telepresence could indicate that the users perceived the virtual environment as reflecting the real world. Prior studies have utilized these two dimensions of telepresence to analyze its effect on flow experience or satisfaction [28].

Furthermore, recent studies focusing on the acceptance of VR or AR have utilized TAM, and they have observed the effect of telepresence on user belief. For example, a study on the acceptance of AR interactive technology, in which consumers were allowed to try on clothing products using AR, confirmed the significant effect of presence on the perceived usefulness and ease of use for both consumers with high and low cognitive innovation [37]. Similarly, Oh and Yoon [38] confirmed the effect of presence on perceived usefulness and perceived ease of use when adopting haptic enabling technology (HET), which allowed users to control a virtual environment using touch.

Therefore, to study the effect of telepresence on user beliefs in the VR construction safety training context, we present the following hypotheses:

H4(a). *Vividness has a positive effect on perceived usefulness.*

H4(b). *Vividness has a positive effect on perceived ease of use.*

H5(a). *Interactivity has a positive effect on perceived usefulness.*

H5(b). *Interactivity has a positive effect on perceived ease of use.*

3.2.2. Risk Perception: Perceived Vulnerability and Severity

Perceived vulnerability and perceived severity are each defined as an individual's perceived probability of a threatening event happening to them and the severity of the damage the event will cause to their life or health, respectively. In this study, these two constructs are defined as the probability of an accident occurring to the construction worker at their workplace, and the damage the accident would do to their health.

Perceived vulnerability and perceived severity are often used in research to study an individual's protective behaviour toward a certain threat. They are also often integrated with TAM as external variables affecting an individual's perceived usefulness toward a health-related technology. For example, Ahadzadeh et al. [39] found that perceived health risk, which is a multi-dimensional construct composed of perceived severity and perceived susceptibility, has a positive effect on perceived usefulness in the context of health-related internet use. Furthermore, Hansen et al. [40] found that perceived risk significantly affected perceived usefulness when studying consumers' intention to use social media for transactions. Dou et al. [41] also confirmed the effect of perceived health threat on perceived usefulness in a study identifying the factors affecting the acceptance of M-health technologies.

Because construction workers are especially vulnerable to life-threatening accidents in the workplace, the level of risk perceived by the worker could have a significant effect on their perceived usefulness of VR safety training. If they consider themselves to be at risk of accidents, there is a higher chance they will think that the training content would be useful in keeping them safe. Therefore, the following hypotheses are presented:

H6. *Perceived vulnerability has a positive effect on perceived usefulness.*

H7. *Perceived severity has a positive effect on perceived usefulness.*

3.3. Training Effectiveness

Training transfer is one of the most widely used criterion for measuring training effectiveness. In several studies, training satisfaction was confirmed to be a significant predictor of training transfer [42,43]. Therefore, by integrating the TAM with the concept of training transfer, the following hypothesis is presented:

H8. *Training satisfaction has a positive effect on training transfer.*

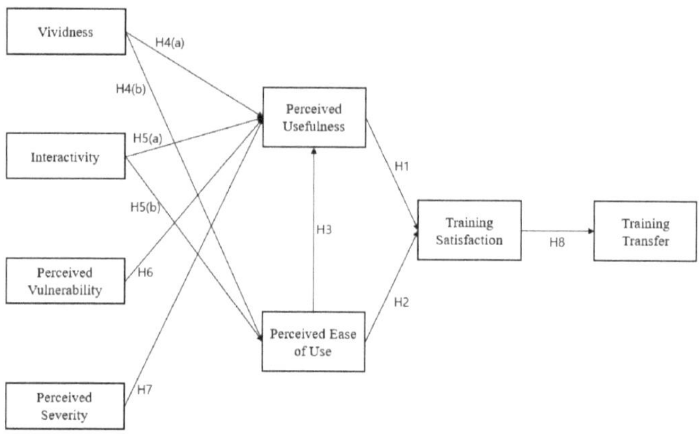

Figure 1. Proposed Research Model.

4. Materials and Methods

4.1. Survey Items

We adopted survey items from prior studies and modified them to fit our research context. The use of existing survey items assures its validity and accuracy since it has been vigorously tested after its development [44]. The items related to the TAM were adopted from Yoon and Kim [45]; Sun et al. [46]; Latif [47]; and Sun et al. [48]. Items for measuring interactivity and vividness were adapted from Kelley et al. [49]; and Yim et al. [50]. Perceived vulnerability and severity were measured using the items adopted from Yoon and Kim [45]; Sun et al. [46]; and Ahadzadeh et al. [39]. Finally, training transfer was measured using items from Gegenfurtner [42]. In addition, the items were revised through a pilot test to ensure content validity. The pilot test was conducted with 10 participants who completed the VR training. Items that did not meet the validity criteria were deleted in the final survey. All items were measured based on a 5-point Likert scale, ranging from 1 for 'strongly disagree' to 5 for 'strongly agree.' The survey items are presented in Table 1.

Table 1. Survey Items.

Variable	Measurement Item
Vividness	VI1. The contents of the VR safety training were very well-defined VI2. The contents of the VR safety training were very clear VI3. The contents of the VR safety training were very detailed VI4. The contents of the VR safety training were very vivid
Interactivity	IN1. I was in control of my navigation through the VR safety training IN2. I was in control of seeing the contents of the VR safety training IN3. I was in control over the pace of the VR safety training IN4. The VR safety training environment responded to my commands quickly and efficiently
Perceived Vulnerability	PV1. I am at risk of suffering from workplace accidents at the construction site PV2. It is likely that I will suffer from workplace accidents at the construction site PV3. It is possible for me to suffer from workplace accidents at the construction site PV4. There is a chance that I will suffer from workplace accidents at the construction site
Perceived Severity	PS1. If I were to suffer from workplace accidents at the construction site, the damage would be severe PS2. If I were to suffer from workplace accidents at the construction site, the damage would be critical PS3. If I were to suffer from workplace accidents at the construction site, the damage would be significant PS4. If I were to suffer from workplace accidents at the construction site, I will have difficulty with my work
Perceived Usefulness	PU1. The VR safety training will be helpful for staying safe at the construction site PU2. The VR safety training is effective for staying safe at the construction site PU3. Upon applying the knowledge and skills obtained from the VR safety training, I will be less likely to be injured at the construction site
Perceived Ease of Use	PEOU1. It is easy for me to complete the VR safety training and apply it to my work PEOU2. I have the ability to complete the VR safety training and fully apply it to my work PEOU3. I am able to complete the VR safety training and apply it to my work without much difficulty
Training Satisfaction	TS1. The VR safety training contents were relevant to the job I perform TS2. The VR safety training increased my understanding of the subject TS3. If I had an opportunity to undergo another safety training using VR, I would gladly do so TS4. Overall, I was very satisfied with the VR safety training
Training Transfer	TT1. I will try to transfer the knowledge and skills obtained from the VR safety training to the construction site TT2. I feel that I am able to use the knowledge and skills gained from the VR safety training at the construction site TT3. The VR safety training prepared me well for applying the related knowledge and skills at the construction site TT4. I will continuously use the knowledge and skills obtained from the safety training at the construction site

4.2. *Sample*

We conducted a survey in April and March 2021 on workers currently working at construction sites in South Korea. The survey was conducted in-person and prior to the survey, all respondents completed a VR safety training wherein they experienced common workplace accidents and were instructed in safe working procedures to prevent such accidents. The VR training was conducted using an Oculus VR HMD and the contents of the training were developed by the Korea Occupational Safety & Health Agency (KOSHA) [51]. An example of the VR screenshot is presented in Figure 2.

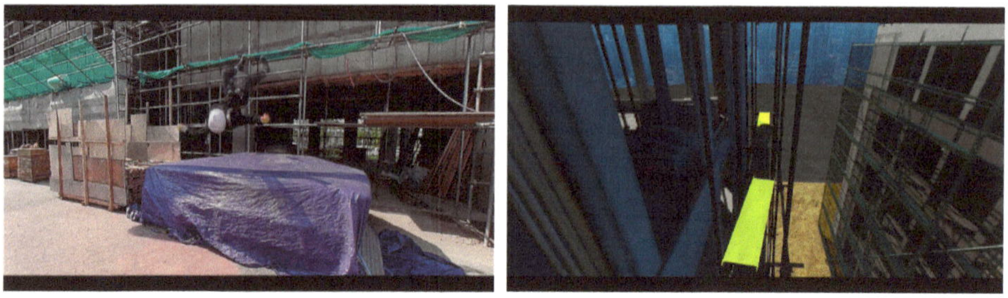

Figure 2. Example VR screenshot of the scaffolding task safety training (Source ref [51], 2019, Korea Occupational Safety & Health Agency).

After eliminating 22 samples with insincere or incomplete responses, a total of 248 samples were used for the final analysis, resulting in a 92% response rate, which is higher than the required rate of 80% [52]. Furthermore, according to Hair et al. [53], for our study to have a statistical power of 80% and a significance level of 5% with a minimum R^2 value of 0.25, it is recommended that we have at least 70 samples. Thus, sample size was not an issue in our study. The demographic characteristics of the respondents are shown in Table 2.

Table 2. Demographic Characteristics.

Classification		Frequency (N = 248)	Percentage (%)
Gender	Male	218	87.9
	Female	30	12.1
Age	20s	15	6.0
	30s	67	27.1
	40s	92	37.1
	50s	61	24.6
	60 and over	13	5.2
Experience in the construction industry	<1 year	18	7.3
	1–5 years	40	16.1
	6–10 years	45	18.1
	11–15 years	63	25.4
	16–20 years	54	21.8
	>20 years	28	11.3
Avg. working hours per day	<3 h	2	0.8
	4–8 h	145	58.5
	9–12 h	96	38.7
	>12 h	5	2.0

5. Results

We conducted partial least squares structural equation modelling (PLS-SEM) using the SmartPLS 3.0 program. PLS-SEM has advantages over traditional analysis methods because it allows for the assessment of measurement error and can predict latent variables using observed variables. In addition, it effectively analyses the causal relationship between several complex variables. Furthermore, compared to CB-SEM, PLS-SEM shows greater statistical power and is applicable when the structural model is complex [54]. Finally, the PLS-SEM method can analyse ordinal data, such as survey data, based on a Likert scale; this was also performed in our study [55].

5.1. Measurement Model Testing

Prior to hypotheses testing, we verified the measurement items by confirming their convergent and discriminant validity. Convergent validity is confirmed when (1) the factor loadings of the survey items exceed 0.7, (2) the average variance extracted (AVE) of the constructs exceeds 0.5, and (3) the composite reliability (CR) and Cronbach's alpha exceed 0.7 [54]. Furthermore, discriminant validity is confirmed if the heterotrait–monotrait ratio of correlations (HTMT) for each construct is lower than 0.9 [54]. As shown in Tables 3 and 4, all the criteria for convergent and discriminant validity were met, confirming the validity of our measurement model.

Table 3. Convergent Validity.

Variable	Factor Loadings	AVE	CR	Cronbach's α
Vividness	0.784, 0.871, 0.888, 0.902	0.744	0.921	0.885
Interactivity	0.881, 0.902, 0.832, 0.790	0.726	0.914	0.875
Perceived Vulnerability	0.903, 0.942, 0.951, 0.954	0.879	0.967	0.954
Perceived Severity	0.967, 0.962, 0.962, 0.948	0.921	0.979	0.971
Perceived Usefulness	0.934, 0.942, 0.907	0.861	0.949	0.919
Perceived Ease of Use	0.936, 0.947, 0.940	0.886	0.959	0.936
Training Satisfaction	0.867, 0.878, 0.888, 0.875	0.769	0.930	0.900
Training Transfer	0.921, 0.925, 0.914, 0.882	0.829	0.951	0.931

Table 4. Discriminant Validity (HTMT).

	VI	IN	PV	PS	PU	PEOU	TS	TT
VI								
IN	0.744							
PV	0.097	0.131						
PS	0.180	0.179	0.556					
PU	0.521	0.443	0.069	0.260				
PEOU	0.487	0.487	0.094	0.185	0.775			
TS	0.701	0.677	0.155	0.171	0.642	0.585		
TT	0.638	0.533	0.069	0.165	0.588	0.588	0.757	

Furthermore, we tested for possible collinearity issues regarding our structural model. As shown in Table 5, all VIF values were less than 3, confirming that collinearity is not an issue [54].

Table 5. Collinearity Test (VIF).

	PU	PEOU	TS	TT
VI	1.903	1.772		
IN	1.867	1.772		
PV	1.408			
PS	1.449			
PEOU	1.362		2.074	
PU			2.074	
TS				1.000

Note: VI: Vividness, IN: Interactivity, PV: Perceived Vulnerability, PS: Perceived Severity, PU: Perceived Usefulness, PEOU: Perceived Ease of Use, TS: Training Satisfaction, TT: Training Transfer.

5.2. Hypotheses Testing

We tested our hypotheses using the PLS-SEM method. A bootstrap resampling procedure was performed to test the significance of the paths. The results, including the path coefficients and the overall explanatory power, are shown in Table 6.

Table 6. Results of the Hypotheses Testing.

Path	Hypotheses	Beta	Results	f^2
PU → TS	H1	0.403 **	Supported	0.125
PEOU → TS	H2	0.254 **	Supported	0.050
PEOU → PU	H3	0.621 **	Supported	0.642
VI → PU	H4(a)	0.160 *	Supported	0.031
VI → PEOU	H4(b)	0.303 **	Supported	0.070
IN → PU	H5(a)	0.008	Not supported	-
IN → PEOU	H5(b)	0.255 **	Supported	0.049
PV → PU	H6	−0.088	Not Supported	-
PS → PU	H7	0.155 *	Supported	0.038
TS → TT	H8	0.698 **	Supported	0.951

Note: * $p < 0.05$, ** $p < 0.001$. Note: VI: Vividness, IN: Interactivity, PV: Perceived Vulnerability, PS: Perceived Severity, PU: Perceived Usefulness, PEOU: Perceived Ease of Use, TS: Training Satisfaction, TT: Training Transfer.

The results of the hypotheses test showed that the effects of interactivity and perceived vulnerability on perceived usefulness were statistically insignificant at $p < 0.05$. Thus, H5(a) and H6 were rejected. However, all the other hypotheses were statistically significant and thus supported. Vividness (β = 0.160), perceived severity (β = 0.155), and perceived ease of use (β = 0.621) had a significant effect on perceived usefulness, whereas vividness (β = 0.303) and interactivity (β = 0.255) significantly affected the perceived ease of use. Moreover, both perceived usefulness (β = 0.403) and perceived ease of use (β = 0.254) significantly affected training satisfaction, which led to training transfer (β = 0.698).

Additionally, while H1, H2, H4(a), H4(b), H5(b), and H7 showed weak effect size (f^2 ≥ 0.02), H3 and H8 showed strong effect size (f^2 ≥ 0.35) [56]. The specific f^2 value of each hypothesis along with its significance is presented in Table 6.

Finally, the explanatory power (R^2) of perceived usefulness (R^2 = 0.559), perceived ease of use (R^2 = 0.258), training satisfaction (R^2 = 0.374), and training transfer (R^2 = 0.487) all exceeded the required threshold of 0.10, proposed by Falk and Miller [57].

6. Discussion and Implications

6.1. Discussion

By empirically testing our research model, this study aimed to identify the specific factors of the VR safety training that affected training transfer in the construction industry, thereby providing guidance for improving the effectiveness of the training. The following are some important findings based on the hypotheses testing results.

First, the constructs of the TAM, which are perceived usefulness, perceived ease of use, and training satisfaction, directly and indirectly act as significant predictors of training transfer. This confirms the usefulness and effectiveness of the TAM in predicting training transfer behaviour when implementing a new technology; moreover, this is consistent with the findings of Park et al. [24] and Granić and Marangunić [58]. Furthermore, the high explanatory power of the TAM constructs also supports the TAM's usefulness in our research.

Second, the two dimensions of telepresence, which are vividness and interactivity, significantly affected the trainees' perceived usefulness and perceived ease of use concerning the VR safety training. Specifically, while vividness influenced both perceived usefulness and perceived ease of use, interactivity directly affected only the perceived ease of use and indirectly affected the perceived usefulness. This result is somewhat consistent with the research of Oh and Yoon [38] and Grabowski et al. [59], which concluded that telepresence experienced while using HET significantly affects the perceived usefulness of HET. Thus, it could be concluded that the telepresence felt during the VR safety training had a significant impact on the trainee's belief regarding the training, which plays a critical role in increasing the effectiveness of the training.

Lastly, of the two external factors regarding the trainee's attitude toward accidents in the workplace, only perceived severity had a significant effect on perceived usefulness.

This is consistent with the result of Ahadzadeh et al. [39], who concluded that perceived health risk, which is a multidimensional construct composed of perceived severity and perceived susceptibility, has an effect on perceived usefulness in the case of health-related internet use. Therefore, instilling a sense of alarm, related to occupational accidents, to the trainees could increase the overall effectiveness of the VR safety training.

6.2. Implications

6.2.1. Theoretical Implications

This study provides an important theoretical contribution in that it analysed the impact of the use of VR technology on the effectiveness of safety training using the TAM as a theoretical basis. By developing a theoretical research model, we were able to overcome the lack of a theory-based approach to the topic of training transfer, which was pointed out by Kontoghiorghes [11]. Our TAM-based research model could be extended to other training/education contexts wherein a new technology is emerging as a training tool.

By analysing the survey data using a SEM-based approach, we were able to understand how the use of VR helps improve the effectiveness of VR safety training. Prior studies that simply compared the results of different training methods failed to explain or provide implications on how to improve effectiveness of a newly introduced method. However, the results of our study could be used for developing and further improving VR safety training content to increase the training effectiveness.

Finally, we utilize the concept of telepresence, which is the key characteristic that distinguishes VR technology from other media. By analysing the effect of the two main dimensions of telepresence, vividness, and interactivity, we were able to understand how each dimension affects the trainee's perception toward the training. The results of our study showed that although both vividness and interactivity are important, the vividness of the VR directly affects both the perceived usefulness and ease of use for the trainee, and these are critical factors that affect the effectiveness of the training.

6.2.2. Managerial Implications

Our study also has meaningful practical implications for VR safety training content developers and training instructors, particularly because the pandemic has caused a dramatic increase in the demand for training methods requiring less face-to-face contact.

The results of our study showed that a trainee's belief and attitude toward VR safety training plays a critical role in enhancing the training effectiveness. These factors are affected by the vividness and interactivity of the VR, along with the trainee's perception of occupational accidents and their own safety.

Therefore, first, content developers should focus on increasing the vividness and interactivity perceived by a trainee to increase the training effectiveness. Because vividness is determined by the sensory breadth and depth perceived by the VR user, developers could use high-definition images captured from a real construction site instead of the currently used animation-based content. Furthermore, newly emerging VR hardware, such as haptic suits that provide a feeling of pressure or vibration based on actions in the virtual environment, could be utilized to provide a richer sensory experience, further increasing vividness.

To increase the interactivity perceived by the trainee, a higher degree of freedom during the VR safety training should be provided to allow users to manipulate the virtual environment in real time. Although response time is not an issue for most VR systems, the current VR training system fails to provide users with a sense of control over the pace, navigation, and content while proceeding through the training. According to a study by Bailenson et al. [60], users who learned physical tasks on a VR training system reported a higher sense of interactivity when they were provided multiple viewing angles of themselves, such as a first-person view and a third-person view, in the virtual environment. Owing to the multiple viewing angles, users easily gained information and real-time feedback regarding their own movements, which gave them a sense of control over the pace and navigation of their own body. Therefore, safety training content developers should provide features that allow users to switch between multiple viewing angles to increase their perceived interactivity, and thus increase training effectiveness.

Furthermore, allowing multiple trainees to interact with each other within the virtual environment could also provide a higher level of freedom and interactivity. The results of Vidal-Balea et al. [61] emphasizes the importance of shared experience among trainees on the effectiveness of an AR-based training. Because the construction industry often requires workers to work cooperatively on a single task, we believe that the development of a social VR training system could significantly improve the effectiveness of the VR safety training. However, to create a realistic social VR environment, advances in related technologies, such as VR cloud and 5G, must be preceded [62].

Both content developers and instructors should focus on increasing a trainee's perceived severity toward accidents at the workplace. This could be achieved by introducing not only accident cases and prevention methods, but also the aftermath of these incidents. Furthermore, the use of VR is likely to increase the severity perceived by the trainees because it provides a more realistic sensation compared with that experienced when simply viewing a training video.

Finally, because training satisfaction positively affects training transfer, instructors should keep track of the trainee's satisfaction level after the training. A survey that obtains trainees' opinion and improves the training based on the obtained feedback could help increase the overall satisfaction level of future trainees. Furthermore, a continuous survey may help eliminate the possibility of the Hawthorne effect, also known as the "novelty effect". The Hawthorne effect, occurs when a user is not experienced or familiar with a new technology, thus resulting in elevated levels of motivation and usability [63]. Since the effect is temporary, a series of surveys would allow instructors to gain a more accurate understanding of the VR training.

7. Conclusions

This study aimed to elucidate how the use of VR helps increase the effectiveness of safety training in the construction industry. We proposed a research model, based on the TAM, to examine the impact of technology- and usage-specific factors of VR safety training on the effectiveness of training. A PLS-SEM analysis of 248 construction workers in Korea was conducted. The results supported most of our hypotheses. Vividness, interactivity, and perceived severity had a significant effect on trainees' beliefs and attitudes concerning the VR safety training. Furthermore, the trainees' satisfaction regarding the training was crucial in increasing the transfer of the skills and knowledge obtained via safety training.

Our findings provide several meaningful implications for improving the effectiveness of a VR-based construction safety training. First, creating an immersive virtual environment that creates a feeling of telepresence is critical for enhancing training effectiveness. This could be achieved by providing various sensory stimulations through the use of haptic suits and other related technologies. Also, an interactive virtual environment with a high degree of freedom must be created. Finally, an effort to keep trainees interested and satisfied must be made by providing updates based on trainee feedback.

Although our study provided meaningful implications, it is not without its limitations. First, our survey was only conducted in Korea. Different countries have different training contents, work practices, and safety regulations. Thus, comparing different cultures may provide a more generalized result and new implications. Another shortcoming of our study is that we analysed a limited number of samples only consisting of construction workers. Future studies could conduct a multi-group analysis between workers and managers, or between construction tasks. Finally, our study fails to consider the possible bias caused by the novelty effect. To mitigate the novelty effect, future studies may need to provide tutorial courses so that the trainee is familiar with the VR before the training begins [64]. Also, a time-series analysis on training effectiveness may provide new implications while eliminating possible bias caused by the novelty effect.

Author Contributions: Conceptualization, J.W.Y. and J.S.P.; methodology, J.W.Y.; software, J.W.Y.; validation, J.S.P.; formal analysis, J.W.Y.; investigation, J.S.P.; resources, H.J.P.; data curation, J.W.Y.; writing—original draft preparation, J.W.Y.; writing—review and editing, J.S.P.; visualization, J.S.P.; supervision, H.J.P.; project administration, H.J.P. All authors have read and agreed to the published version of the manuscript.

Funding: This research received no external funding.

Institutional Review Board Statement: Not applicable.

Informed Consent Statement: Informed consent was obtained from all subjects involved in the study.

Conflicts of Interest: The authors declare no conflict of interest.

References

1. Hussain, R.; Pedro, A.; Lee, D.Y.; Phan, H.C.; Park, C.S. Impact of safety training and interventions on training-transfer: Targeting migrant construction workers. *Int. J. Occup. Saf. Ergon.* **2020**, *26*, 272–284. [CrossRef] [PubMed]
2. The Korea Ministry of Employment and Labor (MoEL). Analysis of Industrial Accidents. 2018. Available online: http://www.moel.go.kr/policy/policydata/view.do?bbs_seq=20191200830 (accessed on 1 February 2021). (In Korean)
3. Zhao, D.; Lucas, J. Virtual reality simulation for construction safety promotion. *Int. J. Inj. Contr. Saf. Promot.* **2015**, *22*, 57–67. [CrossRef] [PubMed]
4. Martínez-Caro, E. Factors affecting effectiveness in e-learning: An analysis in production management courses. *Comput. Appl. Eng. Educ.* **2011**, *19*, 572–581. [CrossRef]
5. Park, C.H.; Jang, G.; Chai, Y.H. Development of a virtual reality training system for live-line workers. *Int. J. Hum.-Comput. Int.* **2006**, *20*, 285–303. [CrossRef]
6. Conges, A.; Evain, A.; Benaben, F.; Chabiron, O.; Rebiere, S. Crisis management exercises in virtual reality. In Proceedings of the 2020 IEEE Conference on Virtual Reality and 3D User Interfaces Abstracts and Workshops (VRW), Atlanta, GA, USA, 22–26 March 2020; pp. 87–92.
7. Xie, B.; Liu, H.; Alghofaili, R.; Zhang, Y.; Jiang, Y.; Lobo, F.D.; Li, C.; Li, W.; Huang, H.; Akdere, M.; et al. A review on virtual reality skill training applications. *Front. Virtual Real.* **2021**, *2*, 645153. [CrossRef]
8. Alzahrani, N.M. Augmented reality: A systematic review of its benefits and challenges in e-learning contexts. *Appl. Sci.* **2020**, *10*, 5660. [CrossRef]
9. Lee, S.M.; Lee, D. "Untact": A new customer service strategy in the digital age. *Serv. Bus.* **2020**, *14*, 1–22. [CrossRef]
10. Sacks, R.; Perlman, A.; Barak, R. Construction safety training using immersive virtual reality. *Constr. Manag. Econ.* **2013**, *31*, 1005–1017. [CrossRef]
11. Kontoghiorghes, C. Factors affecting training effectiveness in the context of the introduction of new technology—A US case study. *Int. J. Train. Dev.* **2001**, *5*, 248–260. [CrossRef]
12. Yamnill, S.; McLean, G.N. Factors affecting transfer of training in Thailand. *Hum. Resour. Dev. Q.* **2005**, *16*, 323–344. [CrossRef]
13. Baldwin, T.T.; Ford, J.K. Transfer of training: A review and directions for future research. *Pers. Psychol.* **1988**, *41*, 63–105. [CrossRef]
14. Lim, D.H.; Morris, M.L. Influence of trainee characteristics, instructional satisfaction, and organizational climate on perceived learning and training transfer. *Hum. Resour. Dev. Q.* **2006**, *17*, 85–115. [CrossRef]
15. Blume, B.D.; Ford, J.K.; Surface, E.A.; Olenick, J. A dynamic model of training transfer. *Hum. Resour. Manag. R.* **2019**, *29*, 270–283. [CrossRef]
16. Davis, F.D. Perceived usefulness, perceived ease of use, and user acceptance of information technology. *MIS Q.* **1989**, *13*, 319–340. [CrossRef]
17. Al-Emran, M.; Mezhuyev, V.; Kamaludin, A. Technology Acceptance Model in M-Learning Context: A Systematic Review. *Comput. Educ.* **2018**, *125*, 389–412. [CrossRef]
18. Riantini, R.E. Adoption of E-Commerce Online to Offline with Technology Acceptance Model (TAM) Approach. In Proceedings of the 2018 4th International Conference on Computer and Information Sciences, Kuala Lumpur, Malaysia, 13–14 August 2018; pp. 1–6.
19. Wang, Y.; Wang, S.; Wang, J.; Wei, J.; Wang, C. An empirical study of consumers' intention to use ride-sharing services: Using an extended technology acceptance model. *Transportation* **2020**, *47*, 397–415. [CrossRef]
20. Venkatesh, V.; Bala, H. Technology acceptance model 3 and a research agenda on interventions. *Decision Sci.* **2008**, *39*, 273–315. [CrossRef]
21. Venkatesh, V.; Davis, F.D. A theoretical extension of the technology acceptance model: Four longitudinal field studies. *Manag. Sci.* **2000**, *46*, 186–204. [CrossRef]
22. Sagnier, C.; Loup-Escande, E.; Lourdeaux, D.; Thouvenin, I.; Valléry, G. User acceptance of virtual reality: An extended technology acceptance model. *Int. J. Hum. Comput. Interact.* **2020**, *36*, 993–1007. [CrossRef]
23. Guner, H.; Acarturk, C. The use and acceptance of ICT by senior citizens: A comparison of technology acceptance model (TAM) for elderly and young adults. *Univers. Access Inf. Soc.* **2020**, *19*, 311–330. [CrossRef]

24. Park, Y.; Son, H.; Kim, C. Investigating the determinants of construction professionals' acceptance of web-based training: An extension of the technology acceptance model. *Autom. Constr.* **2012**, *22*, 377–386. [CrossRef]
25. Steuer, J. Defining virtual reality: Dimensions determining telepresence. *J. Commun.* **1992**, *42*, 73–93. [CrossRef]
26. Radianti, J.; Majchrzak, T.A.; Fromm, J.; Wohlgenannt, I. A systematic review of immersive virtual reality applications for higher education: Design elements, lessons learned, and research agenda. *Comput. Educ.* **2020**, *147*, 103778. [CrossRef]
27. Coyle, J.R.; Thorson, E. The effects of progressive levels of interactivity and vividness in web marketing sites. *J. Advert.* **2001**, *30*, 65–77. [CrossRef]
28. Kim, D.; Ko, Y.J. The impact of virtual reality (VR) technology on sport spectators' flow experience and satisfaction. *Comput. Hum. Behav.* **2019**, *93*, 346–356. [CrossRef]
29. Jang, Y.; Park, E. An adoption model for virtual reality games: The roles of presence and enjoyment. *Telemat. Inform.* **2019**, *42*, 101239. [CrossRef]
30. Wu, H.; Cai, T.; Luo, D.; Liu, Y.; Zhang, Z. Immersive virtual reality news: A study of user experience and media effects. *Int. J. Hum. Comput. Stud.* **2021**, *147*, 102576. [CrossRef]
31. Clark, C.S.; Dobbins, G.H.; Ladd, R.T. Exploratory field study of training motivation: Influence of involvement, credibility, and transfer climate. *Goup. Organ. Manag.* **1993**, *18*, 292–307. [CrossRef]
32. Manis, K.T.; Choi, D. The virtual reality hardware acceptance model (VR-HAM): Extending and individuating the technology acceptance model (TAM) for virtual reality hardware. *J. Bus. Res.* **2019**, *100*, 503–513. [CrossRef]
33. Scherer, R.; Siddiq, F.; Tondeur, J. The technology acceptance model (TAM): A meta-analytic structural equation modeling approach to explaining teachers' adoption of digital technology in education. *Comput. Educ.* **2019**, *128*, 13–35. [CrossRef]
34. Chang, C.T.; Hajiyev, J.; Su, C.R. Examining the students' behavioural intention to use e-learning in Azerbaijan? The general extended technology acceptance model for e-learning approach. *Comput. Educ.* **2017**, *111*, 128–143. [CrossRef]
35. Wu, W.C.; Vu, V.H. Application of Virtual Reality Method in Aircraft Maintenance Service—Taking Dornier 228 as an Example. *Appl. Sci.* **2022**, *12*, 7283. [CrossRef]
36. Nah, F.F.H.; Tan, X.; The, S.H. An empirical investigation on end-users' acceptance of enterprise systems. *Inf. Resour. Manag. J.* **2004**, *17*, 32–53. [CrossRef]
37. Huang, T.L.; Liao, S. A model of acceptance of augmented-reality interactive technology: The moderating role of cognitive innovativeness. *Electron. Commer. Res.* **2015**, *15*, 269–295. [CrossRef]
38. Oh, J.; Yoon, S.J. Validation of haptic enabling technology acceptance model (HE-TAM): Integration of IDT and TAM. *Telemat. Inform.* **2014**, *31*, 585–596. [CrossRef]
39. Ahadzadeh, A.S.; Sharif, S.P.; Ong, F.S.; Khong, K.W. Integrating health belief model and technology acceptance model: An investigation of health-related internet use. *J. Med. Internet. Res.* **2015**, *17*, e45. [CrossRef]
40. Hansen, J.M.; Saridakis, G.; Benson, V. Risk, Trust, and the Interaction of Perceived Ease of Use and Behavioral Control in Predicting Consumers' Use of Social Media for Transactions. *Comput. Hum. Behav.* **2018**, *80*, 197–206. [CrossRef]
41. Dou, K.; Yu, P.; Deng, N.; Liu, F.; Guan, Y.; Li, Z.; Ji, Y.; Du, N.; Lu, X.; Duan, H. Patients' acceptance of smartphone health echnology for chronic disease management: A theoretical model and empirical test. *JMIR Mhealth Uhealth* **2017**, *5*, e177. [CrossRef]
42. Gegenfurtner, A.; Festner, D.; Gallenberger, W.; Lehtinen, E.; Gruber, H. Predicting autonomous and controlled motivation to transfer training. *Int. J. Train. Dev.* **2009**, *13*, 124–138. [CrossRef]
43. Kodwani, A.D. Decoding Training Effectiveness: The Role of Organisational Factors. *J. Workplace Learn.* **2017**, *29*, 200–216. [CrossRef]
44. Hyman, L.; Lamb, J.; Bulmer, M. The use of pre-existing survey questions: Implications for data quality. In Proceedings of the Q2006 European Conference on Quality in Survey Statistics, Cardiff, Wales, UK, 24–26 April 2006; pp. 1–8.
45. Yoon, C.; Kim, H. Understanding computer security behavioural intention in the workplace. *Inform. Technol. People* **2013**, *26*, 401–419. [CrossRef]
46. Sun, Y.; Wang, N.; Guo, X.; Peng, Z. Understanding the acceptance of mobile health services: A comparison and integration of alternative models. *J. Electron. Commer. Res.* **2013**, *14*, 183–200.
47. Latif, K.F. An integrated model of training effectiveness and satisfaction with employee development interventions. *Ind. Commer. Train.* **2012**, *44*, 211–222. [CrossRef]
48. Sun, P.C.; Tsai, R.J.; Finger, G.; Chen, Y.Y.; Yeh, D. What drives a successful e-Learning? An empirical investigation of the critical factors influencing learner satisfaction. *Comput. Educ.* **2008**, *50*, 1183–1202. [CrossRef]
49. Kelley, C.A.; Gaidis, W.C.; Reingen, P.H. The use of vivid stimuli to enhance comprehension of the content of product warning messages. *J. Consum. Aff.* **1989**, *23*, 243–266. [CrossRef]
50. Yim, M.Y.C.; Chu, S.C.; Sauer, P.L. Is augmented reality technology an effective tool for e-commerce? An interactivity and vividness perspective. *J. Interact. Mark.* **2017**, *39*, 89–103. [CrossRef]
51. Korea Occupational Safety & Health Agency. Video-Based VR Content—Scaffolding. 2019. Available online: https://www.kosha.or.kr/kosha/data/mediaBankMain.do?mode=detail&medSeq=40591 (accessed on 1 November 2020). (In Korean).
52. Fincham, J.E. Response rates and responsiveness for surveys, standards, and the Journal. *Am. J. Pharm. Educ.* **2008**, *72*, 43. [CrossRef]
53. Hair, J.F.; Hult, G.T.M.; Ringle, C.M.; Sarstedt, M. *A Primer on Partial Least Squares Structural Equation Modeling (PLS-SEM)*; Sage Publications: Thousand Oaks, CA, USA, 2013.

54. Hair, J.F.; Risher, J.J.; Sarstedt, M.; Ringle, C.M. When to use and how to report the results of PLS-SEM. *Eur. Bus. Rev.* **2019**, *31*, 2–24. [CrossRef]
55. Novikova, S.; Richman, D.; Supekar, K.; Barnard-Brak, L.; Hall, D. NDAR: A model federal system for secondary analysis in developmental disabilities research. *Int. Rev. Res. Dev. Disabil.* **2013**, *45*, 123–153.
56. Cohen, J. *Statistical Power Analysis for the Behavioral Sciences*, 2nd ed.; Lawrence Erlbaum Associates: Hillsdale, NJ, USA, 1988.
57. Falk, R.F.; Miller, N.B. *A Primer for Soft Modeling*; University of Akron Press: Akron, OH, USA, 1992.
58. Granić, A.; Marangunić, N. Technology acceptance model in educational context: A systematic literature review. *Br. J. Educ. Technol.* **2019**, *50*, 2572–2593. [CrossRef]
59. Grabowski, A.; Jankowski, J.; Wodzyński, M. Teleoperated mobile robot with two arms: The influence of a human-machine interface, VR training and operator age. *Int. J. Hum. Comput. Stud.* **2021**, *156*, 102707. [CrossRef]
60. Bailenson, J.; Patel, K.; Nielsen, A.; Bajscy, R.; Jung, S.H.; Kurillo, G. The effect of interactivity on learning physical actions in virtual reality. *Media Psychol.* **2008**, *11*, 354–376. [CrossRef]
61. Vidal-Balea, A.; Blanco-Novoa, O.; Fraga-Lamas, P.; Vilar-Montesinos, M.; Fernández-Caramés, T.M. Creating collaborative augmented reality experiences for industry 4.0 training and assistance applications: Performance evaluation in the shipyard of the future. *Appl. Sci.* **2020**, *10*, 9073. [CrossRef]
62. Muñoz-Saavedra, L.; Miró-Amarante, L.; Domínguez-Morales, M. Augmented and virtual reality evolution and future tendency. *Appl. Sci.* **2020**, *10*, 322. [CrossRef]
63. Miguel-Alonso, I.; Rodriguez-Garcia, B.; Checa, D.; Bustillo, A. Countering the Novelty Effect: A Tutorial for Immersive Virtual Reality Learning Environments. *Appl. Sci.* **2023**, *13*, 593. [CrossRef]
64. Checa, D.; Miguel-Alonso, I.; Bustillo, A. Immersive virtual-reality computer-assembly serious game to enhance autonomous learning. *Virtual Real.* **2021**, 1–18. [CrossRef]

applied sciences

MDPI

Systematic Review

Considering the Consequences of Cybersickness in Immersive Virtual Reality Rehabilitation: A Systematic Review and Meta-Analysis

Xin Li [1], Ding-Bang Luh [1,*], Ruo-Hui Xu [2] and Yi An [1]

[1] School of Art and Design, Guangdong University of Technology, Guangzhou 510090, China; writetoxinli@gmail.com (X.L.); 17806287253@163.com (Y.A.)
[2] City School, Guangzhou Academy of Fine Art, Guangzhou 510006, China; ruohui.xu@vip.163.com
* Correspondence: dingbangluh@gmail.com

Abstract: VR rehabilitation is a rapidly evolving field, with increasing research and development aimed at improving its effectiveness, accessibility, and integration into mainstream healthcare systems. While there are some commercially available VR rehabilitation programs, their adoption and use in clinical practice are still limited. One of the limitations is defined as cybersickness, which is dependent on human contact with virtual reality products. The purpose of this essay is to raise awareness of the associated elements that contribute to cybersickness in rehabilitation using immersive VR. The common factors that influence the amount of cybersickness are user characteristics and device software and hardware. The Simulator Sickness Questionnaire (SSQ) was used as one of the formal models for determining the variables related to virtual reality sickness. The systematic review of the literature and the meta-analysis were chosen by whether the Simulator Sickness Questionnaire in the articles matched the research criteria. Based on PRISMA guidelines, a systematic review of the literature was conducted. Twenty-six publications from the recent past were totaled, comprising 862 individuals with ages ranging from 19 to 95, and 49% were female. The highest overall SSQ mean score for different kinds of symptoms was determined to be 21.058 for brain injuries, with a 95% confidence interval (CI) of 15.357 to 26.760. Time, content, locomotion, control, and display types were other elements that contributed to cybersickness and had significant p-values in the SNK Q-test. The future direction of immersive VR rehabilitation involves the development of immersive and interactive environments that simulate real-world situations, providing patients with a safe and controlled environment in which to practice new skills and movements.

Keywords: cybersickness; immersive virtual reality; rehabilitation; Simulator Sickness Questionnaire (SSQ); systematic review; meta-analysis

Citation: Li, X.; Luh, D.-B.; Xu, R.-H.; An, Y. Considering the Consequences of Cybersickness in Immersive Virtual Reality Rehabilitation: A Systematic Review and Meta-Analysis. *Appl. Sci.* **2023**, *13*, 5159. https://doi.org/10.3390/app13085159

Academic Editors: João M. F. Rodrigues, Calin Gheorghe Dan Neamtu, Radu Comes, Jing-Jing Fang and Dorin-Mircea Popovici

Received: 31 January 2023
Revised: 13 April 2023
Accepted: 18 April 2023
Published: 20 April 2023

1. Introduction

Virtual reality (VR) is a rapidly advancing technology that provides an immersive and interactive digital environment for users to experience computer-generated simulations in a realistic and engaging way. This technology has been developing rapidly in recent years and holds significant potential for various applications, including entertainment, healthcare, education, and business [1,2]. Among these topics, using VR for healthcare has been attracting increasing attention in recent years.

Rehabilitation is crucial in clinical and healthcare scenarios as it enables individuals to regain independence, enhance their quality of life, and reach their full potential in daily activities. Conceptually, rehabilitation is a multifaceted process that aims to restore physical, psychological, and social functioning after a period of illness, injury, or addiction. It takes into account the intricate interplay among biological, psychological, and social factors that may affect a person's capacity to function and achieve their goals. Ultimately, rehabilitation is a process that considers the whole person and their unique circumstances to support them in their journey towards optimal health and well-being.

Manual rehabilitation is deficient in providing consistent and personalized feedback and monitoring. From the user perspective, patients with less motivation and satisfaction mostly result in obsolete applications [3]. What is more, the characteristics of patients may even determine the degree of recovery from physical or physiological sickness [4]. Against this background, many new technologies are seen to be viable options for investigating the possibilities of high-efficiency approaches.

In 2003, Burdea classified virtual reality therapies for rehabilitation as virtual rehabilitation [5]. Since then, virtual rehabilitation has been a significant topic in medical care for the past 20 years. Formally, virtual rehabilitation is a modern approach that utilizes virtual reality technology to deliver therapy, assessment, and training to individuals with various physical and mental conditions. The goal of virtual rehabilitation is to enhance the traditional rehabilitation process by providing an immersive, interactive, and engaging experience that can promote motor and cognitive skills, improve functional outcomes, and enhance the overall quality of life [6,7]. Studying immersive virtual rehabilitation can advance our understanding of the effectiveness and optimal implementation of this novel technology for improving rehabilitation outcomes, particularly in populations with limited access to traditional rehabilitation methods.

Virtual rehabilitation can be divided into different categories based on the types of conditions it aims to address: cognitive impairment, acquired brain damage, and physical inactivity [8–10]. Firstly, cognitive impairment might lead to dementia or apathy. This illness exists with memory, language, and judgment issues that are not severe enough for patients to interfere with daily activities [11]. Different from cognitive impairment, acquired brain injuries might be related to head trauma and increase the risk of neural connection problems. Specific symptoms of brain injuries include stroke or Parkinson's in patients who lack the capacity to care for themselves in daily life [12]. Finally, physical inactivity is more common, and virtual rehabilitation may aid in patients recovering from physical injuries or increase exercise cognitive abilities [13].

Cybersickness is a phenomenon that arises from exposure to immersive virtual environments, causing a range of symptoms, such as nausea, oculomotor, and disorientation. It is a common challenge in VR applications, and its severity can be influenced by several factors. Understanding the underlying mechanisms and factors that contribute to cybersickness is crucial for the development of effective interventions to reduce its impact on users' experience and promote the safe use of VR technology, especially under virtual rehabilitation scenarios. Specifically, we observed that there can be several influencing factors of cybersickness in virtual rehabilitation. One prominent factor is individual susceptibility, i.e., people with different physiques have different degrees of motion sickness reactions. The duration spent on VR equipment also has a great impact on cybersickness. In addition to user demographic differences, there are several device technological aspects that are associated with cybersickness, including software and hardware.

Research in this field of cybersickness tends to concentrate on its various elements, such as its internal and external origins. Meanwhile, the comprehensive review and meta-analyses of recent studies on cybersickness in immersive virtual rehabilitation contexts are still lacking. Cybersickness is entangled with virtual rehabilitation. On one hand, cybersickness can significantly impact the performance of virtual rehabilitation as it can cause symptoms that interfere with the patient's ability to engage effectively in therapy. Nausea, oculomotor, and disorientation can decrease motivation, decrease one's ability to concentrate, and increase fatigue, which can limit the patient's participation in rehabilitation activities. On the other hand, under specific virtual rehabilitation scenarios, the severity of cybersickness might also be different from regular cases. Therefore, it is crucial to study cybersickness in virtual rehabilitation as it helps in understanding the consequences of cybersickness and helps clinicians and researchers develop effective strategies to minimize its impact and optimize the benefits of virtual rehabilitation for patients.

In this paper, we present a systematic review and meta-analysis of the consequences of cybersickness in immersive virtual rehabilitation. Specifically, we adopted the famous Simulator Sickness Questionnaire (SSQ) as a measure of cybersickness, which has four attributes: nausea, oculomotor, disorientation, and overall scores shown in Table 1. There were sufficient literature review and a series of analyses about the questionnaire. A sufficient literature review and a series of analyses were conducted based on the questionnaire. The review specifically summarizes participant demographics, including age range, user symptoms, and usage condition. As mentioned above, brain injuries, cognitive impairment, and physical inactivity are the primary user symptoms. Additionally, the sorts of VR devices for time, content, locomotion, control, and display are taken into account. Our results can provide guidelines for possible directions for improving the experience of immersive VR rehabilitation.

Table 1. Simulator Sickness Questionnaire (SSQ) factors.

Factors	Details
Nausea	General discomfort, increased salivation, sweating, nausea, difficulty concentrating, stomach awareness, burping
Oculomotor	General discomfort, fatigue, headache, eyestrain, difficulty focusing
Disorientation	Difficulty focusing, nausea, fullness of the head, blurred vision, dizzy (eyes open), dizzy (eyes closed)

2. Materials and Methods

2.1. Searching Process

The INPLASY website (http://dx.doi.org/10.37766/inplasy2023.1.0019, accessed on 9 January 2023) has the most recent version of the systematic review procedure. The Preferred Reporting Items for Systematic Reviews and Meta-Analysis (PRISMA) guidelines were used to conduct this systematic review [14], and the checklist is shown in Appendix B. In this article, a systematic literature search was applied to collect journal and conference articles related to cybersickness in virtual rehabilitation. This search process covered the terms as followed: VR OR virtual reality OR HMDs OR virtual environment AND cybersickness OR simulator sickness OR virtual reality sickness AND rehabilitation OR rehab OR brain injuries OR cognitive impairment OR physical inactivity. Based on the PICO model [15], the qualifying requirements were studied (participants, interventions, comparisons, and outcomes). The included papers mainly focused on the implementation of rehabilitation interventions for patients with mental or physical symptoms to alleviate their helplessness. As shown in Figure 1 and described in Section 1, the symptoms can be divided into three types according to the conditions. Pre- and post-experiments were both used to compare the differences between before and after use in the tests of these papers, in which the four attributes of SSQ were employed to measure the subjects' cybersickness scores after virtual rehabilitation.

This research was conducted in November 2022 based on papers selected from several databases: PubMed, Web of Science, Google Scholar, and Scopus. We collected publications by searching the corresponding websites with the keywords mentioned above. The selected papers were all recent publications written in English. "virtual reality," "rehabilitation," "cybersickness," "Simulator Sickness Questionnaire," and "immersive environment" were among the most popular heading phrases. The selection criteria included the following: (1) the subjects utilized the virtual reality product; (2) SSQ scales were used in VR rehabilitation; (3) the papers were formal research papers. On the contrary, articles were excluded if: (1) the products were not virtual reality but mixed reality or augmented reality; (2) the papers were dissertations or reports; (3) the articles did not include SSQ scales or did not emphasize rehabilitation; (4) the standard deviations were missing in the results data.

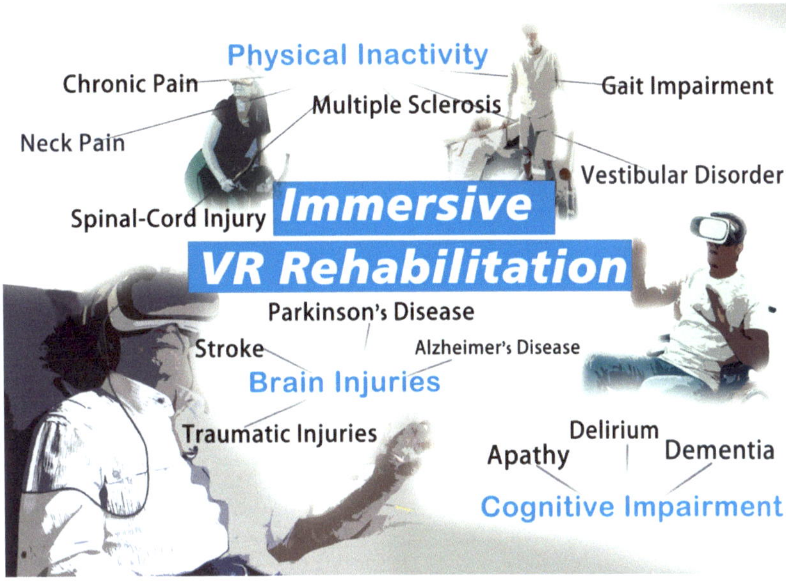

Figure 1. The main symptoms in immersive VR rehabilitation.

Two independent reviewers examined the research's eligibility (XL and DBL in the author list of this paper). Additionally, two reviewers separately conducted a risk-of-bias evaluation (YA and RHX in the author list of this paper). Regarding the SSQ results, the following subscale scores have fixed weights: nausea (9.54), oculomotor (7.58), and disorientation (13.92). Meanwhile, 3.74 is unweighted from the overall score. This is a crucial function in SSQ computing, which might significantly affect the study findings. The whole informative search and selection process is shown in Figure 2, together with the PRISMA principles.

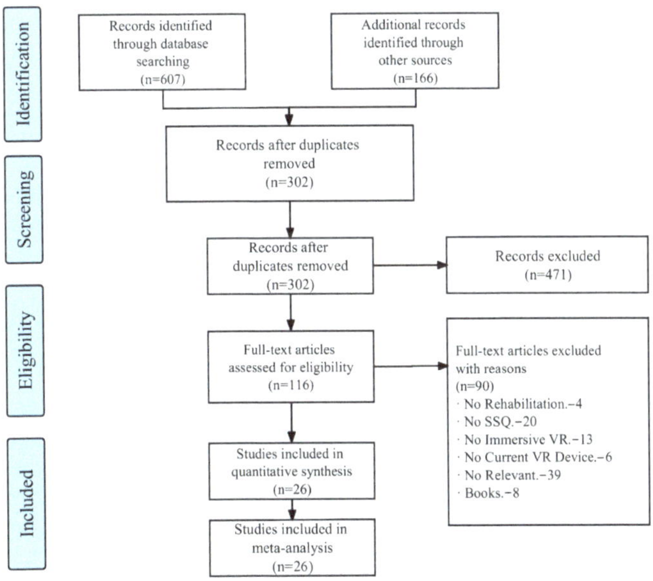

Figure 2. The PRISMA flow diagram for the systematic review detailing the selection process.

2.2. Data Analysis

To conduct our investigation, which mostly relied on meta-analysis, we employed StataSE 14 [16] and Comprehensive Meta-Analysis (CMA) Version 3 [17] for computation. Specifically, three meta-analysis methods were adopted: SNK-test (Q-test), SMD (forest plot), and pooled mean.

Firstly, each subscale was calculated together with the Q-test variable analysis, also known as the conventional test for heterogeneity. W_i is the weighting factor of the ith, and Y_i is the effect size of the ith. M is the average effect size of the number of studies k. In addition, the Q-test in this formula is called the weighted sum of squares (WSS):

$$Q = \sum_{i=1}^{k} W_i (Y_i - M)^2 \quad (1)$$

At the same time, p-values were utilized to compare the Q-value with a chi-squared distribution. This probability, called the p-value, was employed to represent significant differences between the attributes in the study and the SSQ scores, when the value was lower than 0.05.

Secondly, we studied the STD mean difference (SMD). This is a measure of the effect size used in statistics to quantify the difference between the means of two groups or subgroups. When considering subgroups in this study, the SMDs were calculated in the same way by comparing the means of the three subgroups and dividing by the pooled standard deviation. It was important to ensure that the subgroups were well-defined and that any differences between them were appropriately accounted for. The outcomes with differences are presented in forest plots.

Lastly, the pooled mean was calculated by weighting the mean of each study about cybersickness by the sample size and dividing the sum of the weighted means by the sum of the sample sizes across all collected papers. For each of the overall and subscale SSQ scores, the pooled means of various qualities were calculated, which determined the importance of cybersickness. Calculations were carried out for the pooled impact evaluation, with 95% confidence intervals (CI 95%).

The tools and methods mentioned above were utilized to analyze the following factors. (1) Demographic factors. The age range of the patients was divided into three levels: youths under 30, adults between 30 and 60, and seniors above 60. This form of division was made taking into account the cognitive and motor skills of the user. The amount of data regarding gender differences was insufficient. In addition, there were several different types of patient symptoms related to virtual rehabilitation including physical inactivity, moderate cognitive impairment (MCI), acquired brain injuries. Cybersickness-inducing conditions were also included in the majority of article findings. (2) VR software. We mainly considered the exposure time of the VR device and the content of the VR application as software factors. (3) VR hardware. We identified 4 distinct forms of locomotion, 3 different types of control modes, and 2 types of display modes according to the applications in the collected papers. In the next steps, we calculated all of the elements related to cybersickness. Some of the publications had dropout participants, who experienced uncomfortable visual effects.

3. Results

3.1. Study Identification

We found 607 publications in the research articles that met the search criteria. Additionally, there were 166 articles added from other sources to enhance diversity. After that, 471 submissions were eliminated due to having mismatched subject names or abstracts. In further detail, there were no investigations into cybersickness and virtual rehabilitation. A total of 302 papers were successfully evaluated for eligibility. In this eligibility assessment, 116 studies (n = 116) fulfilled the criteria for inclusion, and 26 publications ultimately completed the measurement requirements for the meta-analysis. Inevitably, some participants dropped out of the studies in the middle, but the dropout rate in the selected publications was low. The outcomes of the search tactics are shown in Figure 2. Table 2 lists the 26 articles that used the cybersickness measures in virtual rehabilitation interventions. Of the 26 articles reporting airsickness, more than 5 publications included more than 3 experimental groups. The SSQ scores for the before, after, and modified periods were computed in several papers. Three of the papers compared different patients, including young, elderly, and older with Parkinson's disease, in terms of health. Additionally, one of the publications gathered information from more than 100 participants.

3.2. Study Details

Of the 26 items, 20 had both the SSQ total score and the subscale scores, while only 6 papers contained the total score. Therefore, the SSQ total scores in our study contain 26 items, and the SSQ subscale score values for nausea, oculomotor, and disorientation contain 20 items. The data were taken from articles that may have had various experiment settings in the same article. There were 862 people in total that took part in this study. Analysis of the affiliation shows that five papers originated from the USA, five from Germany, three from Australia, two from Norway, two from France, two from China, and two from Korea. Other affiliations included Switzerland, Italy, Denmark, the Netherlands, Belgium, Ireland, and Poland.

These publications have been featured in journals such as Virtual Reality, Medicine, Neuroscience Letters, and Frontiers in Virtual Reality. The primary study areas of the review papers shown on the WOS platform include "Computer Science" (n = 8), "Rehabilitation" (n = 5), "Engineering" (n = 4), and "Imaging Science & Photographic Technology" (n = 3). Devices including the HTC Vive, Oculus, Samsung, PlayStation, and Sony were used in the study tests.

Concerning the ages of the subjects, the participants ranged in age from teenagers (19 years old) to senior adults (95 years old). The adolescent age range (0–30) had around 311 people, with a mean age of 24.4, while the adult age range (30–60) had more than 200 people, with a mean age of 47.58. Additionally, there were 200 older individuals (over 60), with a mean age of 71.55. The amount of data regarding gender differences was insufficient.

Table 2. Summary of included papers. N denotes number. M denotes male. F denotes female.

No.	Author	N	M	F	Age	Symptom	Induce	Time	Content	Locomotion	Control	Display Type	Equipment
1	Arafat 2017 [18]	16	3	13	37–67 M = 55 (9)	Cognitive impairment	YES	≤15	Exergame	Bicycling	Gesture-based	360° Simulator, 3 DoF	Oculus Rift DK2
2	Arlati 2021 [19]	58	11 22	13 9	M = 72.45 (5.83) M = 70.67 (5.62)	Cognitive impairment	YES	≤15	Exergame	Standing	Controller-based	360° Simulator, 3 DoF	HTC Vive Pro
3	Bovim 2020 [20]	29	6	23	19–40 M = 28.9 (4.8)	Physical inactivity	NO	≤5	Training	Walking	Controller-based	360° Simulator, 6 DoF	HTC Vive
4	Brown 2021 [21]	12	5	7	39–70 M = 56 (9.36)	Physical inactivity	YES	≤5	Exergame	Standing	Gesture-based	360° Simulator, 3 DoF	Oculus Rift CV1
5	Chen 2009 [22]	30	14	16	27–70 M = 53 (2)	Physical inactivity	NO	≤10	Exergame	Walking	Controller-based	360° Simulator, 6 DoF	-
6	Chowdhury 2019 [23]	11	4	7	M = 53.30 (4.87)	Physical inactivity	YES	≤45	Exergame	Sitting	Gesture-based	360° Simulator, 3 DoF	HTC Vive
7	Ciaynska 2022 [24]	45	23	22	19–28 M = 21.69 (2.76)	Physical inactivity	YES	≤30	Exergame	Standing	Controller-based	360° Simulator, 3 DoF	Oculus Quest 1
8	Ham 2018 [25]	21	10	11	19–35 M = 24.19 (4.38)	Brain injuries	YES	n/a	Scene	Walking	Gaze-directed	360° Simulator, 6 DoF	HTC Vive
9	Ham 2019 [26]	45	23	22	19–26 M = 21.82 (1.84)	Physical inactivity	NO	≤15	Training	Walking	Gesture-based	360° Simulator, 6 DoF	HTC Vive
10	Heg 2021 [27]	11	7	4	M = 60 (11)	Physical inactivity	YES	≤15	Scene	Bicycling	Controller-based	360° Simulator, 3 DoF	Oculus Rift CV1
11	Janeh 2019 [28]	15	15	0	M = 67.6 (7)	Brain injuries	YES	≤20	Training	Walking	Controller-based	360° Simulator, 3 DoF	HTC Vive
12	Kern 2019 [29]	36	20	16	19–30 M = 22.68 (2.64)	Physical inactivity	YES	≤15	Training	Walking	Gaze-directed	360° Simulator, 6 DoF	HTC Vive
13	Kim 2017 [30]	33	5 3 3	6 8 8	M = 28 (7) M = 66 (3) M = 65 (7)	Brain injuries	YES	≤30	Training	Walking	Gaze-directed	360° Simulator, 6 DoF	Oculus Rift DK2
14	Lhbetzky 2020 [31]	15	10	5	M = 57 (13.5)	Brain injuries	YES	≤20	Exergame	Walking	Gaze-directed	360° Simulator, 3 DoF	HTC Vive
15	Lheureux 2020 [32]	10	6	4	M = 63.7 (10.6)	Brain injuries	YES	≤15	Training	Walking	-	360° Simulator, 3 DoF	HTC Vive

Table 2. *Cont.*

No.	Author	N	M	F	Age	Symptom	Induce	Time	Content	Locomotion	Control	Display Type	Equipment
16	Maeng 2021 [33]	31 25	8 3	23 22	M = 73.2 (7.3) M = 71.6 (4.4)	Cognitive impairment	YES	≤30	Exergame	Standing	Controller-based	360° Simulator, 6 DoF	Samsung HMD Odyssey
17	Morizio 2022 [34]	38	18	20	19–53 M = 25.2 (8.4)	Brain injuries	NO	≤20	Video	Walking	Gaze-directed	360° Simulator, 3 DoF	HTC Vive
18	Park 2020 [35]	15	6	9	M = 22.60 (1.06)	Cognitive impairment	YES	≤15	Exergame	Standing	Gesture-based	360° Simulator, 3 DoF	PlayStation® VR headset
19	Pot-Kolder 2018 [36]	170	97	73	18–35 M = 25.4 (4.6)	Cognitive impairment	YES	≤20	Video	Standing	Gaze-directed	360° Simulator, 3 DoF	Sony HMZ-T1
20	Salgado 2020 [37]	33	10 8	7 8	M = 30.29 (1.77) M = 30.12 (3.17)	Physical inactivity	YES	≤15	Training	Sitting	Controller-based	360° Simulator, 6 DoF	Oculus Rift DK2
21	Saredakis 2020 [38]	17	7	10	72–95 M = 87.3 (6.3)	Cognitive impairment	YES	≤20	Video	Sitting	Gaze-directed	360° Simulator, 3 DoF	Oculus Go
22	Shah 2022 [39]	14	7	7	60–88 M = 77.57 (7.08)	Physical inactivity	NO	≤15	Exergame	Standing	Gesture-based	360° Simulator, 3 DoF	Oculus Quest 1
23	Tyrrell 2017 [40]	20 14 20	6 11 11	14 8 9	M = 47.15 (11.6) M = 49.64 (13.2) M = 46.5 (12)	Cognitive impairment	YES	≤30	Video	Sitting	Gaze-directed	360° Simulator, 3 DoF	Oculus Rift DK2
24	Vailland 2021 [41]	29	-	-	M = 65	Physical inactivity	YES	n/a	Training	Sitting	Controller-based	360° Simulator, 6 DoF	HTC Vive Pro
25	Vlake 2021 [42]	15	4	11	45–65 M = 54	Cognitive impairment	NO	≤15	Video	Sitting	-	360° Simulator, 3 DoF	-
26	Winter 2021 [43]	14	-	-	M = 52.6 (7.5)	Physical inactivity	YES	≤15	Exergame	Walking	Gaze-directed	360° Simulator, 6 DoF	HTC Vive

Note: items with missing values noted as "-" in Table 2 were excluded.

After a thorough analysis, the primary goal was to compile the SSQ total and subscale scores for the factors that precipitated cybersickness in the field of virtual rehabilitation. The patients' specific demography, VR software, and VR hardware are among the most important aspects of the SSQ scores. Multiple metrics are shown from the systematic review in Tables 2 and 3, and the full names of each abbreviation are included in Appendix A. Figure 3 shows the SSQ total scores forest plot. The Chi-Square Test [44] was then used in this study's statistical analysis. In the virtual rehabilitation scenario, the characteristics of the causes with the highest degree of heterogeneity were collected and are shown in Table 4 (standard deviation in means = 0.343, 95% CI = 0.245–0.440). Tables 5 and 6 and Figure 4 show the results of the pooled mean analysis for the overall score (mean = 19.430, 95% CI: 15.678–23.181), nausea (mean = 17.834, 95% CI: 12.723–22.946), oculomotor (mean = 16.365, 95% CI: 11.512–21.218), and disorientation (mean = 21.096 95% CI: 14.059–28.133).

Group by Subgroup	Study name	Std diff in means	Standard error	Variance	Lower Limit	Upper Limit	Z-Value	p-Value
Brain injuries	Ham 2018	0.288	0.310	0.096	-0.320	0.896	0.930	0.353
	Janeh 2019	-0.074	0.365	0.133	-0.790	0.642	-0.202	0.840
	Kim 2017	1.143	0.266	0.071	0.622	1.663	4.304	0.000
	Lheureux 2020	0.103	0.448	0.200	-0.774	0.980	0.231	0.817
	Lubetzky 2020	0.444	0.370	0.137	-0.281	1.168	1.201	0.230
	Morizio 2022	0.385	0.232	0.054	-0.069	0.839	1.662	0.097
		0.470	0.126	0.016	0.223	0.716	3.728	0.000
Cognitive impairment	Arafat 2017	0.833	0.369	0.136	0.111	1.555	2.260	0.024
	Arlati 2021	0.506	0.189	0.036	0.136	0.876	2.682	0.007
	Maeng 2021	-0.128	0.189	0.036	-0.498	0.243	-0.674	0.500
	Maeng 2021	0.758	0.378	0.143	0.018	1.499	2.006	0.045
	Park 2020	0.366	0.109	0.012	0.152	0.581	3.351	0.001
	Pot-Kolder 2018	0.101	0.343	0.118	-0.572	0.774	0.295	0.768
	Saredakis 2020	0.871	0.201	0.041	0.477	1.266	4.327	0.000
	Vlake 2021	0.557	0.372	0.139	-0.172	1.287	1.497	0.134
		0.407	0.072	0.005	0.266	0.548	5.674	0.000
Physical inactivity	Bovim 2020	-0.307	0.264	0.070	-0.825	0.211	-1.161	0.246
	Brown 2021	0.649	0.419	0.175	-0.172	1.470	1.550	0.121
	Chen 2009	0.128	0.258	0.067	-0.378	0.520	0.497	0.619
	Chow 2019	1.595	0.490	0.240	0.636	2.555	3.258	0.001
	Ciazynska 2022	0.106	0.211	0.045	-0.307	0.520	0.503	0.615
	Ham 2019	1.158	0.228	0.052	0.712	1.605	5.083	0.000
	Heg 2021	1.378	0.474	0.225	0.448	2.308	2.905	0.004
	Kern 2019	-0.379	0.238	0.057	-0.845	0.087	-1.594	0.111
	Salgado 2020	-0.644	0.252	0.064	-1.139	-0.149	-2.551	0.011
	Shah 2022	0.476	0.383	0.147	-0.275	1.227	1.242	0.214
	Vailland 2021	0.214	0.263	0.069	-0.302	0.730	0.812	0.417
	Winter 2021	0.239	0.379	0.144	-0.504	0.982	0.630	0.529
		0.203	0.083	0.007	0.042	0.365	2.466	0.014
Overall		0.343	0.050	0.002	0.245	0.440	6.892	0.000

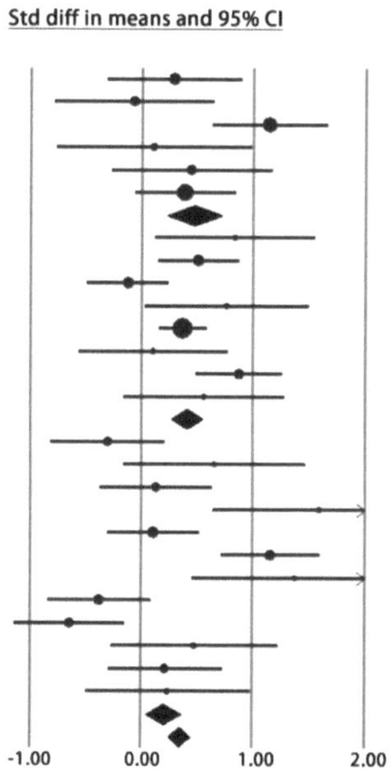

Figure 3. Forest plot of symptom subgroups for SSQ total scores [18–43].

Table 3. Summary of included papers. (Continued).

No.	Author	Measures	Groups	Total SSQ (SD)	Nausea (SD)	Oculomotor (SD)	Disorientation (SD)	Objectives	Results
1	Arafat 2017 [18]	MS, GSR, MSSQ, SSQ	Pre Post	13.090 (12.251) 33.125 (31.730)	10.221 (9.513) 29.301 (29.096)	14.618 (15.581) 27.071 (22.781)	6.960 (11.899) 33.805 (43.922)	How persons with sclerosis experience cybersickness.	Virtual environment-induced cybersickness.
2	Arlati 2021 [19]	SSQ, ITC-SOPI, TAM3	MCI SCD	3.74 (9.35) 11.22 (18.70)	0 (9.54) 0 (9.54)	0 (9.48) 7.58 (18.95)	0 (13.92) 13.92 (27.84)	Evaluating the acceptance and usability of VR environment.	Immersive VR was acceptable and enjoyable for older adults.
3	Bovim 2020 [20]	SSQ, DT	Pre Post	18.2 (22.4) 12.4 (14.6)	11.8 (20.8) 11.3 (16.4)	17.5 (19.1) 6.7 (13.4)	18.4 (26.9) 7.2 (14.5)	Investigating the impact of constraints on gait during treadmill walking in VE.	VE training on a treadmill improved gait and balance control.
4	Brown 2021 [21]	SSQ	Pre Post	10.29 (11.44) 19.39 (6.19)	15.105 (13.184) 23.055 (11.327)	18.318 (19.439) 25.267 (18.908)	2.32 (7.695) 12.76 (34.781)	Investigating cybersickness baseline recordings among a chronic pain population.	Significant differences were found.
5	Chen 2009 [22]	AD-ACL, SSQ	Pre Post	10.54 (9.58) 11.59 (6.47)	14.74 (11.58) 13.36 (11.20)	7.52 (10.17) 6.82 (7.54)	15.19 (24.47) 18.10 (20.80)	Investigating the psychological benefits of VR in rehabilitation.	There were no significant differences between the VR and non-VR groups.
6	Chowdhury 2019 [23]	EDSS, SSQ	Pre Post	13.352 (16.845) 36.876 (12.297)	8.204 (8.586) 25.853 (10.618)	16.221 (24.142) 38.961 (19.784)	7.934 (10.955) 27.84 (11.359)	Investigating a concept called Virtual Ability Simulation (VAS) for people with disability.	VAS enabled participants to perceive the difficulty of the same task more easily.
7	Ciaynska 2022 [24]	SSQ, BioHarness 3.0	Before After	13.65 (10.68) (M) 15.47 (11.41) (F) 15.13 (16.60) (M) 32.98 (17.30) (F)	10.37 (9.22) (M) 9.54 (9.74) (F) 22.40 (12.87) (M) 20.38 (13.05) (F)	14.5 (12.25) (M) 18.26 (14.18) (F) 21.09 (15.33) (M) 34.11 (18.80) (F)	7.87 (10.05) (M) 11.39 (11.42) (F) 15.13 (10.65) (M) 24.68 (22.80) (F)	Examining the differences in the effects of VR 3D HMD gaming on genders.	Significant differences between genders were observed.
8	Ham 2018 [25]	IMI, NASA-TLX, UEQ, SSQ	Pre Post	23.69 (29.76) 33.30 (36.54)	-	-	-	Presenting an immersive VR system for gait rehabilitation after neurological impairments.	The results demonstrated an encouraging user experience and acceptance.
9	Ham 2019 [26]	SSQ, NASA-TLX, IMI, UEQ	Day 1 Day 3	2.89 (3.26) 5.86 (1.59)	-	-	-	Introducing an immersive VR system for gait rehabilitation.	Figuring out the requirements, such as enhancing social communication, interactivity.
10	Heg 2021 [27]	SSQ, SUS, IMI, VEQ, IPI	Pre-test Post-test	4.8 (3.8) 14.5 (9.2)	6.1 (9.8) 25.4 (16.1)	4.1 (5.2) 11.8 (11.3)	5.1 (9.4) 9.3 (13.6)	Encouraging player collaboration on a virtual tandem bike.	Nearly all participants would like to use the system again.
11	Janeh 2019 [28]	MoCA, SSQ, SUS, PDQ-39	Pre Post	16.45 (16.59) 15.21 (17.04)	-	-	-	Finding a VR-based gait manipulation strategy to improve gait symmetry.	Providing rehabilitative training strategies to achieve gait symmetry and prevent FOG.
12	Kern 2019 [29]	SSQ, SAM, IMI, RTLX, UEQ, USEQ, STAI	Pre Post	21.19 (20.87) 14.23 (15.45)	15.63 (16.15) 15.10 (14.49)	21.68 (20.59) 12.42 (16.32)	16.23 (27.54) 11.21 (16.57)	Using VR to enhance motivation during gait rehabilitation.	Providing critical content features in gait rehabilitation.

Table 3. *Cont.*

No.	Author	Measures	Groups	Total SSQ (SD)	Nausea (SD)	Oculomotor (SD)	Disorientation (SD)	Objectives	Results
13	Kim 2017 [30]	Mini-BESTest, CoP, SSQ	Healthy young Healthy old Parkinson's disease	8.3 (10.5) 6.5 (13.0) 27.5 (22.5)	5.8 (7.4) 6.1 (11.2) 20.8 (18.3)	10.2 (12.4) 12.1 (13.2) 21.5 (16.6)	6.5 (13.6) 4.4 (12.4) 28.5 (29.3)	Evaluating the safety of using an HMD for longer bouts of walking.	Older adults with PD were able to use immersive VR during walking without adverse effects.
14	Lhbetzky 2020 [31]	VVAS, DHI, ABC, FSST	(VM) Pre (VM) Post (mTBI) Pre (mTBI) Post	4.75 (4.22) 4.17 (5.06) 13 (11.3) 18.5 (13.4)	-	-	-	Testing the feasibility of a novel VR application (app) for patients with vestibular disorders.	HMD training appeared to be a promising adjunct modality for vestibular rehabilitation.
15	Lheureux 2020 [32]	SSQ	TW (Pre) iVRTW (Post)	15.0 (19.7) 16.8 (14.8)	11.5 (12.6) 17.2 (11.7)	12.1 (15.7) 15.9 (17.7)	16.7 (29.2) 8.4 (9.7)	Comparing PD gait during different conditions.	iVRTW could enhance the effectiveness of TW.
16	Maeng 2021 [33]	CERAD-K, KQOL-AD, GDS, SSQ	Normal group MCI group	16.45 (24.42) 19.90 (29.45)	10.30 (17.61) 14.46 (21.17)	26.16 (37.76) 32.33 (46.91)	10.91 (17.10) 11.24 (19.26)	Introducing a virtual reality-based cognitive training (VRCT) program.	Both groups showed a reduction in discomfort as the VRCT program progressed.
17	Morizio 2022 [34]	SSQ, PQ, SUS	Pre Sess 1 Post Sess 1 Pre Sess 2 Post Sess 2	1.31 (2.53) 3.33 (6.98) 0.80 (2.00) 2.32 (5.53)	-	-	-	Assessing the onset of cybersickness in the health before testing in stroke patients.	The usage of this VR device for gait rehabilitation did not lead to cybersickness.
18	Park 2020 [35]	VRSQ, SSQ	Fixed Moving	7.98 (11.03) 24.43 (28.62)	-	-	-	Investigating how full-immersion VR games cause changes.	Paying a VR game had negative effects on static balance.
19	Pot-Kolder 2018 [36]	SSQ, SUD	Pre Post	32.7 (37.7) 46.7 (38.7)	23.3 (29.2) 40.3 (36.1)	32.7 (33.3) 33.3 (30.6)	27.8 (46.5) 54.0 (51.9)	Investigating the relationship between VR and CS.	CS is expected to decline during treatment.
20	Salgado 2020 [37]	QoE, SSQ, SCR, IBI, HRV	Low (Pre) High (Post)	2.8 (11.2) 16.28 (27.4)	7.75 (16.0) 13.47 (23.6)	−2.36 (12.0) 9.8 (24.4)	2.39 (9.54) 15.71 (21.0)	Presenting a QoE and cybersickness study of wheelchair training simulator.	Simulator with low jerk effect reduced simulator sickness symptoms.
21	Saredakis 2020 [38]	AES, SSQ	Pre Post	12.22 (13.07) 13.46 (11.38)	15.90 (15.99) 17.17 (17.74)	18.70 (21.98) 20.72 (20.75)	7.42 (15.67) 12.06 (14.76)	Assessing whether VR using HMDs could be used to deliver tailored reminiscence therapy.	It is feasible to use VR for therapy to treat symptoms of apathy in older adults.
22	Shah 2022 [39]	SUS, SSQ, GEQ, IMI, VEQ	Pre-test Post-test Change Score	9.08 (11.19) 14.43 (11.29) 5.34 (6.74)	4.77 (10.66) 17.71 (15.23) 12.94 (12.28)	9.75 (10.88) 9.75 (9.25) 0 (4.96)	8.95 (14.51) 9.94 (14.34) 0.99 (3.58)	Motivating elderly individuals to participate in physical exercise and social connectedness.	The participants found the social VR gameplay enjoyable.
23	Tyrrell 2017 [40]	NDI, VSS, VAS, DHI, SS-VAS, SSQ	Control Neck pain Vestibular	21.88 (29.7) 43.20 (31.5) 49.42 (33.4)	24.33 (30.9) 32.91 (29.3) 40.89 (23.5)	12.13 (17.8) 34.11 (21.7) 31.40 (27.1)	23.66 (37.0) 50.11 (46.2) 66.62 (49.5)	This was a cross-sectional, observational study with three populations sought.	Neck pain and vestibular pathology similarly increased rating of SS.

Table 3. *Cont.*

No.	Author	Measures	Groups	Total SSQ (SD)	Nausea (SD)	Oculomotor (SD)	Disorientation (SD)	Objectives	Results
24	Vailland 2021 [41]	SSQ, USE, IPQ	Pre Post	20.44 (22.45) 25.58 (25.52)	13.63 (16.3) 20.61 (25.49)	20.84 (22.84) 20.62 (22.48)	17.9 (25.09) 27.28 (34.69)	Developing a virtual reality-based power wheelchair simulator.	The simulator provoked only slight to moderate cybersickness discomforts.
25	Vlake 2021 [42]	SSQ, IPQ	2D Group VR Group	0.9 (0.3) 3.7 (2.1)	0.9 (0.5) 1.8 (3.8)	0.1 (0.1) 2.1 (1.2)	0.1 (0.1) 2.3 (5.3)	To describe and evaluate the safety and immersiveness of an ICU-specific VR module.	ICU-VR is safe and more immersive than 2D.
26	Winter 2021 [43]	IPQ, SSQ, RTLX, SUS	Pre Post	13.19 (13.34) 17.04 (18.46)	10.34 (11.49) 15.37 (11.47)	12.63 (14.61) 12.84 (19.58)	10.83 (17.00) 17.40 (26.07)	Comparison for VR via HMD, VR via monitor, treadmill training without VR.	Study demonstrated the feasibility of combining treadmill training with VR.

Note: items with missing values noted as "-" in Table 3 were excluded.

Table 4. Statistical analysis results for SSQ Scores.

	Total SSQ Score	Nausea	Oculomotor	Disorientation
Age	Q-value = 0.362 p = 0.835	Q-value = 6.103 p = 0.107	Q-value = 8.870 p = 0.031	Q-value = 1.045 p = 0.790
Symptom	Q-value = 6.628 p = 0.036	Q-value = 8.472 p = 0.037	Q-value = 8.552 p = 0.014	Q-value = 10.724 p = 0.005
Inducement	Q-value = 0.744 p = 0.388	Q-value = 6.602 p = 0.037	Q-value = 10.284 p = 0.001	Q-value = 14.920 p = 0.000
Time	Q-value = 10.181 p = 0.017	Q-value = 14.032 p = 0.003	Q-value = 7.160 p = 0.067	Q-value = 18.070 p = 0.000
Content	Q-value = 9.594 p = 0.048	Q-value = 12.536 p = 0.014	Q-value = 7.990 p = 0.018	Q-value = 26.937 p = 0.000
Locomotion	Q-value = 7.864 p = 0.020	Q-value = 9.355 p = 0.053	Q-value = 7.340 p = 0.059	Q-value = 8.396 p = 0.015
Control	Q-value = 21.936 p = 0.000	Q-value = 14.530 p = 0.002	Q-value = 3.726 p = 0.293	Q-value = 9.222 p = 0.026
Display type	Q-value = 7.660 p = 0.006	Q-value = 21.058 p = 0.000	Q-value = 16.903 p = 0.000	Q-value = 31.741 p = 0.000

Table 5. SSQ total scores.

Attribute	Total SSQ			
	n	%	Mean	95% CI
Age				
0–30	8	30.7	20.508	[13.086, 27.931]
30–60	9	34.6	20.853	[14.138, 27.569]
Above 60	8	30.7	16.036	[12.699, 19.372]
Symptom				
Brain injuries	7	26.9	21.058	[15.357, 26.760]
Cognitive impairment	7	26.9	19.242	[11.294, 27.189]
Physical inactivity	12	46.2	18.156	[12.778, 23.534]
Inducement				
YES	19	73.1	19.430	[15.678, 23.181]
NO	7	26.9	8.519	[5.599, 11.438]
Time				
0–10 min	3	11.5	14.474	[9.165, 19.784]
10–20 min	16	61.5	15.695	[11.559, 19.830]
Above 20 min	5	19.2	26.862	[13.883, 39.841]
Content				
Exergame	11	42.3	21.090	[15.695, 26.484]
Training	8	30.7	16.258	[10.063, 22.453]
Video	4	15.4	35.964	[15.833, 56.095]
Scene	3	11.6	14.446	[6.548, 22.345]
Locomotion				
Sitting	6	23.1	23.044	[10.847, 35.240]
Standing	7	26.9	24.122	[14.779, 33.464]
Walking	11	42.3	13.686	[10.173, 17.199]
Bicycling	2	7.7	22.330	[14.310, 30.349]
Control				
Controller-based	9	34.6	17.537	[12.274, 22.800]
Gesture-based	6	23.1	21.451	[11.341, 31.562]
Gaze-directed	9	34.6	23.953	[12.580, 35.326]
Display Type				
3 DoF	16	61.5	21.307	[14.402, 28.213]
6 DoF	10	38.5	19.114	[14.7005, 23.523]
All studies	26	100	19.430	[15.678, 23.181]

Table 6. SSQ subscale scores.

Attribute	n (%)	Nausea		Oculomotor		Disorientation	
		Mean	95% CI	Mean	95% CI	Mean	95% CI
Age							
0–30	5 (25)	20.212	[15.977, 24.447]	14.222	[8.583, 19.862]	25.868	[15.636, 36.101]
30–60	8 (40)	19.918	[14.020, 25.816]	17.143	[11.752, 22.533]	20.765	[9.722, 31.807]
Above 60	6 (30)	12.806	[8.683, 16.929]	15.859	[12.802, 18.915]	15.527	[10.389, 20.665]
Symptom							
Brain injuries	2 (10)	15.543	[10.253, 20.833]	22.216	[17.006, 27.426]	25.111	[14.646, 35.575]
Cognitive impairment	7 (35)	22.651	[14.995, 30.306]	24.051	[15.766, 32.336]	26.615	[10.778, 42.452]
Physical inactivity	11 (55)	17.014	[14.225, 19.803]	13.333	[7.970, 18.696]	18.174	[14.046, 22.302]
Inducement							
YES	16 (80)	20.429	[13.553, 27.306]	19.366	[13.124, 25.609]	23.395	[16.733, 30.056]
NO	4 (20)	9.597	[5.295, 13.900]	6.136	[3.138, 9.134]	11.602	[5.156, 18.048]
Time							
0–10 min	3 (15)	17.834	[12.723, 22.946]	10.842	[5.741, 15.943]	17.757	[12.083, 23.430]
10–20 min	11 (55)	15.871	[10.636, 21.107]	12.828	[5.655, 20.001]	17.779	[8.491, 27.049]
Above 20 min	5 (25)	24.701	[20.793, 28.610]	24.558	[19.764, 29.351]	27.633	[19.786, 35.480]
Content							
Exergame	9 (45)	16.209	[11.132, 21.286]	18.204	[11.981, 24.428]	18.992	[14.131, 23.852]
Training	6 (30)	16.009	[13.015, 19.002]	12.121	[6.825, 17.417]	19.866	[15.226, 24.507]
Video	4 (20)	32.671	[20.795, 44,546]	21.590	[10.274, 32.907]	31.916	[12.709, 51.123]
Locomotion							
Sitting	6 (30)	19.449	[11.394, 27.504]	17.452	[10.191, 24.712]	21.809	[9.512, 34.106]
Standing	6 (30)	21.466	[15.633, 27.299]	20.162	[10.883, 29.441]	22.378	[12.316, 32.440]
Walking	6 (30)	15.077	[12.680, 17.475]	13.443	[7.806, 19.080]	19.384	[15.276, 23.491]
Bicycling	2 (10)	21.491	[14.254, 28.727]	15.803	[10.315, 31.921]	19.435	[10.218, 27.089]
Control							
Controller-based	8 (40)	13.000	[8.309, 17.691]	10.591	[4.771, 16.410]	17.572	[13.724, 21.421]
Gesture-based	4 (20)	21.888	[15.095, 28.681]	24.669	[10.800, 38.538]	20.369	[8.010, 32.727]
Gaze-directed	5 (25)	21.820	[11.675, 31.966]	19.530	[9.979, 29.081]	30.953	[14.490, 47.416]

Table 6. *Cont.*

Attribute	n (%)	Nausea		Oculomotor		Disorientation	
		Mean	95% CI	Mean	95% CI	Mean	95% CI
Display Type							
3 DoF	12 (60)	19.964	[12.113, 27.814]	19.264	[12.019, 26.509]	22.301	[12.089, 32.513]
6 DoF	7 (35)	14.722	[12.084, 17.360]	12.133	[6.164, 18.102]	17.781	[14.277, 21.286]
All studies	20 (100)	17.834	[12.723, 22.946]	16.365	[11.512, 21.218]	21.096	[14.059, 28.133]

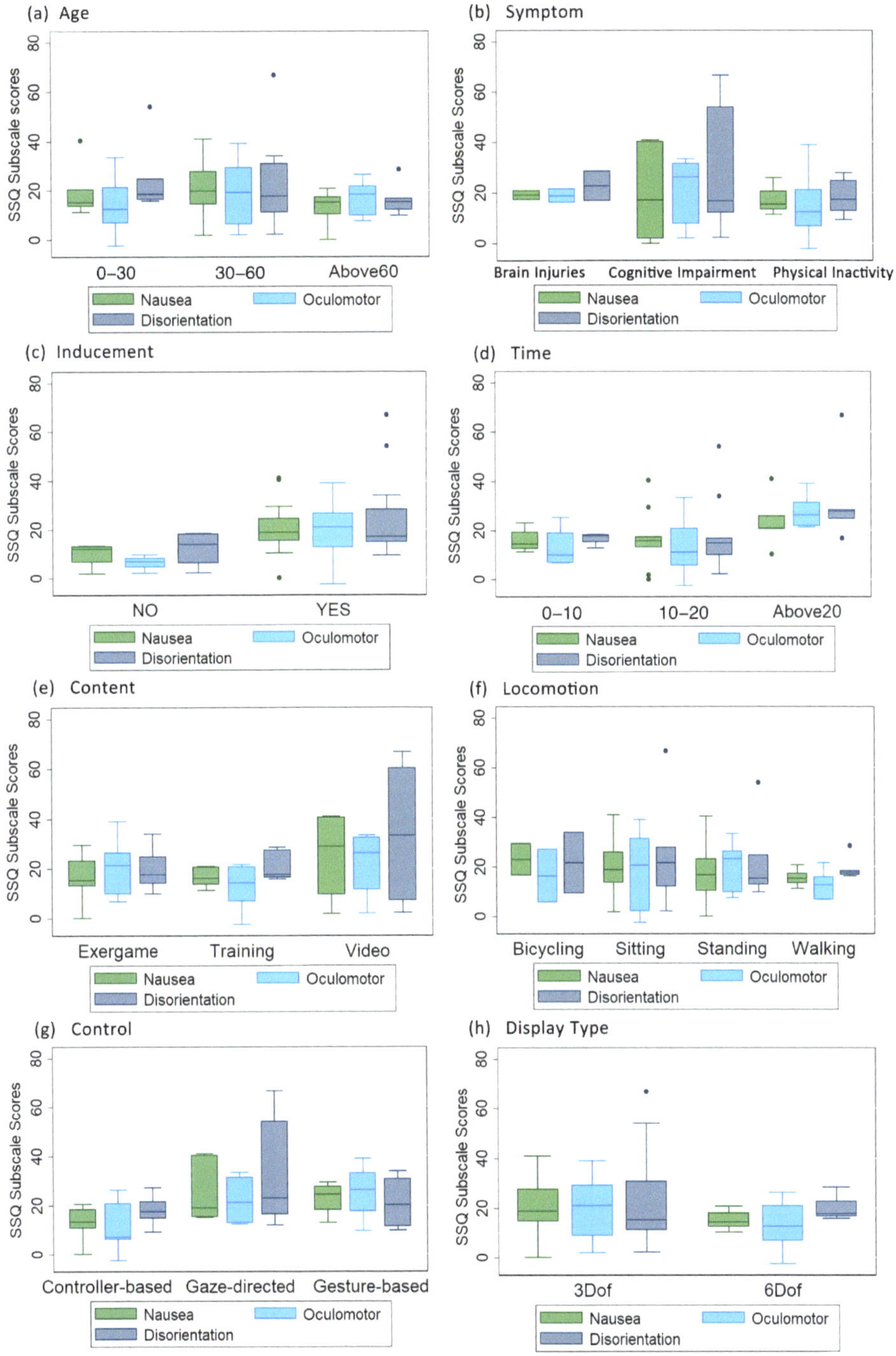

Figure 4. Boxplots for SSQ subscale scores: (**a**) Age, (**b**) Symptom, (**c**) Inducement, (**d**) Time, (**e**) Content, (**f**) Locomotion, (**g**) Control, (**h**) Display Type.

The methodological quality of the research papers was evaluated using the widely adopted risk-of-bias analysis. All of the selected results were assessed according to whether or not the publication included useful SSQ score reference information beneficial to the ongoing endeavor. Publications without subscale scores were considered to have a low level of risk of bias.

3.3. *Subject Characters and VR Cybersickness*

Table 4 shows that the subject's age was not relevant for determining the degree of cybersickness in the VR rehabilitation papers. The age range was divided into three groups, as shown in Table 5: 0–30 (teenagers, n = 8, 30.7%), 30–60 (adults, n = 9, 34.6%), and 60 and older (elderly, n = 8, 30.7%). Adult participants were the most susceptible to cybersickness in the total SSQ scores (mean = 20.853, 95% CI: 14.138–27.569), and after they reached the age of 60, their vulnerability to it gradually declined. Table 6 shows that teens had greater nausea (mean = 20.212, 95% CI: 15.977–24.447) and disorientation (mean = 25.868, 95% CI: 15.636–36.101) experience than adults and the elderly. What is more, adults suffered more serious oculomotor symptoms (mean = 17.143, 95% CI: 11.752–22.533) than the others.

There were variations in the symptoms and conditions among the patients who participated in virtual rehabilitation. The Q-value statistical results in Table 4 show that nausea (Q-value = 8.472, p = 0.037, $p \leq 0.05$ *), oculomotor (Q-value = 8.552, p = 0.014, $p \leq 0.05$ *), and disorientation (Q-value = 10.724, p = 0.005, $p \leq 0.01$ **) symptoms and features of the overall SSQ score (Q-value = 6.628, p = 0.036, $p \leq 0.05$ *) were all statistically significant. In Table 5, we gathered VR rehabilitation cases for our meta-analysis that mostly addressed brain injuries (n = 7, 26.9%), cognitive impairment (n = 7, 26.9%), and physical inactivity (n = 12, 46.2%). According to the calculated pooled mean, cognitive impairment (mean = 19.242, 95% CI: 11.294–27.189) and physical inactivity (mean = 18.156, 95% CI: 12.778–23.534) had lower scores than brain injuries (mean = 21.058, 95% CI: 15.357–26.760). In order to compare different symptoms, the mean scores, standard deviations, and sample sizes of the previous and post-available data were collected. As shown in the forest plot of the subgroup SSQ total scores in Figure 3, in contrast to cognitive impairment (mean = 0.407, 95% CI: 0.266–0.548) and physical inactivity (mean = 0.203, 95% CI: 0.042–0.365), subjects with brain injuries (mean = 0.470, 95% CI: 0.223–0.716) had a higher strictly standardized mean of virtual reality sickness.

We also took the inducement circumstance into consideration. According to Kenndy's publication [45], SSQ total scores between 10 and 15 indicate substantial sickness, those of 15 to 20 indicate cause for serious worry, and those of 20 or more indicate a simulation issue. We used this reference as a benchmark and compared it to the original paper descriptions. By doing this, we formed a judgment on the inducement circumstances of each instance. Based on the result box plots shown in Figure 4, the non-induced data obviously stand out and are lower than the induced group.

3.4. *VR Software and Cybersickness*

In the immersive VR therapies studied, there were three different time durations: 0–10 min (n = 3, 11.5%), 10–20 min (n = 16, 61.5%), and above 20 min (n = 5, 19.5%). From the SNK Q-test, we were able to determine that there was a significant difference between the groups in the duration of VR rehabilitation exposure, which was also reflected in the SSQ scores. The SSQ total scores of times ranging from 0 to 10 min (mean = 14.474), 10 to 20 min (mean = 15.695), and above 20 min (mean = 26.862) are consistent with the trend. In addition, Figure 4 demonstrates that the scores for the three SSQ subscales increased steadily higher over time, excluding the outliers' values. It is evident that prolonged exposure to a virtual environment screen induced feelings of disorientation (mean = 27.633, 95% CI: 19.786–35.454).

Apart from the condition of time, this study included a total of four different types of rehabilitation content: exercise games (n = 11, 42.3%), training (n = 8, 30.7%), videos (n = 4, 15.4%), and scenes (n = 3, 11.6%). In our research, it was clear that video had the highest mean scores on the SSQ's overall and subscale scores (total mean score = 35.964, nausea mean = 32.671, oculomotor mean = 21.590, disorientation mean = 31.916). When compared to the exergame and training contents, the boxplot in Figure 4 thoroughly demonstrates the biggest value interval for video material. Additionally, when compared to the video with the highest score, the exergame's (total mean score = 21.090, 95% CI: 15.695–26.484) mechanism may also heighten the symptoms of cybersickness. Among the four SSQ total score items, the scene (total mean score mean = 14.446, 95% CI: 6.548–22.345) had the lowest coefficients; it exhibited rotational motions along several axes without dynamic influence. Note that since scenes only had SSQ total scores, there are no scene types in Figure 4 and Table 6.

3.5. VR Hardware and Cybersickness

When it comes to hardware factors, in this study, we mainly considered locomotion, control, and display type.

In Table 4, the total SSQ score (Q-value = 7.864, $p = 0.020$, $p \leq 0.05$ *) and disorientation (Q-value = 8.396, $p = 0.015$, $p \leq 0.05$ *) are significantly different among the modes of locomotion. In our study, there were a total of four different modes of locomotion: sitting (n = 6, 23.1%, total mean score = 23.044, 95% CI: 10.847–35.240), standing (n = 7, 26.9%, total mean score = 24.122, 95% CI: 14.779–33.464), walking (n = 11, 42.3%, total mean score = 13.686, 95% CI: 10.173–17.199), and bicycling (n = 2, 7.7%, total mean score = 22.330, 95% CI: 14.310–30.349). Table 6 shows that the bicycling mode had the highest nausea score (mean = 21.491, 95% CI: 14.254–28.727). Meanwhile, standing led to higher oculomotor (mean = 20.162, 95% CI: 10.883–29.441) and disorientation (mean = 22.378, 95% CI: 12.316–32.440) sickness than other locomotion modes. The rankings are shown in Figure 4; the subscale scores of walking were lower than other locomotion.

As for the control aspect, we studied controller-based, gesture-based, and gazed-directed modes. A general controller for virtual rehabilitation equipment in a virtual environment (n = 9, 34.6%, mean = 17.537) was less susceptible to cybersickness. However, there is still proof that the gaze-directed (n = 9, 34.6%, mean = 23.953) and gesture-based control modes (n = 6, 23.1%, mean = 21.451) were significantly more uncomfortable than the typical controller, as shown in the SSQ total scores (Q-value = 21.936, p-value = 0.000, $p \leq 0.001$ ***). Additionally, gesture-based training may have resulted in greater oculomotor (mean = 24.669, 95% CI: 10.800–38.538) and disorientation (mean = 20.369, 95% CI: 8.010–32.727) symptoms. These were brought on by the patients' high vulnerability and high motion degree. The biggest range value in Figure 4 is for gaze-directed. The patient has complete freedom to stare anywhere they choose while traveling with the gaze method. This function causes dizziness and strain on the eyes, which increased the disorientation score (mean = 30.953, 95% CI: 14.490–47.416).

In Table 4, the values for the display types are significant in the total SSQ scores (Q-value = 7.660, $p = 0.006$, $p \leq 0.01$ **), nausea scores (Q-value = 21.058, $p = 0.000$, $p \leq 0.001$ ***), oculomotor scores (Q-value = 16.903, $p = 0.000$, $p \leq 0.001$ ***), and disorientation scores (Q-value = 31.741, $p = 0.000$, $p \leq 0.001$ ***). According to the boxplot, three degrees of freedom (n = 12, 60%) had higher subscale scores on the SSQ than six degrees of freedom (n = 17, 35%).

4. Discussion

The purpose of this systematic review was to gather the current research on cybersickness using SSQ scores, which examine the main consequences of the discomfort experienced. There are many factors related to cybersickness; this paper mainly concentrates on three different aspects, including the subjects' demographics, software factors, and hardware factors.

4.1. Demographic of Cybersickness

The age of subjects may lead to different levels of virtual reality sickness. It has been found that the elderly may experience eye tiredness much more than adults or the young [46]. However, in our research, the comparison of the experiments for age groups showed that the old were not obviously oversensitive when applying virtual rehabilitation. Compared to older people, younger people and adults might be more available for interaction in virtual environments, if there are no big difficulties when using the devices and completing the tests [47]. The scores of the SSQ were also determined by other factors, such as skills, and not just age. When facing difficult missions, such as bicycling or gesture-based movement, older people might be unable to finish the process. More importantly, the SSQ scores for age might be misleading because of the limited number of cases. This conclusion should be proven by more studies from multiple directions in the future.

In virtual rehabilitation scenarios, symptoms are more important and worthy of attention in virtual environment cybersickness.

Firstly, for brain injuries, it has been shown that using immersive virtual rehabilitation as a treatment option may help individuals with brain injuries train their attention [48,49], which may affect the subject's ability to learn new motor skills [50]. Studies on the effects of virtual reality on vital "theta waves" in the hippocampus have been beneficial. For instance, virtual reality improved brain activity associated with memory and learning [51] in the treatment of conditions, including Alzheimer's disease, stroke, traumatic brain injury, and Parkinson's disease. Virtual reality rehabilitation, therefore, offers possible novel treatments for brain injuries, but the cybersickness evaluation scores are so high that product developers should pay more attention to reducing the side effects [52]. Virtual reality provides a secure setting to enhance rehabilitation, particularly with the declining availability of labor and resources in our aging population.

Secondly, for exam users who have cognitive impairment [53], VR-based treatments have been used as health promotion tools to enhance mobility, prevent falls, and train cognitive skills in people who have dementia and those who are at risk of acquiring dementia. According to studies, virtual rehabilitation technology can be used to improve an individual's abilities, such as memory and concentration, and to diagnose attention deficit hyperactivity disorder (ADHD) through hand or body involvement. The development of attention skills may delay cognitive aging [54]. A study at the University of Montreal examined the effects of video games on the grey matter in the area of the brain that supports memory formation, and the results demonstrated the value of exercise games in rehabilitation. All symptoms associated with cognitive impairment pointed to the need for tailored interventions and designed approaches to mitigate the negative effects of cybersickness [55,56].

Finally, a study revealed that virtual rehabilitation improved the effectiveness of VR exercise and particularly aided patients with physical inactivity in improving their physical fitness, muscular strength, and balance [57]. However, there were still flaws in the VR rehabilitation of physical inactivity. For instance, in the case of conducting a mission with a set time frame, the poor efficacy of training increased the amount of cybersickness. VR therapy is beneficial for both youth and the elderly who have gait impairment, vestibular issue, multiple sclerosis, spinal cord injury, neck discomfort, or chronic pain. However, when playing the same exercise game or other rehabilitation assignment simultaneously, a serious disease may cause discomfort and worsen physical or mental conditions [58].

There are individual differences in the severity of cybersickness symptoms based on personal medical conditions. The SSQ scores for individuals with brain injuries, cognitive impairment, and physical inactivity indicate more severe cybersickness symptoms in these groups.

4.2. Software Factors of Cybersickness

It can be concluded that as the exposure time of the VR facility increases, so does cybersickness. However, research on exposure to VR suggests that users can have an adjustment period. After about 15–20 min of exposure to a virtual environment, the parameters will return to baseline levels. Risi [59] discovered that repeated VR device exposures during a two-day period did not lower cybersickness levels. Shah [39] and Heg [27] also demonstrated the probability of SSQ deterioration after adjustment. We could not lessen the amount of cybersickness until consumers adapted to the virtual world, but when the interval was too long, it did not make sense. Furthermore, people with brain injuries are unable to spend an excessive amount of time in an immersive virtual world since doing so might have long-lasting side effects [34]. As a matter of fact, duration is one of the key points that leads to varying degrees of cybersickness, and designers should be more concerned about the interaction time in software engineering.

In addition to the time condition, four different types of rehabilitation contents were included in this study. The degree of cybersickness might be simply described by task performance in different types of content, including exergames, training, video, and scenes [60]. A user of virtual reality feels completely immersed in their surroundings since the environment is computer-generated and contains realistic-looking items and situations. An immersive content experience is totally different from passive reading, such as static PDF, stress immersion, and interaction with text [61]. Interactive polls and quizzes, animated data visualizations and infographics, and 3D images and videos are some of the most popular forms of immersive content. As for exergames and training, there are many types of exercise activities related to rehabilitation, including role play, the use of an omnidirectional treadmill, and others. Video was harder for subjects to get used to and resulted in the highest levels of cybersickness. This phenomenon may be caused by high-intensity training that causes one to lose their sense of direction. It has been suggested that exergames and training has relatively smaller degrees of cybersickness than video content.

4.3. Hardware Factors of Cybersickness

The first hardware factor is locomotion. We can easily infer from the SSQ scores that those strategies with artificial continuous movement led to higher SSQ scores than those with discrete movements [62]. For example, sitting may have had a high SSQ score due to the restrictions on the mobility of bodily movement. When it came to walking, there were two basic types of conditions: walking on a treadmill and walking in a real zone. According to Wilson, natural walking without translation causes less illness from cybersickness than added translation movement. Additionally, as a role player, natural walking resulted in lower SSQ scores than teleportation. Bicycling may also cause a significant amount of cybersickness [63].

For control modes, it is important to note that the gaze-directed samples had higher feelings of discomfort when undergoing the examination. When using the gaze-directed approach, the VR device sets a pointer in the middle of the screen and a target icon (a white cylinder) on the ground in the event that the user's sight crosses the ground. The patient goes to the desired position by pushing a button. This may increase the difficulty of machine control. In contrast, the SSQ scores decreased in controller-based and gesture-based settings, which means that designers should avoid setting gaze-directed control modes.

For the display type, while patients in VR therapy may gaze about in all directions, three DoF cannot be used to get a closer look at anything in the environment. Patients only have access to one perspective, and thus, no matter how they move or swivel their heads in the actual world, they stay still in the virtual one, with higher SSQ scores reflecting the drawback known as visual–vestibular conflict. The visual and vestibular system "disconnect" results in a sensory conflict in 3D space. Therefore, six DoF motion is the foundation of a better VR rehabilitation experience.

4.4. Strengths, Limitations, and Future Works

This paper explores a new area in immersive virtual reality rehabilitation with SSQ score data collected from more than 862 participants. The results show that factors such as symptoms, inducement condition, exposure time, content, and hardware controls vary widely across multiple variants. This article provides a good example for conducting immersive virtual reality rehabilitation research to benefit the rehabilitation industry. Especially in the face of high artificial medical costs, it is impossible to hire more therapists in the digital age.

One limitation of this research is that the number of influencing factors studied is limited. In addition, due to the limited number of papers included, the conclusions of some factors may require further research and proof.

For further studies, researchers can explore more influencing factors. For example, immersive virtual reality rehabilitation can also be further studied in terms of regional differences, VR equipment, interaction modes, and so on. As the market develops, there are more and more requests for better use of virtual rehabilitation. The results show that the SSQ is a useful analytical measure that provides a large amount of valid data. In addition, two variants of the SSQ have been offered for testing cybersickness in recent research and have become popular, which are named the Cybersickness Questionnaire and the Virtual Reality Sickness Questionnaire. These may overcome the shortcomings of the SSQ, which considers virtual reality as the mian object of study.

5. Conclusions

Cybersickness is a common side effect of immersive virtual reality rehabilitation, which can negatively impact a patient's experience and potentially limit the effectiveness of treatment. This research evaluated the cybersickness-related aspects of VR rehabilitation, which was achieved by a systematic review of this field and by conducting a meta-analysis of the SSQ scores. For the demographic factors, the SSQ scores of participants' ages, symptoms, and inducement situations were discussed in this study. We also discussed the VR device software missions' time lengths and contents. As for the hardware aspect, locomotion, control method, and display type were also taken into consideration. These three categories of characteristics exhibited the cybersickness circumstances that affected how smoothly the experiments operated. With the technological revolution taking place against the immersive backdrop, it is beneficial for us to enhance the rehabilitation mode [64]. Furthermore, by better understanding VR technology, we will be able to create equipment that is particularly useful for rehabilitation [65,66].

With proper design and implementation, cybersickness can be minimized, and the benefits of virtual reality rehabilitation can be fully realized. However, it is difficult to draw firm conclusions supporting the use of VR in rehabilitation from small-scale studies, and future directions should focus on more informative or large-scale studies. The FOV, latency, and realism of immersive VR rehabilitation equipment are improving [67]. Given the advancement of technology, the impact of cybersickness should be further assessed [68]. For better product engineering, rehabilitation symptoms require more attention. Overall, while cybersickness can be a significant issue in immersive virtual reality rehabilitation, it should not discourage the use of this technology in healthcare. With careful attention to design and patient needs, virtual reality can provide a valuable tool for rehabilitation and improved patient outcomes.

Author Contributions: Conceptualization, X.L.; methodology, X.L.; software, Y.A.; validation, D.-B.L., Y.A.; formal analysis, X.L.; investigation, R.-H.X.; resources, X.L.; data curation, X.L.; writing—original draft preparation, X.L.; writing—review and editing, X.L.; visualization, X.L.; supervision, D.-B.L.; project administration, D.-B.L. All authors have read and agreed to the published version of the manuscript.

Funding: This research received no external funding.

Conflicts of Interest: The authors declare no conflict of interest.

Appendix A

Abbreviations	Description	Abbreviations	Description
AD-ACL	Activation–Deactivation Adjective Check List	AES	Apathy Evaluation Scale
CCT	Computerized Cognitive Training	CERAD-K	A Korean version of the Consortium to Establish a Registry for Alzheimer's Disease Assessment
CET	Cognitive Evaluation Theory	DHI	Dizziness Handicap Inventory
IMI	Intrinsic Motivation Inventory	DOF	Degrees of Freedom
EDQ	Equipment and Display Questionnaire	GMS	Global Motivation Scale
ITC-SOPI	International Test Commission—Sense of Presence Inventory	ICU-VR	ICU-specific VR
HMD	Head-Mounted Display	KQOL-AD	Korean Version of Quality of Life—Alzheimer's Disease
GEQ	Game Experience Questionnaire	GDS	Geriatric Depression Scale
MCI	Mild Cognitive Impairment	GSR	Galvanic Skin Response
NDI	Neck Disability Index	NASA-TLX	NASA Task Load Index
QoE	Quality of Experience	RAGT	Robot-Assisted Gait Training
VEQ	Virtual Embodiment Questionnaire	SoP	Sense of Presence
SP	Spatial Presence	RTLX	Raw Task Load Index
SMET	Submaximal Tourniquet Effort Test	PAS	Psychogeriatric Assessment Scale
QoE	Quality of Experience	SCR	Skin Conductance Response
PQ	Presence Questionnaire	VRSQ	Virtual Reality Symptom Questionnaire
UEQ	Experience Questionnaire	USEQ	User Satisfaction Evaluation Questionnaire
SS-VAS	Simulator Sickness Visual Analog Scale	VRISE	VR Sickness or Virtual Reality-Induced Symptoms and Effects
SSQ	Simulator Sickness Questionnaire	SUS	System Usability Scale
VSS	Visual Symptoms Scale	VRCT	Virtual Reality-Based Cognitive Therapy
VAS	Visual Analog Scale	TAM	Technology Acceptance Model

Appendix B

Section and Topic	Item	Checklist Item	Location Where Item Is Reported
		TITLE	
Title	1	Identify the report as both systematic review and meta-analysis.	Page 1
		ABSTRACT	
Structure summary	2	Provide a structured summary including, as applicable: background; objectives; data sources; study eligibility criteria, participants, and interventions; study appraisal and synthesis methods; results; conclusions and implications of key findings.	Page 1
		INTRODUCTION	
Rationale	3	Describe the rationale for the review in the context of what is already known.	Page 2
Objectives	4	Provide an explicit statement of questions being addressed with reference to participants, interventions, comparisons, outcomes, and study design (PICOS).	Page 2–4
		METHODS	
Eligibility criteria	5	Present the systematic review registration number. And specify the inclusion and exclusion criteria for the review and how studies were grouped for the syntheses.	Page 4
Information sources	6	Specify all databases, registers, websites, organizations, reference lists and other sources searched or consulted to identify studies.	Page 4
Search strategy	7	Present the full search strategies for all databases, registers and websites, including any filters and limits used.	Page 4–5
Selection process	8	Specify the methods used to decide whether a study met the inclusion criteria of the review, including how many reviewers screened each record and each report retrieved, whether they worked independently, and if applicable, details of automation tools used in the process.	Page 5
Data collection process	9	Specify the methods used to collect data from reports, including how many reviewers collected data from each report, whether they worked independently, any processes for obtaining or confirming data from study investigators.	Page 5
Data items	10	List and define all outcomes for which data were sought. Specify whether all results that were compatible with each outcome domain in each study were sought (e.g., for all measures, time points, analyses).	Page 5
Study risk of bias assessment	11	Specify the methods used to assess risk of bias in the included studies, including details of the tool(s) used, how many reviewers assessed each study and whether they worked independently, and if applicable, details of automation tools used in the process.	Page 5
Effect measures	12	Specify for each outcome the effect measure(s) (e.g., risk ratio, mean difference) used in the synthesis or presentation of results.	Page 5
Synthesis methods	13	Describe any methods used to explore possible causes of heterogeneity among study results (e.g., subgroup analysis, meta-regression).	Page 5–6
Reporting bias assessment	14	Describe any methods used to assess risk of bias due to missing results in a synthesis (arising from reporting biases).	Page 5–6
Certainty assessment	15	Describe any methods used to assess certainty (or confidence) in the body of evidence for an outcome.	Page 6
		RESULTS	
Study selection	16	Describe the results of the search and selection process, from the number of records identified in the search to the number of studies included in the review, ideally using a flow diagram.	Page 7 Figure 2
Study characteristics	17	Cite each included study and present its characteristics.	Page 7
Risk of bias in studies	18	Present assessments of risk of bias for included study.	Page 14
Results of individual studies	19	For all outcomes, present, for each study: (a) summary statistics for each group (where appropriate) and (b) an effect estimate and its precision (e.g., confidence/credible interval), ideally using structured tables or plots.	Tables 2 and 3

Section and Topic	Item	Checklist Item	Location Where Item Is Reported
Results of syntheses	20	Present results of all statistical syntheses conducted. As meta-analysis was done, present for each the summary estimate and its precision (e.g., confidence/credible interval) and measures of statistical heterogeneity. Comparing the groups and describing the direction of the effect.	Figures 3 and 4 Tables 4–6
Reporting biases	21	Present results of any assessment of risk of bias across studies (see Item 18).	Page 14
		DISCUSSION	
Discussion	22	Provide a general interpretation of the results in the context of other evidence and implications of the results for practice, policy, and future research.	Page 20
		OTHER INFORMATION	
Registration and protocol	23	Provide registration information for the review, including register name and registration number, or state that the review was not registered.	NA
Support	24	Describe sources of financial or non-financial support for the review, and the role of the funders or sponsors in the review.	NA
Competing interests	25	Declare any competing interests of review authors.	NA
Availability of data, code and other materials	26	Report which of the following are publicly available and where they can be found: template data collection forms; data extracted from included studies; data used for all analyses; analytic code; any other materials used in the review.	NA

From: Page MJ, McKenzie JE, Bossuyt PM, Boutron I, Hoffmann TC, Mulrow CD, et al. The PRISMA 2020 statement: an updated guideline for reporting systematic reviews. BMJ 2021;372:n71. doi: 10.1136/bmj.n71. For more information, visit: http://www.prisma-statement.org/, accessed on 9 January 2023.

References

1. Tan, T.F.M.; Li, Y.; Lim, J.S.F.; Gunasekeran, D.V.M.; Teo, Z.L.M.; Ng, W.Y.F.; Ting, D.S. Metaverse and Virtual Health Care in Ophthalmology: Opportunities and Challenges. *Asia-Pac. J. Ophthalmol.* **2022**, *11*, 237–246. [CrossRef] [PubMed]
2. Kye, B.; Han, N.; Kim, E.; Park, Y.; Jo, S. Educational applications of metaverse: Possibilities and limitations. *J. Educ. Evaluation Health Prof.* **2021**, *18*, 32. [CrossRef] [PubMed]
3. Monardo, G.; Pavese, C.; Giorgi, I.; Godi, M.; Colombo, R. Evaluation of Patient Motivation and Satisfaction During Technology-Assisted Rehabilitation: An Experiential Review. *Games Health J.* **2021**, *10*, 13–27. [CrossRef]
4. Petri, K.; Feuerstein, K.; Folster, S.; Bariszlovich, F.; Witte, K. Effects of Age, Gender, Familiarity with the Content, and Exposure Time on Cybersickness in Immersive Head-mounted Display Based Virtual Reality. *Am. J. Biomed. Sci.* **2020**, *12*, 107–121. [CrossRef]
5. Burdea, G.C. Virtual rehabilitation–benefits and challenges. *Methods Inf. Med.* **2003**, *42*, 519–523.
6. Rose, T.; Nam, C.S.; Chen, K.B. Immersion of virtual reality for rehabilitation—Review. *Appl. Ergon.* **2018**, *69*, 153–161. [CrossRef]
7. Calabrò, R.S.; Cerasa, A.; Ciancarelli, I.; Pignolo, L.; Tonin, P.; Iosa, M.; Morone, G. The arrival of the metaverse in neurorehabilitation: Fact, fake or vision? *Biomedicines* **2022**, *10*, 2602. [CrossRef]
8. Kurz, A.; Pohl, C.; Ramsenthaler, M.; Sorg, C. Cognitive rehabilitation in patients with mild cognitive impairment. *Int. J. Geriatr. Psychiatry A J. Psychiatry Late Life Allied Sci.* **2009**, *24*, 163–168. [CrossRef]
9. Teasell, R.; Bayona, N.; Marshall, S.; Cullen, N.; Bayley, M.; Chundamala, J.; Villamere, J.; Mackie, D.; Rees, L.; Hartridge, C.; et al. A systematic review of the rehabilitation of moderate to severe acquired brain injuries. *Brain Inj.* **2007**, *21*, 107–112. [CrossRef]
10. Zelle, D.M.; Klaassen, G.; Van Adrichem, E.; Bakker, S.J.; Corpeleijn, E.; Navis, G. Physical inactivity: A risk factor and target for intervention in renal care. *Nat. Rev. Nephrol.* **2017**, *13*, 152–168. [CrossRef]
11. Kim, O.; Pang, Y.; Kim, J.-H. The effectiveness of virtual reality for people with mild cognitive impairment or dementia: A meta-analysis. *BMC Psychiatry* **2019**, *19*, 219. [CrossRef]
12. Cullen, N.; Chundamala, J.; Bayley, M.; Jutai, J. The efficacy of acquired brain injury rehabilitation. *Brain Inj.* **2007**, *21*, 113–132. [CrossRef]
13. Dębska, M.; Polechoński, J.; Mynarski, A.; Polechoński, P. Enjoyment and Intensity of Physical Activity in Immersive Virtual Reality Performed on Innovative Training Devices in Compliance with Recommendations for Health. *Int. J. Environ. Res. Public Health* **2019**, *16*, 3673. [CrossRef]
14. Takkouche, B.; Norman, G. Prisma statement. *Epidemiology* **2011**, *22*, 128. [CrossRef]
15. Eriksen, M.B.; Frandsen, T.F. The impact of patient, intervention, comparison, outcome (PICO) as a search strategy tool on literature search quality: A systematic review. *J. Med. Libr. Assoc.* **2018**, *106*, 420–431. [CrossRef]
16. Rebenitsch, L.; Owen, C. Individual variation in susceptibility to cybersickness. In Proceedings of the 27th annual ACM Symposium on User Interface Software and Technology, Honolulu, HI, USA, 5–8 October 2014; pp. 309–317.
17. Bruck, S.; Watters, P.A. Estimating Cybersickness of Simulated Motion Using the Simulator Sickness Questionnaire (SSQ): A Controlled Study. In Proceedings of the 2009 6th International Conference on Computer Graphics, Imaging and Visualization, Tianjin, China, 11–14 August 2009; pp. 486–488. [CrossRef]

18. Arafat, I.M. Cybersickness in Persons with Multiple Sclerosis. Ph.D. Thesis, The University of Texas at San Antonio, San Antonio, TX, USA, 2019.
19. Arlati, S.; Di Santo, S.G.; Franchini, F.; Mondellini, M.; Filiputti, B.; Luchi, M.; Ratto, F.; Ferrigno, G.; Sacco, M.; Greci, L. Acceptance and Usability of Immersive Virtual Reality in Older Adults with Objective and Subjective Cognitive Decline. *J. Alzheimer's Dis.* **2021**, *80*, 1025–1038. [CrossRef]
20. Bovim, L.P.; Gjesdal, B.E.; Mæland, S.; Aaslund, M.K.; Bogen, B. The impact of motor task and environmental constraints on gait patterns during treadmill walking in a fully immersive virtual environment. *Gait Posture* **2020**, *77*, 243–249. [CrossRef]
21. Brown, P.; Powell, W. Pre-Exposure Cybersickness Assessment Within a Chronic Pain Population in Virtual Reality. *Front. Virtual Real.* **2021**, *2*, 67. [CrossRef]
22. Chen, C.-H.; Jeng, M.-C.; Fung, C.-P.; Doong, J.-L.; Chuang, T.-Y. Psychological benefits of virtual reality for patients in rehabilitation therapy. *J. Sport Rehabil.* **2009**, *18*, 258–268. [CrossRef]
23. Chowdhury, T.; Ferdous, S.; Peck, T.; Quarles, J. Virtual ability simulation: Applying rotational gain to the leg to increase confidence during physical rehabilitation. In Proceedings of the ICAT-EGVE 2019-International Conference on Artificial Reality and Telexistence and Eurographics Symposium on Virtual Environments, Tokyo, Japan, 11–13 September 2019.
24. Ciążyńska, J.; Janowski, M.; Maciaszek, J. Effects of a Modern Virtual Reality 3D Head-Mounted Display Exergame on Simulator Sickness and Immersion Under Specific Conditions in Young Women and Men: Experimental Study. *JMIR Serious Games* **2022**, *10*, e41234. [CrossRef]
25. Hamzeheinejad, N.; Straka, S.; Gall, D.; Weilbach, F.; Latoschik, M.E. Immersive Robot-Assisted Virtual Reality Therapy for Neurologically-Caused Gait Impairments. In Proceedings of the 2018 IEEE Conference on Virtual Reality and 3D User Interfaces (VR), Tuebingen/Reutlingen, Germany, 18–22 March 2018; pp. 565–566. [CrossRef]
26. Hamzeheinejad, N.; Roth, D.; Götz, D.; Weilbach, F.; Latoschik, M.E. Physiological effectivity and user experience of immersive gait rehabilitation. In Proceedings of the 2019 IEEE Conference on Virtual Reality and 3D User Interfaces (VR), Osaka, Japan, 23–27 March 2019; pp. 1421–1429.
27. Høeg, E.R.; Bruun-Pedersen, J.R.; Cheary, S.; Andersen, L.K.; Paisa, R.; Serafin, S.; Lange, B. Buddy biking: A user study on social collaboration in a virtual reality exergame for rehabilitation. *Virtual Real.* **2021**, *27*, 1–18. [CrossRef]
28. Janeh, O.; Fründt, O.; Schönwald, B.; Gulberti, A.; Buhmann, C.; Gerloff, C.; Steinicke, F.; Pötter-Nerger, M. Gait Training in Virtual Reality: Short-Term Effects of Different Virtual Manipulation Techniques in Parkinson's Disease. *Cells* **2019**, *8*, 419. [CrossRef] [PubMed]
29. Kern, F.; Winter, C.; Gall, D.; Kathner, I.; Pauli, P.; Latoschik, M.E. Immersive Virtual Reality and Gamification Within Procedurally Generated Environments to Increase Motivation During Gait Rehabilitation. In Proceedings of the 26th IEEE Conference on Virtual Reality and 3D User Interfaces, VR 2019, Osaka, Japan, 25–29 March 2017; pp. 500–509. [CrossRef]
30. Kim, A.; Darakjian, N.; Finley, J.M. Walking in fully immersive virtual environments: An evaluation of potential adverse effects in older adults and individuals with Parkinson's disease. *J. Neuroeng. Rehabil.* **2017**, *14*, 1–12. [CrossRef] [PubMed]
31. Lubetzky, A.V.; Kelly, J.; Wang, Z.; Gospodarek, M.; Fu, G.; Sutera, J.; Hujsak, B.D. Contextual sensory integration training via head mounted display for individuals with vestibular disorders: A feasibility study. *Disabil. Rehabil. Assist. Technol.* **2020**, *17*, 74–84. [CrossRef]
32. Lheureux, A.; LeBleu, J.; Frisque, C.; Sion, C.; Stoquart, G.; Warlop, T.; Detrembleur, C.; Lejeune, T. Immersive Virtual Reality to Restore Natural Long-Range Autocorrelations in Parkinson's Disease Patients' Gait During Treadmill Walking. *Front. Physiol.* **2020**, *11*, 572063. [CrossRef]
33. Maeng, S.; Hong, J.P.; Kim, W.-H.; Kim, H.; Cho, S.-E.; Kang, J.M.; Na, K.-S.; Oh, S.-H.; Park, J.W.; Bae, J.N.; et al. Effects of Virtual Reality-Based Cognitive Training in the Elderly with and without Mild Cognitive Impairment. *Psychiatry Investig.* **2021**, *18*, 619–627. [CrossRef]
34. Morizio, C.; Compagnat, M.; Boujut, A.; Labbani-Igbida, O.; Billot, M.; Perrochon, A. Immersive Virtual Reality during Robot-Assisted Gait Training: Validation of a New Device in Stroke Rehabilitation. *Medicina* **2022**, *58*, 1805. [CrossRef]
35. Park, S.; Lee, G. Full-immersion virtual reality: Adverse effects related to static balance. *Neurosci. Lett.* **2020**, *733*, 134974. [CrossRef]
36. Pot-Kolder, R.; Veling, W.; Counotte, J.; Van Der Gaag, M. Anxiety Partially Mediates Cybersickness Symptoms in Immersive Virtual Reality Environments. *Cyberpsychology Behav. Soc. Netw.* **2018**, *21*, 187–193. [CrossRef]
37. Salgado, D.P.; Flynn, R.; Naves, E.L.M.; Murray, N. The Impact of Jerk on Quality of Experience and Cybersickness in an Immersive Wheelchair Application. In Proceedings of the 2020 Twelfth International Conference on Quality of Multimedia Experience, Athlone, Ireland, 26–28 May 2020; pp. 1–6. [CrossRef]
38. Saredakis, D.; Keage, H.A.; Corlis, M.; Loetscher, T. Using Virtual Reality to Improve Apathy in Residential Aged Care: Mixed Methods Study. *J. Med. Internet Res.* **2020**, *22*, e17632. [CrossRef]
39. Shah, S.H.H.; Karlsen, A.S.T.; Solberg, M.; Hameed, I.A. A social vr-based collaborative exergame for rehabilitation: Codesign, development and user study. *Virtual Real.* **2022**, 1–18. [CrossRef]
40. Tyrrell, R.; Sarig-Bahat, H.; Williams, K.; Williams, G.; Treleaven, J. Simulator sickness in patients with neck pain and vestibular pathology during virtual reality tasks. *Virtual Real.* **2017**, *22*, 211–219. [CrossRef]

41. Vailland, G.; Devigne, L.; Pasteau, F.; Nouviale, F.; Fraudet, B.; Leblong, E.; Babel, M.; Gouranton, V. VR based Power Wheelchair Simulator: Usability Evaluation through a Clinically Validated Task with Regular Users. In Proceedings of the 2021 IEEE Virtual Reality and 3D User Interfaces, Lisbon, Portugal, 27 March–1 April 2021; pp. 420–427. [CrossRef]
42. Vlake, J.H.B.; Wils, E.-J.M.; van Bommel, J.M.; Korevaar, T.I.M.M.; Gommers, D.M.; van Genderen, M.E.M. Virtual Reality Tailored to the Needs of Post-ICU Patients: A Safety and Immersiveness Study in Healthy Volunteers. *Crit. Care Explor.* **2021**, *3*, e0388. [CrossRef]
43. Winter, C.; Kern, F.; Gall, D.; Latoschik, M.E.; Pauli, P.; Käthner, I. Immersive virtual reality during gait rehabilitation increases walking speed and motivation: A usability evaluation with healthy participants and patients with multiple sclerosis and stroke. *J. Neuroeng. Rehabil.* **2021**, *18*, 1–14. [CrossRef]
44. Tallarida, R.J.; Murray, R.B.; Tallarida, R.J.; Murray, R.B. Chi-square test. *Man. Pharmacol. Calc. Comput. Programs* **1987**, 140–142.
45. Kennedy, R.; Drexler, J.; Compton, D.; Stanney, K.; Lanham, D.; Harm, D. Configural scoring of simulator sickness, cybersickness and space adaptation syndrome: Similarities and differences. *Virtual Adapt. Environ. Appl. Implic. Hum. Perform. Issues* **2003**, *2003*, 247.
46. Dilanchian, A.T.; Andringa, R.; Boot, W.R. A Pilot Study Exploring Age Differences in Presence, Workload, and Cybersickness in the Experience of Immersive Virtual Reality Environments. *Front. Virtual Real.* **2021**, *2*, 736793. [CrossRef]
47. Xu, W.; Liang, H.-N.; Yu, K.; Baghaei, N. Effect of gameplay uncertainty, display type, and age on virtual reality exergames. In Proceedings of the 2021 CHI Conference on Human Factors in Computing Systems, Yokohama, Japan, 8–13 May 2021; pp. 1–14.
48. Pietrzak, E.; Pullman, S.; McGuire, A. Using Virtual Reality and Videogames for Traumatic Brain Injury Rehabilitation: A Structured Literature Review. *Games Health J.* **2014**, *3*, 202–214. [CrossRef]
49. Rose, F.D.; Brooks, B.M.; Rizzo, A.A. Virtual Reality in Brain Damage Rehabilitation: Review. *CyberPsychology Behav.* **2005**, *8*, 241–262. [CrossRef]
50. Patel, M.; Snyder, A.R.; Baham, M.; Sheridan, C.A.; Brown, A.; Asarnow, R.; Babikian, T.; Choe, M.; Giza, C. Brief Autonomic Assessment in Concussion Clinic. *Neurology* **2020**, *95*, S4–S5. [CrossRef]
51. Huang, H.-M.; Rauch, U.; Liaw, S.-S. Investigating learners' attitudes toward virtual reality learning environments: Based on a constructivist approach. *Comput. Educ.* **2010**, *55*, 1171–1182. [CrossRef]
52. Moraes, T.M.; Zaninotto, A.L.; Neville, I.S.; Hayashi, C.Y.; Paiva, W.S. Immersive virtual reality in patients with moderate and severe traumatic brain injury: A feasibility study. *Health Technol.* **2021**, *11*, 1035–1044. [CrossRef]
53. Coyle, H.; Traynor, V.; Solowij, N. Computerized and Virtual Reality Cognitive Training for Individuals at High Risk of Cognitive Decline: Systematic Review of the Literature. *Am. J. Geriatr. Psychiatry* **2014**, *23*, 335–359. [CrossRef] [PubMed]
54. Cushman, L.A.; Stein, K.; Duffy, C.J. Detecting navigational deficits in cognitive aging and Alzheimer disease using virtual reality. *Neurology* **2008**, *71*, 888–895. [CrossRef]
55. Tuena, C.; Serino, S.; Stramba-Badiale, C.; Pedroli, E.; Goulene, K.M.; Stramba-Badiale, M.; Riva, G. Usability of an Embodied CAVE System for Spatial Navigation Training in Mild Cognitive Impairment. *J. Clin. Med.* **2023**, *12*, 1949. [CrossRef]
56. Mondellini, M.; Arlati, S.; Gapeyeva, H.; Lees, K.; Märitz, I.; Pizzagalli, S.L.; Otto, T.; Sacco, M.; Teder-Braschinsky, A. User Experience during an Immersive Virtual Reality-Based Cognitive Task: A Comparison between Estonian and Italian Older Adults with MCI. *Sensors* **2022**, *22*, 8249. [CrossRef]
57. García-Muñoz, C.; Cortés-Vega, M.-D.; Heredia-Rizo, A.M.; Martín-Valero, R.; García-Bernal, M.-I.; Casuso-Holgado, M.J. Effectiveness of vestibular training for balance and dizziness rehabilitation in people with multiple sclerosis: A systematic review and meta-analysis. *J. Clin. Med.* **2020**, *9*, 590. [CrossRef]
58. Norouzi-Gheidari, N.; Hernandez, A.; Archambault, P.S.; Higgins, J.; Poissant, L.; Kairy, D. Feasibility, Safety and Efficacy of a Virtual Reality Exergame System to Supplement Upper Extremity Rehabilitation Post-Stroke: A Pilot Randomized Clinical Trial and Proof of Principle. *Int. J. Environ. Res. Public Health* **2019**, *17*, 113. [CrossRef]
59. Risi, D.; Palmisano, S. Effects of postural stability, active control, exposure duration and repeated exposures on HMD induced cybersickness. *Displays* **2019**, *60*, 9–17. [CrossRef]
60. Servotte, J.-C.; Goosse, M.; Campbell, S.H.; Dardenne, N.; Pilote, B.; Simoneau, I.L.; Guillaume, M.; Bragard, I.; Ghuysen, A. Virtual reality experience: Immersion, sense of presence, and cybersickness. *Clin. Simul. Nurs.* **2020**, *38*, 35–43. [CrossRef]
61. Chandra, A.N.R.; El Jamiy, F.; Reza, H. A Systematic Survey on Cybersickness in Virtual Environments. *Computers* **2022**, *11*, 51. [CrossRef]
62. Saint-Aubert, J.; Cogné, M.; Bonan, I.; Launey, Y.; Lécuyer, A. Influence of user posture and virtual exercise on impression of locomotion during vr observation. *IEEE Trans. Vis. Comput. Graph.* **2022**, *14*, 8. [CrossRef]
63. Mittelstaedt, J.; Wacker, J.; Stelling, D. Effects of display type and motion control on cybersickness in a virtual bike simulator. *Displays* **2018**, *51*, 43–50. [CrossRef]
64. Petrigna, L.; Musumeci, G. The Metaverse: A New Challenge for the Healthcare System: A Scoping Review. *J. Funct. Morphol. Kinesiol.* **2022**, *7*, 63. [CrossRef]
65. Yang, J.O.; Lee, J.S. Utilization exercise rehabilitation using metaverse (vr· ar· mr· xr). *Korean J. Sport Biomech.* **2021**, *31*, 249–258.
66. Garavand, A.; Aslani, N. Metaverse phenomenon and its impact on health: A scoping review. *Inform. Med. Unlocked* **2022**, *32*, 101029. [CrossRef]

67. Garrido, L.E.; Frías-Hiciano, M.; Moreno-Jiménez, M.; Cruz, G.N.; García-Batista, Z.E.; Guerra-Peña, K.; Medrano, L.A. Focusing on cybersickness: Pervasiveness, latent trajectories, susceptibility, and effects on the virtual reality experience. *Virtual Real.* **2022**, *26*, 1347–1371. [CrossRef]
68. Stanney, K.; Lawson, B.D.; Rokers, B.; Dennison, M.; Fidopiastis, C.; Stoffregen, T.; Weech, S.; Fulvio, J.M. Identifying Causes of and Solutions for Cybersickness in Immersive Technology: Reformulation of a Research and Development Agenda. *Int. J. Human-Comput. Interact.* **2020**, *36*, 1783–1803. [CrossRef]

sensors MDPI

Article

Integration of Virtual Reality in the Control System of an Innovative Medical Robot for Single-Incision Laparoscopic Surgery

Florin Covaciu [1], Nicolae Crisan [2], Calin Vaida [1,*], Iulia Andras [2], Alexandru Pusca [1], Bogdan Gherman [1], Corina Radu [3], Paul Tucan [1], Nadim Al Hajjar [4] and Doina Pisla [1,*]

1 Research Center for Industrial Robots Simulation and Testing—CESTER, Technical University of Cluj-Napoca, 400114 Cluj-Napoca, Romania
2 Department of Urology, "Iuliu Hatieganu" University of Medicine and Pharmacy, 400012 Cluj-Napoca, Romania
3 Department of Internal Medicine, "Iuliu Hatieganu" University of Medicine and Pharmacy, 400012 Cluj-Napoca, Romania
4 Department of Surgery, "Iuliu Hatieganu" University of Medicine and Pharmacy, 400012 Cluj-Napoca, Romania
* Correspondence: calin.vaida@mep.utcluj.ro (C.V.); doina.pisla@mep.utcluj.ro (D.P.); Tel.: +40-264-401684 (D.P.)

Abstract: In recent years, there has been an expansion in the development of simulators that use virtual reality (VR) as a learning tool. In surgery where robots are used, VR serves as a revolutionary technology to help medical doctors train in using these robotic systems and accumulate knowledge without risk. This article presents a study in which VR is used to create a simulator designed for robotically assisted single-uniport surgery. The control of the surgical robotic system is achieved using voice commands for laparoscopic camera positioning and via a user interface developed using the Visual Studio program that connects a wristband equipped with sensors attached to the user's hand for the manipulation of the active instruments. The software consists of the user interface and the VR application via the TCP/IP communication protocol. To study the evolution of the performance of this virtual system, 15 people were involved in the experimental evaluation of the VR simulator built for the robotic surgical system, having to complete a medically relevant task. The experimental data validated the initial solution, which will be further developed.

Keywords: surgical robot; virtual reality; control; simulator; single-incision laparoscopic surgery

Citation: Covaciu, F.; Crisan, N.; Vaida, C.; Andras, I.; Pusca, A.; Gherman, B.; Radu, C.; Tucan, P.; Al Hajjar, N.; Pisla, D. Integration of Virtual Reality in the Control System of an Innovative Medical Robot for Single-Incision Laparoscopic Surgery. *Sensors* **2023**, *23*, 5400. https://doi.org/10.3390/s23125400

Academic Editors: Bijan Shirinzadeh, Calin Gheorghe Dan Neamtu, Radu Comes, Jing-Jing Fang and Dorin-Mircea Popovici

Received: 7 April 2023
Revised: 18 May 2023
Accepted: 5 June 2023
Published: 7 June 2023

1. Introduction

Applications using surgical robots are increasingly used in hospitals, found in an approximately 5%, although they were unequally distributed. Currently, these applications have multiple uses, such as abdominal, thoracic, neurosurgical, brachytherapy, pelvic procedures, and so on [1,2]. These values are quite different from one country to another based on financial stability, with a large increase in the number of surgical robots in the private medical sector. The skills of doctors play a vital role in performing surgical tasks through improved medical outcomes, patient safety, sensitivity, and increased accuracy. Just as aviation and military simulators have become standard for personnel training, so too may they have become for the surgical profession. Surgical interventions are performed with the help of robotic systems to support the surgeon perform these interventions with higher dexterity and faster responses to intraoperative complications [3].

The first robots used in surgical applications targeted specific parts of the intervention dealing with bone perforation in orthopedic surgery. In the 1990s, several robotic devices were introduced for simple tasks, such as the manipulation of the laparoscopic camera. A cornerstone in robotic surgery was the development of the first two full robotic platforms,

Zeus and DaVinci, which, controlled from a master console, enabled the surgeon to perform the entire surgery by manipulating a set of instruments handled by the slave robotic platform. Following medical and commercial success, the da Vinci robotic platform has slowly spread throughout the world, even becoming a gold standard in many minimally invasive procedures. It must be pointed out that from a medical point of view, the robotic platform is a highly dexterous and accurate advanced tool with zero autonomy, with the entire procedure being performed by the surgeon [4].

Medically, surgical procedures evolved, also aiming to provide maximum therapeutic efficiency while minimizing the damage of healthy tissues. Thus, from classical, open surgery, in the 1980s, an important step was taken towards minimally invasive procedures, followed by the newer techniques which aim to perform the surgery through the anatomic orifices of the body, i.e., natural-orifice transluminal endoscopic surgery (NOTES) or through a unique access port, i.e., single-incision laparoscopic surgery (SILS) [5].

SILS is a developing technique due to its limitations in terms of surgeon ergonomics, instrument crossing, and limited working volume, but most of these negative aspects can be eliminated using a robotic platform dedicated to this task.

Surgeons need to develop their skills by practicing on robotic training systems that emphasize complex surgical scenarios, evaluations, and challenges for these skills. Such surgical training systems are available in two variants, namely: The first training approach is a classic method which involves the use of actual physical robotic systems on human phantoms, cadavers and then real patients (under the supervision of an expert in robotic surgery). This approach has a high cost and limited accessibility because a physical robotic system is and a mentor are needed to guide the future surgeon, while for live surgeries a second console must be used. The second training approach is a relatively new technique that uses VR to create simulators for robotic surgical training as a method to improve the robotic assisted surgical skills; it is derived from the gaming industry and with the technological progress it is now able to encompass high detail environments, relevant for advanced training programs. Furthermore, by using VR simulators, modifiable levels of difficulty and challenges can be used, where surgeons can also learn to manage unpredictable events [6]. Thus, these simulators are able to properly train surgeons before entering the operating room and working with patients. A second, very important advantage of these simulators is the preplanning of complex cases, when the digital twin of the patient is loaded and studied before the actual surgery to establish the most efficient approach [7]. Besides this, these simulators offer possibilities to implement new learning methods in a revolutionary way, yielding optimization of the acquisition of skills and their evaluation, leading to an overall risk reduction, enhanced medical outcomes, and efficient handling of any intraoperative complications.

This article describes a study in which a virtual reality simulator is developed for a medical robotic system for single-incision laparoscopic surgery (SILS). The novel character of this research consists of the implementation of a new robotic system in a VR environment and the use of multiple control strategies to perform the surgical act. This enables validation of the robotic structure before the experimental model is built, enabling its optimization based on the reported experience by the testers. The use of combined control modalities is also assessed. The robotic system consists of a parallel robotic module designed to manipulate a platform which carries three independent robotic modules for the manipulation of the specific instruments used in SILS procedures. The manipulation of the slave robotic system is carried out from a master console that embeds different end-effectors: a wristband multi-sensor used to actuate the active instruments and a set of voice commands proven to be a valid interaction solution for the laparoscopic camera [8]. For the validation of the surgical task involving the manipulation of the surgical instruments into the body of a virtual patient, a user must reach specific (predefined) points. The procedure time is recorded to be used as an efficiency indicator of the training process. The article is structured as follows: after the introduction, the next section provides the literature review, followed by the Materials and Methods section in Section 3. Section 4 presents the results and discussion, followed by Section 5 in which a summary and conclusions are given.

2. Literature Review

In the current literature, multiple applications can be found that use VR to create a highly immersive three-dimensional virtual environment that is used as a learning tool for systems found in the real environment. An example of such an application is found in a study that focused on developing/improving skills in robotic surgery using VR to train medical doctors in multidisciplinary surgery [9]. The study used the DaVinci simulator and included 24 exercises. The study was conducted over a period of 12 months, with the learning platform providing automated performance metrics and tracking learner progress. To complete the curriculum, a pre-test and post-test were required for the 21 students who participated in the study. After completing the curriculum, trainees reported improvements in their ability to operate the robotic system, and post-test scores were significantly higher than pre-test scores. Iop et. al. presented a systematic review of research related to VR in neurosurgery, with an emphasis on education. Five databases including thirty-one studies were investigated in this study after a thorough review process. This study focused on performance and user experience, showing that this technology has the potential to improve neurosurgical education using a wide range of both objective information and subjective metrics [10]. Korayem et al. discussed the possibility of using the Leap Motion Controller to directly control surgical robot arms and laparoscopic scissors during surgical procedures [11]. In [12], the authors performed a study where they trained 30 participants on how to configure a robotic arm in an environment that mimics the clinical setup. These participants were divided into three groups: one group was trained with paper-based instructions, one was trained with video-based instructions, and one was trained with VR-based instructions. By comparing the three methods, it emerged that the participants who used VR for learning gained a better understanding of the spatial awareness skills needed to achieve the desired robotic arm positioning. Mishra et al. presented a study that searched and reviewed articles showing numerous applications of VR/augmented reality (AR) in neurosurgery. These applications included their utility in the areas of diagnosis for complex vascular interventions, correction of spinal deformities, resident training, procedural practice, pain management, and rehabilitation of neurosurgical patients [13]. Covaciu et al. develop upper-limb rehabilitation simulators using VR [14,15]. Korayem et al. performed a study in which a vision-based contactless user interface named the Leap Motion Controller was presented. The device can track the speed, position, and orientation of the surgeon's hand, being also able to detect the gestures and movements of each finger and then transfer data to the computer. Via this controller, a robotic arm that has a laparoscope attached is controlled [16]. Ehrampoosh et al. presented a new force-sensing instrument that facilitates teleoperated robotic manipulation and semi-automates the suturing task. The end-effector mechanism of the instrument has a rotating degree of freedom to generate the ideal needle-insertion trajectory and to pass the needle through its curvature [17]. In [18], a modular 3-degrees-of-freedom (3DoF) force sensor that easily integrates with an existing minimally invasive surgical instrument was presented. Abad et al. presented a haptic exoskeleton that attaches to the hand, consisting of five 4×4 miniaturized fingertip actuators (eighty actuators in total) to provide cutaneous feedback in laparoscopic surgeries, allowing the user to feel sensations in the form of vibrations produced by the actuators [19]. In [20], a hybrid parallel robot, called PARASURG 9M, was presented, consisting of a positioning and orientation module, with a kinematically constraint remote center of motion (RCM) and a dexterous active instrument with wide orientation angles for the distal head. A study was presented in [21] that demonstrated improvement in the performance of robotic surgery for beginners after training on a virtual reality simulator called RobotiX Mentor VR. The skills acquired during training are relevant to the use of the real robot in clinical practice because they have been transferred to a realistic model (avian tissue model). VR has also been used in the development of ankle rehabilitation simulators for people who suffered strokes. By attaching sensors to the limb, this simulator can interact with a real person. The data that are taken from the sensors are sent to an intelligent module to create new levels of exercises and control of the robotic rehabilitation structure in the virtual environment using machine learning [22]. VR is also used in the development of simulators in the control of a drone [23]. Luca et al. accomplished a study illustrating the potential of training using VR in spine surgery [24]. In [25], a meta-analysis was conducted in which it was shown that VR improves efficiency in trainee surgical practice. This study aimed to compare virtual reality with traditional training approaches, determining if it can complement or replace the training model. Performing research of the literature, 24 studies were highlighted that provided essential data. The results of the study suggested a positive effect that was observed during training with the VR simulator for controlling the laparoscope. Furthermore, this study highlighted that VR training emphasized crucial aspects for adequate surgical performance. Different VR systems offer multiple levels of difficulty, providing the student the opportunity to develop basic laparoscopic skills. Trochimczuk et al. carried out a study in which the concept of a novel telemanipulator for minimally invasive surgery was presented, and numerical analysis was carried out to validate the performance of the main system [26]. In [27,28], a review was made regarding the robots used in laparoscopic surgery. In [29], a study which mainly proposed to provide context for remote control of laparoscopic devices to improve the performance of minimally invasive surgical interventions was presented, so that all patients can have access to qualified surgeons even if they are in another region. First, with the help of the leap motion controller, the fine movements of the surgeons' hands, the position and gesture of the fingers, and an awareness of the changes in the corresponding angles and coordinates, which were necessary at every moment, are acquired. To control the laparoscopic gripper, a 5-DOF robotic arm is built that is controlled using data from the Leap Motion sensor. Batty et al. presented the implementation of an environment estimation and force prediction methodology to mitigate system communication time delays for efficient implementation of haptic feedback in a minimally invasive robotic surgical system [30]. Mao et al. examined the current literature on the effectiveness of VR simulators regarding surgical skills in medical students, residents, and surgical staff. By examining the literature, it was concluded that trainees who used VR demonstrated an improvement in surgical skills, especially compared to those who used traditional non-VR methods [31]. In [32], a study was conducted that aimed to investigate the satisfaction of medical students regarding the training in robotic surgery offered at the Medical University of Varna, Bulgaria with the Da Vinci skills simulator. The results suggested that training in this field can be achieved even at the student level, using robotic surgery in realistic scenarios. Lamblin et al. conducted a study at the University of Lyon, France, in which they enrolled 26 junior specialist trainees to perform laparoscopic salpingectomy exercises on a VR simulator called LapSim. Junior trainees demonstrated that they improved their surgical skills following these exercises [33]. In [34], a study was conducted to evaluate the benefit of training with virtual reality simulation. The study was conducted at the ALEXEA (Alexandria Endoscopy Association) Center, in collaboration with the Department of Gynecology and Obstetrics, University Hospital, Campus Kiel Schleswig Holstein, Germany. The laparoscopy virtual reality simulator used was LapSim. The study concluded that virtual simulation could help teach basic skills in the early stages of training and provide a good simulation for procedural functioning for resident training. The virtual simulation demonstrated significant results in most parameters by a reduction in operating time, improvement in tissue handling, coordination of instruments, and reduction in the incidence of complications, resulting in an improvement in patient safety.

3. Materials and Methods

The innovative robotic system, PARA-SILS-ROB, was built based on the "master–slave" architecture, common for any surgical robotic system. This implies "zero" autonomy for the robot itself, all decisions and operations being performed by the surgeon. The master console includes all the necessary elements to enable full control of the surgical instruments, a task achieved through the slave robotic system. The VR simulation environment presented in this paper acts, from the user point of view, as a virtual master console where interfaces can be tested, user skills can be enhanced, and the slave robotic system, embedded as a digital twin, can be optimized in parallel before its actual development.

In Figure 1, the general architecture of the "master–slave" training system and its "virtual" counterparts are illustrated. The master console consists of the IMU sensor (having an accelerometer, gyroscope, and magnetometer); the voice control module, which is used to select the controlled module of the slave robotic system; other various elements of the VR environment (e.g., the viewing camera); and the graphical user interface (GUI) used as a backup solution of the IMU system and to provide additional parameters' selection. The slave robotic system consists of three modules: the 6-DOF parallel robot, used to position the mobile platform (MP), on which the 1-DOF laparoscope module (for laparoscope insertion) and the two 3-DOF active instruments orientation and insertion modules, used to guide the active SILS instruments, are placed. According to medical protocol [35], the 6-DOF task is used to perform instruments' modules registration, namely to control the mobile platform and position it at the SILS port, so that the remote center of motion (RCM) of the three mechanisms match the three corresponding trocar ports. After the registration, the MP is used for the orientation of the laparoscope, while the active instruments are controlled via the two 3-DOF modules. A virtual patient is placed within the VR environment, and a fuzzy logic system is developed to monitor their vital signs (heart rate, temperature, and oxygen level) and to generate specific alarms displayed on the operator GUI.

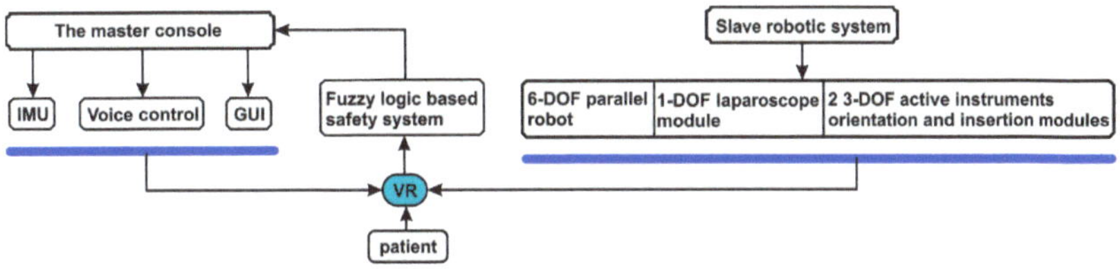

Figure 1. The SILS master–slave training system.

With focus on the VR environment, the next paragraph describes in detail the main components of the system from a hardware, software, and interconnectivity point of view.

3.1. The Slave Robotic System

The parallel robotic structure (Figure 2) has six degrees of freedom (DOF) with a modular construction consisting of three identical kinematic chains positioned along the sides of an equilateral triangle, connected to a mobile platform through three spherical joints. On the platform, three independent modules are embedded, each of them handing one instrument: the central module is a 1-DOF mechanism that performs the insertion/retraction of the endoscopic camera, while the lateral modules are two mechanisms with 3-DOF that have the role of achieving independent orientation of the mounted active instruments on the platform. The complete slave robotic structure contains the following main components:

- robot rigid frame;
- operating table;
- kinematic chain 1;
- kinematic chain 2;
- kinematic chain 3;
- instrument orientation module 1;
- active instrument 1;
- instrument orientation module 2;
- active instrument 2;
- endoscopic camera.

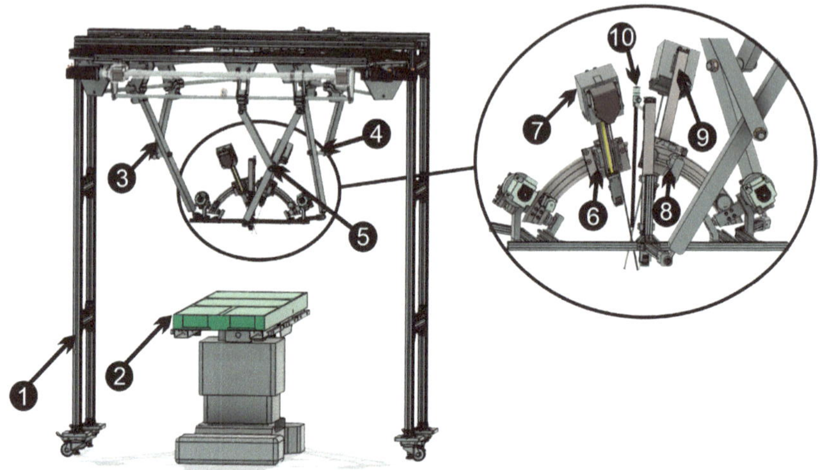

Figure 2. The parallel robotic structure and operating table: 1—framework; 2—operating table; 3—kinematic chain 1; 4—kinematic chain 2; 5—kinematic chain 3; 6—instrument orientation module 1; 7—active instrument 1; 8—instrument orientation module 2; 9—active instrument 2; 10—endoscopic camera.

3.2. Singularity Analysis and Workspace of Parallel Robotic Structure

Robot singularity and workspace analyses are achieved to determine potential configurations where the mechanism could gain or lose degrees of freedom (becoming uncontrollable) and the operational working volume of the robotic structure in order to ensure safe conditions for the patient [36,37]. Singularity analysis of the 3-R-PRR-PRS parallel structure with a triangular frame and 6-DOF (Figure 3) is performed based on the kinematic model [38] of the structure, the CAD model being generated in the Siemens NX software, while the singularity positions of the structures are generated without assigning numerical values for the geometric parameters. Siemens NX software can also be used for finite element analysis (FEA) to determine the maximum deformation and the distribution of deformation [39], one of the critical factors in ensuring the safety operations of robotic systems working in the proximity of people [40]. Starting from the kinematic chain of the robot (Figure 3), the following are defined: LC_1, LC_2, and LC_3 are the three kinematic chains (type R-PRR-PRS) that are actuated by the prismatic joints, namely q_1, q_2, q_3, q_4, and q_5, q_6. Each chain contains other three passive revolute joints: R_{11}, R_{12}, and R_{13} for LC_1; R_{21}, R_{22}, and R_{23} for LC_2; and R_{31}, R_{32}, and R_{33} for LC_3. Each kinematic chain is connected through a passive spherical joint (S_1, S_2, S_3) with the mobile platform, having the following geometric parameters: l_0 represents the distance between the actuation axes, while l_1 and l_2 represent the mechanical links that compose the kinematic chains.

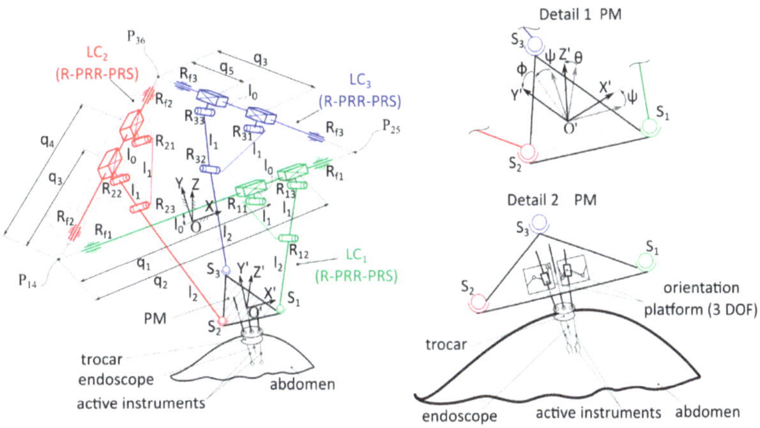

Figure 3. Kinematic diagram of the 6-DOF parallel robot type 3-R-PRR-PRS with triangular frame [41].

Following the solution of the kinematic model of the 3-R-PRR-PRS robot (with a triangular frame), the six expressions that represent the characteristic equations of the mechanism (Equation (1)) are determined, which are then be used to calculate the Jacobi matrices A and B [42].

$$\begin{aligned}
f_1 &= q_1 - q_2 + 2 \cdot l_1 \cdot \sqrt{1 - \frac{d_1^2}{(l_1+l_2)}} = 0 \\
f_2 &: q_2 - \sqrt{(l_1+l_2)^2 - d_1^2} - d_{14_S1} = 0 \\
f_3 &: q_3 - q_4 + 2 \cdot l_1 \cdot \sqrt{1 - \frac{d_2^2}{(l_1+l_2)^2}} = 0 \\
f_4 &: q_4 - \sqrt{(l_1+l_2)^2 - d_2^2} - d_{36_S2} = 0 \\
f_5 &: q_5 - q_6 + 2 \cdot l_1 \cdot \sqrt{1 - \frac{d_3^2}{(l_1+l_2)^2}} = 0 \\
f_6 &: q_6 - \sqrt{(l_1+l_2)^2 - d_3^2} - d_{25_S3} = 0
\end{aligned} \tag{1}$$

Because the characteristic equations (Equation (1)) were defined to contain expressions in which the six active joints, qi, i = 1 … 6, are free terms of the first degree, the expression of matrix B is a very simple one, described in Equation (2). The determinant of matrix B is as follows: det(B) = 1, which leads to the statement that there are no singularities of type I.

$$B = \begin{bmatrix} 1 & -1 & 0 & 0 & 0 & 0 \\ 0 & 1 & 0 & 0 & 0 & 0 \\ 0 & 0 & 1 & -1 & 0 & 0 \\ 0 & 0 & 0 & 1 & 0 & 0 \\ 0 & 0 & 0 & 0 & 1 & -1 \\ 0 & 0 & 0 & 0 & 0 & 1 \end{bmatrix} \tag{2}$$

The determinant of matrix B is as follows: det(B) = 1, which leads to the statement that we have no singularities of type I. The determinant of matrix A has a complex form which, due to its large dimensions, is be illustrated in an explicit form. Applying several transformations and simplifications, this could be written as a product of 14 factors, which can be analyzed independently to determine type II singularity conditions:

$$\det(A) = \prod_{i=1}^{14} F_i \tag{3}$$

The first factor has a numerical expression (Equation (4)), introducing no singularity conditions:

$$F_1 = 108 \tag{4}$$

Factors 4, 5, and 7 are terms that depend exclusively on geometric parameters, which can only theoretically become zero as all geometric parameters of the robot that represent lengths have positive values (Equation (7)):

$$F_6 = l^3, F_7 = l_1^3, F_9 = \frac{1}{(l_1 + l_2)^6} \tag{5}$$

Further analysis of the other factors reveals that some have very complex expressions and, as such, they are analyzed. Therefore, factor 2 in its initial form has 1698 terms and degree 21, which is then transformed through combinatorial mathematical operations and brought to a more compact form, consisting of three terms, two of which are simple expressions, while the third has 330 of terms and degree 11. The first two resulting terms are as follows:

$$F_{2\_1} = -1, F_{2\_2} = \cos(\theta) \tag{6}$$

If the first term does not introduce singularities, the second term introduces a singularity for $0 = \pm\frac{\pi}{2}$, but this singularity is outside the operational workspace of the robot, for which, under special conditions, $\theta \in \left[-\frac{\pi}{3}, \frac{\pi}{3}\right]$, and during the procedure, after inserting the instruments into the patient's body, $\theta \in \left[-\frac{\pi}{6}, \frac{\pi}{6}\right]$.

For the evaluation of the polynomial equation defined by the third factor, MATLAB script was developed to evaluate the value of the function in the robot's workspace, looking for the following information:

- Zero equality;
- Very small values of the evaluation result, which could suggest proximity to a singularity zone;
- Changes in the sign of the equation from one value to another, which could illustrate crossing through zero.

The results of these evaluations are presented below, where two examples are highlighted. In one, the values of the independent coordinates of the characteristic point of the mobile platform are varied, and in the second, its rotation angles varied between $\left[-\frac{\pi}{6} \div \frac{\pi}{6}\right]$:

Case 1. Based on the graphical representation of the F_{2_3} values (computed with respect to the variation of the linear coordinates of the TCP), no points were identified in the robot workspace where the value of the factor was zero or close to zero. The range of variation was as follows:

$$\begin{array}{r} \min(F_{2\_3}) = -2.2353 \cdot 10^9 \\ \max(F_{2\_3}) = 2.4313 \cdot 10^9 \\ \min(|F_{2\_3}|) = 1.1629 \cdot 10^4 \end{array} \tag{7}$$

Case 2. Based on the graphical representation of the F_{2_3} values illustrated in Figure 4 (computed with respect to the variation of the linear coordinates of the TCP), no points were identified in the robot's workspace where the value of the factor F_{2_3} was zero or close to zero. The range of variation was:

$$\begin{array}{r} \min(F_{2\_3}) = -1.3435 \cdot 10^{10} \\ \max(F_{2\_3}) = 1.2066 \cdot 10^{10} \\ \min(|F_{2\_3}|) = 2.9878 \cdot 10^4 \end{array} \tag{8}$$

Sign changes occurred only when switching from one set of input data values to another, which were generated between the minimum and maximum values. Thus, it can be stated that this term does not introduce singularities into the robot's workspace.

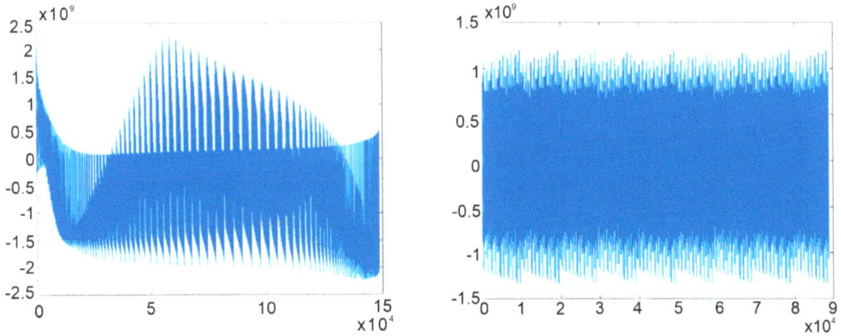

Figure 4. Graphical representation of the values of the term F_{2_3} for the two cases.

The third factor is presented below:

$$F_3 = 3 \cdot l \cdot \sin(\psi) \cdot \sin(\theta) \cdot \sin(\varphi) - 3 \cdot l \cdot \cos(\varphi) \cdot \cos(\psi) + 3\sqrt{3} \cdot l \cdot \cos(\varphi) \cdot \sin(\psi) \cdot \sin(\theta) + 6\sqrt{3} \cdot l_{instr} \cdot \cos(\theta) \cdot \sin(\psi) + \sqrt{3} \cdot l \cdot \cos(\theta) \cdot \sin(\varphi) + 3\sqrt{3} \cdot l \cdot \cos(\psi) \cdot \sin(\varphi) + 9 \cdot L_{pf} + 3 \cdot l \cdot \cos(\varphi) \cdot \cos(\theta) - 6\sqrt{3} \cdot Y_E - 6 \cdot l_{instr} \cdot \sin(\theta) - 6 \cdot X_E \quad (9)$$

In this case, all the calculated values are positive for the entire operational workspace of the robot, which indicates that this term does not introduce singularities.

The fourth factor is presented below:

$$F_4 = -3 \cdot l \cdot \sin(\psi) \cdot \sin(\theta) \cdot \sin(\varphi) + 3 \cdot l \cdot \cos(\varphi) \cdot \cos(\psi) + 3\sqrt{3} \cdot l \cdot \cos(\varphi) \cdot \sin(\psi) \cdot \sin(\theta) - 6\sqrt{3} \cdot l_{instr} \cdot \cos(\theta) \cdot \sin(\psi) + \sqrt{3} \cdot l \cdot \cos(\theta) \cdot \sin(\varphi) + 3\sqrt{3} \cdot l \cdot \cos(\psi) \cdot \sin(\varphi) + 3 \cdot L_{pf} - 3 \cdot l \cdot \cos(\varphi) \cdot \cos(\theta) + 6\sqrt{3} \cdot Y_E - 6 \cdot l_{instr} \cdot \sin(\theta) - 6 \cdot X_E \quad (10)$$

In a similar way, the calculated values are entirely positive for the entire operational workspace of the robot, which indicates that this term does not introduce singularities either.

The fifth factor is presented next, with similar behavior to the previous two.

$$F_5 = 2l \cdot \sqrt{3} \cdot \cos(\theta) \cdot \sin(\varphi) + 6 \cdot l_{instr} \cdot \sin(\theta) + 3 \cdot L_{pf} + 6 \cdot X_E \quad (11)$$

The terms F_8 and F_{10}, similar in content (but too bulky to represent), have similar behavior with no negative values for the entire operational workspace of the robot.

$$T^*_{11} = 2l \cdot \sqrt{3}(\sin(\varphi)\sin(\theta) l_{instr}\cos(\theta) + \sin(\varphi)(\cos(\psi)Z_E - \sin(\psi)Y_E)\sin(\theta)) + 2l \cdot \sqrt{3}(\cos(\varphi)(\cos(\psi)Y_E + \sin(\psi)Z_E)) + \left(-\cos(\varphi)^2 l^2 + l^2 - 3{l_{instr}}^2\right)\cos(\theta)^2 - 6l_{instr}(\cos(\psi)Z_E - \sin(\psi)Y_E)\cos(\theta) - l^2 - 3{Y_E}^2 - 3(Z_E + l_1 + l_2)(Z_E - l_1 - l_2) \quad (12)$$

The term T^*_{11} represents the irreducible expression in the term T_{11} that was again analyzed with respect to the operational workspace of the robot without registering values close to zero or changes in sign, with all values being positive.

In the analysis of the term after simplifications, the following expression of the form is obtained:

$$Exp = \sqrt{\left(T^*_{12}\right)^2} \quad (13)$$

Expression (12) yields elimination of the square root and raising to the power of 2 because the equation resolves the set of real numbers. Analysis of the remaining term, T^*_{12}, shows that it only takes positive values for all points considered in the operational space of the robot, with similar behavior encountered in the case of the next factor of the determinate, F_{13}.

By careful analysis, the last factor, F_{14} has the following form (14):

$$F_{14} = \frac{1}{\sqrt{(F_5)^2}} \quad (14)$$

By solving this equation in the set of real numbers, it leads to the simplification of the two factors, which leads to their elimination from the final expression of the determinant of matrix A.

Thus, it can be concluded that for the operational space of the robot, which takes into account the orientation angles for the platform around the X and Y axes in the domain $\left[-\frac{\pi}{6} \div \frac{\pi}{6}\right]$, we have no singularity points, therefore ensuring safety conditions for the patient.

The workspace of the 3-R-PRR-PRS robot was generated using the inverse geometric model. The working space of the robot was calculated starting from the following geometric values of the main elements of the robot structure: l_{PM} = 760 mm; L_{FP} = 1260 mm; l_1 = 375 mm; and l_2 = 400 mm. Using a MATLAB script that embeds the inverse geometric model of the robot structure. Different configurations of the mobile platform attached to the robot structure were generated to study the following:

- The configuration with respect to the angle (φ), which was demonstrated in [42], to greatly influence the workspace size (Figure 5);
- The total workspace of the robot with respect to the required orientation angles for the endoscopic camera, namely:$\psi, \theta \in [-45^\circ \div 45^\circ]$.

In Figure 5, the workspace of the robot is evaluated for a vertical position of the laparoscopic camera (used for the initial steps of the procedure—when the camera is inserted into the patient), and it can be easily seen that the robot ensures the most efficient workspace when the angle (φ) is around the value of -60°.

Figure 6 illustrates the total workspace of the robot with respect to the SILS procedure where the coordinates of the endoscopic camera and the angles ψ and θ vary between minimum and maximum values, preserving the angle (φ) at the optimum value of -60°. Additionally, for validation, a second workspace is modelled with the angle (φ) at the "classical" value of 0°. The number of valid points for $\varphi = -60^\circ$ is 13.3 times higher than for $\varphi = 0^\circ$, which points out the importance of using an efficient configuration for the robot platform (visible even from the density of points).

3.3. The Master Console

The master console consists of a set of hardware and software elements, which are used to control the slave robotic system. Through the different hardware interfaces, the user generates motion commands for the active instruments, which are processed by the software programs, generating the necessary movements at the level of the robot modules while providing real-time feedback through the endoscopic camera.

3.3.1. The Multi-Modal Master Control Architecture

The block diagram (Figure 7) shows the interconnection of the logical components in the control system. Control of the surgical robotic system can be performed through a device attached to the user's forearm. This device contains a three-sensor module that includes a gyroscope, an accelerometer, and a magnetometer, and fusion of the three sensors is carried out for precise positioning. The control device is equipped with an ESP32 microcontroller used for data acquisition from the sensor module, and these data are sent to the user interface via the TCP/IP protocol to be processed. Voice recognition is used to change the control modules for the robotic system.

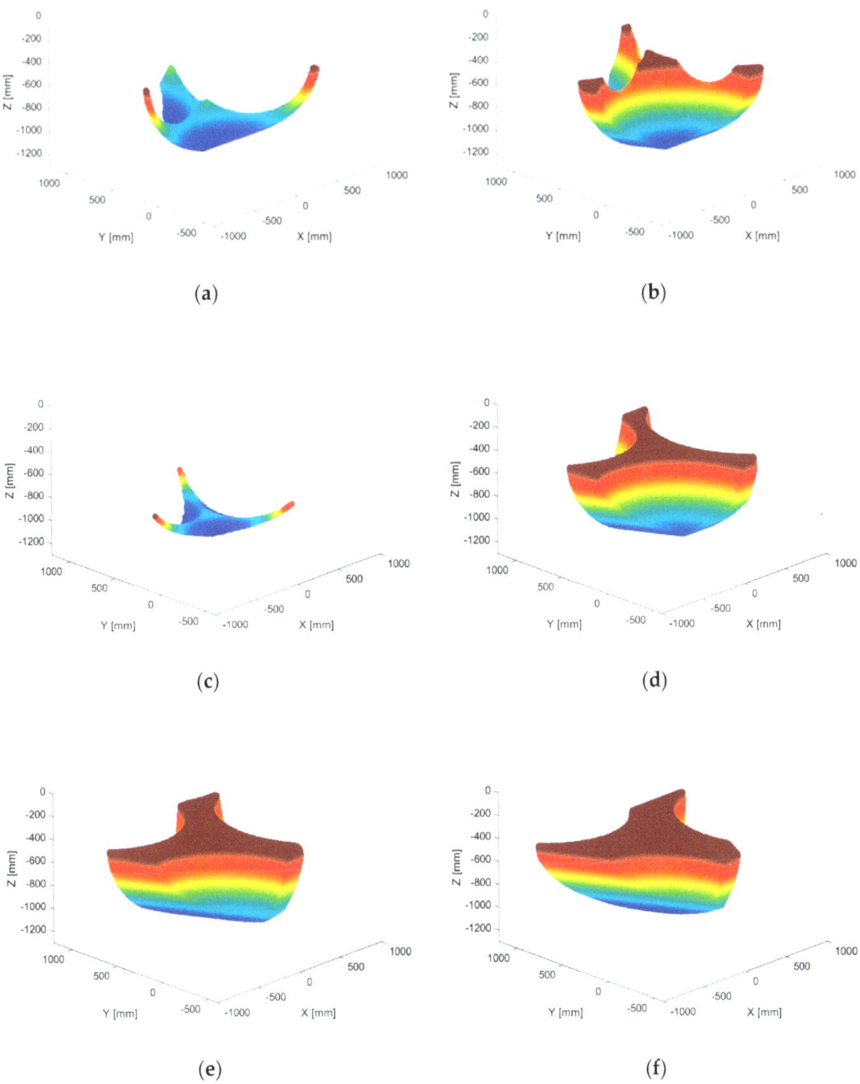

Figure 5. Workspace analysis of the 3-R-PRR-PRS parallel robot. (**a**) $\psi = 0°$, $\theta = 0°, \varphi = 0°$; (**b**) $\psi = 0°$, $\theta = 0°, \varphi = -30°$; (**c**) $\psi = 0°$, $\theta = 0°, \varphi = 30°$; (**d**) $\psi = 0°$, $\theta = 0°, \varphi = -45°$; (**e**) $\psi = 0°$, $\theta = 0°, \varphi = -60°$; (**f**) $\psi = 0°$, $\theta = 0°, \varphi = -75°$.

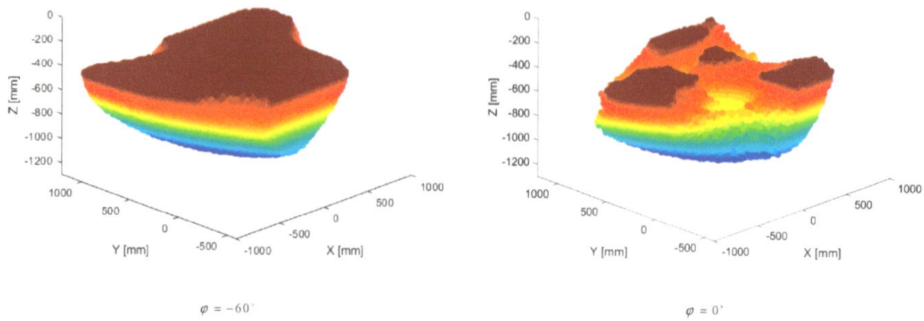

Figure 6. The total workspace of the 3-R-PRR-PRS parallel robot for φ= −60° versus φ = 0°.

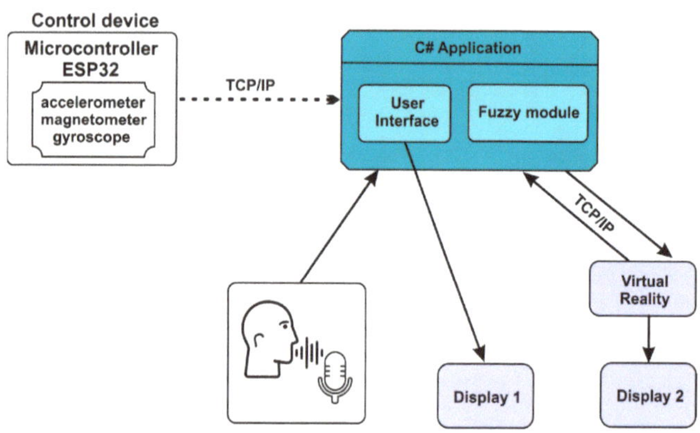

Figure 7. Interconnection of components.

The control device (Figure 8) attached to the user's forearm contains the following components:

- Absolute orientation sensor, which includes an accelerometer, magnetometer, and a gyroscope, model IMU BNO055 [43];
- Microcontroller ESP32 [44];
- Power supply: 5V DC.

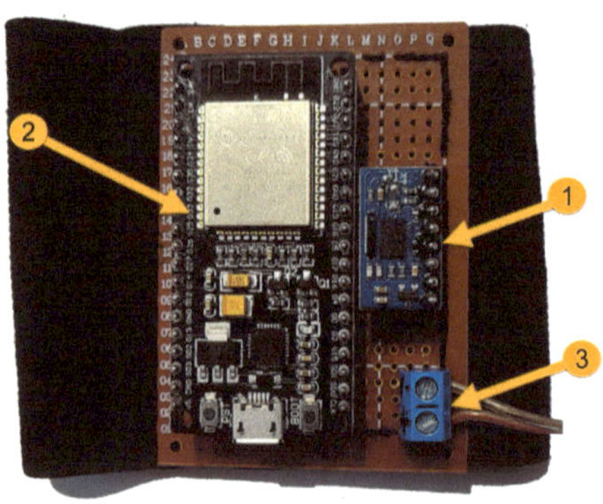

Figure 8. Control device: 1—Absolute orientation sensor, model IMU BNO055, 2—Microcontroller ESP32, 3—Power supply: 5V DC.

3.3.2. Software Application Development

The software applications are developed using two programming languages, namely C# (C Sharp) and Arduino. The Arduino programming language is used to implement the program that is stored on the ESP32 microcontroller for the control device (Figure 8) that attaches to the upper limb of the person controlling the surgical robotic system. The program stored on the ESP32 microcontroller receives data from the sensors embedded in the control device and encodes them in the format supported by the C# application, developed using the Visual Studio program. Data transmission from the microcontroller to the C# application occurs only when there is a change in the values provided by the sensors, being transmitted using the Wi-Fi network protocol. Both the user application and the VR application were written using the C# programming language, and the VR simulator was developed in the Unity development environment. Figure 9 shows the architecture of this application and how to establish communication between programs.

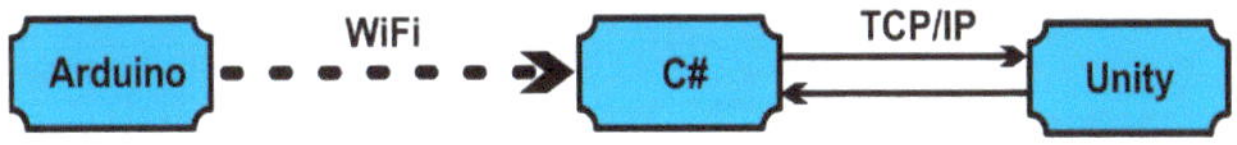

Figure 9. Software architecture.

C# Software Analysis

A graphical depiction of the facilities offered by the software application can be made using UML diagrams [45]. In Figure 10, the use case diagram that indicates the functionalities of the software application implemented using C# programming language is presented [46]. This UML diagram is structured as follows:

- Eleven use cases that represent the functionalities of the C# software application.
- Three actors:
    - The user or the external entity that interacts with the C# application.
    - Script implemented in Arduino.
    - Unity virtual reality application.
- Relations between the user and the use cases and relations between the use cases.

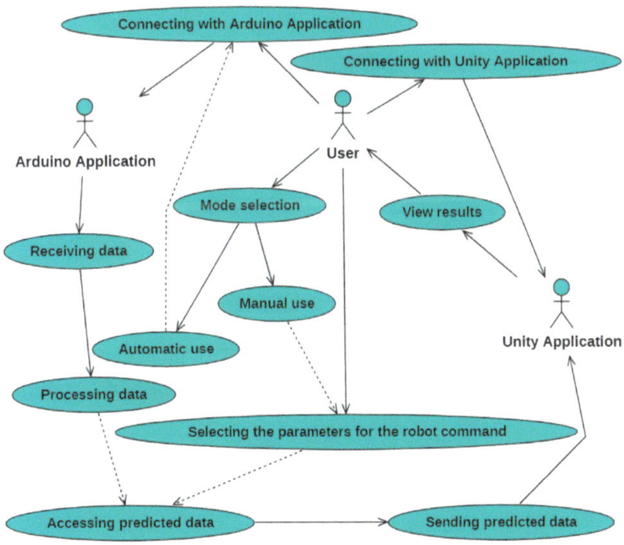

Figure 10. UML use case diagram.

Starting from the functionalities presented in the use case diagram, five classes were designed and implemented, between which there are composition relations. The UML class diagram [47,48] represented in Figure 11 presents these five classes, the relation between them, and the used C# standard packages. These five classes are as follows:

- **GUI** class: enables the user to interact with the C# application. In order to realize the graphic interface for the user, eight classes from the System.Windows.Forms package are used.
- **ArduinoConnexion** class: establishes connection with the Arduino script and the transmission of the data acquired from the sensors.
- **UnityConnexion** class: establishes the connection with the virtual application developed in Unity.
- **FuzzyModule** class: implements a specific artificial intelligence algorithm [49], based on the fuzzy technique, to control the robot. For this purpose, three classes from the AForge.Fuzzy package are used: FuzzySet, TrapezoidalFunction, and InferenceSystem.
- **C#Main** class: constitutes the principal class of the C# application, consisting of four objects, i.e., one object of each previously presented class.

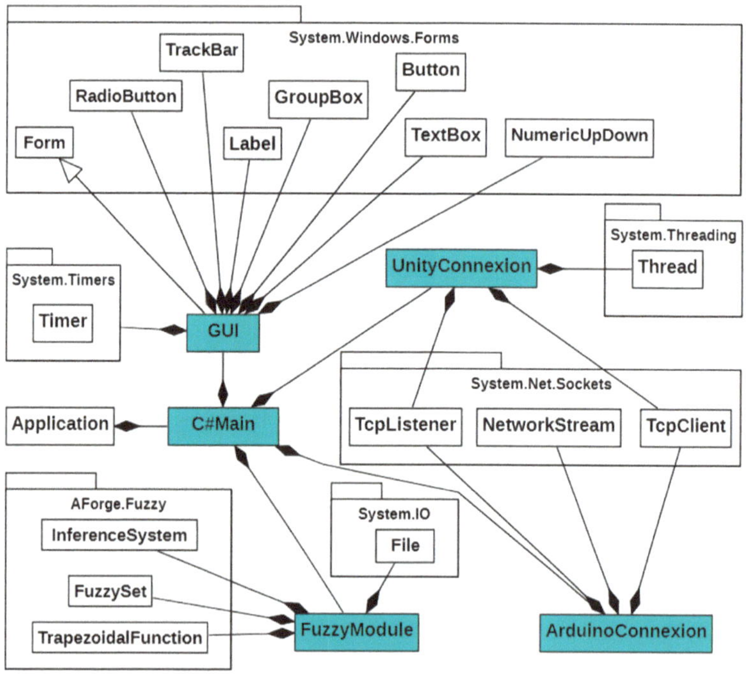

Figure 11. UML class diagram.

User Interface

The user interface was developed to control the surgical robotic system embedded in a virtual environment using VR technologies. The robotic system can be controlled via the user interface in two main modes:

- manually, by means of buttons and sliders on the user interface;
- automatically, using a control device equipped with sensors that attaches to the user's upper limb, combined with voice control.

The user interface was developed based on the features specified in the use case diagram, and the steps for using the interface are described in this section. For manual control, it is necessary to press the "Manual" button (Figure 12 (1)), which enables the manual control tools and disables the automatic controls for the user interface. The following commands are used for manual control:

- To establish the connection between the user interface and the virtual reality application through the TCP/IP protocol, the "ConnectVRApp" button must be pressed (Figure 12 (2));
- Data transmission between the user interface and the virtual reality application starts only after pressing the "StartApp" button (Figure 12 (2));
- Control of the robotic system is performed by means of sliders (Figure 12 (3)), as follows:
  - **Laparoscope insertion**: insert the laparoscope (Figure 2 (9)) into the virtual patient's body;
  - **Control orientation instrument 1**: control the orientation of instrument 1 (Figure 2 (5));
  - **Insert instrument 1**: inserting instrument 1 into the body of the virtual patient (Figure 2 (6));
  - **Control orientation instrument 2**: control the orientation of instrument 2 (Figure 2 (7));
  - **Insert instrument 2**: inserting instrument 2 into the body of the virtual patient (Figure 2 (8));
  - **Kinematic chain control**: are controlled the kinematic chains of the robotic system structure (Figure 2 (3–5));
- For visualization in the virtual reality application from several angles, five viewing cameras can be set (Cam1...Cam5), and organ visualization in the virtual patient's body is enabled by pressing the "ON" button (Figure 12 (4));
- By means of the sliders, the user can control the robotic system to insert the laparoscope and the two active instruments within a recorded time in defined points that are positioned on the kidneys, and when the three points are reached, the stopwatch stops and the elapsed time is recorded in a file (Figure 12 (5));
- Setting values for three virtual sensors (heart rate (HR), temperature, and oxygen(SpO_2)) that are attached to the virtual patient (Figure 12 (6));
- Fields in which messages are displayed for monitor virtual sensor values and collisions when inserting instruments into the virtual patients.

Automatic control is enabled in the user interface by pressing the "Automatic" button, which in turn disables the manual control tools. Switching the user interface to the automatic control mode can be carried out through the following steps:

- In order to create the connection between the microcontroller and the C# application (user interface) found on the computer via the Wi-Fi network protocol, the "ConnectionESP32" button must be pressed, and from that moment the "DisconnectionESP32" (Figure 13 (2)) status appears on the button on a red background;
- By pressing the "Start" button, the "Stop" status appears on the button (Figure 13 (2)), and from that moment the data from the microcontroller are transmitted to the C# application. For optimal functioning of the sensors, they are calibrated by moving the sensors of the device attached to the user's upper limb on three axes; when the calibration is successfully executed in the "Calibration status" field, the status "ON" (Figure 13 (2)) appears on a yellow background. After the calibration is successfully accomplished, the sensors can be used to control the robotic system.
- In order to make a connection between the C# application and the virtual reality application via the TCP/IP protocol, the "ConnectVRApp" button must be pressed, and the virtual reality application starts, and from that moment the connection is created, and the status of the button reads "Disconnection" on a red background (Figure 13 (3)). In order to make data communication in both directions between the C# application and the virtual reality application, the "StartApp" button must be

pressed, and from that moment the data communication starts, and the status of the button becomes "Stop" on a red background (Figure 13 (3)).

- In order to be able to use the control device with sensors that are attached to the user's upper limb, the "Start Control Speech rec." button must be pressed, and after pressing the button, its color changes to yellow-green (Figure 13 (4)). Pressing the button starts the stopwatch (Figure 13 (5)) and activates voice recognition commands that are combined with the sensors' device commands to control the robotic system from within the virtual reality application. When activating the command via voice recognition, the color of the activated button changes from blue to yellow (Figure 13 (4)). The following describes these commands as follows:
    - **KCC** are controlled the kinematic chains of the robotic system structure (Figure 2 (3–5));
    - **Lap**: laparoscope control (Figure 2 (9));
    - **CM 1**: the module for controlling the rotation and insertion of the instrument 1 (Figure 2 (5,6));
    - **CM 2**: the module for controlling the rotation and insertion of the instrument 2 (Figure 2 (7,8));
    - **Stop C**: Stop control of the robotic system (Figure 13 (4));
    - **Cam 1 ... Cam5**: Five viewing cameras are used for different angles in the virtual reality application (Figure 13 (4));
    - **Organs Visualization ON**: command used to visualize the internal organs of the virtual human patient (Figure 13 (4));

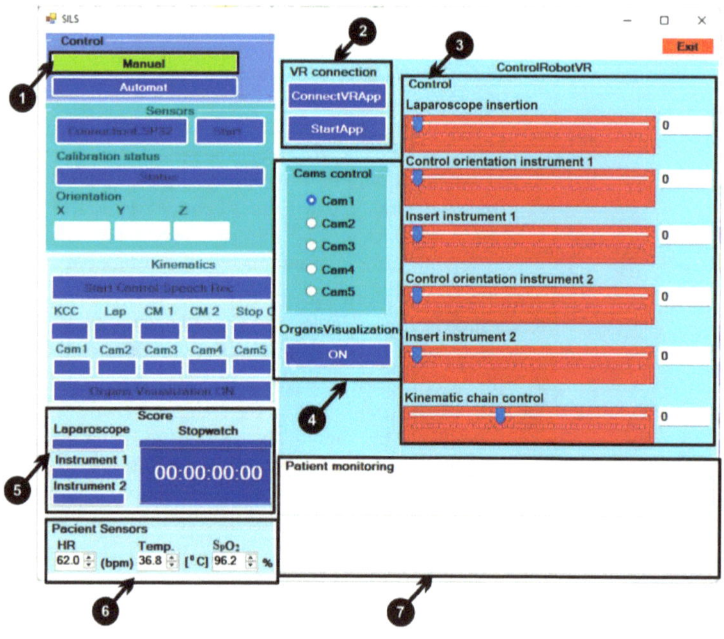

Figure 12. User interface: manual control.

- Upon touching each point positioned on the kidney by the laparoscope and the two active instruments, one LED lights up, and when both points have been successfully touched, the stopwatch stops (Figure 13 (5)), and the time is recorded in a file.
- Field for setting sensor (Figure 13 (6)) values (heart rate, temperature, and oxygen) that are attached to the virtual human patient;

- Field where messages are displayed regarding the condition of the virtual human patient from a medical point of view (Figure 13 (7)) by monitoring using three sensors (heart rate, temperature, and oxygen). In this field, messages alerting the user of the robotic system regarding the detection of collisions that may occur between the active instruments and the internal organs of the virtual human patient during the surgical procedure are also displayed.

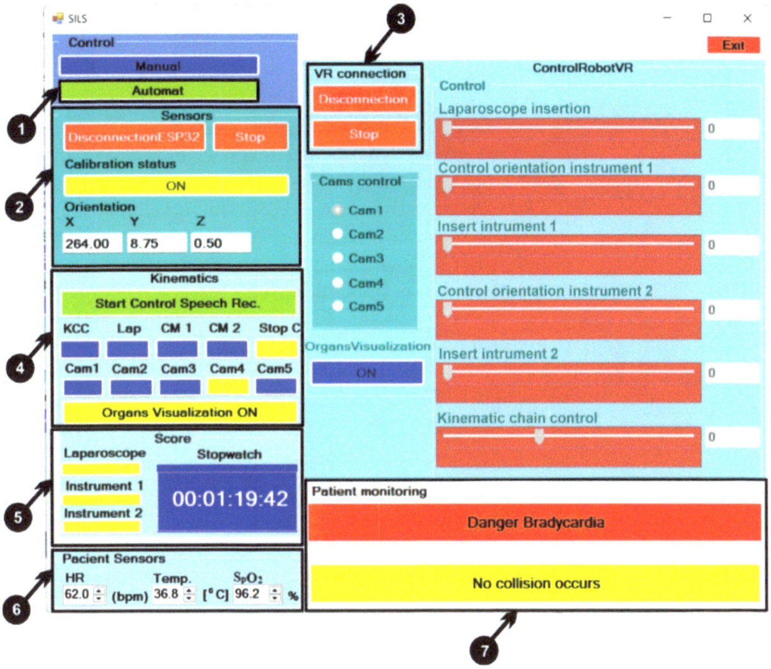

Figure 13. User interface: automatic control.

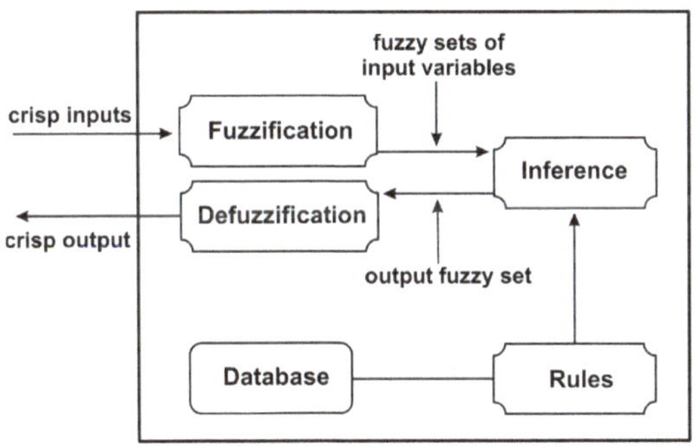

Figure 14. Block diagram of a fuzzy logic system.

Program for ESP32 Microcontroller

The embedded script for the ESP32 microcontroller was programmed and developed in an open-source programming environment called Arduino software (IDE) in the Arduino programming language. The following libraries were required in order to write the control script for the microcontroller:

- utility/imumaths.h: library for mathematical methods;

- Adafruit_Sensor.h, Adafruit_BNO055.h: library for BNO055 sensor use;
- Wi-Fi.h: library use for Wi-Fi network protocol;
- Wire.h: library for communication of ESP32 microcontroller with BNO055 IMU sensor.

After the C# application is connected to the Arduino script and while the connection is active, the data from the sensors are processed by the ESP32 script and encoded into a format supported by the C# application so that it can be sent later.

3.3.3. Artificial Intelligence Based on Fuzzy Logic for Detecting and Avoiding Unforeseen Events

Artificial intelligence agents based on fuzzy logic are used to create systems that detect and avoid unforeseen events. Fuzzy logic systems are an approach to variable processing that resembles human reasoning, with an approach that mimics human decision making. Fuzzy systems make an extension of classical sets by associating a function that returns a value between 1 and 0. Where it is difficult to implement a traditional control system, fuzzy logic can intervene. A block diagram of the fuzzy logic system can be seen in Figure 14. To activate rules, a fuzzification process is designed which transposes numerical expressions into fuzzy sets, which in turn associate fuzzy sets, corresponding to linguistic values. Rule manipulation is implemented by the inference motor which applies transformation of rule sets to fuzzy sets. To make a transformation from fuzzy sets to numerical values, the defuzzification process is used [50].

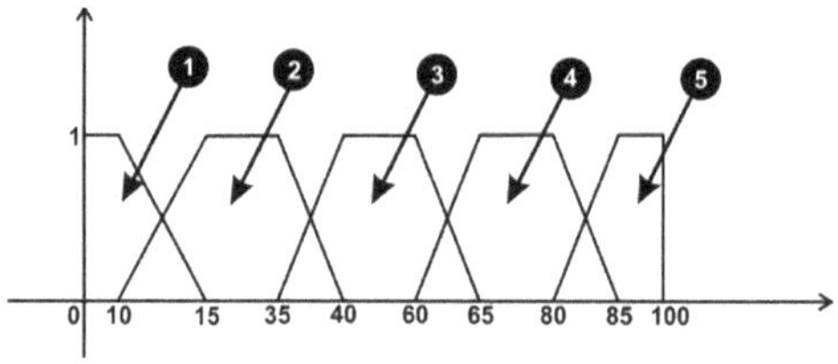

Figure 15. Fuzzy sets corresponding to events related to sensors.

To implement the fuzzy logic system, an open-source library called AForce.NET was used, implemented using the C# programming language. The scope of such a system in the entire surgical robotic application is to provide relevant information about the patient, considering the ongoing surgical operation. For this surgery application, two fuzzy logic systems were used as follows:

- For the first system, three virtual sensors (heart rate, body temperature, and blood oxygen level) were attached to the virtual patient and configured in such a way as to obtain distinct information about the patient's biological signals by emitting visual signals of alarm (Figure 13 (7)) if these parameters are about to change in such a way that the patient's life is endangered. Furthermore, a series of relationships between the parameters of these signals was created, starting from the premise that the change in the values of a signal can lead to the change in the values of another biological signal important for the safety of the patient, for example, the decrease in the level of oxygen in the blood can lead to tachycardia. The system can be integrated as suggestive behavior in the control of the robotic system, considering that any change in the patient's medical condition can reconfigure the command the robot receives. The system architecture consists of three inputs: heart rate signal, temperature, and blood oxygen level. For prediction, the system has an output to display future events, as can be seen in Figure 15.

  The five output variables (Figure 15) are interpreted by the system as follows:

1. Between values 0 and 10, the output is "Danger Bradycardia";
2. Between values 15 and 35, the output is "Bradycardia Alert!";
3. Between values 40 and 60, the output is "Biological signals are within normal parameters";

4. Between values 65 and 80, the output is "Tachycardia Alert!";
5. Between values 85 and 100, the output is "Danger Tachycardia".

- The second fuzzy system is used to detect collisions between the active tools and the organs of the virtual human patient (Figure 16). During the control of the robotic system when the three instruments are inserted into the body of the virtual human patient, these instruments may touch other organs than the desired ones and, as such, sets of rules are implemented that alert the user of the robotic system through messages (Figure 13 (7)) when an unwanted collision with another organ is happening or is about to happen.

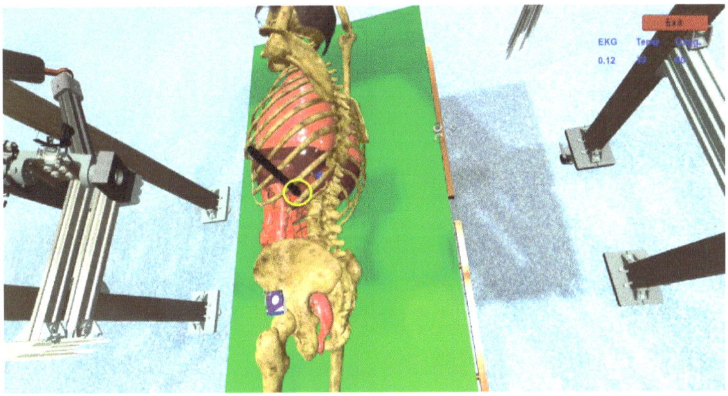

Figure 16. Laparoscope insertion.

The architecture of the system consists of two inputs: collision ribs and collision internal organs. For prediction, the system contains an output for displaying events, as can be seen in Figure 17.

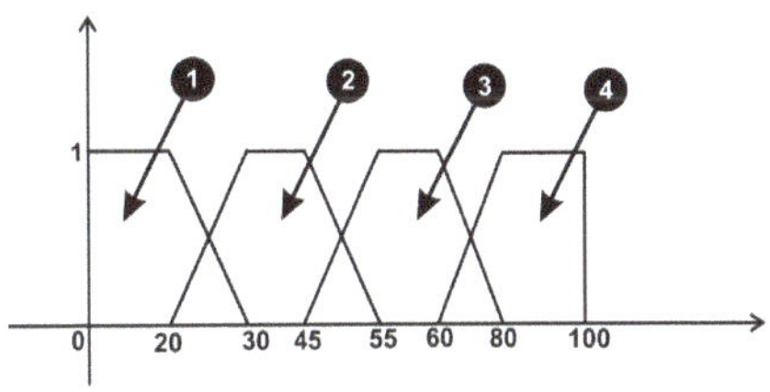

Figure 17. Fuzzy sets corresponding to events related to organs collision.

The four output variables (Figure 17) are interpreted by the system as follows:

1. Between values 0 and 20, the output is "No collision occurs";
2. Between values 30 and 45, the output is "Danger: Rib collision!";
3. Between values 55 and 60, the output is "Danger: Organ collision!";
4. Between values 80 and 100, the output is "Danger: Rib and Organ collision!".

3.3.4. Virtual Reality Application

The parallel robotic system from virtual reality is designed to manipulate instruments using the single-incision laparoscopic surgery (SILS) procedure. This procedure represents a very good alternative for most minimally invasive procedures, offering a reduced hospitalization time [51], a shorter recovery time, and better aesthetic results compared to other procedures [52]. The virtual robotic system is controlled via the user interface by combining two types of controls. Before starting the VR application, the user attaches the control device to their wrist (Figure 2) and performs the calibration. To start the application from the user interface, the automatic control mode must be selected and the connection between the ESP32 microcontroller and user interface must be established. Pressing the "Start Control Speech Rec." button activates the ability to control the robotic system through the following commands by voice recognition:

- **KCC**: the background becomes yellow, and the user can control the kinematic chain of the robotic structure (Figures 2–4) by rotating the upper limb in the horizontal plane (parallel to the xOz plane) around the axis Oy (Figure 18a);
- **Lap**: the command is activated by voice recognition, the background becomes yellow (Figure 13 (4)), and the user can control the insertion and removal of the laparoscope (Figure 2 (9)) by a movement of rotating the upper limb in the vertical plane (parallel with the plane yOz) around the axis Ox of the upper limb (Figure 18b,c);
- **CM 1**: the background becomes yellow (Figure 13 (4)), and the user can control rotation module 1 (Figure 2 (5)) by a rotation movement of the upper limb in the vertical plane (parallel to the plane yOz) around the Ox axis (Figure 18e). After positioning rotation mode 2, the user can insert and remove active instrument 2 (Figure 2 (6)) through a movement of rotation of the upper limb in the vertical plane (parallel to the yOz plane) around the axis Ox of the upper limb (Figure 18b,c);
- **CM 2**: the background becomes yellow (Figure 13(4)), and the user can control rotation module 2 (Figure 2 (7)) through a movement of rotation of the upper limb in the vertical plane (parallel to the plane yOz) around the Ox axis (Figure 18,f). After positioning rotation mode 2, the user can insert and remove active instrument 2 (Figure 2 (8)) through a movement of rotation of the upper limb in the vertical plane (parallel to the yOz plane) around the axis Ox of the upper limb (Figure 18b,c);
- **Stop C**: the background becomes yellow (Figure 13 (4)), and the user stops controlling the robotic system;
- **Cam1 . . . Cam5**: the background becomes yellow, and the user can change the viewing angle of the cameras;
- **Organs Visualization ON**: the background becomes yellow (Figure 13 (4)), and through this command the user can visualize the internal organs of the virtual human patient.

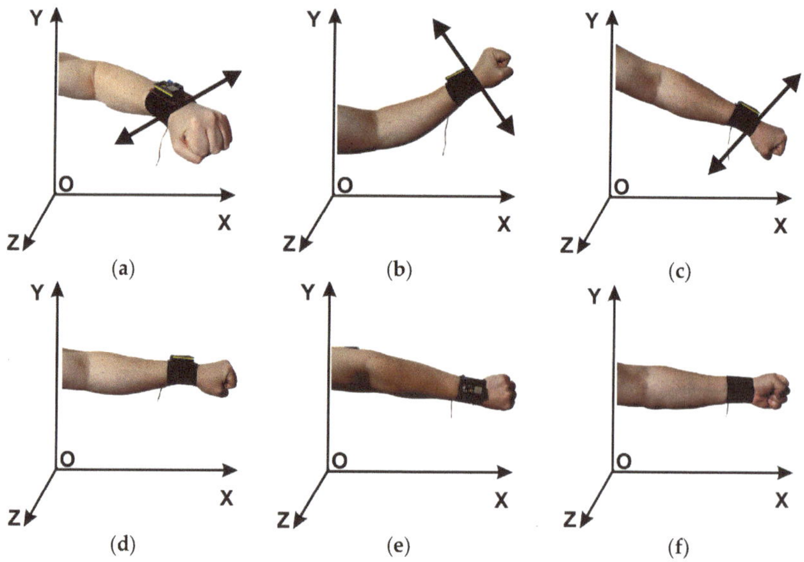

Figure 18. Rotation of the upper limb. (**a**) Around the Oy axis. (**b**–**f**) Around the Ox axis.

When operating the robotic surgical system, the user must insert two active instruments and a laparoscope through a trocar that is positioned on the body of a virtual human patient (Figure 19a). Before the instruments can be manipulated, it is necessary to make a setting for three virtual sensors: heart rate, temperature, and oxygen from the "Patient Sensors" field (Figure 13 (6)). By changing the values of the sensors on the user interface in the "Patient monitoring" field, messages appear (Figure 13 (7)) in order to warn the user of the robotic system about possible medical problems. When manipulating the laparoscope and the two active instruments, accidental contact with internal organs can happen. These events are monitored by the fuzzy algorithm which reports any such event. For the user to be able to monitor the performance while operating the robotic system, three spheres are introduced that the user must touch with the laparoscope and the two active instruments (Figure 19b) while recording the time. When the targeted sphere is touched, the color of the background element changes to yellow for the three instruments (Figure 13 (5)). When the user successfully touches the spheres with the corresponding instruments, the timer is stopped.

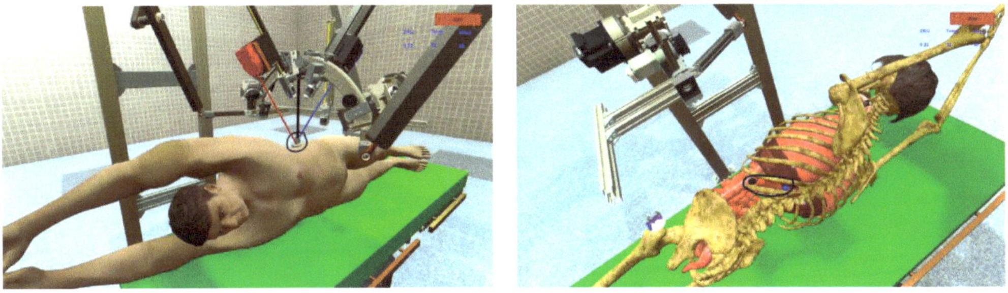

(a) (b)

Figure 19. Operating the robotic surgical system. (**a**) Insertion of instruments through a trocar; (**b**) points to be reached by instruments.

4. Results and Discussion

4.1. Experimental Validation

4.1.1. Participants

Fifteen healthy subjects (nine men and six women with a mean age of 31 years) participated in the experimental study after giving their informal written consent. To perform the experiment, all participants used their dominant upper limb and a headset with a microphone to control the robotic surgical system. Only two subjects knew the intention of the experiment, and the other subjects had no prior practice in controlling the surgical robotic system. Demographic details of the participants are shown in Table 1.

4.1.2. Performance Evolution

In this study, the performance of each participant included in the experiment is analyzed. Before controlling the surgical robotic system, each participant attached a bracelet with sensors to their wrist (Figure 8).

The goal for the participants in this experiment was to operate the robotic system in such a way as to insert the two active instruments and the laparoscope through the trocar (Figure 19a) into the body of the virtual patient and reach three target areas marked by three spheres (each sphere is assigned to an instrument). When inserting the instruments, to be able to visualize the contact with the spheres, the "Organs Visualization ON" command is activated on the user interface (Figure 13 (4)), and from that moment the internal organs of the virtual human patient can be seen. Successful contact between the instrument and the target sphere is indicated on the user interface through an associated element by changing the background from blue to yellow (Figure 13 (5)). When the three spheres are touched by the three instruments, the timer stops, and the elapsed time is recorded in a file. Figure 20 presents the performance of each participant in the experiment.

Table 1. Demographic details specific to the participants included in the experiment.

Subject	Age	Gender
1	42	m
2	25	f
3	22	f
4	43	m
5	35	m
6	36	m
7	43	f
8	24	f
9	22	m
10	43	m
11	26	m
12	23	f
13	30	m
14	24	f
15	27	m

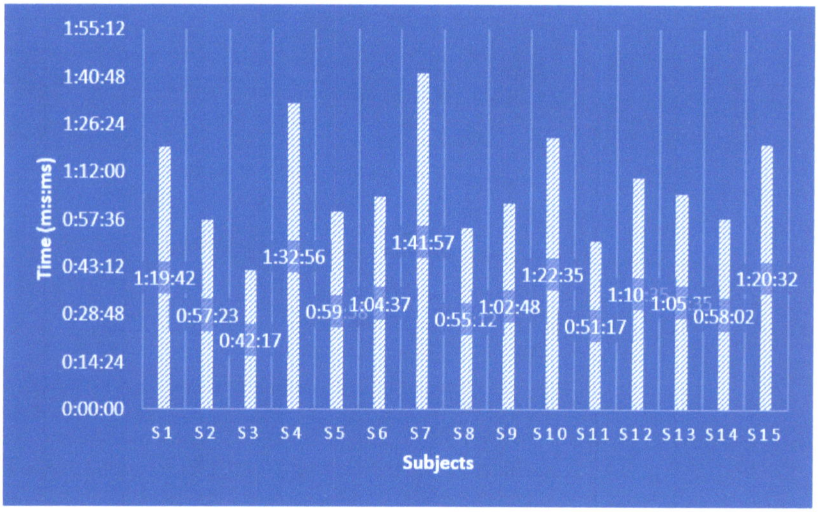

Figure 20. Performance results of users of the surgical robotic system.

5. Summary and Conclusions

This article presents a study for the development of a virtual reality simulator of a robotic system for single-incision laparoscopic surgery (SILS). The VR environment represents an efficient solution for the validation of different features of the robot and the assessment of different interfaces that can be used for slave robot control, as well as an efficient training environment for young surgeons. By also integrating a "digital twin" of the innovative robotic structure, dimensional optimization can be achieved by running different medically relevant scenarios.

The theoretical study on the singularities of the slave robotic platform demonstrated its feasibility for the surgical act in terms of safety in operation. Workspace analysis enabled the identification of the most efficient configuration of the robotic system to maximize its operational working volume.

From the master console, the user can interact with the virtual robotic system using either voice commands or a wristband attached to the forearm. While voice commands have been previously used in surgery, the use of a wristband is a new approach. The team aims to evaluate the stability of the solution, the user acceptance, and the learning curve to determine the feasibility of this approach. The VR platform also supports the loading of simulated patient data (heart rate, temperature, and oxygen level), which can reproduce different critical situations. In the first iteration of the VR simulator, a demonstrative exercise was implemented to test the user performance, to test the acceptance levels with respect to the wristband utilization, and to assess the motion capabilities of the robotic system.

Regarding future improvements, the assessment of accuracy during the use of the VR simulator by the users will be considered. A special set of simulated incidents during different stages of the procedure is also targeted for implementation to assess the reaction of surgeons in critical, unexpected conditions [53].

6. Patents

Pisla, D., Birlescu I., Vaida C., Tucan P., Gherman B., Plitea N.: Family of modular parallel robots with active translational joints for single-incision laparoscopic surgery, OSIM A00733/03.12.2021.

Author Contributions: Conceptualization, F.C. and D.P.; methodology, C.V.; software, F.C.; validation, F.C., D.P. and C.V.; formal analysis, N.C., A.P., C.R., N.A.H. and I.A.; investigation, A.P.; resources, D.P.; data curation, B.G.; writing—original draft preparation, F.C.; writing—review and editing, F.C., D.P. and C.V.; visualization, P.T.; supervision, D.P.; project administration, D.P.; funding acquisition, D.P. All authors have read and agreed to the published version of the manuscript.

Funding: This work was supported by a grant of the Ministry of Research, Innovation and Digitization, CNCS/CCCDI–UEFISCDI, project number PCE171/2021-Challenge within PNCDI III, and project POCU/380/6/13/123927–ANTREDOC, "Entrepreneurial competencies and excellence re-search in doctoral and postdoctoral studies programs", a project co-funded by the European Social Fund through the Human Capital Operational.

Informed Consent Statement: Not applicable.

Data Availability Statement: Data sharing is not applicable to this article.

Conflicts of Interest: The authors declare no conflict of interest.

References

1. Benway, B.M.; Bhayani, S.B.; Rogers, C.G.; Dulabon, L.M.; Patel, M.N.; Lipkin, M.; Wang, A.J.; Stifelman, M.D. Robot Assisted Partial Nephrectomy Versus Laparoscopic Partial Nephrectomy for Renal Tumors: A Multi-Institutional Analysis of Perioperative Outcomes. *J. Urol.* **2009**, *182*, 866–873. [CrossRef] [PubMed]
2. Tucan, P.; Vaida, C.; Horvath, D.; Caprariu, A.; Burz, A.; Gherman, B.; Iakab, S.; Pisla, D. Design and Experimental Setup of a Robotic Medical Instrument for Brachytherapy in Non-Resectable Liver Tumors. *Cancers* **2022**, *14*, 5841. [CrossRef] [PubMed]
3. Plitea, N.; Hesselbach, J.; Vaida, C.; Raatz, A.; Pisla, D.; Budde, C.; Vlad, L.; Burisch, A.; Senner, R. Innovative development of surgical parallel robots. *Acta Electron. Mediamira Sci. Cluj Napoca* **2007**, *4*, 201–206.
4. Pugin, F.; Bucher, P.; Morel, P. History of robotic surgery: From AESOP® and ZEUS® to da Vinci®. *J. Visc. Surg.* **2011**, *148*, 3–8. [CrossRef] [PubMed]
5. Arkenbout, E.A.; Henselmans, P.W.J.; Jelínek, F.; Breedveld, P. A state of the art review and categorization of multi-branched instruments for NOTES and SILS. *Surg. Endosc.* **2015**, *29*, 1281–1296. [CrossRef]
6. Vasudevan, M.K.; Isaac, J.H.R.; Sadanand, V.; Muniyandi, M. Novel virtual reality based training system for fine motor skills: Towards developing a robotic surgery training system. *Int. J. Med. Robot. Comput. Assist. Surg.* **2020**, *16*, 1–14. [CrossRef]
7. Hagmann, K.; Hellings-Kuß, A.; Klodmann, J.; Richter, R.; Stulp, F.; Leidner, D. A Digital Twin Approach for Contextual Assistance for Surgeons During Surgical Robotics Training. *Front. Robot. AI* **2021**, *8*, 1–14. [CrossRef]
8. Vaida, C.; Pisla, D.; Plitea, N.; Gherman, B.; Gyurka, B.; Graur, F.; Vlad, L. Development of a Voice Controlled Surgical Robot. In *New Trends in Mechanism Science. Mechanisms and Machine Science*; Pisla, D., Ceccarelli, M., Husty, M., Corves, B., Eds.; Springer: Berlin/Heidelberg, Germany, 2010; Volume 5, pp. 567–574.

9. Gleason, A.; Servais, E.; Quadri, S.; Manganiello, M.; Cheah, Y.L.; Simon, C.; Preston, E.; Graham-Stephenson, A.; Wright, V. Developing basic robotic skills using virtual reality simulation and automated assessment tools: A multidisciplinary robotic virtual reality-based curriculum using the Da Vinci Skills Simulator and tracking progress with the Intuitive Learning platform. *J. Robot. Surg.* **2022**, *16*, 1313–1319. [CrossRef]
10. Iop, A.; El-Hajj, V.G.; Gharios, M.; de Giorgio, A.; Monetti, F.M.; Edström, E.; Elmi-Terander, A.; Romero, M. Extended Reality in Neurosurgical Education: A Systematic Review. *Sensors* **2022**, *22*, 6067. [CrossRef]
11. Korayem, M.; Vahidifar, V. Detecting hand's tremor using leap motion controller in guiding surgical robot arms and laparoscopic scissors. *Measurement* **2022**, *204*, 1–11. [CrossRef]
12. Mehrfard, A.; Fotouhi, J.; Forster, T.; Taylor, G.; Fer, D.; Nagle, D.; Armand, M.; Navab, N.; Fuerst, B. On the effectiveness of virtual reality-based training for surgical robot setup. *Comput. Methods Biomech. Biomed. Eng. Imaging Vis.* **2020**, *9*, 1–10. [CrossRef]
13. Mishra, R.; Narayanan, M.D.; Umana, G.E.; Montemurro, N.; Chaurasia, B.; Deora, H. Virtual Reality in Neurosurgery: Beyond Neurosurgical Planning. *Int. J. Environ. Res. Public Health* **2022**, *19*, 1719. [CrossRef] [PubMed]
14. Covaciu, F.; Pisla, A.; Vaida, C.; Gherman, B.; Pisla, D. Development of a Virtual Reality Simulator for a Lower Limb Rehabilitation Robot. In Proceedings of the IEEE International Conference on Automation, Quality and Testing, Robotics (AQTR), Cluj-Napoca, Romania, 21–23 May 2020.
15. Covaciu, F.; Gherman, B.; Pisla, A.; Carbone, G.; Pisla, D. Rehabilitation System with Integrated Visual Stimulation. In Proceedings of the European Conference on Mechanism Science, Cluj-Napoca, Romania, 7–10 September 2020.
16. Korayem, M.; Madihi, M.; Vahidifar, V. Controlling surgical robot arm using leap motion controller with Kalman filter. *Measurement* **2021**, *178*, 109372. [CrossRef]
17. Ehrampoosh, A.; Shirinzadeh, B.; Pinskier, J.; Smith, J.; Moshinsky, R.; Zhong, Y. A Force-Feedback Methodology for Teleoperated Suturing Task in Robotic-Assisted Minimally Invasive Surgery. *Sensors* **2022**, *22*, 7829. [CrossRef] [PubMed]
18. Chua, Z.; Okamura, A.M. A Modular 3-Degrees-of-Freedom Force Sensor for Robot-Assisted Minimally Invasive Surgery Research. *Sensors* **2023**, *23*, 5230. [CrossRef]
19. Abad, A.C.; Reid, D.; Ranasinghe, A. A Novel Untethered Hand Wearable with Fine-Grained Cutaneous Haptic Feedback. *Sensors* **2022**, *22*, 1924. [CrossRef]
20. Pisla, D.; Gherman, B.; Plitea, N.; Gyurka, B.; Vaida, C.; Vlad, L.; Graur, F.; Radu, C.; Suciu, M.; Szilaghi, A.; et al. PARASURG hybrid parallel robot for minimally invasive surgery. *Chirurgia* **2011**, *106*, 619–625.
21. Martin, J.R.; Stefanidis, D.; Dorin, R.P.; Goh, A.C.; Satava, R.M.; Levy, J.S. Demonstrating the effectiveness of the fundamentals of robotic surgery (FRS) curriculum on the RobotiX Mentor Virtual Reality Simulation Platform. *J. Robot. Surg.* **2020**, *15*, 187–193. [CrossRef]
22. Covaciu, F.; Pisla, A.; Iordan, A.-E. Development of a Virtual Reality Simulator for an Intelligent Robotic System Used in Ankle Rehabilitation. *Sensors* **2021**, *21*, 1537. [CrossRef]
23. Covaciu, F.; Iordan, A.-E. Control of a Drone in Virtual Reality Using MEMS Sensor Technology and Machine Learning. *Micromachines* **2022**, *13*, 521. [CrossRef]
24. Luca, A.; Giorgino, R.; Gesualdo, L.; Peretti, G.M.; Belkhou, A.; Banfi, G.; Grasso, G. Innovative Educational Pathways in Spine Surgery: Advanced Virtual Reality–Based Training. *World Neurosurg.* **2020**, *140*, 674–680. [CrossRef]
25. Portelli, M.; Bianco, S.; Bezzina, T.; Abela, J. Virtual reality training compared with apprenticeship training in laparoscopic surgery: A meta-analysis. *R. Coll. Surg. Engl.* **2020**, *102*, 672–684. [CrossRef] [PubMed]
26. Trochimczuk, R.; Łukaszewicz, A.; Mikołajczyk, T.; Aggogeri, F.; Borboni, A. Finite element method stiffness analysis of a novel telemanipulator for minimally invasive surgery. *Simulation* **2019**, *95*, 1015–1025. [CrossRef]
27. Kawashima, K.; Kanno, T.; Tadano, K. Robots in laparoscopic surgery: Current and future status. *BMC Biomed. Eng.* **2019**, *1*, 1–6. [CrossRef] [PubMed]
28. Longmore, S.K.; Naik, G.; Gargiulo, G.D. Laparoscopic Robotic Surgery: Current Perspective and Future Directions. *Robotics* **2020**, *9*, 42. [CrossRef]
29. Korayem, M.; Vosoughi, R.; Vahidifar, V. Design, manufacture, and control of a laparoscopic robot via Leap Motion sensors. *Measurement* **2022**, *205*, 1–13. [CrossRef]
30. Batty, T.; Ehrampoosh, A.; Shirinzadeh, B.; Zhong, Y.; Smith, J. A Transparent Teleoperated Robotic Surgical System with Predictive Haptic Feedback and Force Modelling. *Sensors* **2022**, *22*, 9770. [CrossRef]
31. Mao, R.Q.; Lan, L.; Kay, J.; Lohre, R.; Ayeni, O.R.; Goel, D.P.; de Sa, D. Immersive Virtual Reality for Surgical Training: A Systematic Review. *J. Surg. Res.* **2021**, *268*, 40–58. [CrossRef]
32. Kalinov, T.; Georgiev, T.; Bliznakova, K.; Zlatarov, A.; Kolev, N. Assessment of students' satisfaction with virtual robotic surgery training. *Heliyon* **2023**, *9*, 1–8. [CrossRef]
33. Lamblin, G.; Thiberville, G.; Druette, L.; Moret, S.; Couraud, S.; Martin, X.; Dubernard, G.; Chene, G. Virtual reality simulation to enhance laparoscopic salpingectomy skills. *J. Gynecol. Obstet. Hum. Reprod.* **2020**, *49*, 101685. [CrossRef]
34. Elessawy, M.; Mabrouk, M.; Heilmann, T.; Weigel, M.; Zidan, M.; Abu-Sheasha, G.; Farrokh, A.; Bauerschlag, D.; Maass, N.; Ibrahim, M.; et al. Evaluation of Laparoscopy Virtual Reality Training on the Improvement of Trainees' Surgical Skills. *Medicina* **2021**, *57*, 130. [CrossRef] [PubMed]

35. Gherman, B.; Vaida, C.; Pisla, D.; Plitea, N.; Gyurka, B.; Lese, D.; Glogoveanu, M. Singularities and Workspace Analysis for a Parallel Robot for Minimally Invasive Surgery. In Proceedings of the IEEE International Conference on Automation, Quality and Testing, Robotics (AQTR), Cluj-Napoca, Romania, 28–30 May 2010.
36. Wenger, P.; Chablat, D. A Review of Cuspidal Serial and Parallel Manipulators. *ASME J. Mech. Robotics.* **2023**, *15*, 040801. [CrossRef]
37. Pisla, D.; Plitea, N.; Videan, A.; Prodan, B.; Gherman, B.; Lese, D. Kinematics and design of two variants of a reconfigurable parallel robot. In Proceedings of the ASME/IFToMM International Conference on Reconfigurable Mechanisms and Robots, London, UK, 24 July 2009.
38. Franklin, C.S.; Dominguez, E.G.; Fryman, J.D.; Lewandowski, M.L. Collaborative robotics: New era of human–robot cooperation in the workplace. *J. Saf. Res.* **2020**, *74*, 153–160. [CrossRef] [PubMed]
39. Tucan, P.; Vaida, C.; Plitea, N.; Pisla, A.; Carbone, G.; Pisla, D. Risk-Based Assessment Engineering of a Parallel Robot Used in Post-Stroke Upper Limb Rehabilitation. *Sustainability* **2019**, *11*, 2893. [CrossRef]
40. Merlet, J.-P. *Parallel Robots*, 2nd ed.; Springer: Berlin/Heidelberg, Germany, 2006.
41. Pisla, D.; Gherman, B.; Tucan, P.; Birlescu, I.; Pusca, A.; Rus, G.; Pisla, A.; Vaida, C. Application oriented modelling and simulation of an innovative parallel robot for single incision laparoscopic surgery. In Proceedings of the ASME, St. Louis, MI, USA, 14–17 August 2022; pp. 1–10.
42. Pisla, D.; Pusca, A.; Tucan, P.; Gherman, B.; Vaida, C. Kinematics and workspace analysis of an innovative 6-dof parallel robot for SILS. *Proc. Rom. Acad.* **2022**, *23*, 279–288.
43. Available online: https://ro.mouser.com/new/bosch/bosch-bno55-sensor/ (accessed on 5 January 2022).
44. Available online: https://www.espressif.com/sites/default/files/documentation/esp32_datasheet_en.pdf (accessed on 5 January 2022).
45. Iordan, A.E.; Covaciu, F. Improving Design of a Triangle Geometry Computer Application using a Creational Pattern. *Acta Tech. Napoc. Ser.-Appl. Math. Mech. Eng.* **2020**, *63*, 73–78.
46. Iordan, A.E. Optimal solution of the Guarini puzzle extension using tripartite graphs. *IOP Conf. Ser. Mater. Sci. Eng.* **2019**, *477*, 1–8. [CrossRef]
47. Levitin, A. Algorithmic Puzzles: History, Taxonomies, and Applications in Human Problem Solving. *J. Probl. Solving* **2017**, *10*, 1. [CrossRef]
48. Iordan, A. Development of Interactive Software for Teaching Three-Dimensional Analytic Geometry. In Proceedings of the 9th International Conference on Distance Learning and Web Engineering, Budapest, Hungary, 3–5 September 2009.
49. Panoiu, M.; Panoiu, C.; Iordan, A.; Ghiormez, L. Artificial neural networks in predicting current in electric arc furnaces. *IOP Conf. Ser. Mater. Sci. Eng.* **2014**, *57*, 1–7. [CrossRef]
50. Dumitrescu, C.; Ciotirnae, P.; Vizitiu, C. Fuzzy Logic for Intelligent Control System Using Soft Computing Applications. *Sensors* **2021**, *21*, 2617. [CrossRef]
51. Dong, B.; Luo, Z.; Lu, J.; Yang, Y.; Song, Y.; Cao, J.; Li, W. Single-incision laparoscopic versus conventional laparoscopic right colectomy: A systematic review and meta-analysis. *Int. J. Surg.* **2018**, *55*, 31–38. [CrossRef] [PubMed]
52. Pisla, D.; Carami, D.; Gherman, B.; Soleti, G.; Ulinici, I.; Vaida, C. A novel control architecture for robotic-assisted single incision laparoscopic surgery. *Rom. J. Tech. Sci. Appl. Mech.* **2021**, *66*, 141–162.
53. Aydın, A.; Ahmed, K.; Abe, T.; Raison, N.; Van Hemelrijck, M.; Garmo, H.; Ahmed, H.U.; Mukhtar, F.; Al-Jabir, A.; Brunckhorst, O.; et al. Effect of Simulation-based Training on Surgical Proficiency and Patient Outcomes: A Randomised Controlled Clinical and Educational Trial. *Eur. Urol.* **2021**, *81*, 385–393. [CrossRef] [PubMed]

sensors

MDPI

Article

Research on the Perceived Quality of Virtual Reality Headsets in Human–Computer Interaction

Yongzhong Yang, Linling Zhong *, Shihui Li and Aixian Yu

Department of Business Administration, Business School, Sichuan University, Chengdu 610207, China
* Correspondence: zhonglinling@stu.scu.edu.cn

Abstract: The progress of commercial VR headsets largely depends on the progress of sensor technology, the iteration of which often means longer research and development cycles, and also higher costs. With the continuous maturity and increasing competition of VR headsets, designers need to create a balance among user needs, technologies, and costs to achieve commercial competition advantages. To make accurate judgments, consumer feedback and opinions are particularly important. Due to the increasing maturity in the technology of commercial VR headsets in recent years, the cost has been continuously decreasing, and potential consumers have gradually increased. With the increase in consumer demand for virtual reality headsets, it is particularly important to establish a perceptual quality evaluation system. The relationship between consumer perception and product quality determined by evaluations of experience is improving. Using the research method implemented in this work, through semi-structured interviews and big data analysis of VR headset consumption, the perceptual quality elements of VR headsets are proposed, and the order of importance of perceptual quality attributes is determined by questionnaire surveys, quantitative analysis, and verification. In this study, the perceptual quality elements, including technical perceptual quality (TPQ) and value perceptual quality (VPQ), of 14 types of VR headsets were obtained, and the importance ranking of the VR headsets' perceptual quality attributes was constructed. In theory, this study enriches the research on VR headsets. In practice, this study provides better guidance and suggestions for designing and producing VR headsets so that producers can better understand which sensor technology has met the needs of consumers, and which sensor technology still has room for improvement.

Keywords: sensor technology; human–computer interaction; VR headsets; consumption big data; perceived quality; perceived quality framework; PQAIR

Citation: Yang, Y.; Zhong, L.; Li, S.; Yu, A. Research on the Perceived Quality of Virtual Reality Headsets in Human–Computer Interaction. *Sensors* **2023**, *23*, 6824. https://doi.org/10.3390/s23156824

Academic Editors: Radu Comes, Dorin-Mircea Popovici, Calin Gheorghe Dan Neamtu and Jing-Jing Fang

Received: 13 June 2023
Revised: 16 July 2023
Accepted: 28 July 2023
Published: 31 July 2023

1. Introduction

With the rise of emerging technologies such as 5G, artificial intelligence, and virtual reality, the development of intelligent wearable devices has been accelerated. Human–computer interaction has been widely used in people's daily lives. It brings great convenience while profoundly changing people's work, entertainment, and lifestyles. The relationship between humans and machines has entered the era of human–computer interaction; rather than constituting a single way for human beings to obtain information from computers, we are gradually realizing the development of this relationship into a two-way accurate transmission of information [1]. VR headsets can provide people with a wealth of entertainment and professional applications and are an important device to help people participate in the era of human–computer interaction. The current, rapid development of computer technology, image processing, multimedia technology, sensors, and network technology has brought new possibilities for virtual reality technology. People can interact with the virtual world with experiences that seem more real than they were previously [2]. When people wear VR headsets, they can be in a three-dimensional world, giving them a new sense of reality [3]. To achieve an immersive effect, the application of various sensor technologies is very important. In recent years, research into VR headsets has focused more on the optimization of various sensing technologies such as distance sensors, tactile sensors, and force sensors. These studies have verified the necessity and feasibility of technological progress from a technical point of view. However, few studies have discussed and verified the rationality of the optimization of various sensing technologies from the perspective of consumers. In the face of increasingly fierce competition in the market, this paper believes that researchers and producers need to pay more attention to consumers' opinions and feedback while studying the iteration of sensor technology.

According to TrendForce, a data website, global VR headset equipment shipments reached about 8.58 million units in 2022, and it is predicted that global VR headset equipment shipments will soar to 10.35 million units in 2023, an increase of 20.6% over the same period in the prior year. Based on the theory of perceptual quality, this study aims to determine the importance ranking of the perceptual quality attributes of VR headsets, and provide a reference for manufacturers to design and manufacture VR headsets from consumers' perceived quality.

2. Literature Review

2.1. Research on VR Headsets

At present, the research on VR headsets can be roughly divided into two directions: one is the technologies used and the other is the applications.

In relation to VR headset technologies, VR headsets are the integration products of software and hardware technologies. For example, they integrate computer graphics, digital image processing, multimedia technology, sensor technology, artificial intelligence and other software technologies [4]. Through VR headsets, users can interact with computer-generated visual outputs, such as visualization options and animations, which float in front of the user. Many scholars have studied the visual system of VR headsets, because the visual system is the core element [5]. For example, Lu discusses how to improve the VR eye tracking system to achieve better tracking results [6]. Xu discusses how to improve the performance of tactile sensors and force sensors for wearable devices, including VR headsets [7]. Dempsey and Rossz study the software and hardware technologies of VR headsets as a whole by evaluating the HTC Vive and Razer OSVR HDK, respectively [8,9].

The research on the applications of VR headsets is another direction of study in the academic world, which includes the analysis of VR technologies' current applications as well as its prospects in these fields, such as medical care, games, education, sports, fashion, tourism, and so on. In the medical field, for instance, VR technology has been used as a treatment for PTSD [10] and for rehabilitation training after a stroke [11]. Three-dimensional gaming is an important field of VR applications, and the evolution of the game also plays a certain role in promoting the development of VR technology. More games are evolving in the direction of VR technology [12]. In the field of education, VR headsets have the advantage of breaking the limitations of time, space, and resources. Through human–computer interaction and immersive experience, a student's imagination is stimulated, and teaching is realized by playing. Furthermore, VR headsets can avoid some experimental operation risks [13]. VR headsets can also help athletes to carry out dynamic balance and reaction time [14]. Chen combines VR technology with MTM (MadetoMeasure) which allows people to try on clothes at home [15]. If you want to travel, you can experience global cultural heritage through VR headsets staying at home [16].

2.2. Research on the Co-Occurrence Map of VR Headsets Based on Sensor Technology

Sensor technology is one of the core technologies of VR headsets. VR headsets on the market usually have sound sensors, IMU (Inertial Measurement Unit), distance sensors, Hall sensors, tactile sensors, mechanical sensors, optical sensors, and so on.

In this paper, the Citespace software was used to search for papers on the Web of Science over the past ten years, which are listed on SCI, SSCI, and AHCI, and are related to "VR Headset". A total of 823 related articles were retrieved. The co-occurrence map of sensor technology based on VR headsets was obtained by selecting sensor technology-related keywords from 291 keywords which are classified based on the 823 articles, as shown in Figure 1:

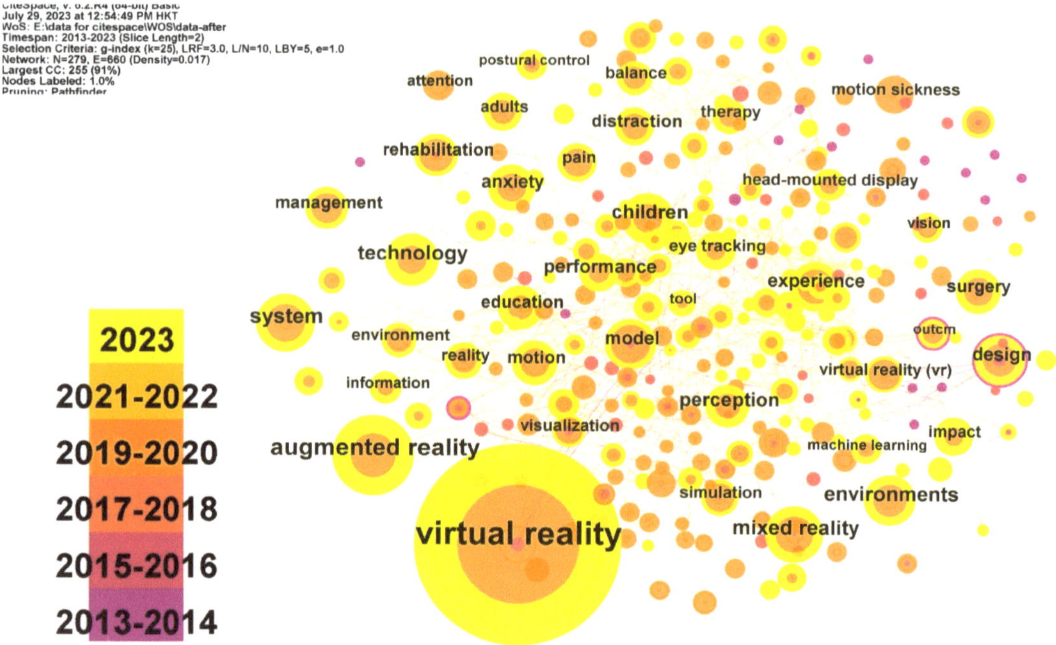

Figure 1. Research on Co-occurrence Map of VR Headsets Based on Sensor Technology.

In the co-occurrence map, the higher the frequency of the keywords, the larger the text; and the thicker the ligature between nodes, the stronger the correlation between keywords. Virtual reality in the map is the keyword with the highest frequency. In addition, keywords related to sensor technology are mainly concentrated on vision, eye tracking, walking, movements, and audio. This paper further studies the articles contained in general descriptions such as "design" and "sense". It is found that in the past 10 years, the research on the sensor of VR headsets mainly focuses on the following three categories:

(1) Distance Sensor: Mainly based on the prediction technology of an inertial measurement unit (IMU) sensor [17], the asynchronous time difference (ATW) [18], and the MEMS ultrasonic sensing technology.

(2) Tactile and Mechanical Sensors: Tactile and mechanical sensors for the Human–Machine Interface (HMI), which include piezoresistive sensors, capacitive sensors, piezoelectric sensors, triboelectric sensors, and wearable skin integrated with tactile and mechanical sensors [7]. It also includes TGI space–time control that can sense hot and cold pain [19].

(3) Optical Sensors: Most of them are optical sensors in head-mounted displays (HMD), and also include a precision task head-mounted projector HMP [20]. In addition, there are few research articles on sound sensors and temperature sensors (mainly used to ensure the stability of Cpu operation) in the field of VR headsets.

2.3. Perceived Quality

Olson and Jacoby (1972), the first scholars who proposed perceived quality, defined perceived quality as a method to evaluate product quality [21]. Wheatley (1981) further proposed that perceived quality was not only an evaluation of product quality but also an evaluation of service quality [22]. Zeithaml (1988) then held that perceived quality was about consumers' perception of a product's price, quality, and value, and was a judgment of the overall superiority of the product [23,24]. Perceived quality is the evaluation of the overall excellence or advantages of the product; that is, the evaluation of a product [25]. The evaluation results come from comparing actual quality with expected quality. When the product quality is better than the product's expectations, the perceived quality is good [26]. The evaluation includes the product's performance and consumers' overall perception of the overall quality of the product; that is, whether a product or service is superior [27], including a subjective quality evaluation based on product packaging, price, and consumer purchase experience [28].

2.4. Perceived Quality Framework

Scholars are currently committed to quantifying the perceived quality of a product or service and its attributes and building its perceived quality framework. Perceived quality elements are the basis of the framework of perceived quality. In terms of how to explore the perceived quality elements of products, according to the clue utilization theory, Olson (1972) proposed quantifying the quality of products or services from internal cues and external cues [21]. The former mainly relies on the physical elements of the products and services; the latter relies on nonphysical elements derived from products or services. Many scholars have proposed different frameworks composed of multiple cue dimensions. Dodds (1991) proposed a five-dimensional (reliability, workmanship, quality, dependability, and durability) perceived quality framework [29]. Robert (1978) held that the most commonly used clues for consumers to choose products are advertising image, individual needs, price, and experience [30]. Zeithaml (2000) proposed six dimensions (usability, multifunctionality, durability, performance, serviceability, and reputation) of the perceived quality framework [23]. Stylidis and Wickman (2019) further put forward the two-dimensional-type theory of perceived quality–technical perceived quality (TPQ) and value-based perceived quality (VPQ), which expands the subject of perceived quality from consumers to producers. TPQ is more inclined to the inherent attributes of products and services. VPQ is more related to the external attributes of products and services such as brand image, product reputation, customer emotional judgment, values, advertising, and after-sales service [31].

2.5. Big Data for Online Consumption Reviews

In 2001, the scholar Chatterjee put forward the concept of online review for the first time. Online consumer review refers to the online shopping evaluation of purchased goods or services based on an e-commerce platform after consumers buy products [32]. Online consumption review has the characteristics of wide dissemination, measurable information, and reliable reality and plays an important role and value in many aspects such as consumers and enterprises [33]. Commodity review is an important kind of consumer feedback data, constituting the link between products and consumers, which implies valuable consumer feedback information. How to mine information beneficial to product design, production, and sales from comment data has become the focus of scholars [34].

2.6. Perceived Quality Elements

Perceived quality is a general view of product performance and overall quality; that is, whether the product is superior [27]. These general views are composed of subjective quality evaluations of factors such as product packaging, price, and consumer purchase experience. The perceived quality factors of different products are different, because the product itself can convey different attributes. For analysis on one same product, different researchers adopt different methods and perspectives, which can uncover different perceived quality factors. For example, the perceived quality factors of automobiles that Stylidis analyzed are the qualities of process, aesthetics, physical function, geometry, operating sound, materials, lighting, dynamic and static noise, surface finish, spray paint cover, and so on [35]. The elements excavated by Yang are: modeling design, static perception, operational perception, and dynamic experience [36]. Although there is no research on the perceived quality elements of VR headsets in academic circles, research on consumers' reviews of VR headsets has emerged. For instance, Amanda believes that a wider perspective can give users a better feeling [37]. The tracking technology of VR headsets can enhance the user's visual immersion when using the device [38], while Tarr discussed the consumers' social experiences of VR headsets [39]. However, the comprehensive study of the overall perceived quality elements of VR headsets remains to be studied by scholars.

3. Materials and Methods

To obtain the elements of VR headsets' perceptual quality more comprehensively, this study adopts a two-dimensional perceived quality theory proposed by Stylidis and Wickman (2019) to build a framework of perceived quality [31]. In the research method—a hybrid research metho—a combination of qualitative and quantitative analysis was used. Based on different coexistence goals, different research methods can be embedded in the same research design.

Quantitative analysis:

(1) Organize semi-structured interviews to obtain the preliminary perceived quality elements and framework of a VR headset.
(2) Collect huge numbers of VR headset consumers' reviews from different websites and obtain the high-frequency words after cleaning the dirty data.
(3) Through the Delphi method, experts can classify the high-frequency words of VR headsets and improve the perceived quality framework.

Qualitative analysis:

(4) Use Likert ten scale to design the importance ranking questionnaire of perceived quality elements.
(5) Distribute, collect, and analyze the questionnaires.
(6) Obtain the final importance ranking of VR headset perceived quality elements.

Research roadmap is shown in Figure 2:

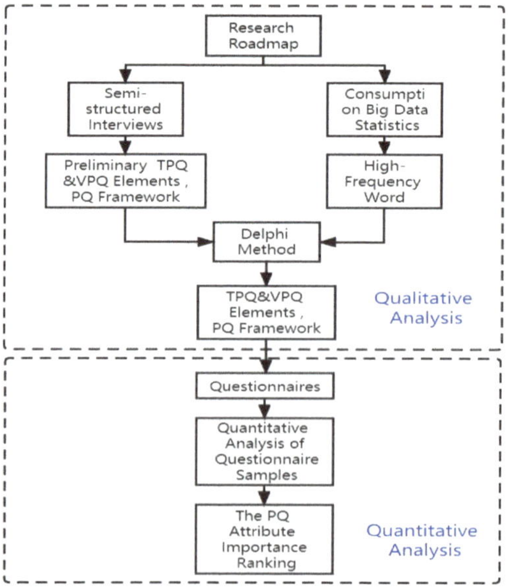

Figure 2. Research roadmap.

3.1. Semi-Structured Interviews

Found through industry conferences and online forums, 22 professionals were invited to participate in semi-structured interviews. All of them have experienced VR headsets for more than two years. There were more men than women as interviewees, and most of them were young and middle-aged people. About half of the interviewees were industry practitioners and half were consumers. The specific information of the interviewees is shown in Table 1.

Table 1. Basic information of interviewees in semi-structured interviews.

Characteristics	Grouping	Number of People	Percentage
Gender	Male	17	77.27%
	Female	5	22.73%
Age	18–24 years old	3	13.64%
	25–35 years old	11	50.00%
	36–45 years old	6	27.27%
	46–55 years old	2	9.09%
Personnel Type	Industry expert	5	22.73%
	Senior VR enthusiasts	4	18.18%
	Internet industry experts	3	13.64%
	VR headsets consumers	10	45.45%

The semi-structured interviews, mainly face-to-face include individual interviews and group interviews (no more than five people). The process is as follows:

(1) One day before the interview, the interviewers distributed the same interview guide to the interviewees and informed them that the interview would be conducted according to the content of the interview guide. The respondents were asked to familiarize themselves with the questions in the interview guide.

(2) Based on the Behavioral Event Interview (BEI) developed by Dr. McClelland, this interview collected detailed information on the specific behaviors and psychological activities of the interviewees in representative events by asking a series of questions [40]. Through a comparative analysis of the collected information, key elements can be found. According to BEI, combined with the specific situation of VR headsets, the interviewers developed the following interview guide:
   - ① What do you think of the quality of the VR headset?
   - ② What memorable events do you have when using the VR headset?
   - ③ In your opinion, what aspects of the quality of the VR headset must be guaranteed?
   - ④ What needs to be improved in the quality of the VR headset?
   - ⑤ What is the most satisfactory thing when you use the VR headset?
   - ⑥ What is the most unsatisfactory thing when you use the VR headset?
   - ⑦ What other attributes do you think high-quality VR headsets should have in the future?

(3) In the interview, firstly the interviewers introduce the purpose of the interview to the interviewees and explain freedom of speech in that the interview contents are only used for this academic research.

(4) One interviewer talked to the interviewee about the questions in the interview guide, and the other interviewer wrote down the contents of the conversation.

(5) The interview recordings were transcribed into text and the results were proofread.

(6) Grounded theory was used in this study. Grounded theory is a scientific and rigorous qualitative research method, which was first proposed by Glaser and Strauss in 1967 [41]. Through grounded research, the interview records were coded, analyzed, and iteratively synthesized to obtain 11 preliminary perceived quality elements of VR headsets. Rooted theory studies flow charts is shown in Figure 3:

(7) TPQ is more inclined to the inherent attributes of products and services. VPQ is more related to the external attributes of products and services, such as brand image, product reputation, customer emotional judgment, value, advertising, and after-sales service [31]. The organizers divided the initial perceived quality elements of the 11 VR headsets into TPQ and VPQ. The results shown in Table 2 are as follows:
(8) The organizers further classified the initial perceived quality elements of 11 VR headsets, and divided them into three levels, as shown in Table 3:

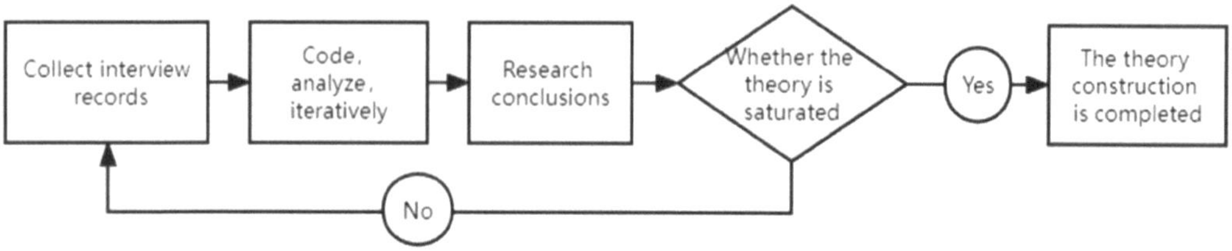

Figure 3. Rooted theory studies flow charts.

Table 2. Preliminary perceived quality elements of VR headsets.

Elements	TPQ	Elements	VPQ
1	Visual angle	1	Immersion
2	Resolution	2	Dizziness
3	Refresh rate	3	After-sales service
4	Hardware compatibility	4	Brand reputation
5	VR resource quality		
6	Tracking accuracy		
7	Battery life		

Table 3. Preliminary perceived quality framework of VR headsets.

Level I	Level II	Level III
Sight	Picture clarity	Visual angle
		Resolution
	Picture fluency	Refresh rate
		Tracking accuracy
Somatosensory	Positive feeling	Immersion
	Negative feelings	Dizziness
Durability	Hardware durability	Battery life
	Durable software	VR resource quality
Usability	Hardware usability	Hardware compatibility
Sociality	Goodwill	Brand reputation
	Service	After-sales service

3.2. Big Data Statistics on Consumption

Product comments are significant consumer feedback data. They are the link between products and consumers, implying valuable consumer feedback information [34]. This step focused on mining information beneficial to product design, production, and sales from a large amount of review data.

3.2.1. VR Headsets Consumption Big Data Collection

To understand the elements of the VR headsets' quality framework more comprehensively and objectively, this study screened consumer reviews of mainstream VR headset products with more than 100 reviews on Taobao, JDOM, Amazon, and other major e-commerce platforms. A total of 56,419 reviews were collected (as of 30 March 2023). Comments covered 15 brands and 35 models, as shown in Table 4:

Table 4. Brands and models of VR headsets.

No.	Brand	Product Model
1	DP	DPVR E3
2		DPVR E4
3	GOOVIS	GOOVIS G2-X
4		GOOVIS G3
5		GOOVIS Lite
6		GOOVIS Pro-X
7	HP	HP Reverb G2
8	HTC	HTC Vive CE
9		HTC Vive Cosmos
10		HTC Vive Focus3
11		HTC Vive Pro 1.0
12		HTC Vive Pro 2.0
13		HTC ViveFlow
14	HUAWEI	HUAWEI VR GIASS
15	iQIYI	iQIYI 2Pro
16		iQIYI 4KVR
17		iQIYI Dream Pro
18	Microsoft	Microsoft HoloLens 2
19	NOLO	NOLO X1 6DoF
20	Oculus/Meta	Oculus/Meta Quest 2
21		Oculus/Meta Quest 2 Pro
22		Oculus/Meta Rift S
23	Pico	Pico 4
24		Pico 4 Pro
25		Pico Neo2 Lite
26		Pico Neo3
27	Pimax	Pimax 8KX DMAS
28		Pimax Vision 8K Plus
29		Pimax Vision 8KX
30	SAMSUNG	SAMSUNG Gear 4KVR
31	Skyworth	Skyworth-S801
32		Skyworth-S802
33		Skyworth-V901
34	Valve	Valve Index1.0
35		Valve Index2.0

3.2.2. Big Data Cleaning for Data on VR Headset Consumption

In this study, UTF-8 was used in the coding format. For all crawling data, non-text parts were removed, including new line characters, punctuation marks, web links, HTML tags, etc., and regular expressions were used to filter them. Comments that were too short or did not contribute to the study were deleted from 56,419 samples. In addition, during the process of data collation, the application template comments published by a suspected robot were deleted. After cleaning up the above data, 31,075 of the remaining valid comment data were further processed. Flow chart showing big data cleaning for VR headset consumption data is shown in Figure 4:

3.2.3. Word Frequency Analysis of VR Headsets' Consumption Big Data Based on TF-IDF

The word frequency can reflect the importance of this word in the text and present the content of the text provider's attention [42]. By extracting those high-frequency words from the consumers' reviews of VR headsets, we can obtain the focus of consumers on VR headsets, which can deeply explore the perceived quality framework of VR headsets.

Term frequency–inverse document frequency (TF-IDF) is a common statistical method. TF is the frequency of words in the traditional sense, meaning the frequency of a word in the text. IDF is "inverse text frequency", which means that when a word appears very frequently in all texts, such as a preposition or a modal auxiliary, it may not be as important as some less frequent words. With Jieba participle software data segmentation and, subsequently, Rost software for word segmentation of data statistics, the study obtained consumers' assessments of VR headsets through high-frequency words. Cloud diagram showing high-frequency words is shown in Figure 5:

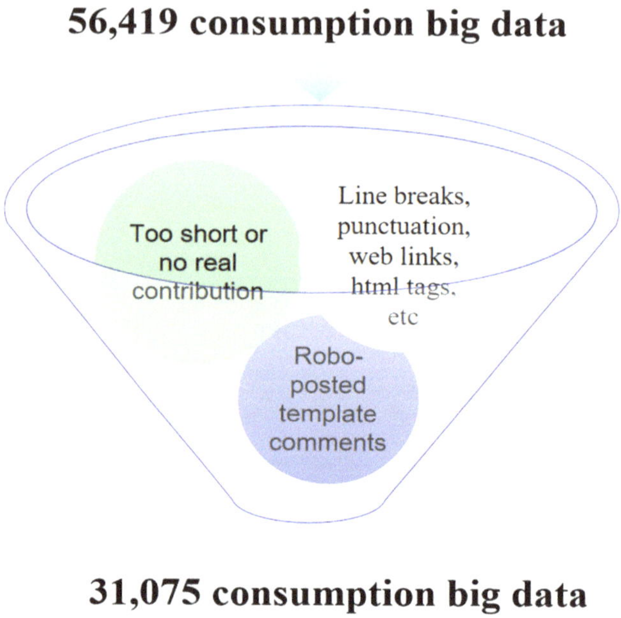

Figure 4. Flow chart showing big data cleaning for VR headset consumption data.

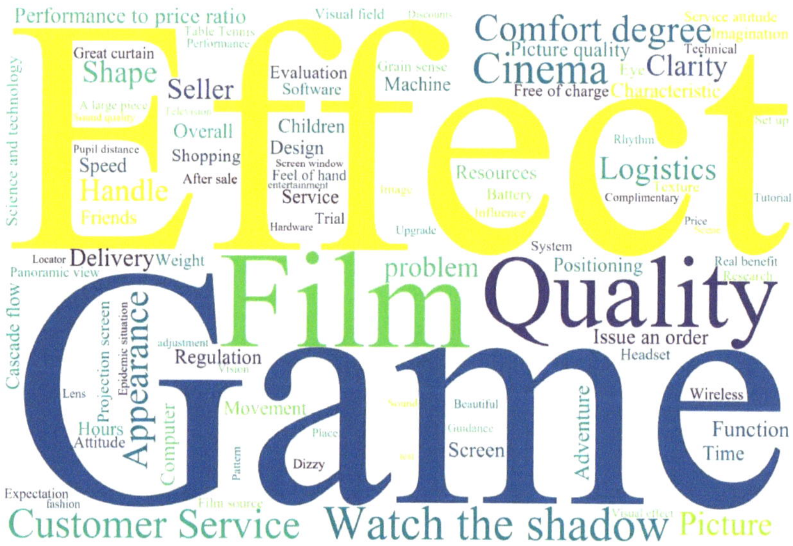

Figure 5. Cloud diagram showing high-frequency words.

3.3. Classification of High-frequency Words by the Delphi Method

By screening, cleaning, and merging high-frequency words, this study produced a high-frequency vocabulary list of the top 100 ranking words related to VR headset consumption. A total of 22 interviewees who had previously participated in semi-structured interviews were invited to form an expert group and asked to evaluate these high-frequency words and categorize them into the preliminary perceptual quality framework. High-frequency words related to VR headset use are shown in Table 5:

Table 5. High-frequency words related to VR headset use.

No.	Words	Frequency	No.	Words	Frequency
1	Game	7787	51	Trial	429
2	Effect	7571	52	Great curtain	428
3	Film	4209	53	Headset	424
4	Quality	3930	54	Wireless	422
5	Watch the shadow	3829	55	Texture	408
6	Cinema	3271	56	Visual field	400
7	Customer Service	2909	57	Service attitude	397
8	Comfort degree	2397	58	Grain sense	382
9	Appearance	2210	59	Feel of hand	380
10	Picture	1836	60	System	354
11	Logistics	1729	61	Panoramic view	349
12	Handle	1609	62	After sale	334
13	Shape	1608	63	Influence	324
14	Clarity	1472	64	Expectation	321
15	problem	1369	65	Technical	318
16	Seller	1366	66	Research	318
17	Delivery	959	67	Film source	313
18	Performance to price ratio	922	68	Table Tennis	301
19	Adventure	910	69	Dizzy	296
20	Function	903	70	Set up	293
21	Screen	837	71	Real benefit	286
22	Issue an order	795	72	Image	275
23	Picture quality	767	73	A large piece	272
24	Computer	754	74	Rhythm	266
25	Regulation	753	75	Lens	259
26	Resources	746	76	Performance	256
27	Time	745	77	Beautiful	247
28	Characteristic	745	78	Guidance	245
29	Speed	742	79	Epidemic situation	242
30	Overall	741	80	Place	242
31	Positioning	709	81	Visual effect	238
32	Service	688	82	Complimentary	231
33	Movement	684	83	Tutorial	231
34	Friends	678	84	Sound	229
35	Hours	678	85	Upgrade	225
36	Machine	675	86	Vision	224
37	Children	666	87	Pattern	223
38	Cascade flow	658	88	fashion	221
39	Design	655	89	Pupil distance	220
40	Evaluation	563	90	adjustment	207
41	Shopping	562	91	Television	202
42	Science and technology	536	92	Price	200
43	Projection screen	521	93	Discounts	197
44	Weight	500	94	Scene	196
45	Free of charge	485	95	test	194
46	Software	485	96	Sound quality	192
47	Eye	478	97	entertainment	187
48	Imagination	455	98	Screen window	186
49	Attitude	453	99	Hardware	185
50	Battery	439	100	Locator	184

The organizer collected and summarized the classification results of all interviewees in the first round and then sent them to each interviewee, asking them to compare their different opinions with others in the first round of evaluation, modify their opinions and judgments, and form the results of the second round of evaluation. The organizer then collected and summarized the results of the second round of evaluation of all interviewees and sent them to each interviewee, asking them to compare their different opinions with others in the second round of evaluation, modify their opinions and judgments, and form the results of the third round of evaluation. Finally, after three rounds of assessment, none of the interviewees changed their opinions. Organizers summarized the results of the third round of evaluation, and they integrated and unified the naming of the results, classifying words such as "friends" and "children" into the same category; however, some respondents used words such as "socializing", while others used words such as "social relation". The organizer returned to the original consumption review information, combed the content when referring to friends, children, and other words, and found that most of these words were mentioned enough times to evaluate feelings towards VR headsets with friends and children. Therefore, the organizer determined that this category would be labeled as "socializing". After the final evaluation results were integrated with Tables 2 and 3, a list of the perceived quality elements (Table 6) and the VR headsets' perceived quality framework (Table 7) screened by industry experts and consumers was obtained. Table 6 added five new elements: Multifunctionality, Pupillary distance regulation, Equipment weight, Material, and Socializing. There were 6 items in Level I of Table 7, and Compatibility was added. There were 12 items in Level II, newly including the Myopia application, Wear suitable, Software durability, and Interaction.

Table 6. Perceived quality elements of VR headsets.

Elements	TPQ	Elements	VPQ
1	Visual angle	1	Immersion
2	Resolution	2	Dizziness
3	Refresh rate	3	After-sales service
4	Hardware compatibility	4	Brand reputation
5	Multifunctionality	5	VR resource quality
6	Tracking accuracy	6	Socializing
7	Pupillary distance regulation		
8	Battery life		
9	Equipment weight		
10	Material		

Table 7. Perceived quality framework of VR headsets.

Level I	Level II	Level III
Sight	Picture clarity	Visual angle
		Resolution
	Picture fluency	Refresh rate
		Tracking accuracy
Somatosensory	Positive feeling	Immersion
	Negative feeling	Dizziness
Compatibility	Myopia application	Pupillary distance regulation
	Wear suitable	Equipment weight
Durability	Hardware durability	Material
		Battery life
	Software durability	VR resource quality
Usability	Hardware usability	Hardware compatibility
		Multifunctionality
Sociality	Goodwill	Brand reputation
	Service	After-sale service
	Interaction	Socializing

3.4. PQAIR of VR Headsets

Bi (2004) proposed a set of processes according to the order of many elements that affect the formation and degree of customer-perceived quality: firstly, study the significant stages and elements; then, determine the critical elements of customer-perceived quality from the customer perspective [43]. This study ranked the importance of perceived quality attributes of VR headsets by analyzing the questionnaire results.

3.4.1. Questionnaire Design

The Likert scale is a compound measurement developed by American social psychologist Likert in 1932. It attempts to improve the level of measurement in social research by using standardized answer classifications in a questionnaire survey and to determine the relative intensity of different items. The Richter scale is a single stimulus–response model (single stimulus–response format). Under the single stimulus–response model, subjects need to judge whether the topic description agrees with their characteristics according to the description of topic and then choose the degree of conformity with themselves on the Richter scale, which usually ranges from very disagreeable to very agreeable.

To ensure the smooth progress of the survey, during the process of questionnaire design, the interviewees' answer experience was fully considered during the question design process. Because there were many items in the main part of the questionnaire, to ensure the reliability of the analysis and to obtain better results, a level 10 Rickett scale (10-point Likert scale) was used to indicate the extent to which investigators pay attention to the project (1 was the lowest and 10 was the most significant).

3.4.2. Questionnaire Distribution and Collection

The questionnaire was mainly administered offline and online and was completed by VR industry practitioners, VR enthusiasts, and consumers. The interviewees who participated in the survey had either purchased or learned about VR products. A total of 383 questionnaires were distributed. After further screening, 340 valid questionnaires were obtained, with an effective rate of 88.77%. The demographic data of the respondents to the questionnaire are presented in Tables 8 and 9.

Table 8. PQAIR of VR Headsets.

Visual angle	1	2	3	4	5	6	7	8	9	10
Resolution	1	2	3	4	5	6	7	8	9	10
Refresh rate	1	2	3	4	5	6	7	8	9	10
Hardware compatibility	1	2	3	4	5	6	7	8	9	10
VR resource quality	1	2	3	4	5	6	7	8	9	10
Multifunctionality	1	2	3	4	5	6	7	8	9	10
Tracking accuracy	1	2	3	4	5	6	7	8	9	10
Pupillary distance regulation	1	2	3	4	5	6	7	8	9	10
Battery life	1	2	3	4	5	6	7	8	9	10
Equipment weight	1	2	3	4	5	6	7	8	9	10
Material	1	2	3	4	5	6	7	8	9	10
Socializing	1	2	3	4	5	6	7	8	9	10
Immersion	1	2	3	4	5	6	7	8	9	10
Dizziness	1	2	3	4	5	6	7	8	9	10
Brand reputation	1	2	3	4	5	6	7	8	9	10
After-sale service	1	2	3	4	5	6	7	8	9	10

Table 9. Demographics of the PQAIR of VR headsets questionnaire.

Characteristic	Grouping	Frequency	Percentage
Gender	Male	234	68.82%
	Female	106	31.18%
Age	Under 18 years old	28	8.24%
	18–24 years old	91	26.76%
	25–35 years old	134	39.41%
	36–45 years old	69	20.29%
	46–55 years old	18	5.29%
Monthly income (RMB)	Less than 500 dollars	32	9.41%
	500–715 dollars	43	12.65%
	715–1000 dollars	79	23.24%
	1000–1285 dollars	87	25.59%
	1285 dollars and above	99	29.12%
Education level	High school or below	29	8.53%
	Junior college	95	27.94%
	Undergraduate	166	48.82%
	Graduate students and above	50	14.71%

3.4.3. Quantitative Analysis of Questionnaire Samples

Cronbach's α coefficient is one of the most commonly used reliability indicators, indicating the consistency of scores between items in a scale. The Cronbach's α coefficient of the questionnaire took advantage of the scale module of the SPSS 11.5 software. The SPSS reliability analysis results are presented in Table 10.

Table 10. The overall reliability analysis of the questionnaire.

Reliability Statistics	
Cronbach's Alpha	**N of Items**
0.844	16

From the reliability statistics, it can be concluded that the analysis results were acceptable.

The modified correlation coefficient (CITC) was used in the reliability analysis to purify the measurement indicators, detect the impact of each element on the overall reliability, and find elements with problems in the questionnaire design. Then, the study used Cronbach's α coefficient to test the reliability of the questionnaire again. When using CITC-modified reliability screening items, the following criteria were used to identify problematic elements:

The revised item correlation coefficient CITC (the correlation coefficient between each item score and the remaining item score) was less than 0.3; if the item was deleted, the α value, indicating overall reliability, increased.

CITC analysis was performed on all 16 items. The reliability analysis results for all indicators are presented in Table 11.

From the analysis results of the CITC index, the CITC value of most items was higher than the standard value of 0.3. Among them, the CITC value of pupillary distance regulation was 0.200, and the CITC value of hardware compatibility was 0.064. The CITC values of the two items were less than the standard value of 0.3 and, after deleting these two items, the overall Cronbach's α value improved. According to the CITC deletion principle, this indicator can be deleted. After deletion, the results for Cronbach's α are displayed in Table 12.

After analyzing the two items, pupillary distance regulation and hardware compatibility were deleted. Their CITC values were lower than the certified value. This can be explained by the mean variance of 340 valid questionnaires of these two items, as shown in Table 13.

Table 11. Analysis of the items' CITC reliability.

Item-Total Statistics				
	Scale Mean if Item Deleted	Scale Variance if Item Deleted	Corrected Item-Total Correlation	Cronbach's Alpha if Item Deleted
Visual_angle	87.83	169.231	0.333	0.841
Pupillary_distance_regulation	88.78	168.279	0.2	0.854
Resources	86.24	155.422	0.724	0.822
Brand_reputation	87.22	155.264	0.784	0.82
Resolution	87.54	164.119	0.413	0.837
Immersion	85.43	159.414	0.676	0.825
After_sales_service	87.66	154.085	0.607	0.826
Material	88.71	152.648	0.647	0.824
Multifunctionality	89.44	165.22	0.407	0.838
Refresh_rate	87.64	160.029	0.437	0.836
Tracking_accuracy	86.94	163.252	0.406	0.838
Equipment_weight	87.84	167.182	0.391	0.838
Dizziness	87.59	156.543	0.615	0.826
Baterry_life	88.08	162.569	0.472	0.834
Socializing	89.02	163.793	0.418	0.837
Hardware_compatibility	88.12	177.365	0.064	0.856

Table 12. Revised overall reliability statistics.

Reliability Statistics	
Cronbach's Alpha	N of Items
0.868	14

Table 13. Mean and variance statistics of deleted items.

Item Statistics			
	Mean	Std. Deviation	Number
Pupillary_distance_regulation	4.83	1.995	340
Hardware_compatibility	5.48	1.588	340

As for pupillary distance regulation, the interviewees disagreed, and they judged the importance of this item based on the basis of whether they were myopic. As a result, interviewees without myopia thought this item was not significant, while those with myopia thought it was significant. The survey results are subjective, and this item is not suitable for questionnaire design.

For hardware compatibility, interviewees also showed large differences. We speculate that the reason may be that the condition of the hardware owned by interviewees was quite different; e.g., the hardware configuration of the host was different. Some hosts are compatible with each other. These kind of interviewees are not troubled by poor compatibility.

On the premise of reliability, the study further used the KMO test and Bartlett spherical test to analyze the structural validity of the questionnaire samples. The results are as presented in Table 14.

Table 14. KMO test and Bartlett spherical test.

KMO and Bartlett's Test		
Kaiser–Meyer–Olkin Measure of Sampling Adequacy.		**0.861**
Bartlett's Test of Sphericity	Approx. Chi-Square	2705.056
	Df	91
	Sig.	0

The KMO test is used to test the partial correlation of variable construction. The closer the KMO test value is to 1, the better the structural validity is. If the KMO test value is less than 0.5, the structural validity of the questionnaire sample is considered unacceptable. The KMO test value of the questionnaire sample after deleting the question item was 0.861, which indicated that the selected structural sample was suitable for factor analysis.

If the result of the Bartlett spherical test is less than 0.005, the spherical hypothesis is rejected, which indicates that there is a strong correlation between variables. The spherical test result of this questionnaire sample was 0; thus, we can infer that the questionnaire possessed good structural validity.

With the results of the Cronbach's α coefficient, KMO test, and Bartlett spherical test, we concluded that the design and results of the hypothetical variables in the questionnaire were consistent and credible.

4. Results

According to the scores for the importance of each index in the questionnaire sample, we used the mean analysis method of perceived quality attribute importance ranking (PQAIR) to rank the VR headsets from high to low, as shown in Table 15.

Table 15. PQAIR of VR headsets (after removing distortion elements).

Rank	Element	Attribute	Mean Value	Variance	N
1	Immersion	Somatosensory	8.18	1.264	340
2	VR resource quality	Durability	7.36	1.396	340
3	Tracking accuracy	Sight	6.67	1.612	340
4	Brand reputation	Sociality	6.39	1.311	340
5	Resolution	Sight	6.06	1.526	340
6	Dizziness	Somatosensory	6.01	1.538	340
7	Refresh rate	Sight	5.96	1.76	340
8	After-sale service	Sociality	5.95	1.7	340
9	Visual angle	Sight	5.77	1.337	340
10	Equipment weight	Compatibility	5.77	1.344	340
11	Battery life	Durability	5.53	1.482	340
12	Material	Durability	4.89	1.693	340
13	Socializing	Sociality	4.58	1.537	340
14	Multifunctionality	Usability	4.17	1.482	340

The PQAIR of the studied VR headsets can be obtained through the study of questionnaire samples. The average value of each element represents the average score of the element in the whole questionnaire sample. The higher the score, the higher the importance of attributes. Variance reflects the difference between each sample and the mean value. The higher the variance is, the greater the fluctuation of the element in the whole questionnaire sample; that is to say, the greater the difference between different interviewees for the element. The mean variance statistics are based on all 340 valid questionnaires.

5. Discussion

In the PQAIR of VR headsets, somatosensory immersion is the most important factor for manufacturers and consumers, because the VR headsets are essentially a system designed to improve immersion by installing wide field displays within the user's line of sight [44]. Somatosensory dizziness ranks sixth in importance; somatosensory dizziness refers to the limitation of VR headsets in terms of possible network disease, which may lead to headaches, nausea, and other symptoms. There are several terms for this phenomenon: motion sickness, simulator disease, and virtual reality disease [45]. When we compiled the big data statistics on the e-commerce website, we found that users frequently used words such as "immersive experience" when making positive comments while, when making negative comments, they often described their dizziness and discomfort after using VR headsets.

In addition to the somatosensory attributes, the line-of-sight attribute is an important attribute that affects the quality of perception. The elements following the line-of-sight attribute, in terms of importance, included tracking accuracy (third), resolution (fifth), refresh rate (seventh), and visual angle (ninth). Tracking accuracy in VR headsets usually means that the system can accurately capture the trajectory of the consumers' heads. In many VR headset game usage scenarios, the movement of the head determines the direction and location in which the consumers can see the virtual scene. If the tracking accuracy is low and there is a mismatch between vision and the vestibule system, users who wear VR headsets will feel dizzy [46]. The difference between the motion time captured by the consumers through the sensor and when the image appears on the headsets makes the motion-to-photon (MTP) and offset feel stronger. The long MTP delay is a significant reason for why consumers feel sick and carsick [47]. The higher the resolution of the product, the sharper, more detailed, and more realistic the image displays. The refresh rate is also known as the frame rate (frames per second), which refers to the number of refresh times of images on the screen. The refresh rate of the mainstream VR headsets in the current market is generally between 80–120 Hz. The higher the resolution, the smoother and more realistic the virtual reality experience. Whether watching movies or playing games, resolution and refresh rate are significant guarantees for providing consumers with a high-quality visual experience. Visual angle determines the angle of the visible area when the consumer uses the VR headsets; it determines the range of images that the consumer can see. The wider the image range, the stronger the consumer's immersion. One eye has a field of view of about 160 degrees (lateral) times 130 degrees (vertical). The combined binocular field of view is about 200 degrees (laterally) multiplied by 130 degrees (vertically); the overlap is 120 degrees. The perspective of the VR headsets on the market is generally between 80 degrees and 120 degree, and the visual angle of some products, such as the Pimax Vision 8K, can even reach 200 degrees. Tethered VR headsets and all-in-one VR headsets, as wearable devices, have a small optical display in front of at least one wearer's eyes [48]. Visual experience interaction is the most basic human–computer interaction experience between VR headsets and consumers. Therefore, to improve the experience of human–computer interaction, VR headsets must pay attention to consumers' positive sight experience when using VR headsets.

From the perspective of sociality, including brand reputation (fourth in rank), after-sale service (ranked eight), and socializing (ranked thirteenth), the brand of VR headsets has a positive impact on product value creation [49], and a good brand reputation can significantly enhance the perceived value of VR headsets. For this kind of technology product, in addition to the purchase evaluation of the product on electronic commerce websites, consumers can find commodity evaluations and consumer experiences on domestic social media platforms such as WeChat and Weibo as well as on word-of-mouth websites such as Meituan Dianping. In addition to offline VR headset exhibitions, video sites such as Bilibili and YouTube are significant channels for accumulating brand reputation. The impact of the after-sale service on consumers is mainly reflected in the warranty strategies provided for different products. When consumers choose foreign brands, the impact of the after-sale service is especially more notable. Within the same country, different brands often have little difference in after-sales service strategies. The elements of VR headsets in socializing are mainly focused on VR social networks and the VR online game scene. Currently, VR headsets are combined with social network services and consumers can interact in VR-based social network services (SNS) as avatars [50]. Furthermore, some VR-based chat products have been created, but the majority of interviewees in this study had not learned about these products; most of the knowledge surrounding socializing focused on VR online game scenarios. In the VR online game scene, the socializing element has not received a great deal of attention. On the one hand, the interviewees think that the mainstream VR headsets in the current market are more mature in the network online, and the online speed and online delay usually depend on the network situation of the consumers, rather than the VR headsets themselves. On the other hand, in VR online games, socializing depends more on the optimization of the game itself than on the VR device. In summary, with regard to socializing, products with good brand reputations often have better perceived quality, which is also the element that consumers pay more attention to when choosing VR products; consumers pay more attention to products with a warranty period compared to products without one. Products that can provide stable quality assurance for some time have more advantages. Human–computer interaction is highly correlated with service experience [51]. The service experience before and after the use of VR headsets also affects the experience of the consumer's human–computer interaction. For socializing, many people use VR headsets for social interaction, which increases the scene of human–computer interaction while increasing the fun of the use of products, but consumers generally believe that socializing depends more on the network environment and VR multi-person interaction software optimization, rather than VR headsets themselves, with interviewees believing that different VR headsets make little difference in socializing.

Regarding durability, this paper studied durable software and hardware durability, in which durable software (ranked second) mainly refers to VR resource quality, while hardware durability includes battery life (ranked eleventh) and material (ranked twelfth). In this study, VR resource quality ranked second and was a significant part of the perceived quality of VR headsets. The human–computer interaction between consumers and VR headsets is concentrated in three major content areas: VR videos, VR games, and VR industry applications. Different brands usually have their resources exclusively in VR videos and VR games. When consumers choose different brands of VR headsets, they tend to pay more attention to the exclusive VR resources of the brand, which are only available in the corresponding brand's App Store. These exclusive VR resources tend to have high game quality, and players who like these games must purchase the corresponding VR headset to play these exclusive games, which are not carried by the app stores for other brands. Experiencing the unique content brought by VR technology is also the purpose of interpersonal interaction between consumers and VR headsets. VR videos and VR games are the human–computer interaction scenes most frequently used by consumers. However, the VR industry is still in the stage of rapid development. Industries such as tourism and education, sports entertainment, real estate, medical treatment, etc., have now begun to try applying VR technology, e.g., Stewart Birrell (2022) using a tethered VR headset device to allow participants to use controller navigation in the virtual environment of urban airports [52]. Virtual reality technology is now used to treat sensorimotor disorders in medical environments [53]. These industry applications represent the future development direction of VR headsets, which will become more comfortable and more suitable for multiple environments. The aspects of hardware durability, battery life, and material had some influence on the perceived quality of the interviewees. The battery life of mainstream VR headsets is generally about three hours while, in general, the interviewees usually use VR headsets continuously for between half an hour and one hour.

More than half of the interviewees said they had a more obvious sense of fatigue after half an hour of continuous use, and after more than one hour of continuous use, there was often a certain degree of discomfort; thus, three hours of battery life is usually adequate for consumers. The influence of material on durability is more focused on the performance of product features such as anti-fall, being waterproof, etc. To reduce the weight of VR headsets, most VR headsets use plastic fuselage, which also poses a higher challenge to the anti-fall ability of the product. However, due to the use of the environment, many interviewees also said that the material is not an element they focus on. In this study, interviewees paid more attention to durable software than the impact of hardware durability on perceived value. The perceived quality element of compatibility equipment weight only ranked 10th but was indicated to improve comfort. Sai Akhil Penumudi (2020) demonstrated that improper neck flexion torque and musculoskeletal load will cause discomfort when consumers use VR equipment [54]. Neck joint torque is significantly affected by mass and compatibility, which increases with the weight of VR headsets [55]. Therefore, equipment weight overload will cause musculoskeletal discomfort for consumers, affecting their personal interaction experience. In the study, interviewees generally said that the impact of equipment weight on compatibility was more focused on the ergonomic design of products. VR headsets with good equipment weight tend to be more comfortable to wear, and longer use does not easily produce fatigue; on the other hand, products with poor equipment weight are more likely to be uncomfortable to wear.

Finally, the perceived quality element of multifunctionality in usability ranked last. The study found that almost all interviewees had some knowledge of PC and mobile operations, which enabled them to be started faster when using VR headsets. At the same time, the UI interface of most of the operating systems used in VR headsets is flattened, which makes both the menu bar and icon display more intuitive, making it easy for consumers to find most of the features they want. Although some new VR industry applications or games still have a learning threshold for consumers, multifunctionality also creates more possibilities for VR headset consumers. For example, Woojoo Kim (2022) proposed VR headsets without additional equipment to satisfy consumers who wish to obtain experiential effects in virtual reality text input [56]. The development of multifunctionality in VR headsets is key to their future application scenarios and potential, and interviewees generally have a high degree of tolerance for it. Combined with the conclusions of this study, it can be further seen that in the field of commercial VR headsets, immersion, tracking accuracy, dizziness, and other elements related to distance sensing technology are more concern by consumers, while in optical sensing technology, consumers pay more attention to resolution, refresh rate, and visual angle. For tactile and mechanical sensors, consumers have not paid much attention, which means that the effect of technology investment in this area on promoting consumer purchases is not significant.

6. Conclusions

This paper discusses the importance ranking of the perceived quality factors of VR headsets, aiming to discuss and verify the rationality of the optimization of various sensing technologies from the perspective of the market and consumers. Different from most previous research perspectives, this study innovatively combines TPQ, VPQ, and big data statistical analysis technology, not only taking the views of VR headset industry experts and designers into consideration, but also considering the consumers' attitudes towards the VR headsets to study the perceived quality elements. Through this study, we obtained the importance ranking of different perceived quality elements. We concluded the importance ranks of different perceived quality factors in this research. For VR headset products, these quality factors include not only the future optimization direction of sensing technology but also the improvement suggestions about marketing, after-sales service, and so on. This is of great significance for VR headset manufacturers and designers to create market-competitive VR headsets.

In future research, we will continue to focus on the perceived quality of wearable devices, not only the VR headsets. There are two research directions in the future: one is to expand the research of consumer big data to the global e-commerce platform, strive to obtain a wider range of consumers' feedback on VR headsets, then analyze the consumer perception through machine learning algorithms; the other is to further subdivide the user groups and usage scenarios for the user's optimization suggestions for distance sensing technology and optical sensing technology, and study the sensitivity and acceptable range of specific users for various sensors in specific scenarios.

Author Contributions: Conceptualization, L.Z., S.L. and A.Y., methodology, Y.Y. and L.Z., software, Y.Y. and L.Z., validation, L.Z. and A.Y., formal analysis, Y.Y. and L.Z., investigation, Y.Y. and L.Z., resources, S.L. and A.Y., data curation, Y.Y. and L.Z., writing—original draft preparation, Y.Y. and L.Z., writing—review and editing, Y.Y., L.Z., S.L. and A.Y., visualization, S.L., supervision, S.L. and A.Y., project administration, Y.Y., funding acquisition, Y.Y. All authors have read and agreed to the published version of the manuscript.

Funding: This work is partially supported Sichuan University project funding 2023ZDPY-05 and Grant 18 AGL024 of the National Social Science Foundation's key project 'Value Management of Cultural Creativity Research, China.

Institutional Review Board Statement: Not applicable.

Informed Consent Statement: Written informed consent was obtained from all participants involved in the study.

Data Availability Statement: The data presented in this study are available on request from the corresponding author.

Conflicts of Interest: The authors declare no conflict of interest.

References

1. Li, J. Construction of Science Communication Model based on Human-computer interaction technology in 5G era. *Media Today* **2002**, *30*, 95–99.
2. Liu, X.X.; Zhang, J.; Hou, G.X.; Wang, Z.A. Virtual Reality and Its Application in Military. *IOP Conf. Ser. Earth Environ. Sci.* **2018**, *37*, 662–667. [CrossRef]
3. Lu, L. Research on the application of Virtual Reality Technology (VR) in the design of sample room. *Chang. Inf. Commun.* **2020**, *6*, 3.
4. Li, Z.R. Significance and Status quo of Virtual reality research. *Sci. Technol. Inf.* **2009**, *4*, 220.
5. Radianti, J.; Majchrzak, T.A.; Fromm, J.; Wohlgenannt, I. A systematic review of immersive virtual reality applications for higher education: Design elements, lessons learned, and research agenda. *Comput. Educ.* **2020**, *147*, 103778. [CrossRef]
6. Lu, S.; Li, R.; Jiao, J.; Kang, J.; Zhao, N.; Li, M. An Eye Gaze Tracking Method of Virtual Reality Headset Using A Single Camera and Multi-light Source. *J. Phys. Conf. Ser.* **2020**, *1518*, 012020. [CrossRef]
7. Xu, J.; Pan, J.; Cui, T.; Zhang, S.; Yang, Y.; Ren, T.-L. Recent Progress of Tactile and Force Sensors for Human–Machine Interaction. *Sensors* **2023**, *23*, 1868. [CrossRef]
8. Dempsey, P. The Teardown: HTC Vive virtual reality headset. *Eng. Technol.* **2016**, *11*, 70–71. [CrossRef]
9. Ross, D. The Teardown: Razer OSVR HDK 2 virtual reality headset. *Eng. Technol.* **2016**, *11*, 80–81.
10. Jonathan, N.T.; Bachri, M.R.; Wijaya, E.; Ramdhan, D.; Chowanda, A. The efficacy of virtual reality exposure therapy (VRET) with extra intervention for treating PTSD symptoms. *Procedia Comput. Sci.* **2023**, *216*, 252–259. [CrossRef]
11. Demeco, A.; Zola, L.; Frizziero, A.; Martini, C.; Palumbo, A.; Foresti, R.; Buccino, G.; Costantino, C. Immersive Virtual Reality in Post-Stroke Rehabilitation: A Systematic Review. *Sensors* **2023**, *23*, 1712. [CrossRef] [PubMed]
12. Hsu, K.S. Application of a Virtual Reality Entertainment System with Human-Machine Sensor Device. *J. Appl. Sci.* **2011**, *11*, 2145–2153. [CrossRef]
13. Fang, J. Research on the development status of VR Education in China. *Times Educ.* **2016**, *21*, 200.
14. Kesilmis, I. The Effect of Using Virtual Reality Headset on Dynamic Balance and Reaction Time of Handball Players. *Ambient. Sci.* **2020**, *7*, 20–27. [CrossRef]
15. Chen, L. Application Analysis of VR Technology in Clothing Customization. In *Progress in Textile Science and Technology*; China Textile Industry Association: Chengdu, China, 2008; pp. 87–89.
16. Mokhtar, M.B. Virtual Reality Usability and Accessibility for Cultural Heritage Practices: Challenges Mapping and Recommendations. *Electronics* **2021**, *10*, 397.
17. LaValle, S.M.; Yershova, A.; Katsev, M.; Antonov, M. Head tracking for the Oculus Rift. In Proceedings of the 2014 IEEE International Conference on Robotics and Automation (ICRA), Hong Kong, China, 31 May–7 June 2014.
18. Evangelakos, D.; Mara, M. Extended TimeWarp latency compensation for virtual reality. In Proceedings of the 20th ACM SIGGRAPH Symposium on Interactive 3D Graphics and Games, Redmond, WA, USA, 27–28 February 2016; pp. 193–194. [CrossRef]
19. Saga, S.; Kimoto, R.; Kaguchi, K. Spatiotemporal Thermal Control Effects on Thermal Grill Illusion. *Sensors* **2022**, *23*, 414. [CrossRef]
20. Mamone, V.; Ferrari, V.; D'amato, R.; Condino, S.; Cattari, N.; Cutolo, F. Head-Mounted Projector for Manual Precision Tasks: Performance Assessment. *Sensors* **2023**, *23*, 3494. [CrossRef]
21. Olson, J.C.; Jacoby, J. Resrarch of Perceiving Quality. *J. Emerg. Concepts Mark.* **1972**, *9*, 220–226.
22. Wheatley, J.J.; Chiu, J.; Goldman, A. Physical Quality, Price, And Perceptions of Product Quality: Implications for Retailers. *J. Retail.* **1981**, *57*, 100–116.
23. Zeithaml, V.A.; Berry, L.L.; Parasuraman, A. Communication and Control Processes in the Delivery of Service Quality. *J. Mark.* **1988**, *52*, 35–48. [CrossRef]
24. Valarie, A.; Zeithaml, V.A. Consumer Perceptions of Price, Quality, and Value: A Means-End Model and Synthesis of Evidence. *J. Mark.* **1988**, *52*, 2–22.
25. Tsiotsou, R. The role of perceived product quality and overall satisfaction on purchase intentions. *Int. J. Consum. Stud.* **2006**, *30*, 207–217. [CrossRef]
26. Gronroo, C. From Marketing Mix to Relationship Marketing: Towards a Paradigm Shift in Marketing. *Asia-Aust. Mark. J.* **1994**, *2*, 4–20. [CrossRef]

27. Wu, P.X. The impact of perceived quality and perceived risk on private brand purchase intention. *China's Circ. Econ.* **2012**, *26*, 83–89.
28. Gao, Z.; Jiang, R.C. The Effects of Consumption Scenario and perceived Quality on Product Premium: An Empirical Study Based on Vending machines. *J. Beijing Technol. Bus. Univ. (Soc. Sci. Ed.)* **2020**, *35*, 15–27.
29. Dodds, W.B.; Monroe, K.B.; Grewal, D. Effects of Price, Brand, and Store Information on Buyers' Product Evaluations. *J. Mark. Res.* **1991**, *28*, 307–319. [CrossRef]
30. Burnkrant, R.E. Cue utilization in product perception. *J. Consum. Res.* **1978**, *5*, 724–729.
31. Stylidis, K.; Wickman, C.; Söderberg, R. Defining Perceived Quality in the Automotive Industry: An Engineering Approach. *Procedia CIRP* **2015**, *36*, 165–170. [CrossRef]
32. Chatterjee, P. Online Reviews: Do Consumers Use Them? *Adv. Consum. Res.* **2001**, *28*, 129–134.
33. Decker, R.; Trusov, M. Estimating aggregate consumer preferences from online product reviews. *Int. J. Res. Mark.* **2010**, *27*, 293–307. [CrossRef]
34. Zhang, L.; Wu, L.; Mattila, A.S. Online Review. *J. Travel Res.* **2015**, *7*, e3–e5.
35. Stylidis, K.; Wickman, C.; Söderberg, R. Perceived quality of products: A framework and attributes ranking method. *J. Eng. Des.* **2019**, *31*, 37–67. [CrossRef]
36. Yang, W. Application of perceived Quality in the Development of Passenger car products. *Beijing Automob.* **2016**, *1*, 36–40.
37. Haskins, A.J.; Mentch, J.; Botch, T.L. Active vision in immersive, 360° real-world environments. *Sci. Rep.* **2020**, *10*, 14304. [CrossRef] [PubMed]
38. Han, X.H.; Xu, M.; Shao, J.Y. Application research of VR glasses suitable for mass fitness. *Comput. Knowl. Technol.* **2021**, *17*, 126–128.
39. Tarr, B.; Slater, M.; Cohen, E. Synchrony and social connection in immersive Virtual Reality. *Sci. Rep.* **2018**, *8*, 3693. [CrossRef]
40. McClelland, D.C. Testing for competence rather than for "intelligence". *Am. Psychol.* **1973**, *28*, 1–14. [CrossRef]
41. Wagner, H.R.; Glaser, B.G.; Strauss, A.L. The Discovery of Grounded Theory: Strategies for Qualitative Research. *Soc. Forces* **1967**, *46*, 555. [CrossRef]
42. Rossolatos, G. Negative brand meaning co-creation in social media brand communities: A laddering approach using NVivo. *Psychol. Mark.* **2019**, *36*, 1249–1266. [CrossRef]
43. Bi, X.M. Research on Customer Perceived Quality. *J. Huazhong Agric. Univ. (Soc. Sci. Ed.)* **2004**, *3*, 42–45.
44. Azuma, R.; Baillot, Y.; Behringer, R.; Feiner, S.; Julier, S.; MacIntyre, B. Recent advances in augmented reality. *IEEE Comput. Graph. Appl.* **2001**, *21*, 34–47. [CrossRef]
45. Sawada, T.; Uda, H.; Suzuki, A.; Tomori, K.; Ohno, K.; Iga, H.; Okita, Y.; Fujita, Y. The Pilot Study of the Hazard Perception Test for Evaluation of the Driver's Skill Using Virtual Reality. *Electronics* **2021**, *10*, 1114. [CrossRef]
46. Choi, S.-W.; Lee, S.; Seo, M.-W.; Kang, S.-J. Time Sequential Motion-to-Photon Latency Measurement System for Virtual Reality Head-Mounted Displays. *Electronics* **2018**, *7*, 171. [CrossRef]
47. Hazarika, A.; Rahmati, M. Towards an Evolved Immersive Experience: Exploring 5G- and Beyond-Enabled Ultra-Low-Latency Communications for Augmented and Virtual Reality. *Sensors* **2023**, *23*, 3682. [CrossRef]
48. Bal, M.; Benders, J.; Dhondt, S.; Vermeerbergen, L. Head-worn displays and job content: A systematic literature review. *Appl. Ergon.* **2021**, *91*, 103285. [CrossRef] [PubMed]
49. Utami, H.N.; Sadeli, A.H.; Perdana, T. Customer value creation of fresh tomatoes through branding and packaging as customer perceived quality. *J. Int. Soc. Southeast Asian Agric. Sci.* **2016**, *22*, 123–136.
50. Schroeder, R. Social Interaction in Virtual Environments: Key Issues, Common Themes, and a Framework for Research. In *The Social Life of Avatars*; Computer Supported Cooperative Work Book Series; Springer: London, UK, 2002; pp. 1–18. [CrossRef]
51. Tung, V.W.S.; Law, R. The potential for tourism and hospitality experience research in human-robot interactions. *Int. J. Contemp. Hosp. Manag.* **2017**, *29*, 2498–2513. [CrossRef]
52. Birrell, S.; Payre, W.; Zdanowicz, K.; Herriotts, P. Urban air mobility infrastructure design: Using virtual reality to capture consumer experience within the world's first urban airport. *Appl. Ergon.* **2022**, *105*, 103843. [CrossRef]
53. Faity, G.; Sidahmed, Y.; Laffont, I.; Froger, J. Quantififcation and Rehabilitation of Unilateral Spatial Neglect in Immersive Virtual Reality: A Validation Study in Healthy Subjects. *Sensors* **2023**, *23*, 3481. [CrossRef]
54. Penumudi, S.A.; Kuppam, V.A.; Kim, J.H.; Hwang, J. The effects of target location on musculoskeletal load, task performance, and subjective discomfort during virtual reality interactions. *Appl. Ergon.* **2019**, *84*, 103010. [CrossRef]
55. Chihara, T.; Seo, A. Evaluation of physical workload affected by mass and center of mass of head-mounted display. *Appl. Ergon.* **2018**, *68*, 204–212. [CrossRef] [PubMed]
56. Kim, W.; Xiong, S. Pseudo-haptics and self-haptics for freehand mid-air text entry in VR. *Appl. Ergon.* **2022**, *104*, 103819. [CrossRef] [PubMed]

sensors

Article

Exploring Gaze Dynamics in Virtual Reality through Multiscale Entropy Analysis

Sahar Zandi * and Gregory Luhan

Department of Architecture, Texas A&M University, College Station, TX 77843, USA; gregory.luhan@tamu.edu
* Correspondence: sahar.zandi@tamu.edu

Abstract: This study employs Multiscale Entropy (MSE) to analyze 5020 binocular eye movement recordings from 407 college-aged participants, as part of the GazeBaseVR dataset, across various virtual reality (VR) tasks to understand the complexity of user interactions. By evaluating the vertical and horizontal components of eye movements across tasks such as vergence, smooth pursuit, video viewing, reading, and random saccade, collected at 250 Hz using an ET-enabled VR headset, this research provides insights into the predictability and complexity of gaze patterns. Participants were recorded up to six times over a 26-month period, offering a longitudinal perspective on eye movement behavior in VR. MSE's application in this context aims to offer a deeper understanding of user behavior in VR, highlighting potential avenues for interface optimization and user experience enhancement. The results suggest that MSE can be a valuable tool in creating more intuitive and immersive VR environments by adapting to users' gaze behaviors. This paper discusses the implications of these findings for the future of VR technology development, emphasizing the need for intuitive design and the potential for MSE to contribute to more personalized and comfortable VR experiences.

Keywords: virtual reality; time series analysis; eye movements; multiscale entropy; user experience; human sensing

Citation: Zandi, S.; Luhan, G. Exploring Gaze Dynamics in Virtual Reality through Multiscale Entropy Analysis. *Sensors* **2024**, *24*, 1781. https://doi.org/10.3390/s24061781

Academic Editors: Calin Gheorghe Dan Neamtu, Radu Comes, Jing-Jing Fang and Dorin-Mircea Popovici

Received: 21 January 2024
Revised: 1 March 2024
Accepted: 8 March 2024
Published: 10 March 2024

1. Introduction

In the changing world of innovation, augmented reality (AR) and virtual reality (VR) technologies are making a powerful impact. They are revolutionizing interaction, visualization, and immersion in industries. These technologies have the ability to transform entertainment by creating gaming experiences and interactive media. They also have the potential to revolutionize education and training through simulated environments. Moreover, they are enhancing care through therapy and reshaping the retail industry with interactive shopping experiences. At the heart of these technologies lies eye tracking, a method that captures a user's gaze within a virtual environment. By understanding and responding to where users look, eye tracking technology significantly improves interactivity and personalization in AR/VR experiences. This leads to engaging and effective user experiences [1–6].

In the realm of healthcare, VR technologies have shown promise in enhancing surgical planning and patient outcomes. For instance, Innocente et al. demonstrated the application of Mixed Reality for Total Hip Arthroplasty Assessment, offering surgeons advanced visualization tools to evaluate and predict post-operative results [7]. This application exemplifies the transformative potential of VR and AR in medical procedures, aligning with our findings on the impact of VR on user experience. Similarly, Su et al. (2022) discuss the use of mixed-reality technology in total knee arthroplasty, highlighting its advantages in complex surgical procedures [8]. Furthermore, Zavala-González et al. (2022) conducted a randomized controlled trial on the effectiveness of adding virtual reality to physiotherapeutic treatment in patients with total hip arthroplasty, showcasing the potential of virtual reality in enhancing rehabilitation outcomes [9]. These studies exemplify the diverse applications of technology in orthopedic surgery and rehabilitation, emphasizing the role of innovative solutions in improving patient care and outcomes.

However despite the progress and widespread acceptance of AR/VR technologies, there are still obstacles that need to be overcome in order to fully utilize their potential and ensure sustainable growth. One major concern in the realm of VR is user comfort. Extended exposure to VR environments can cause discomfort and sensory overload commonly referred to as VR sickness. This condition is characterized by symptoms such as nausea, headaches, and disorientation. Addressing this challenge highlights the importance of creating VR experiences that are not immersive but also comfortable and safe, for users [10–16].

Maintaining user engagement poses another challenge in virtual reality (VR) applications. As the initial excitement of VR diminishes, it becomes increasingly crucial to sustain user interest and captivation over time. This challenge underscores the importance of creating adaptive content and interface designs that cater to user preferences and behaviors, ensuring a continuous level of engagement and immersion. Furthermore, optimizing interface design for seamless navigation and interaction is essential to provide users with an enjoyable VR experience. Recent works, such as the study by Cannavò et al. [17] on the automatic generation of affective 3D virtual environments from 2D images, highlight the significance of design considerations in retaining users and determining the success of VR applications [18–21].

Industry leaders such as Meta (previously known as Facebook) along with their Oculus VR systems, Netflix, and Amazon are at the forefront of advancing VR experiences. One of the challenges in this field is finding a balance between the costs involved in creating avatars that enable a sense of embodiment and the need for hardware to track and render natural movements. Meta specifically needs to strike a balance between achieving convincing motion and visual accuracy to maintain a feeling of presence while ensuring accessibility and scalability across their VR platforms, for consumers. Recent research also emphasizes the significance of understanding user behavior eye movement in order to create user-centric VR experiences [22–24].

To address these challenges, our study adopts Multiscale Entropy (MSE) analysis, a computational technique initially developed by Javaherian et al. [25]. MSE analysis offers a unique perspective on time series data by dissecting it into non-overlapping windows, revealing patterns and correlations at various scales. Applied to the eye movement data obtained from the GazeBaseVR dataset [26,27], which provides a comprehensive and longitudinal perspective on eye movement behavior in various VR tasks and stimuli, MSE analysis enables us to explore the intricate dynamics of eye movement patterns. This dataset captures the eye movements of participants engaged in a series of diverse and dynamic tasks, including vergence, smooth pursuit, video viewing, self-paced reading, and random saccades, collectively referred to as 'VRG', 'PUR', 'VID', 'TEX', and 'RAN'. These tasks encompass a wide range of stimuli and activities typical in VR environments, making the dataset an invaluable resource for our study [28,29].

In our research, we specifically focus on the horizontal (θ_H) and vertical (θ_V) components of eye movement, quantified in degrees of visual angle (dva). These components are essential as they provide insights into the intricate dynamics of eye movements in VR. The utilization of MSE analysis allows us to quantify the complexity of these eye movement patterns, offering valuable insights into their predictability and dynamics across different VR tasks and stimuli [26].

By using Mean Squared Error (MSE) on this dataset our study aims to uncover the aspects of eye movements, in different tasks and stimuli. This will help us understand how users interact with and respond to virtual reality (VR) environments. These valuable insights will play a role in addressing the challenges mentioned earlier such as user comfort, engagement, and optimizing interface design. Moreover, they have the potential to drive advancements by allowing us to explore MSE analysis findings for informing VR interface and content design resulting in intuitive, engaging, and comfortable user experiences.

Additionally, our research strives to provide suggestions and insights for leaders, in the tech industry. This will assist them in overcoming challenges related to VR production and delivery aligning with the needs and goals of these companies while contributing to the advancement and refinement of VR technologies.

In conducting this study, the paper enhances understanding of eye movement behavior in virtual reality environments and provides practical insights that drive innovation and improvement in the VR industry. The subsequent sections detail the methodology of Multiscale Entropy (MSE) analysis, present findings from this approach, and discuss implications for VR design and user experience. Specifically, the Methodology section outlines the dataset used and the steps taken in the MSE analysis. The Results section presents the complexity patterns observed in eye movements across different VR tasks. The Discussion interprets these findings in the context of current challenges faced by leaders in the tech industry, offering strategic insights and recommendations. Finally, the Conclusion and Future Work summarize the study's key contributions and propose directions for further research, emphasizing the potential for collaborative efforts with the tech industry.

2. Methodology

2.1. Dataset Description

The dataset utilized in this study, referred to as GazeBaseVR, is a large-scale longitudinal binocular eye-tracking dataset collected at a high frequency of 250 Hz using an eye-tracking enabled virtual reality (VR) headset. For an in-depth description of the dataset, including the VR application used and the purpose of data collection, readers are referred to Lohr et al. (2023) [26]. The GazeBaseVR dataset includes 5020 binocular recordings from a diverse population of 407 college-aged participants, recorded up to six times each over a 26-month period. Each session included a series of five different eye-tracking (ET) tasks designed to elicit various eye movements and behaviors. These tasks were a vergence task, horizontal smooth pursuit task, video-viewing task, self-paced reading task, and random oblique saccade task. These tasks were selected to simulate a wide range of visual experiences in VR, from focusing on specific objects at varying depths to engaging in activities that mimic everyday visual behaviors, providing a comprehensive assessment of eye movement patterns. This comprehensive set of tasks was carefully selected to cover a broad spectrum of eye movements and to provide insights into both the micro-movements and overall behavioral patterns of the participants' eye movements in a virtual reality environment.

The dataset's longitudinal nature, with multiple recordings of the same individuals over an extended period, provides a unique opportunity to investigate not just the variability and commonalities in eye movements across individuals and tasks but also changes and trends over time, whether due to learning, adaptation, or other long-term factors.

Furthermore, the diversity of the participant pool in terms of demographics and the detailed recording of participant details make this dataset particularly valuable for investigating factors such as the impact of demographic variables on eye movement behavior and the potential for personalized or adaptive VR experiences based on eye movement patterns.

From a technical perspective, the data were captured using SensoMotoric Instrument's eye-tracking virtual reality head-mounted display (ET-HMD) based on the HTC Vive. This device tracks both eyes at a nominal sampling rate of 250 Hz with a high spatial accuracy and precision, ensuring detailed and reliable eye movement data. The dataset provides an extensive range of metrics, including gaze direction vectors and positional data, which can be used to derive various eye movement characteristics.

In our study, we specifically focus on the horizontal (x) and vertical (y) components of the eye rotation, denoted as θ_H and θ_V, respectively, in terms of degrees of visual angle (dva). These components are crucial for understanding the direction and extent of eye movements, especially in the context of interactive VR environments where users are constantly engaging with dynamic content. The conversion of the direction vector $\mathbf{v} = [x, y, z]$ into these components is performed using the following equations:

$$\theta_H = \frac{180}{\pi} \arctan 2\left(x, \sqrt{y^2 + z^2}\right) \tag{1}$$

$$\theta_V = \frac{180}{\pi} \arctan 2(y, z) \tag{2}$$

The "z" component in this vector represents the depth axis in a three-dimensional coordinate system, indicating the depth at which a user is looking into the screen or virtual environment. This depth component is essential for calculating the exact direction of gaze in the 3D space of VR, providing a comprehensive understanding of eye movement behavior.

These equations provide a standardized way of quantifying eye movement in terms of horizontal and vertical rotation angles, facilitating the analysis of eye movement patterns and the application of Multiscale Entropy (MSE) analysis to assess the complexity and predictability of eye movements across different VR tasks [26,27].

2.2. Analysis of Multiscale Entropy

A system's time series data can be affected by various noises that stem from its interaction with the surrounding environment. These noises can introduce short-term correlations that falsely appear as long-term effects in the time-series analysis. Therefore, it is crucial to mitigate the impact of these noises and the associated short-term correlations. This is achieved through a process known as coarse graining. In this process, a time series with N data points $(y_1, y_2, \ldots, y_N)$ is divided into equal-length, non-overlapping segments called windows, each of length λ. Within each window, the data points are averaged to produce a new time series with reduced granularity as follows:

$$y_p^{(\lambda)} = \frac{1}{\lambda} \sum_{q=1}^{\lambda} y_{(p-1)\lambda+q} \tag{3}$$

This results in a new series composed of the averaged data points $(y_1^{(\lambda)}, \ldots, y_{N_\lambda}^{(\lambda)})$, where λ serves as the scaling factor. The restructured data can then be represented by vectors of m dimensions as shown below:

$$Y_m^{(\lambda)}(p) = (y_p^{(\lambda)}, \ldots, y_{p+m-1}^{(\lambda)}) \tag{4}$$

The subsequent step involves counting the number of vector pairs whose mutual distance is less than a specified value r. This quantity is denoted as $n_m(r, \lambda)$. This counting is also performed for vectors of dimension $m+1$, denoted as $n_{m+1}(r, \lambda)$. The measure of complexity, known as sample entropy, is then computed with the following formula:

$$S_e(m, r, \lambda) = -\log\left(\frac{n_{m+1}(r, \lambda)}{n_m(r, \lambda)}\right). \tag{5}$$

Given that $n_{m+1}(r, \lambda) \leq n_m(r, \lambda)$, it follows that S_e is non-negative. A graph plotting sample entropy against the scale factor illustrates the correlation ranges present in the time series. This comprehensive procedure is referred to as multiscale entropy (MSE) analysis [25].

2.3. Computational Methodology

The Multiscale Entropy (MSE) analysis of the eye movement data was conducted using a Python script that leverages libraries such as NumPy for numerical operations and Matplotlib for visualizing the entropy trends. The script's core consists of functions specifically designed to perform coarse graining, calculate sample entropy, and compile multiscale entropy across varying scales for a comprehensive understanding of complexity in eye movement data. The choice of Python and these libraries was driven by their robustness, efficiency, and widespread use in scientific computing, ensuring reliability and reproducibility of our results.

As illustrated in Figure 1, the computational process of Multiscale Entropy (MSE) analysis involves several key steps. Starting with the initialization of the process for each file in the dataset, it proceeds with loading the data specifically from the 'x' and 'y' columns indicative of the horizontal and vertical gaze positions. Parameters for the MSE analysis are set according to standard practices and preliminary analysis to ensure robustness and relevance of the results. The time series data are then coarse grained at multiple scales, upon which sample entropy is calculated to quantify the complexity at each scale. Finally, these complexity measures are compiled across all scales to visualize and analyze the variation of eye movement complexity. The coarse graining and sample entropy calculations are guided by specific equations, integral to understanding the underlying mechanics of this analysis.

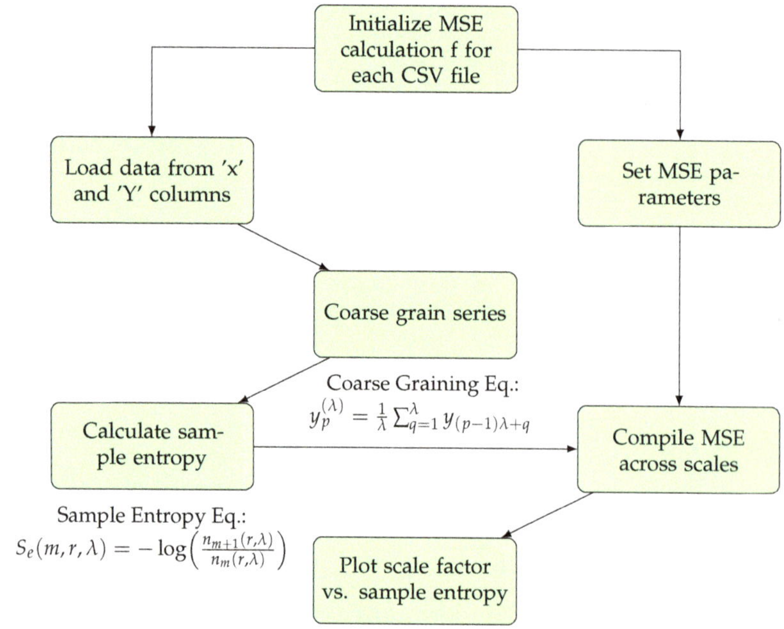

Figure 1. Flowchart illustrating the MSE calculation process with included equations.

2.4. Rationale Behind Parameters and Approach

The selection of parameters for Multiscale Entropy (MSE) analysis, particularly the `max_scale` parameter set to 20, is instrumental in dissecting the complexity and predictability of eye movements within virtual reality (VR) environments. This value is chosen based on a balance between capturing a broad range of temporal scales and maintaining computational efficiency. A `max_scale` of 20 typically covers the spectrum from rapid, short-term dynamics to more extended patterns of engagement without overly smoothing the data, thus preserving the detailed behavior inherent in the eye movement recordings. This careful calibration allows for a nuanced examination of eye movement behavior across these scales, revealing insights into immediate reactions and prolonged engagement patterns. The choice is further supported by empirical testing and alignment with standard practices in time-series analysis, ensuring that the scale range is both practical and effective for capturing the complexities of eye movement in VR environments.

Interpreting MSE Analysis: Interpretations of MSE plots draw upon complex signal analyses, aligning with methodologies used in various scientific studies. These interpretations help us understand the diverse nature of eye movements, from short-term adjustments to long-term strategies [30–33].

- **Rising Trends (Increasing Sample Entropy with Scale Factor):** Gradual increases in sample entropy across scales can indicate adaptive or exploratory behavior, reflecting users' continuous engagement and adjustment to the complexities of the VR environment. This pattern may denote a dynamic and enriching interaction, where the gaze behavior becomes progressively complex and unpredictable, suggesting deepening engagement or increasing task difficulty.
- **Fluctuating Trends (Variable Sample Entropy):** Fluctuations in sample entropy highlight moments of transition in cognitive demand or strategy. Peaks in entropy may indicate periods of heightened complexity or adaptation to new stimuli, whereas valleys suggest more predictable or habitual gaze patterns. Such variability is crucial for understanding how users interact with changing content or complexities within the VR environment.
- **Steady Trends (Consistent Sample Entropy across Scale Factors):** A consistent level of sample entropy across scales suggests a uniform cognitive load or a continuous level of interaction complexity. This trend may indicate that users have reached an equilibrium in their gaze behavior, efficiently balancing exploration and exploitation of visual information in the VR environment. It might also suggest that the VR task or experience is consistently engaging users at a stable level throughout.

Comprehensive Insights from MSE Analysis: The understanding of these trends provides deeper insights into the cognitive load, user engagement, and possible avenues for VR experience enhancement as follows:

- Datasets with rising trends and fluctuations might indicate a constantly adapting and highly engaged user, with significant moments of cognitive demand interspersed with periods of routine interaction.
- Steady trends can suggest a balanced and consistent level of interaction, possibly pointing towards efficient user navigation or well-calibrated task demands within the VR environment.
- The absence of declining trends in our analysis indicates that users do not typically exhibit decreasing complexity or increasing predictability in their gaze patterns across the studied tasks, highlighting the consistent challenge or engagement presented by the VR tasks.

Scale Factor and Sample Entropy: Both the scale factor and sample entropy are pivotal in MSE analysis. The scale factor, a dimensionless number, determines the granularity of the time series analysis, affecting the temporal resolution and interpretability of complexity patterns. Specifically, it represents the level of coarse-graining applied to the time series data, signifying the extent to which data points are averaged together. A scale factor of 1 indicates no coarse-graining, thus reflecting the original data, while higher-scale factors imply a progressive averaging of data points, highlighting broader, long-term patterns.

Sample entropy, also a dimensionless measure, quantifies the regularity and unpredictability within the time series across scales. As a statistical tool, it offers insights into the complexity inherent in the eye movement data. A decrease in entropy at larger scale factors typically implies increasing predictability and regularity over longer periods, while an increase might indicate more complex and less predictable patterns, reflecting changes in cognitive demand or task complexity. Together, these metrics provide a comprehensive understanding of the intricate dynamics of eye movements in VR environments, reflecting the cognitive processes and engagement levels of users.

3. Results and Discussion

Understanding the intricacies of eye movement behavior in virtual reality (VR) environments is crucial for enhancing user experience and interface design. This study applies Multiscale Entropy (MSE) analysis to dissect the complexity of eye movements, specifically focusing on the horizontal (x) and vertical (y) components of gaze position. MSE, a robust method for quantifying the complexity and predictability of time series data, is particularly well suited for exploring the nuanced patterns of eye movement in various VR tasks.

By analyzing these components across different scales, the study reveals insights into the dynamic nature of gaze behavior and its implications for VR interaction. The following subsections present the key findings from the MSE analysis, highlighting the distinct complexity patterns observed in eye movements across a series of VR tasks. Through these results, the study aims to shed light on the multifaceted nature of human gaze in virtual environments and contribute to the optimized design and development of VR systems.

3.1. *Multiscale Entropy Analysis of Eye Movements in the VRG Task*

Task Context: The vergence (VRG) task involves eye movements where participants adjust their gaze to focus on objects at varying depths within the virtual environment, simulating a 3D experience. This task is critical for depth perception and fundamental to a realistic and immersive virtual environment.

MSE Findings: Multiscale Entropy (MSE) analysis was performed on both the horizontal (x) and vertical (y) components of eye movements during the VRG task. Figure 2 illustrates the sample entropy across different scale factors for the horizontal and vertical gaze positions, respectively. The sample entropy was plotted across different scale factors for both gaze positions, illustrating the complexity and predictability of eye movements as participants engaged in depth-adjusting tasks.

Interpretation:

Horizontal Component (x) Analysis: For the horizontal component, the rising trends in sample entropy across nearly all datasets indicate an increase in complexity and unpredictability of gaze patterns as the scale factor increases. The patterns resembling $y = \ln(x)$ suggest an adaptive or exploratory behavior, reflecting continuous engagement and adjustment by the users to the depth variations in the VR environment. The slight positive slope observed in the rest of the datasets, similar to $y = \frac{1}{n}x$, although indicative of a rising trend, suggests a more gradual increase in complexity, possibly due to a more steady or predictable aspect of the vergence task.

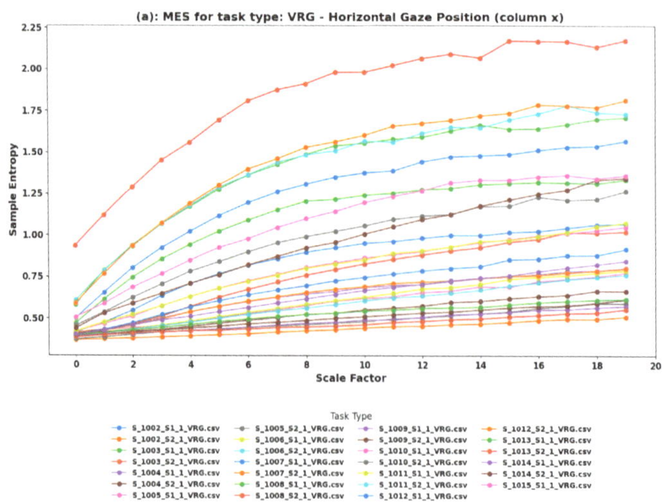

Figure 2. *Cont.*

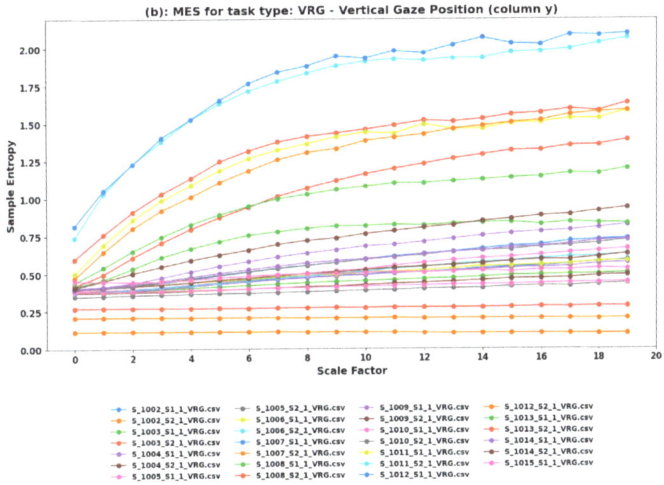

Figure 2. Multiscale Entropy analysis of eye movements in the VRG Task. (**a**) Horizontal and (**b**) Vertical Gaze Position. The VRG task involves vergence eye movements, where participants adjust their gaze to focus on objects at varying depths, simulating a 3D environment in VR.

Vertical Component (y) Analysis: In the vertical component, the datasets split into two distinct behaviors: approximately half exhibiting a logarithmic increase, indicating adaptive behavior as seen in the horizontal component, and the other half displaying a steady trend, suggesting a uniform cognitive load or a consistent level of interaction complexity. The consistent sample entropy across scales in these steady trend datasets might imply that for certain aspects of the VRG task, users maintain a stable gaze behavior, efficiently balancing exploration and exploitation of depth information presented in the virtual environment.

Comprehensive Insights from VRG Task Analysis: The observed MSE trends for the VRG task provide valuable insights into how users interact with and adapt to 3D virtual environments. Rising trends across most datasets, especially in the horizontal component, underscore the dynamic and engaging nature of the task, prompting users to continuously adjust their gaze strategy. The variability in entropy, particularly the distinction between rising and steady trends in the vertical component, highlights the complexity of depth perception and the different strategies users might employ to navigate 3D spaces. These findings emphasize the need for VR content design to consider the varying cognitive loads and interaction complexities inherent in depth-oriented tasks, aiming to optimize user comfort and enhance the overall immersive experience.

Implications for VR Content Design and User Experience: Understanding the complexity patterns in eye movements during vergence tasks can inform the design of more intuitive and comfortable VR experiences. By aligning VR content and interface design with the natural tendencies of human ocular activity in 3D environments, developers can create more immersive and engaging applications that cater to the depth perception needs of users. Furthermore, recognizing the adaptive behaviors and stable interaction trends in eye movements can help optimize the balance between visual challenge and user comfort, contributing to the reduction of VR sickness and enhancing long-term user engagement.

3.2. *Multiscale Entropy Analysis of Eye Movements in the VID Task*

Task Context: The Video Viewing (VID) task is a central component of virtual reality (VR) experiences, involving participants watching diverse video content. This immersive activity requires users to maintain sustained attention and engagement, as they visually explore and react to dynamic visual scenes. Understanding how gaze behavior adapts during video viewing is crucial for enhancing user experience and optimizing content design in cinematic or narrative VR settings.

MSE Findings: For the VID task, Multiscale Entropy (MSE) analysis was conducted on the horizontal (x) and vertical (y) components of eye movements. Figure 3 showcases the sample entropy across different scale factors for horizontal and vertical gaze positions, respectively. The analysis produced plots showing sample entropy across various scale factors for both gaze positions, reflecting the complexity and predictability of eye movements as participants interacted with video content.

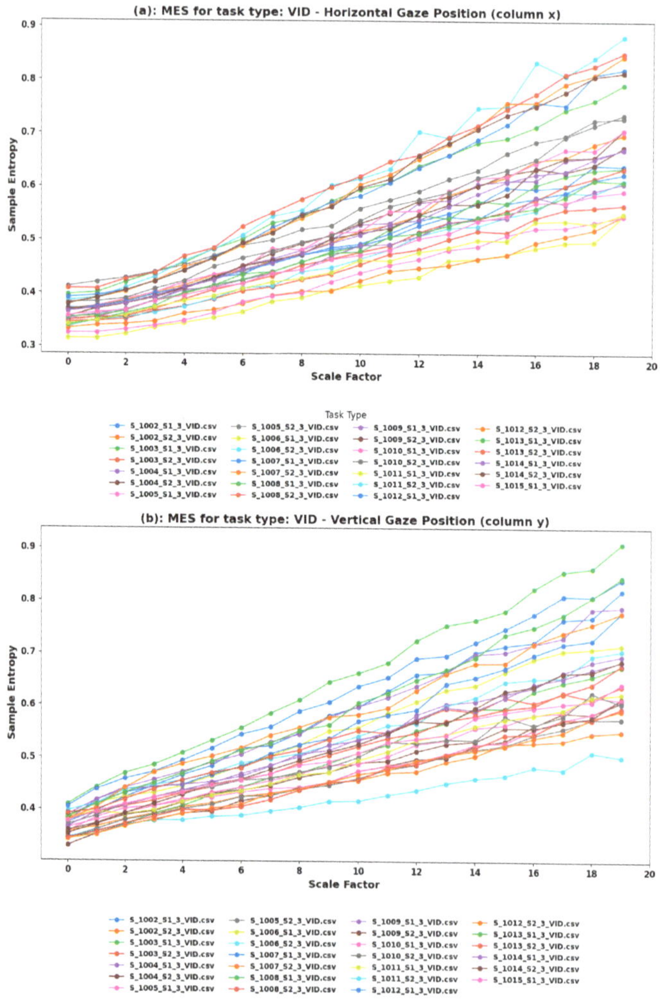

Figure 3. Multiscale Entropy analysis of eye movements in the VID Task. (**a**) Horizontal and (**b**) Vertical Gaze Position. The VID task involves participants watching videos, a common activity in VR, focusing on understanding how gaze behavior changes during passive viewing.

Interpretation:

Linearly Rising Trends: Both the horizontal and vertical components exhibit linearly rising trends in sample entropy with different slopes. This consistent increase across the scale factors suggests that as the viewing time extends, the complexity of gaze patterns also increases. The variation in slopes between the horizontal and vertical components could indicate different levels or types of engagement and visual exploration. For instance, steeper slopes may represent periods of more intense visual exploration or engagement with the content, possibly during dynamic or rapidly changing scenes.

Comprehensive Insights from VID Task Analysis: The MSE analysis of eye movements during the VID task underscores the dynamic interaction between viewers and video content in VR environments. The linearly rising trends across most datasets highlight the ongoing adaptation and engagement of viewers with the content, providing a quantitative measure of how video narratives and visual stimuli influence gaze behavior. These insights can drive the development of more captivating and immersive VR video experiences, ensuring that content remains engaging and aligned with the viewer's natural gaze dynamics.

Implications for Content Design and User Experience: These findings have significant implications for VR video content creators. Understanding the nature of gaze complexity during video viewing can help in identifying key moments for narrative or visual shifts to maintain or enhance viewer engagement. For example, creators might introduce changes in content at points where the entropy trend suggests a decrease in engagement or predictability, thereby reinvigorating viewer attention and interest.

3.3. Multiscale Entropy Analysis of Eye Movements in the PUR Task

Task Context: The pursuit (PUR) task is a crucial component in understanding user interaction in virtual reality (VR), particularly focusing on smooth pursuit eye movements. Participants track moving targets, a fundamental activity for simulating realistic scenarios in interactive and gaming environments. This task is vital for examining the mechanisms of visual tracking and how individuals maintain focus on dynamic objects within VR.

MSE Findings: Multiscale Entropy (MSE) analysis was performed on both the horizontal (x) and vertical (y) components of eye movements during the PUR task. Figure 4 illustrates the sample entropy across different scale factors for the horizontal and vertical gaze positions, respectively. The analysis yielded entropy trends across various scale factors, reflecting the complexity and predictability of eye movements as participants engaged in tracking moving targets.

Interpretation:

Horizontal Component—Logistic Function Trends: The horizontal eye movements exhibited trends similar to logistic functions with varying heights, indicating a saturation effect in the complexity of eye movements.

Vertical Component—Logarithmic and Steady Trends: Vertical eye movements predominantly displayed a logarithmic increase in complexity, suggesting a continuous adaptation or increasing challenge in tracking the vertical motion of targets. A few datasets exhibited steady trends, which might indicate consistent tracking behavior or uniform task difficulty across those particular sessions.

Comprehensive Insights from PUR Task Analysis: The MSE trends in the PUR task provide a detailed account of how users engage with moving targets in VR. The logistic-like patterns in horizontal movements suggest a bounded complexity, perhaps due to the capabilities of the human visual system or the specific nature of the task. On the other hand, the logarithmic trends in vertical movements reflect a more nuanced adaptation process, with users possibly exerting more effort or strategy in tracking vertical motion.

Implications for VR Content Design and User Experience: Understanding these intricate patterns of eye movement can inform the design of VR content, particularly in scenarios requiring object tracking or interaction with moving elements. Designers and developers might consider the limitations and capabilities reflected in the logistic function trends when creating moving targets or interactive elements, ensuring that these are within comfortable tracking ranges for users. Additionally, the varying complexity in vertical tracking might influence how vertical motion is incorporated into VR experiences, balancing challenge and comfort to enhance overall engagement and minimize discomfort or disorientation.

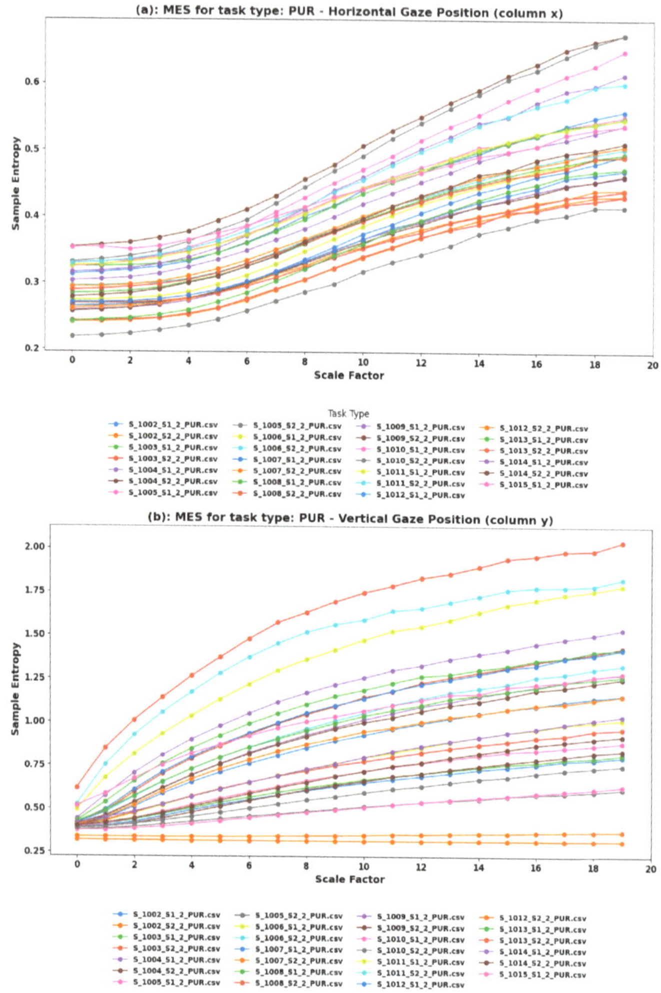

Figure 4. Multiscale Entropy analysis of eye movements in the PUR task. (**a**) Horizontal and (**b**) Vertical Gaze Position. In the PUR task, subjects engage in smooth pursuit movements, following moving objects with their eyes, which is essential for tracking moving stimuli in VR.

3.4. Multiscale Entropy Analysis of Eye Movements in the TEX Task

Task Context: The text reading (TEX) task simulates the act of reading within a virtual environment, an essential component in educational and informational VR applications. This task involves participants reading text presented in the VR space, requiring saccadic movements and fixations similar to those in real-world reading scenarios. Understanding the complexity of these eye movements is vital for creating VR systems that support effective and comfortable reading experiences.

MSE Findings: In the TEX task, Multiscale Entropy analysis was applied to both the horizontal (x) and vertical (y) components of eye movements associated with reading. The analysis yields distinct patterns of sample entropy across different scale factors for both gaze positions. Figure 5 represents the sample entropy across different scale factors for horizontal and vertical gaze positions, respectively. Horizontally, there is a trend of linearly rising entropy with minor fluctuations, indicative of the systematic left-to-right eye movement typical of reading in many languages. Vertically, most datasets show a rising trend with more pronounced fluctuations, reflecting the varied complexity as eyes move down the page or screen and possibly adjust to different lengths of text or formatting changes.

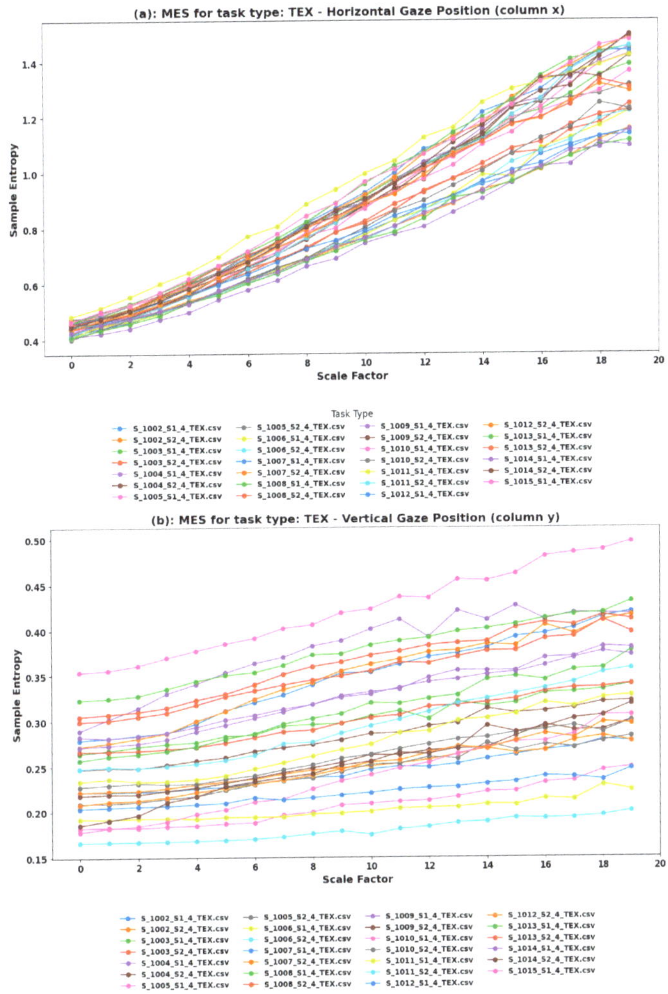

Figure 5. Multiscale Entropy analysis of eye movements in the TEX task. (**a**) Horizontal and (**b**) Vertical Gaze Position. The TEX task represents reading text in VR, a scenario that involves distinct eye movement patterns due to the linear nature of text and frequent line shifts.

Interpretation: The MSE trends observed in the TEX task shed light on the nuanced complexity of eye movements during VR reading activities. In the horizontal component, the mostly linearly rising trend with little fluctuations suggests a consistent, though slightly increasing, complexity in eye movement as the text progresses, likely due to accumulating cognitive load or adapting strategies for text navigation. The presence of minor fluctuations might also indicate variations in line lengths, word complexity, or punctuation that momentarily alter the reading rhythm.

For the vertical component, the varying slopes and more pronounced fluctuations in rising trends suggest a diverse range of strategies or challenges as users navigate between lines or paragraphs. This variability might reflect differences in text layout, the effort required to adjust to new lines, or the cognitive processing of section breaks or paragraph endings. A few datasets showing a more steady trend might represent users with more uniform reading strategies or perhaps simpler text structures that elicit more consistent eye movement patterns.

In both cases, the MSE analysis illustrates the complex landscape of reading behavior in VR, offering valuable insights for designing VR content and interfaces that accommodate the natural reading process. By aligning text presentation with the observed entropy trends, developers can enhance readability, reduce cognitive load, and improve user comfort and engagement with textual content in VR.

Implications for VR Content Design and User Experience: Understanding the entropy patterns in reading-related eye movements enables VR content developers to optimize text layout, pacing, and interaction in educational and informational applications. The insights from the horizontal and vertical components of eye movement can inform decisions about font size, line spacing, and the placement of textual elements to align with natural reading patterns and minimize discomfort or disorientation. Furthermore, recognizing the variability in individual reading strategies, as suggested by the different slopes and fluctuations in entropy, underscores the need for customizable or adaptive reading interfaces that can accommodate a range of user preferences and capabilities.

3.5. Multiscale Entropy Analysis of Eye Movements in the RAN Task

Task Context: The random saccades (RAN) task captures the eye movements when participants are required to swiftly and randomly shift their gaze between various points within the VR environment. This task simulates the erratic and spontaneous eye movements that occur as users navigate through and respond to unpredictable or rapidly changing virtual scenarios. Assessing the complexity of these movements is essential for understanding user navigational strategies and responsiveness in a dynamic VR landscape.

MSE Findings: Multiscale Entropy analysis applied to the RAN task's eye movements, both horizontal (x) and vertical (y), shows a pattern of rising entropy, depicted in Figure 6. The entropy progression in both components, characterized by a generally linear rise with similar slopes across different datasets, suggests a consistent increase in complexity as the scale factor increases. This uniformity in the trend across datasets might indicate a standardized response to the random saccades required in the task, reflecting the users' adaptation to the unpredictability inherent in the activity.

Interpretation: The MSE findings from the RAN task offer insights into the nature of eye movements during random, quick shifts of gaze in VR. The consistently rising entropy across scales in both horizontal and vertical components suggests that participants exhibit a gradual increase in complexity in their eye movements, possibly as a reflection of ongoing adaptation to the unpredictability and dynamism of the task. This adaptation might be indicative of users' efforts to optimize their gaze strategy to efficiently deal with random stimuli, maintaining a level of readiness to shift focus swiftly and accurately.

The similar slopes in the linear rise of entropy among datasets imply a commonality in the approach users take to handle random saccades in VR. This could be due to the nature of the task, which requires a general alertness and readiness to move the gaze randomly, leading to a uniform increase in complexity across users.

Comprehensive Insights from RAN Task Analysis: The RAN task's analysis underscores the importance of understanding spontaneous and random eye movements in VR, as they are indicative of how users might navigate and respond to unstructured or unpredictable environments. Insights from this task can inform the design of VR experiences that require users to be alert and ready to change focus quickly, such as in certain gaming scenarios or training simulations where rapid situational awareness is critical.

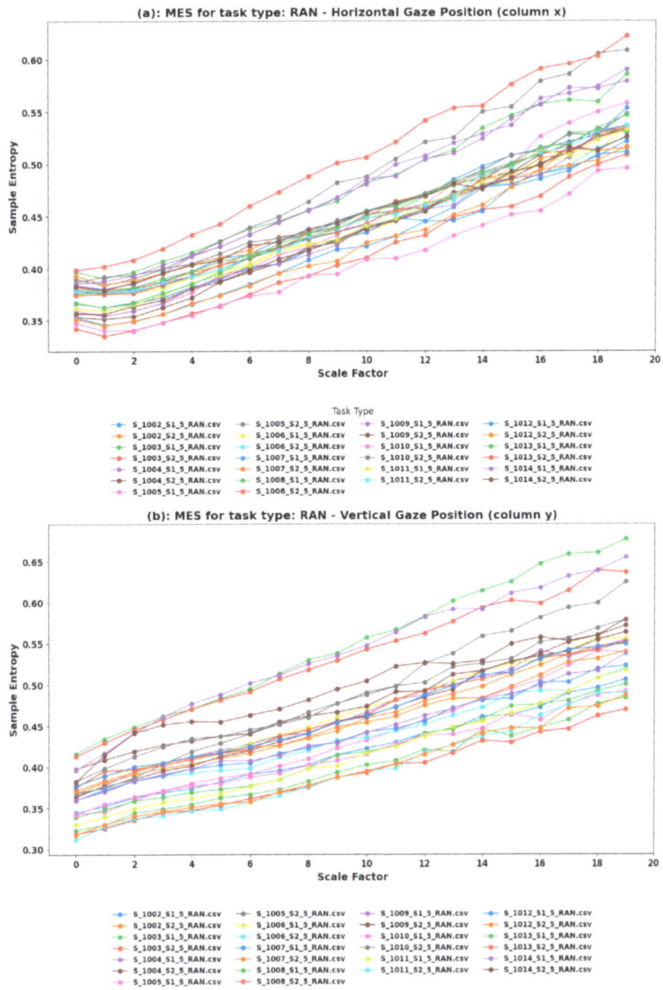

Figure 6. Multiscale Entropy analysis of eye movements in the RAN task. (**a**) Horizontal and (**b**) Vertical Gaze Position. In the RAN task, participants perform random saccades, simulating unpredictable eye movements as they might occur in a dynamic and unstructured VR environment.

Implications for VR Content Design and User Experience: Understanding the consistent increase in complexity in eye movements during random saccades tasks can help VR designers create environments that are attuned to the naturalistic movements of users. By recognizing the characteristics of eye movement in unpredictable scenarios, VR experiences can be optimized to accommodate or even leverage these natural behaviors, enhancing user navigation, orientation, and overall engagement with the content. Moreover, insights into the uniform strategies employed by users across different datasets may assist in standardizing certain aspects of VR design, ensuring a coherent and user-friendly experience even in the most dynamic and unstructured virtual scenarios.

3.6. Deciphering Eye Movement Dynamics

The MSE analysis reveals diverse patterns in eye movements, reflecting users' cognitive states and adaptability within VR environments. The absence of declining trends suggests users may be consistently engaged or adapting to the complexities of VR tasks.

Rising, fluctuating, and steady trends indicate different user interactions, each providing insights into how participants navigate and respond to VR environments. These patterns highlight the need for adaptive VR systems that are responsive to the intricate behaviors of users.

3.7. Insights into User Comfort from MSE Analysis

Our study's Multiscale Entropy (MSE) analysis of eye movements across various VR tasks provides critical insights that can significantly contribute to enhancing user comfort in VR environments. By examining the complexity of eye movements, we can identify potential triggers of discomfort and devise strategies to mitigate these issues. For instance, tasks that exhibit high complexity in eye movements may signal a higher cognitive load or visual stress, potentially leading to discomfort or VR sickness.

Specifically, the analysis revealed that certain VR tasks, such as the PUR (pursuit) and RAN (random saccades) tasks, show pronounced complexity in eye movement patterns. This complexity could indicate that users are required to constantly adapt their gaze, potentially leading to eye strain or fatigue over extended periods. To address this, VR content designers can consider integrating more natural gaze paths and reducing the frequency of abrupt visual changes in these tasks. Moreover, implementing dynamic difficulty adjustments based on real-time MSE analysis of eye movements can help maintain user engagement without overwhelming them, thereby enhancing comfort.

Furthermore, our findings suggest that steady trends in eye movement complexity, observed in tasks like the TEX (text reading) task, could be leveraged to design VR experiences that align with natural eye movement patterns, minimizing the risk of discomfort. By tailoring content to match these naturalistic patterns, VR experiences can become more intuitive and less taxing on the user, promoting longer and more comfortable usage.

Incorporating adaptive interfaces that respond to the MSE analysis of a user's eye movements can also offer personalized comfort adjustments. For example, interfaces could automatically adjust text size, brightness, or even the pace of content based on real-time analysis, ensuring a comfortable viewing experience tailored to individual user needs.

Overall, the application of MSE analysis in understanding and optimizing eye movement dynamics in VR opens up new avenues for creating more comfortable and engaging virtual environments. By closely aligning VR design with the natural complexities of human eye movements, we can significantly reduce discomfort and enhance the overall user experience. Future research should continue to explore the relationship between eye movement complexity and user comfort, fostering the development of VR technologies that prioritize user well-being.

3.8. Comparative Analysis with Existing Research

Our study contributes to the burgeoning field of VR and eye movement analysis by providing insights into the complexity of gaze patterns in VR environments. Previous research, including Mallari et al.'s systematic review on VR's impact on chronic pain [34], highlights VR's potential in enhancing user experiences. Riva et al. [35] and Chiquet et al. [36] have further elucidated the benefits of VR in various therapeutic and wellness contexts, underscoring the versatility of VR applications. Wu et al.'s work [37] on VR in clinical settings adds to the understanding of VR's applicability across different domains.

Expanding on these foundations, our application of Multiscale Entropy (MSE) analysis to VR gaze data offers a novel perspective on user engagement and cognitive load. Parsons (2015) [38], Kourtesis et al. (2019) [39], and Tashjian et al. (2017) [40] emphasize the importance of immersive and interactive VR experiences for cognitive research and therapeutic interventions. Our findings resonate with these studies by demonstrating how MSE analysis can be used to assess and enhance the VR experience, contributing to a deeper understanding of user behavior in VR environments.

Moreover, recent studies by Tang et al. [41] and Sipatchin et al. [42] highlight the critical role of eye-tracking in VR for cognitive assessments and clinical applications. By integrating

MSE analysis with eye-tracking data, our research aligns with the broader trajectory of leveraging VR technology to create immersive, beneficial, and user-centric experiences.

4. Conclusions

This study advances our understanding of eye movement behavior in virtual reality (VR) through Multiscale Entropy (MSE) analysis. By dissecting the complexity of eye movements across various VR tasks, we highlight the potential of MSE to contribute to more intuitive and immersive VR environments. The nuanced insights into gaze behavior provided by this analysis are invaluable for enhancing user experience and interface design in VR technology.

4.1. Contributions

We conducted a comprehensive investigation into the complexity of eye movement patterns in VR using MSE analysis. Our meticulous analysis of the horizontal and vertical components of eye movements across a range of VR tasks—including vergence, smooth pursuit, video viewing, reading, and random saccades—revealed distinct complexity patterns. These patterns, characterized by logarithmic, logistic, rising, and steady behaviors, contribute to a deeper understanding of gaze predictability and complexity in VR. Our findings offer valuable insights for optimizing VR interfaces and enhancing user experiences by adapting to dynamic user interactions.

4.2. Future Work

The continued exploration of MSE and its applications in VR is crucial for unlocking the full potential of this technology for users worldwide. A collaborative approach between academia and industry will accelerate innovation and ensure that VR technology evolves in tandem with our understanding of user needs and preferences. Future research should focus on the following:

- Investigating a broader range of VR tasks and long-term user interactions to provide a more comprehensive understanding of how entropy trends manifest in different contexts.
- Exploring the implications of these findings for enhancing user comfort and engagement in VR, aiming to support the development of more personalized and immersive experiences.
- Integrating complex signal analysis like MSE into VR research, recognizing the potential for transformative impacts on technology and user interaction.

These directions for future research underscore the importance of a nuanced approach to studying VR interactions, with the goal of creating more engaging and sustainable VR environments.

Author Contributions: Conceptualization, S.Z.; methodology, S.Z.; software, S.Z.; validation, S.Z.; formal analysis, S.Z.; investigation, S.Z.; data curation, S.Z.; writing—original draft preparation, S.Z.; writing—review and editing, S.Z. and G.L.; visualization, S.Z.; supervision, G.L.; project administration, G.L. All authors have read and agreed to the published version of the manuscript.

Funding: Sahar Z. would like to express her sincere gratitude to the College of Architecture and Gregory A. Luhan, Department Head of Architecture at Texas A&M University, for providing financial support and research assistantship (grant #248012) during the past four years.

Institutional Review Board Statement: Not applicable.

Informed Consent Statement: Not applicable.

Data Availability Statement: Data and Python code for reproducing the experiments reported in this article are available upon request. Please contact Sahar Zandi at sahar.zandi@tamu.edu for access.

Acknowledgments: Sahar Z. is grateful to Shahriar Esmaeili for his assistance and guidance in understanding the Multiscale Entropy Analysis (MSE) concepts, which significantly contributed to the development of the Python code used in this study.

Conflicts of Interest: The authors declare no conflicts of interest.

Abbreviations

The following abbreviations are used in this manuscript:

MSE	Multiscale Entropy
AR	Augmented Reality
VR	Virtual Reality
VRG	vergence task
VID	video-viewing atsk
PUR	pursuit task
TEX	text-reading task
RAN	random saccades task

References

1. Billinghurst, M.; Clark, A.; Lee, G. A survey of augmented reality. *Found. Trends Hum. Comput. Interact.* **2015**, *8*, 73–272. [CrossRef]
2. Rizzo, A.; Koenig, S.T. Is clinical virtual reality ready for primetime? *Neuropsychology* **2017**, *31*, 877. [CrossRef] [PubMed]
3. Clay, V.; König, P.; Koenig, S. Eye tracking in virtual reality. *J. Eye Mov. Res.* **2019**, *12*. [CrossRef] [PubMed]
4. Mihelj, M.; Novak, D.; Beguš, S. *Virtual Reality Technology and Applications*; Springer: Dordrecht, The Netherlands, 2014.
5. Kaewrat, C.; Boonbrahm, P.; Sahoh, B. The Design and Development of a Foot-Detection Approach Based on Seven-Foot Dimensions: A Case Study of a Virtual Try-On Shoe System Using Augmented Reality Techniques. *Informatics* **2023**, *10*, 48. [CrossRef]
6. Zandi, S. Revival of the Silk Road using the applications of AR/VR and its role on cultural tourism. *arXiv* **2023**, arXiv:2304.10545.
7. Innocente, C.; Piazzolla, P.; Ulrich, L.; Moos, S.; Tornincasa, S.; Vezzetti, E. Mixed Reality-Based Support for Total Hip Arthroplasty Assessment. In Proceedings of the International Joint Conference on Mechanics, Design Engineering & Advanced Manufacturing, Ischia, Italy, 1–3 June 2022; pp. 159–169.
8. Su, S.; Lei, P.; Wang, C.; Gao, F.; Zhong, D.; Hu, Y. Mixed reality technology in total knee arthroplasty: An updated review with a preliminary case report. *Front. Surg.* **2022**, *9*, 804029. [CrossRef] [PubMed]
9. Zavala-González, J.; Martínez, D.; Gutiérrez-Espinoza, H. Effectiveness of adding virtual reality to physiotherapeutic treatment in patients with total hip arthroplasty. A randomized controlled trial. *Clin. Rehabil.* **2022**, *36*, 660–668. [CrossRef] [PubMed]
10. Chang, E.; Kim, H.T.; Yoo, B. Virtual reality sickness: A review of causes and measurements. *Int. J. Hum. Comput. Interact.* **2020**, *36*, 1658–1682. [CrossRef]
11. Won, J.; Kim, Y.S. A new approach for reducing virtual reality sickness in real time: Design and validation study. *JMIR Serious Games* **2022**, *10*, e36397. [CrossRef] [PubMed]
12. Parida, K.; Bark, H.; Lee, P.S. Emerging thermal technology enabled augmented reality. *Adv. Funct. Mater.* **2021**, *31*, 2007952. [CrossRef]
13. Zandi, S.; Luhan, G.A. Exploring User Interactions in AR/VR Interfaces: A Simulation-Based Study. In Proceedings of the 2023 International Conference on Electrical, Computer and Energy Technologies (ICECET), Cape Town, South Africa, 16–17 November 2023; pp. 1–6. [CrossRef]
14. Dwivedi, Y.K.; Hughes, L.; Baabdullah, A.M.; Ribeiro-Navarrete, S.; Giannakis, M.; Al-Debei, M.M.; Dennehy, D.; Metri, B.; Buhalis, D.; Cheung, C.M.; et al. Metaverse beyond the hype: Multidisciplinary perspectives on emerging challenges, opportunities, and agenda for research, practice and policy. *Int. J. Inf. Manag.* **2022**, *66*, 102542. [CrossRef]
15. Palumbo, A. Microsoft HoloLens 2 in medical and healthcare context: State of the art and future prospects. *Sensors* **2022**, *22*, 7709. [CrossRef] [PubMed]
16. Zandi, S. Sustainable and Resilient Systems for Intergenerational Justice. *arXiv* **2021**, arXiv:2102.09122.
17. Cannavo, A.; D'Alessandro, A.; Daniele, M.; Giorgia, M.; Congyi, Z.; Lamberti, F. Automatic generation of affective 3D virtual environments from 2D images. In Proceedings of the 15th International Conference on Computer Graphics Theory and Applications (GRAPP 2020), Valetta, Malta, 27–29 February 2020; pp. 113–124.
18. Buttussi, F.; Chittaro, L. Effects of different types of virtual reality display on presence and learning in a safety training scenario. *IEEE Trans. Vis. Comput. Graph.* **2017**, *24*, 1063–1076. [CrossRef] [PubMed]
19. Huang, K.T.; Ball, C.; Francis, J.; Ratan, R.; Boumis, J.; Fordham, J. Augmented versus virtual reality in education: An exploratory study examining science knowledge retention when using augmented reality/virtual reality mobile applications. *Cyberpsychol. Behav. Soc. Netw.* **2019**, *22*, 105–110. [CrossRef] [PubMed]
20. Logan, D.E.; Simons, L.E.; Caruso, T.J.; Gold, J.I.; Greenleaf, W.; Griffin, A.; King, C.D.; Menendez, M.; Olbrecht, V.A.; Rodriguez, S.; et al. Leveraging virtual reality and augmented reality to combat chronic pain in youth: Position paper from the interdisciplinary network on virtual and augmented technologies for pain management. *J. Med. Internet Res.* **2021**, *23*, e25916. [CrossRef] [PubMed]
21. Demeco, A.; Zola, L.; Frizziero, A.; Martini, C.; Palumbo, A.; Foresti, R.; Buccino, G.; Costantino, C. Immersive virtual reality in post-stroke rehabilitation: A systematic review. *Sensors* **2023**, *23*, 1712. [CrossRef] [PubMed]

22. Haley, A.C.; Thorpe, D.; Pelletier, A.; Yarosh, S.; Keefe, D.F. Inward VR: Toward a Qualitative Method for Investigating Interoceptive Awareness in VR. *IEEE Trans. Vis. Comput. Graph.* **2023**, *29*, 2557–2566. [CrossRef] [PubMed]
23. Anastasaki, I.; Drosatos, G.; Pavlidis, G.; Rantos, K. User Authentication Mechanisms Based on Immersive Technologies: A Systematic Review. *Information* **2023**, *14*, 538. [CrossRef]
24. Jia, F.; Wang, W.; Yang, J.; Li, T.; Song, G.; Xu, Y. Effectiveness of Rectangular Cartogram for Conveying Quantitative Information: An Eye Tracking-Based Evaluation. *ISPRS Int. J. Geo-Inf.* **2023**, *12*, 39. [CrossRef]
25. Javaherian, M.; Mollaei, S. Multiscale Entropy Analysis of Gravitational Waves. *Adv. High Energy Phys.* **2021**, *2021*, 6643546. [CrossRef]
26. Lohr, D.; Aziz, S.; Friedman, L.; Komogortsev, O.V. GazeBaseVR: A large-scale, longitudinal, binocular eye-tracking dataset collected in virtual reality. *Sci. Data* **2023**, *10*, 177. [CrossRef] [PubMed]
27. Griffith, H.; Lohr, D.; Abdulin, E.; Komogortsev, O. GazeBase, a large-scale, multi-stimulus, longitudinal eye movement dataset. *Sci. Data* **2021**, *8*, 184. [CrossRef] [PubMed]
28. D'Amelio, A.; Patania, S.; Bursic, S.; Cuculo, V.; Boccignone, G. Using Gaze for Behavioural Biometrics. *Sensors* **2023**, *23*, 1262. [CrossRef] [PubMed]
29. Yin, J.; Sun, J.; Li, J.; Liu, K. An Effective Gaze-Based Authentication Method with the Spatiotemporal Feature of Eye Movement. *Sensors* **2022**, *22*, 3002. [CrossRef]
30. Costa, M.; Goldberger, A.L.; Peng, C.K. Multiscale entropy analysis of biological signals. *Phys. Rev.* **2005**, *71*, 021906. [CrossRef] [PubMed]
31. Richman, J.S.; Moorman, J.R. Physiological time-series analysis using approximate entropy and sample entropy. *Am. J. Physiol. Heart Circ. Physiol.* **2000**, *278*, H2039–H2049. [CrossRef] [PubMed]
32. Ahmed, M.U.; Mandic, D.P. Multivariate multiscale entropy analysis. *IEEE Signal Process. Lett.* **2011**, *19*, 91–94. [CrossRef]
33. Humeau-Heurtier, A. The multiscale entropy algorithm and its variants: A review. *Entropy* **2015**, *17*, 3110–3123. [CrossRef]
34. Mallari, B.; Spaeth, E.K.; Goh, H.; Boyd, B.S. Virtual reality as an analgesic for acute and chronic pain in adults: A systematic review and meta-analysis. *J. Pain Res.* **2019**, *12*, 2053–2085. [CrossRef]
35. Riva, G.; Wiederhold, B.K.; Mantovani, F. Neuroscience of virtual reality: From virtual exposure to embodied medicine. *Cyberpsychol. Behav. Soc. Netw.* **2019**, *22*, 82–96. [CrossRef]
36. Chiquet, S.; Martarelli, C.S.; Mast, F.W. Eye movements to absent objects during mental imagery and visual memory in immersive virtual reality. *Virtual Real.* **2021**, *25*, 655–667. [CrossRef]
37. Wu, H.Y.; Robert, F.; Fafet, T.; Graulier, B.; Passin-Cauneau, B.; Sassatelli, L.; Winckler, M. Designing Guided User Tasks in VR Embodied Experiences. *Proc. ACM Hum. Comput. Interact.* **2022**, *6*, 1–24. [CrossRef]
38. Parsons, T.D. Virtual reality for enhanced ecological validity and experimental control in the clinical, affective and social neurosciences. *Front. Hum. Neurosci.* **2015**, *9*, 660. [CrossRef] [PubMed]
39. Kourtesis, P.; Collina, S.; Doumas, L.A.; MacPherson, S.E. Technological competence is a pre-condition for effective implementation of virtual reality head mounted displays in human neuroscience: A technological review and meta-analysis. *Front. Hum. Neurosci.* **2019**, *13*, 342. [CrossRef] [PubMed]
40. Tashjian, V.C.; Mosadeghi, S.; Howard, A.R.; Lopez, M.; Dupuy, T.; Reid, M.; Martinez, B.; Ahmed, S.; Dailey, F.; Robbins, K.; et al. Virtual reality for management of pain in hospitalized patients: Results of a controlled trial. *JMIR Ment. Health* **2017**, *4*, e7387. [CrossRef] [PubMed]
41. Tang, Z.; Liu, X.; Huo, H.; Tang, M.; Qiao, X.; Chen, D.; Dong, Y.; Fan, L.; Wang, J.; Du, X.; et al. Eye movement characteristics in a mental rotation task presented in virtual reality. *Front. Neurosci.* **2023**, *17*, 1143006. [CrossRef] [PubMed]
42. Sipatchin, A.; Wahl, S.; Rifai, K. Eye-tracking for clinical ophthalmology with virtual reality (vr): A case study of the htc vive pro eye's usability. *Healthcare* **2021**, *9*, 180. [CrossRef]

applied sciences

MDPI

Article

Examining and Comparing the Effectiveness of Virtual Reality Serious Games and LEGO Serious Play for Learning Scrum

Aldo Gordillo *, Daniel López-Fernández and Jesús Mayor

Computer Science Department, Universidad Politécnica de Madrid, 28040 Madrid, Spain; daniel.lopez@upm.es (D.L.-F.); jesus.mayor@upm.es (J.M.)
* Correspondence: a.gordillo@upm.es

Abstract: Significant research work has been undertaken related to the game-based learning approach over the last years. However, a closer look at this work reveals that further research is needed to examine some types of game-based learning approaches such as virtual reality serious games and LEGO Serious Play. This article examines and compares the effectiveness for learning Scrum and related agile practices of a serious game based on virtual reality and a learning activity based on the LEGO Serious Play methodology. The presented study used a quasi-experimental design with two groups, pre- and post-tests, and a perceptions questionnaire. The sample was composed of 59 software engineering students, 22 of which belonged to group A, while the other 37 were part of group B. The students in group A played the virtual reality serious game, whereas the students in group B conducted the LEGO Serious Play activity. The results show that both game-based learning approaches were effective for learning Scrum and related agile practices in terms of learning performance and motivation, but they also show that the students who played the virtual reality serious game outperformed their peers from the other group in terms of learning performance.

Keywords: game-based learning; virtual reality; educational games; serious games; technology-enhanced learning; LEGO Serious Play; Scrum; agile methodologies

Citation: Gordillo, A.; López-Fernández, D.; Mayor, J. Examining and Comparing the Effectiveness of Virtual Reality Serious Games and LEGO Serious Play for Learning Scrum. *Appl. Sci.* **2024**, *14*, 830. https://doi.org/10.3390/app14020830

Academic Editors: Calin Gheorghe Dan Neamtu, Radu Comes, Jing Fang and Dorin-Mircea Popovici

Received: 20 November 2023
Revised: 15 January 2024
Accepted: 17 January 2024
Published: 18 January 2024

1. Introduction

A considerable effort has been and continues to be devoted to search for new alternatives to improve and complement traditional learning methodologies. In recent years, game-based learning has become one of the most promising learning approaches due to its potential to increase not only students' motivation but also students' learning. As evidenced by several recent literature reviews [1–7], a plethora of studies reported successful game-based learning experiences. This evidence allows the conclusion that, when game-based learning is suitably applied, it can lead to enhancements in both students' motivation and learning outcomes.

However, although a lot of research work has been conducted in the game-based learning field, a closer look at this work reveals that not all types of game-based learning approaches have been extensively investigated. For example, despite there being plenty of studies examining the educational use of videogames [1–7], much less research has been conducted to examine the use of educational videogames based on virtual reality or game-based learning activities based on LEGO Serious Play.

This article examines and compares the instructional effectiveness of a virtual reality serious game and a learning activity based on the LEGO Serious Play methodology. In particular, the study reported in this article examined and compared the use of the two approaches for learning the Scrum framework and some agile practices commonly adopted by Scrum teams. In this regard, it should be noted that, nowadays, Scrum is by far the most widely employed agile methodology in the industry [8] and is part of many degree programs, especially in software engineering. The research questions addressed by this article are as follows:

- RQ1: Are virtual reality serious games effective in terms of knowledge acquisition and motivation for learning Scrum?
- RQ2: Are activities based on LEGO Serious Play effective in terms of knowledge acquisition and motivation for learning Scrum?
- RQ3: Are virtual reality serious games more effective than activities based on LEGO Serious Play in terms of knowledge acquisition and motivation for learning Scrum?

The article is organized into six sections. The next section reviews the existing literature on virtual reality serious games, LEGO Serious Play, and Scrum training. Section 3 details the research methodology, including a description of the virtual reality serious game and the LEGO Serious Play activity that were employed. The results are presented and discussed in Sections 4 and 5, respectively. Finally, Section 6 outlines the conclusions of the article and suggests future works that could be undertaken.

2. Related Work

2.1. Serious Games Based on Virtual Reality

As evidenced by recent literature reviews, virtual reality is being widely used for educational purposes in many knowledge fields and industrial sectors because this technology contributes to improve knowledge acquisition and skills development, engages and motivates learners, and enhances the whole learning experience [9–11].

Some works have reported the use of virtual reality serious games by practitioners in professional contexts, including games to simulate medical operations [12], operate control panels in power plants [13], and conduct psychological exposure therapies [14]. Furthermore, some works have reported the use of this kind of game in educational settings, including games for learning languages and culture [15], physics [16], engineering [17], and topics related to computer science such as computer programming [18]. In this regard, it should be pointed out that the authors of the present contribution recently presented ScrumVR [19–21], which is the virtual reality serious game examined in this article.

In addition to ScrumVR, other virtual reality serious games aimed to teach the Scrum framework have been reported in the literature [22–24]. In the game presented by Caserman et al. [22], the player controls a Scrum Master that must guide their team throughout a Sprint. Radhakrishnan and Koumaditis [23] proposed the creation of a multiplayer virtual reality environment for simulating Sprints. However, a full implementation or validation of this system was not reported in that work. In a more recent work, Visescu et al. [24] presented ScrumSim, a multiplayer simulation in which players, with the assistance of two avatars who play the roles of the Scrum Master and the Product Owner, interact with a virtual reality environment, perform tasks, and receive feedback on their performance. Although ScrumSim has been used in real-world settings, a formal evaluation has not yet been reported.

2.2. LEGO Serious Play

LEGO Serious Play [25] is a learning methodology initially designed to teach professionals in a playful and active way soft skills such as leadership, communication, and conflict resolution. However, in the last decades this methodology has evolved substantially [26] and it is being applied in higher education across many knowledge fields. Indeed, LEGO Serious Play activities have been used in fields as diverse as marketing [27], arts [28], industrial engineering [29], and systems engineering [30]. These contributions indicate that LEGO Serious Play can be used not only to learn soft skills, but also to learn specific competences in many fields of knowledge, including software engineering.

Several LEGO Serious Play activities have been designed to teach concepts related to software engineering. A very prolific author in this area is Kurkovsky [31–35], whose works present activities to teach requirements engineering [31,32], complex systems dependability [31], component integration, and software interface design [33], Test-Driven Development (TDD) [34], and Scrum [35]. The conclusion of these contributions is that this learning methodology is useful to learn specific competences about software engineering, develop soft skills, and improve students' motivation. In the same vein, some authors of the present contribution reported in [36] another LEGO Serious play which proved to be highly appealing and motivating from the students' perspective and effective to learn about software life-cycle models and software development activities.

Another remarkable LEGO Serious play activity in the software engineering field is LEGO City, which was conceived by Krivitsky [37] and serves to teach the Scrum framework. In his book [37], this author presents guidelines to conduct the activity as well as empirical experiences reporting positive outcomes. Beyond the experiences described by Krivitsky himself, this activity has been adapted and replicated by other researchers in professionals and higher education contexts. For example, ref. [38] used the LEGO City activity with professionals of Croatian IT companies, ref. [39] with students of a computer science degree delivered by the University of Pernambuco (Brazil), and ref. [40] with students of a software project management master degree delivered by the Aalto University (Finland). In every case, the authors found out that the LEGO City activity was very well appreciated by the participants and highly effective to learn about Scrum. Another interesting experience is the one reported by [41], who adapted the LEGO City activity to be performed remotely using online whiteboards and real-time communication tools. Similarly, ref. [42] adapted a LEGO Serious Play activity aimed at teaching Scrum to be used with Minetest, an open-source variant of the Minecraft game.

2.3. *Scrum Training*

As described in the previous subsections, virtual reality serious games [19–24] and LEGO Serious Play activities [35,37–42] have been used to deliver Scrum training. Moreover, other noteworthy alternatives have been used for this purpose, including serious video games not based on virtual reality [43–45], physical games [46–48], agile project management tools [49], and classroom exercises [50].

Scrum-X [43] is a game developed in Microsoft Excel 365 with VBA programming designed to teach Scrum to graduates and professionals in which players can manage software projects. Another serious video game for learning Scrum is Virtual Scrum [45]. In this game, players can explore and interact with a virtual world that simulates the room of a Scrum team. In [44], an online Scrum simulation conducted by using the multiplayer video game "Don't Starve Together", Trello, and Discord is presented. In addition to video games, some physical games aimed at teaching Scrum have been designed such as the card games PlayScrum [46] and "Don't Break the Build" [47]. Another physical game to teach Scrum was proposed by [48]. In this game, players organized in groups must build paper boats, hats, and planes following the Scrum framework.

Another approach that has been adopted for Scrum training is the planning and monitoring of software projects through agile project management tools such as Taiga [49]. Lastly, it is also worth mentioning that some classroom exercises have been proposed for introducing Scrum. For example, ref. [50] proposed "Play Ball", an exercise targeted to undergraduates that only requires 20–30 hand-size balls per team and that aims to introduce students to basic Scrum concepts and allow them to practice self-organization.

3. Research Methodology

The study presented in this article used a quasi-experimental design with two groups (A and B), pre- and post-tests, and a perceptions questionnaire. The goal of the study was to empirically examine and compare the effectiveness in terms of knowledge acquisition and motivation of two game-based interventions for learning Scrum and related agile practices: one in which participants played a virtual reality serious game and another based on LEGO Serious Play in which participants built a part of a city by using LEGO blocks. The students in group A played the virtual reality serious game, whereas the students in group B conducted the LEGO Serious Play activity.

3.1. Sample

This study involved the participation of 59 students in total. Group A was comprised of 22 students with a median age of 22.3 (SD = 2.3): 15 males, 5 females, and 2 students who preferred not to indicate their gender. Group B was comprised of 37 students with a median age of 22.5 (SD = 4.8): 32 males and 5 females. All students who participated in this study were enrolled in a project management course at Universidad Politécnica de Madrid. This project management course is worth 6 ECTS (European Credit Transfer System) credits (so it requires 150–180 h of student work) and all students in their fourth year of the Bachelor's Degree in software engineering are required to take it. The course covers the fundamentals and common practices of project management and introduces software project management using traditional and agile approaches.

3.2. Procedure

First, all participating students gave informed consent to participate in the study. Then, these students were split into two groups. Random assignment was not possible because some of the students had already played the serious game the previous academic year in a different course. Therefore, the students who had never played the serious game were assigned to group A and the remaining students were assigned to group B. Once the groups were established, all the participating students were given 10 min for completing a pre-test. Once this test was completed, students in group A played the virtual reality serious game over 40–45 min after spending 15 min attending to the teachers' instructions and setting up their devices; whereas students in group B conducted the LEGO Serious Play activity, which lasted around one hour. Then, all students were given 10 min for completing the post-test. Finally, students completed the perceptions questionnaire. The whole intervention, including the tests and the questionnaire, lasted around one hour and a half in both groups. All participating students completed both the pre- and post-test, as well as the perceptions questionnaire.

3.3. Methods and Instruments

The pre-test consisted of 10 theoretical questions encompassing the Scrum framework and related agile practices, including user stories, MoSCoW, story points, and Planning Poker. The questions were aligned with the official Scrum Guide 2020 [51] and the resources provided by the Agile Alliance [52]. Each question had four options, only one of which was correct. Correct answers were worth +1 point each, whereas incorrect answers were worth -0.33 points each. Thus, the pre-test was scored from 0 to 10. The post-test was composed by the same 10 questions included in the pre-test and was scored in the same way as this test. In this regard, it should be clarified that, with the aim of preventing students from memorizing answers, correct answers and additional feedback were only revealed to the students after the time to complete the post-test had expired. Moreover, in order to discourage copying and other unexpected misconduct, the students' final course grade remained unaffected by either their post-test scores or their pre-test scores.

The questionnaire distributed to all participants at the end of the intervention to collect their perceptions was developed ad hoc for this study. This questionnaire was comprised of two demographic questions (age and gender), a set of statements to be rated on a Likert scale ranging from one (strongly disagree) to five (strongly agree), and an open-ended question that allowed respondents to provide comments. The Likert items of the questionnaire are included in Section 4 together with the results. The questionnaire distributed to both groups was identical, except for item 18, which was exclusively included in the questionnaire given to the students in group A. This particular item aimed to inquire whether these students had experienced any dizziness while using the virtual reality serious game.

3.4. Materials: Virtual Reality Serious Game

The virtual reality serious game examined in this article is called ScrumVR and aims to instruct the player in the Scrum framework and some related agile practices in an immersive and effective way. ScrumVR is a first-person game in which the main character is a developer who starts to work in a software company that joins a Scrum team. During the game, the player receives explanations, interacts with other members of the Scrum team, engages actively in the Scrum events, contributes to the development of Scrum artifacts, and employs diverse agile techniques, including MoSCoW and Planning Poker. Screenshots of certain key events taking place throughout the game are shown in Figure 1.

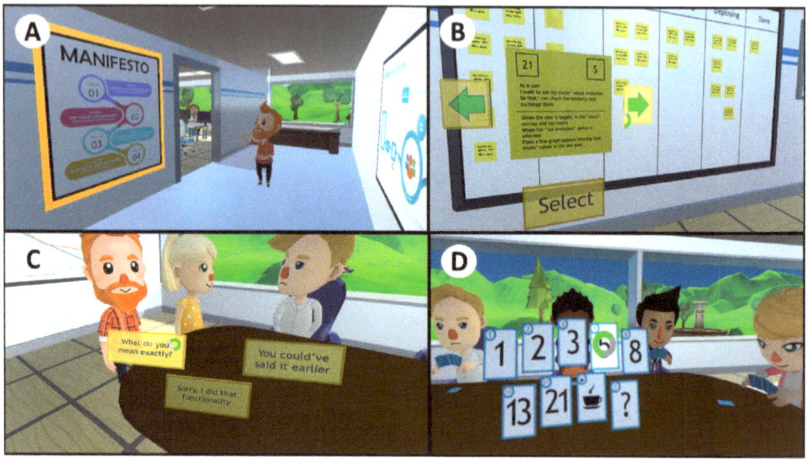

Figure 1. (**A**) The Scrum Master explains the foundation of agile methodologies. (**B**) The player chooses a user story. (**C**) The player talks with the Product Owner. (**D**) The player selects a card during a Planning Poker.

From a didactic standpoint, the game is narrated linearly, and it is divided into four chapters of approximately the same duration. Completing the four chapters requires the player to spend around 40–45 min. Each chapter is aimed at achieving certain learning objectives in such a way that the player learns how the Scrum framework works. Table 1 presents a summary of the main topics covered by each chapter of ScrumVR.

Table 1. Main topics covered by ScrumVR.

Chapter	Topics
1: Introduction	Agile and Scrum foundation. The role of the Scrum Master. How to operate a Kanban board.
2: Daily Scrum	Performance of a Daily Meeting in Scrum. How to select user stories based on their priority and size estimation. How to interpret a burndown chart.
3: Sprint Review and Sprint Retrospective	The role of the Product Owner. Performance of a Sprint Review. Performance of a Sprint Retrospective. How to analyze the Sprint performance using a burndown chart.
4: Sprint Planning	Performance of a Sprint Planning. How to define user stories. How to prioritize user stories using MoSCoW. How to estimate the size of user stories using Planning Poker and story points.

Regarding its technical characteristics, ScrumVR was developed using the Unity game engine and was conceived to be played by using Android devices equipped with a simple cardboard. One of the most remarkable points in the development of this educational application is the selected locomotion method. Since ScrumVR was designed for mobile devices, where positional tracking is not available, it was decided to use the on-rails guided locomotion method [53] in order to fully guide the player's movement and minimize the cybersickness feeling. Therefore, the players can look in all directions by rotating the head but do not have the freedom to move wherever they want, thus avoiding distractions and, consequently, facilitating the achievement of the established learning objectives. Additionally, positional sound [54] was used to guide the players to look in the most convenient direction throughout the experience. Another technical feature that was used for guiding the attention of the players was the use of illumination [55].

Another key technical feature of ScrumVR is the use of diegetic menus to allow the player to select an element by looking at it for a certain period of time. Whenever the player can perform an action in the game, a reticle that can be moved by rotating the head is displayed on the screen. When the reticle is placed over a selectable element, it starts to visually indicate the waiting time required to select that element. The diegetic menus used by ScrumVR allow the player to make decisions (see Figure 1C) and engage in agile techniques with other characters by playing mini-games (see Figure 1B,D). These mini-games were developed using a finite state machine model where all possible answers have an associated narrative feedback. Thereby, the learning experience is enriched with feedback generated according to the player's actions. More technical details about ScrumVR can be found at [19,20].

3.5. Materials: LEGO Serious Play Activity

The LEGO Serious Play activity assessed in this article aims to teach in an active and engaging way the Scrum framework and some related agile practices, including MoSCoW and Planning Poker. This activity was designed based on the LEGO City activity, which was initially conceived by Krivitsky [37] as explained in the related work section.

In the LEGO Serious Play activity, students work in teams of 4–6 members and each team assumes the role of a Scrum team belonging to a certain organization and working on a project whose goal is to build a part of a city (e.g., a neighborhood, a zoo, or a motor vehicle fleet). One student of each team assumes the role of the Product Owner, another student of the team assumes the role of the Scrum Master, and the remaining students of the team assume the role of the developers.

Each part of the city consists of a set of LEGO constructions. Therefore, each Scrum team has to build a part of a city by using the Scrum framework as methodology and LEGO pieces as materials. At the beginning of the activity, the Product Owner of each team is provided with a set of user story cards. Each of these cards includes a user story that describes a LEGO construction following the classic role–feature–benefit pattern, as well as two empty boxes in order to allow students to write the priority and estimated size of the user story (see Figure 2). During the activity, the LEGO constructions should be built by the developers (and only by the developers) using LEGO pieces according to their corresponding user stories and the LEGO construction manuals (see Figure 3). These manuals can also be used by the developers in order to estimate the size of the user stories.

The LEGO Serious Play activity consisted of the following phases:

1. Preparation. Students were divided into teams of 4–6 people and each team appointed a Product Owner and a Scrum Master. Then, each team received a starting pack comprised of the following elements: three instruction manuals (one for the Product Owner, one for the Scrum Master, and one for the developers), a LEGO box with pieces and construction manuals, a set of user story cards, and a kit of Planning Poker cards (see Figure 4). After that, each student read the instructions corresponding to his/her role (Product Owner, Scrum Master, or developer).

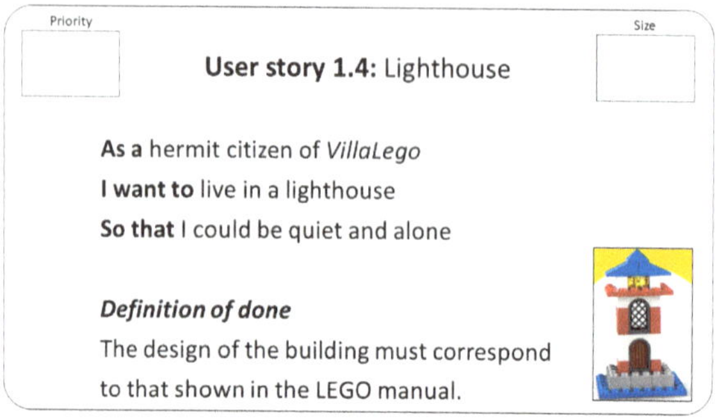

Figure 2. Example of a user story card.

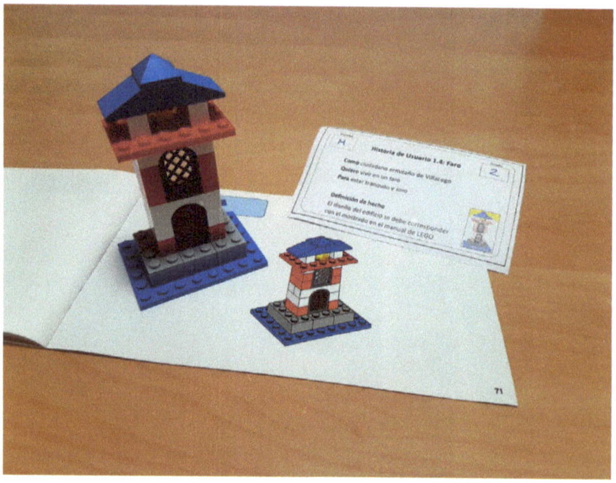

Figure 3. Example of a LEGO construction.

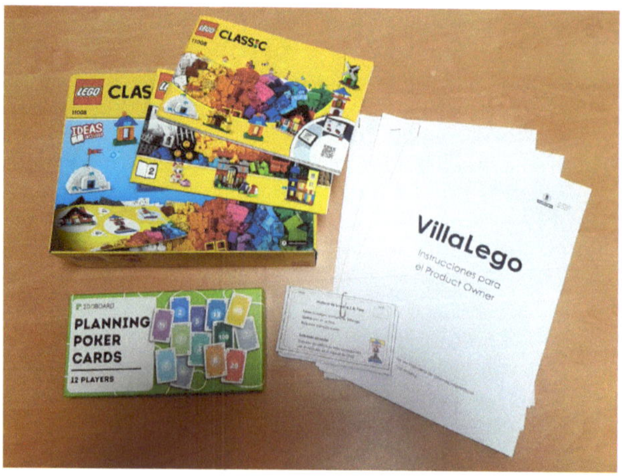

Figure 4. LEGO Serious Play activity starting pack.

2. Product backlog prioritization. The Product Owner prioritized the user stories using the MoSCoW technique. The Scrum Master was allowed to help the Product Owner

in applying this prioritization technique. Meanwhile, students playing the role of developers continued to familiarize themselves with its instructions.

3. Sprint planning. The Product Owner explained the client needs to the rest of the Scrum team and then all students defined a goal for the current Sprint. Then, the developers selected user stories to be included in the current Sprint in a consensual manner with the Product Owner. During this process, the size of the selected user stories was estimated by the developers using story points and Planning Poker.
4. Sprint execution. Once the Sprint planning event was over, students were given a total of 20 min for this phase. Each team had to hold two Daily Scrums during the Sprint: one at the beginning of this phase and another one 10 min later. During the Sprint, the students assuming the role of developers worked on building LEGO constructions in order to complete user stories, whereas the Product Owner was in charge of validating these constructions (i.e., the increments). The Scrum Master was accountable for the Scrum framework being adopted correctly, that is, as defined in the Scrum Guide.
5. Sprint review. The students held a Sprint review at the end of the Sprint, in which they presented the results of the Sprint (i.e., the LEGO constructions that were completely built during it) to the teachers, who acted as clients in this event. Furthermore, students discussed about what to do on the next Sprints.
6. Sprint Retrospective. After the Sprint review, students held a Sprint retrospective, in which they discussed what went well during the Sprint, what problems arose, and how these problems were or were not solved. Moreover, students reflected on their performance during the Sprint by using a burndown chart and identified at least one improvement for the next Sprint.

3.6. Data Analysis

The learning performance was determined as the difference between post-test and pre-test scores. A Shapiro–Wilk test of normality determined that not all collected data were normally distributed and hence non-parametric methods were employed. Within each group, the Wilcoxon signed-ranks test for paired samples was utilized to compare the post-test and pre-test scores, while the Mann–Whitney U test was employed to conduct comparisons between groups. In all comparisons, the correlation coefficient r was employed as the measure of effect size. Following Cohen's guidelines [56], an r value between 0.1 and 0.3 indicates a small effect size, between 0.3 and 0.5 it indicates a medium effect size, while an r value of 0.5 or greater signifies a large effect size. Finally, the mean (M) and the standard deviation (SD) were employed to analyze the results of the perceptions questionnaire. Moreover, the Spearman correlation analysis was performed to explore the relationships among the items of the perceptions questionnaire. The data collected and analyzed in this study are provided in the Supplementary Materials.

4. Results

4.1. Learning Performance

Table 2 shows the pre- and post-test scores achieved by the students in group A (who played the virtual reality game) and group B (who played the LEGO Serious Play activity). The learning performance, determined by the difference between post-test scores and pre-test scores, exhibited statistical significance in both groups. Its effect size was large ($r = 0.59$) in group A and medium ($r = 0.35$) in group B. These figures indicate that the two game-based learning approaches were effective in terms of knowledge acquisition.

When pre-test scores between groups were compared, a statistically significant difference with a medium effect size (p-value = 0.01; $r = 0.35$) was found in favor of group B. On the contrary, the difference between post-test scores obtained by both groups was non-statistically significant and had a less than small effect size (p-value = 0.50; $r = 0.09$). These results indicate that students in group A had less prior knowledge on Scrum and agile practices than their counterparts in group B but that, after the intervention, all students had similar knowledge on this matter regardless of their group. The comparison of learning performance between groups shows that there is a statistically significant difference with a medium effect size (p-value = 0.02, r = 0.30) in favor of group A. In view of this fact, it can be concluded that the serious game based on virtual reality used by the students in group A was more effective in terms of knowledge acquisition than the activity based on LEGO Serious Play conducted by the students in group B.

Table 2. Pre- and post-test scores.

Group	Pre-Test		Post-Test		Learning Performance		Wilcoxon Signed-Ranks Test for Paired Samples	
	M	SD	M	SD	M	SD	p-Value	Effect Size (r)
A (N = 22)	3.9	1.8	7.3	1.3	3.5	2.3	<0.01	0.59
B (N = 37)	5.3	2.5	6.8	2.2	1.5	2.6	<0.01	0.35

4.2. Students Perceptions

On the one hand, Table 3 shows the Likert items of the questionnaire that were used to collect the students' perceptions toward the game-based learning interventions. On the other hand, Table 4 shows the results of the questionnaire for both groups, including the rating difference between groups for each item.

Table 3. Likert items of the questionnaire.

Item	
1	My overall opinion of the activity is positive.
2	The activity helped me learn.
3	The activity was appealing and motivating.
4	The activity made learning fun.
5	The activity was immersive.
6	The activity was easy to complete.
7	I needed help to complete the activity.
8	The activity was well organized.
9	The activity is useful to learn about Scrum.
10	The activity is useful to learn about the roles defined by Scrum.
11	The activity is useful to learn about the events defined by Scrum.
12	The activity is useful to learn about the artifacts defined by Scrum.
13	The activity is useful to learn about the Planning Poker technique.
14	The activity is useful for learning about the MoSCoW technique.
15	In the future, I would like to conduct activities similar to the one I have conducted in other courses.
16	I prefer learning through activities such as the one I conducted for learning through traditional teaching methodologies.
17	The activity is a good complement to traditional teaching methodologies.
18 *	I did not experience any dizziness during the activity.

* Item 18 was included only for group A.

Overall, the students in both groups had a very positive opinion of the game-based learning activity that was performed in its group and found it beneficial for their learning, as well as motivating, fun, immersive, and well organized. Moreover, in both groups, most students thought the activity was easy to complete and stated that they did not need help to do so. Regarding self-perceived learning effectiveness, in both groups a vast majority of students considered the activity to be useful for learning about Scrum in general and, specifically, for learning about the roles, events, and artifacts defined by Scrum, as well as about two agile practices often used by Scrum teams: MoSCoW, and Planning Poker. Finally, students in both groups were generally in favor of using similar activities in future courses, either as a substitute for traditional teaching or as a complement to it.

Table 4. Results of the questionnaire.

Item	A Group		B Group		Mann–Whitney U Test	
	M	SD	M	SD	*p*-Value	Effect Size (r)
1	4.6	0.8	4.8	0.6	0.42	0.10
2	4.6	0.6	4.6	0.7	0.87	0.02
3	4.4	0.9	4.7	0.5	0.25	0.15
4	4.5	0.8	4.7	0.7	0.27	0.14
5	4.4	0.9	4.7	0.6	0.20	0.17
6	4.7	0.5	4.4	0.7	0.07	0.24
7	1.5	1.2	2.2	1.1	<0.01	0.45
8	4.8	0.4	4.5	0.6	0.07	0.23
9	4.7	0.5	4.6	0.7	0.34	0.12
10	4.5	0.8	4.6	0.5	0.74	0.04
11	4.8	0.4	4.6	0.6	0.47	0.09
12	4.4	0.8	4.4	0.8	0.87	0.02
13	4.9	0.3	4.7	0.6	0.30	0.13
14	4.7	0.4	4.3	1.0	0.15	0.19
15	4.7	0.6	4.7	0.6	0.97	0.00
16	3.8	1.3	4.4	1.1	0.09	0.22
17	4.7	0.5	4.8	0.5	0.54	0.08
18	3.5	1.5	-	-	-	-

With respect to the question about dizziness, included only in the questionnaire administered to the students in group A, 7 out of 22 (32%) students reported experiencing some kind of dizziness while using the virtual reality serious game. In this regard, it should be indicated that all participating students were able to complete the activity without major issues. Furthermore, the Spearman correlation analysis was run and no statistically significant correlations were found between dizziness and the intention to use similar virtual reality games in the future or any other item of the perceptions questionnaire.

The average ratings given by the students in both groups were very similar for most questionnaire items. In fact, the effect size of the difference between group ratings was found to be less than small and non-statistically significant at the 0.05 level for all items except for items 6, 7, 8, and 16. For the items 6, 8, and 16 the effect size was small and non-statistically significant. The item 7 (needed help) was the only one for which the difference was found to be statistically significant at the 0.05 level. The effect size of this difference was found to be medium to large (r = 0.45) and indicates that, although in general terms students in both groups agreed that they did not need help to complete the activity, the students in group A agreed more strongly on this statement in comparison with their counterparts. In general, the comments provided by the participating students through the administered questionnaire were in line with the outcomes of the Likert items in both groups. Several students expressed in their comments the innovative nature of both activities and expressed gratitude to the course instructors for organizing them. In group A, some students explained that they felt some dizziness and eyestrain during the use of the virtual reality serious game. In group B, students suggested to increase the time of the activity and to incorporate more Sprints.

5. Discussion

The results of this article show that the two game-based learning interventions examined were effective in terms of both knowledge acquisition and motivation. These results are consistent with the current body of research on game-based learning [1–7], which suggests that this methodology is capable of producing positive impacts on student performance and motivation. More specifically, the results obtained for the virtual reality serious game are consistent with those of previous assessments of this game [19–21]. Regarding the results obtained for the LEGO Serious Play activity, it is worth remarking that they are aligned with those of [37–40], who also examined the use of a LEGO Serious Play activity for learning Scrum and found that it was beneficial for the students' learning.

Although student perceptions were very similar for the two interventions, students in group A (who played the virtual reality serious game) outperformed their counterparts in group B (who conducted the LEGO Serious Play activity) in terms of knowledge acquisition. In this regard, it is worth pointing out that the students in group A had less prior knowledge on Scrum and agile practices than those in group B. A possible explanation for this fact is that students in group B had played the virtual reality serious game in the previous academic year in a different course so they received extra training on Scrum and agile practices compared to their peers. The results also show that, in spite of this difference in prior knowledge on Scrum and related agile practices, students in both groups had similar knowledge on this matter after the intervention.

Regarding students' perceptions, it should be remarked that most students found both game-based learning interventions motivating, fun, immersive, easy to complete, and adequately organized, as well as beneficial for their learning. In regard to this latter finding, it is worth pointing out that the students' reports of self-perceived learning effectiveness were aligned with the results of the pre- and post-tests and clearly evidence that both interventions were useful for learning about the core concepts of Scrum including its roles, events, and artifacts, as well as for learning about agile practices frequently used by Scrum teams such as MoSCoW and Planning Poker.

Another interesting finding of this article is that the participating students were generally in favor of conducting similar game-based learning activities in future courses, either as a complement to traditional teaching or as a substitute of traditional teaching. In this regard, it should be noted that the use of such activities as a complement to traditional learning methodologies seems to have greater acceptance among students using them as a replacement. The students who conducted the LEGO Serious Play activity agreed more strongly on these statements than their counterparts, which is a noteworthy but not statistically significant difference between groups. A reasonable explanation for this fact could have been that a significant percentage (32%) of the students who played the virtual reality serious game reported experiencing some kind of dizziness during the intervention. However, all participating students were able to complete the activity without major issues and no statistically significant correlation was found between dizziness and the intention to use similar virtual reality games in the future or any other item of the perceptions questionnaire. Therefore, it can be concluded that students' perceptions toward the virtual reality serious game were not affected by dizziness and that dizziness was not severe in any case.

The only statistically significant difference between groups in terms of student perceptions was that the students who played the virtual reality serious game reported that they did not need help to a greater extent than their counterparts. This is an expected finding, since the serious game is a resource that was designed for self-learning whereas the LEGO Serious Play activity was designed to be conducted in class under the supervision of the teaching staff. Notwithstanding, according to the results of the student questionnaire, most students who participated in the LEGO Serious Play activity did not need help. This finding suggests that the provided instructions, although having room for improvement, were found suitable in most cases.

6. Conclusions

This article empirically examined and compared the effectiveness for learning Scrum and related agile practices of a serious game based on virtual reality and a learning activity based on the LEGO Serious Play methodology by means of a quasi-experiment with two groups, pre- and post-tests, and a perceptions questionnaire. The reported results show that both game-based learning approaches were effective in terms of knowledge acquisition and motivation, as well as showing that the students who played the virtual reality serious game outperformed their peers, who conducted a LEGO Serious Play activity, in terms of knowledge acquisition. Therefore, the results of the article suggest that game-based learning using virtual reality serious games or LEGO Serious Play is a suitable option for educators who are willing to teach in an innovative and playful way agile methodologies such as Scrum.

Although previous works examined the use of virtual reality serious games for learning Scrum [19–24], as well as the use of LEGO Serious Play for this same purpose [35,37–42], to the knowledge of the authors this is the first work that performed a comparison between these two game-based learning approaches. Therefore, this article makes a novel contribution by providing, for the first time, evidence on the learning effectiveness of virtual reality serious games compared to LEGO Serious Play. Furthermore, the results reported in this article contribute to a better understanding of the benefits and drawbacks of these two game-based learning approaches.

It should be taken into account that, in spite of providing solid evidence of the effectiveness of virtual reality serious games and LEGO Serious Play, the study presented in this article has some important limitations. First, no random sampling was used because students had to be divided based on whether or not they had played the virtual reality serious game in the past. Second, the study was focused on the evaluation of a single virtual reality serious game and a single LEGO Serious Play activity and the sample size was small (22 for group A and 37 for group B), so the conclusions should be treated with caution. Third, the study examined the learning effectiveness in the short term, but not in the long term. Another noteworthy limitation is that certain aspects of the game-based learning experiences such as enjoyment, motivation, and immersion could have been explored in more detail by extending the perceptions questionnaire to cover additional criteria (e.g., [57]) and by using other evaluations instruments such as the GAMEX scale [58], the Game Engagement Questionnaire [59], the Game Experience Questionnaire [60], or the Igroup Presence Questionnaire [61]. Therefore, an interesting direction for future work is to make further comparisons addressing these aspects in more depth.

An interesting finding of this article was that most students preferred to learn through virtual reality serious games or LEGO Serious Play activities rather than through traditional teaching methods. However, no comparison was conducted between these game-based learning approaches and traditional teaching using control and experimental groups. Thus, future works should conduct this type of comparison, preferably through randomized control trials. Other interesting future works could be to examine the long-term impacts of these approaches through longitudinal studies, as well as to examine them with different games, technologies, instructional designs, and knowledge areas.

Supplementary Materials: The following supporting information can be downloaded at: https://www.mdpi.com/article/10.3390/app14020830/s1, the data collected and analyzed in this study are available as Supplementary Material File.

Author Contributions: Conceptualization, A.G., D.L.-F. and J.M.; methodology, A.G. and D.L.-F.; software, D.L.-F. and J.M.; formal analysis, A.G.; investigation, A.G. and D.L.-F.; resources, A.G. and D.L.-F.; writing—original draft preparation, A.G., D.L.-F. and J.M.; writing—review and editing, A.G., D.L.-F. and J.M. All authors have read and agreed to the published version of the manuscript.

Funding: This work was supported in part by Universidad Politécnica de Madrid (UPM) through the educational innovation projects under Grant IE22.6104 and Grant IE23.6104.

Institutional Review Board Statement: Ethical review and approval were waived for this study due to the fact that the study only involved the collection of information via surveys and educational tests and all information collected was anonymized so that the identity of the participants cannot be ascertained.

Informed Consent Statement: Informed consent was obtained from all subjects involved in the study.

Data Availability Statement: The data collected and analyzed in this study are available as Supplementary Material. The authors will request after publication that these data be published under an open license in e-cienciaDatos—https://edatos.consorciomadrono.es (accessed on 17 November 2023).

Conflicts of Interest: The authors declare no conflict of interest.

References

1. Udeozor, C.; Toyoda, R.; Russo Abegão, F.; Glassey, J. Digital games in engineering education: Systematic review and future trends. *Eur. J. Eng. Educ.* **2022**, *48*, 321–339. [CrossRef]
2. Karakoç, B.; Eryılmaz, K.; Turan Özpolat, E.; Yıldırım, İ. The effect of game-based learning on student achievement: A meta-analysis study. *Technol. Knowl. Learn.* **2020**, *27*, 207–222. [CrossRef]
3. Tokac, U.; Novak, E.; Thompson, C.G. Effects of game-based learning on students' mathematics achievement: A meta-analysis. *J. Comput. Assist. Learn.* **2019**, *35*, 407–420. [CrossRef]
4. Hussein, M.H.; Ow, S.H.; Cheong, L.S.; Thong, M.-K.; Ale Ebrahim, N. Effects of digital game-based learning on elementary science learning: A systematic review. *IEEE Access* **2019**, *7*, 62465–62478. [CrossRef]
5. Boyle, E.A.; Hainey, T.; Connolly, T.M.; Gray, G.; Earp, J.; Ott, M.; Lim, T.; Ninaus, M.; Ribeiro, C.; Pereira, J. An update to the systematic literature review of empirical evidence of the impacts and outcomes of computer games and serious games. *Comput. Educ.* **2016**, *94*, 178–192. [CrossRef]
6. Hainey, T.; Connolly, T.M.; Boyle, E.A.; Wilson, A.; Razak, A. A systematic literature review of games-based learning empirical evidence in primary education. *Comput. Educ.* **2016**, *102*, 202–223. [CrossRef]
7. Bodnar, C.A.; Anastasio, D.; Enszer, J.A.; Burkey, D.D. Engineers at play: Games as teaching tools for undergraduate engineering students. *J. Eng. Educ.* **2016**, *105*, 147–200. [CrossRef]
8. Digital.ai. *15th State of Agile Report*; Digital.ai: Raleigh, NC, USA, 2021; Available online: https://info.digital.ai/rs/981-LQX-968/images/SOA15.pdf (accessed on 17 November 2023).
9. Verma, P.; Kumar, R.; Tuteja, J.; Gupta, N. Systematic review of virtual reality & its challenges. In Proceedings of the 3rd International Conference on Intelligent Communication Technologies and Virtual Mobile Networks (ICICV 2021), Tirunelveli, India, 4–6 February 2021; pp. 434–440.
10. Radhakrishnan, U.; Koumaditis, K.; Chinello, F. A systematic review of immersive virtual reality for industrial skills training. *Behav. Inf. Technol.* **2021**, *40*, 1310–1339. [CrossRef]
11. Kurniawan, C.; Rosmansyah, Y.; Dabarsyah, B. A Systematic Literature Review on Virtual Reality for Learning. In Proceedings of the 2019 5th International Conference on Wireless and Telematics, ICWT 2019, Yogyakarta, Indonesia, 25–26 July 2019.
12. Zhang, J.; Chang, J.; Yang, X.; Zhang, J.J. Virtual reality surgery simulation: A survey on patient specific solution. In *Next Generation Computer Animation Techniques, Proceedings of the Third International Workshop, AniNex 2017, Bournemouth, UK, 22–23 June 2017*; Lecture Notes in Computer Science (including subseries Lecture Notes in Artificial Intelligence and Lecture Notes in Bioinformatics); Springer: Cham, Switzerland, 2017; Volume 10582, pp. 220–233.
13. Hernandez, Y.; Ramirez, M.P. Virtual reality systems for training improvement in electrical distribution substations. In Proceedings of the IEEE 16th International Conference on Advanced Learning Technologies, ICALT 2016, Austin, TX, USA, 25–28 July 2016; pp. 75–76.
14. Stănică, I.-C.; Dascalu, M.-I.; Moldoveanu, A.; Bodea, C.-N.; Hostiuc, S. A survey of virtual reality applications as psychotherapeutic tools to treat phobias. In Proceedings of the 12th International Scientific Conference eLearning and Software for Education, Bucharest, Romania, 21–22 April 2016.
15. Cheng, A.; Yang, L.; Andersen, E. Teaching language and culture with a virtual reality game. In Proceedings of the Conference on Human Factors in Computing Systems, Denver, CO, USA, 6–11 May 2017; pp. 541–549.
16. Rivas, D.; Alvarez, M.V.; Guerrero, F.; Grijalva, D.; Loor, S.; Espinoza, J.; Vayas, G.; Huerta, M. Virtual reality applied to physics teaching. In Proceedings of the 2017 9th International Conference on Education Technology and Computers, Barcelona, Spain, 20–22 December 2017; pp. 27–30.
17. Kamińska, D.; Sapiński, T.; Wiak, S.; Tikk, T.; Haamer, R.E.; Avots, E.; Helmi, A.; Ozcinar, C.; Anbarjafari, G. Virtual reality and its applications in education: Survey. *Information* **2019**, *10*, 318. [CrossRef]
18. Pirker, J.; Dengel, A.; Holly, M.; Safikhani, S. Virtual Reality in Computer Science Education: A Systematic Review. In Proceedings of the 26th ACM Symposium on Virtual Reality Software and Technology, Virtual Event, Canada, 1–4 November 2020.
19. Mayor, J.; López-Fernández, D. Scrum VR: Virtual reality serious video game to learn Scrum. *Appl. Sci.* **2021**, *11*, 9015. [CrossRef]
20. López-Fernández, D.; Mayor, J.; Perez, J.; Gordillo, A. Learning and Motivational Impact of Using a Virtual Reality Serious Video Game to Learn Scrum. *IEEE Trans. Games* **2023**, *15*, 430–439. [CrossRef]
21. Lopez-Fernandez, D.; Mayor, J.; Garcia-Perez, M.; Gordillo, A. Are virtual reality serious video games more effective than web video games? *IEEE Comput. Graph. Appl.* **2023**, *43*, 32–42. [CrossRef]
22. Caserman, P.; Gobel, S. Become a Scrum Master: Immersive virtual reality training to learn Scrum framework. In *Serious Games*; Ma, M., Fletcher, B., Göbel, S., Hauge, J.B., Marsh, T., Eds.; Springer: Cham, Switzerland, 2020; pp. 34–48.
23. Radhakrishnan, U.; Koumaditis, K. Teaching Scrum with a Virtual Sprint Simulation: Initial design and considerations. In Proceedings of the 26th ACM Symposium on Virtual Reality Software and Technology, Virtual Event, Canada, 1–4 November 2020; pp. 1–2.

24. Visescu, I.; Blindu, A.; Radhakrishnan, U.; Kadenic, M.; Chinello, F.; Koumaditis, K. Teaching project management in a virtual environment: The Virtual Scrum Simulator (ScrumSim). In Proceedings of the 2022 Nordic Human-Computer Interaction Conference, Aarhus, Denmark, 8–12 October 2022; pp. 1–2.
25. LEGO Serious Play. Available online: https://www.lego.com/themes/serious-play/background (accessed on 17 November 2023).
26. Roos, J.; Victor, B. How It All Began: The Origins Of LEGO® Serious Play®. *Int. J. Manag. Appl. Res.* **2018**, *5*, 326–343. [CrossRef]
27. Dann, S. Facilitating co-creation experience in the classroom with Lego Serious Play. *Australas. Mark. J.* **2018**, *26*, 121–131. [CrossRef]
28. James, A.R. Lego Serious Play: A three-dimensional approach to learning development. *J. Learn. Dev. High. Educ.* **2013**, *6*. [CrossRef]
29. Hansen, P.K.; O'Connor, R. Innovation and learning facilitated by play. In *Encyclopedia of the Sciences of Learning*; Springer: Boston, MA, USA, 2012; pp. 1569–1570.
30. Nielsen, C.B.; Adams, P. Active learning via LEGO MINDSTORMS in Systems Engineering education. In Proceedings of the 2015 IEEE International Symposium on Systems Engineering (ISSE), Rome, Italy, 28–30 September 2015; IEEE: Piscataway, NJ, USA, 2015; pp. 489–495.
31. Kurkovsky, S. Teaching software engineering with LEGO serious play. In Proceedings of the 2015 ACM Conference on Innovation and Technology in Computer Science Education, Vilnius, Lithuania, 4–8 July 2015; pp. 213–218.
32. Kurkovsky, S.; Ludi, S.; Clark, L. Active learning with LEGO for software requirements. In Proceedings of the 50th ACM Technical Symposium on Computer Science Education (SIGCSE 2019), Minneapolis, MN, USA, 27 February 2019; Association for Computing Machinery: New York, NY, USA, 2019; pp. 218–224.
33. Kurkovsky, S. Using LEGO to teach software interfaces and integration. In Proceedings of the 23rd Annual ACM Conference on Innovation and Technology in Computer Science Education, Larnaca, Cyprus, 2–4 July 2018; pp. 371–372.
34. Kurkovsky, S. A LEGO-based approach to introducing test-driven development. In Proceedings of the 2016 ACM Conference on Innovation and Technology in Computer Science Education, Arequipa, Peru, 9–13 July 2016; pp. 246–247.
35. Kurkovsky, S. A simple game to introduce Scrum concepts. In Proceedings of the 51st ACM Technical Symposium on Computer Science Education (SIGCSE 2020), Portland, OR, USA, 11–14 March 2020; p. 1321.
36. López-Fernández, D.; Gordillo, A.; Ortega, F.; Yague, A.; Tovar, E. LEGO® Serious Play in Software Engineering Education. *IEEE Access* **2021**, *9*, 103120–103131. [CrossRef]
37. Krivitsky, A. *lego4scrum: A Complete Guide. A Great Way to Teach the Scrum Framework and Agile Thinking*; Self-published by Alexey Krivitsky: Kyiv, Ukraine, 2017.
38. Velić, M.; Padavić, I.; Dobrović, Ž. Metamodel of Agile Project Management and the Process of Building with LEGO® Bricks. In Proceedings of the 23rd Central European Conference on Information and Intelligent Systems (CECIIS 2012), Varazdin, Croatia, 19–21 September 2012; pp. 481–493.
39. Gama, K. An experience report on using LEGO-based activities in a software engineering course. In Proceedings of the XXXIII Brazilian Symposium on Software Engineering, Salvador, Brazil, 23–27 September 2019; pp. 289–298.
40. Paasivaara, M.; Heikkilä, V.; Lassenius, C.; Toivola, T. Teaching students Scrum using LEGO blocks. In Proceedings of the 36th International Conference on Software Engineering, Hyderabad, India, 31 May–7 June 2014; pp. 382–391.
41. Gama, K.; Oliveira, H. An experience report on teaching Scrum principles in a playful way through distant collaboration with online whiteboards. In Proceedings of the XXXVI Brazilian Symposium on Software Engineering (SBES '22), Virtual, 5–7 October 2022; pp. 143–152.
42. Steghofer, J.-P.; Burden, H. One block on top of the other: Using Minetest to teach Scrum. In Proceedings of the 2022 IEEE/ACM 44th International Conference on Software Engineering: Software Engineering Education and Training, Pittsburgh, PA, USA, 25–27 May 2022; pp. 176–186.
43. Lee, W.L. SCRUM-X: An interactive and experiential learning platform for teaching Scrum. In Proceedings of the 7th International Conference on Education, Training and Informatics (ICETI 2016), Orlando, FL, USA, 8–11 March 2016; pp. 192–197.
44. Christensen, E.L.; Paasivaara, M. Respond to change or die: An educational Scrum simulation for distributed teams. In Proceedings of the ACM/IEEE 44th International Conference on Software Engineering: Software Engineering Education and Training, Pittsburgh, PA, USA, 25–27 May 2022; pp. 235–246.
45. Rodriguez, G.; Soria, Á.; Campo, M. Virtual Scrum: A teaching aid to introduce undergraduate software engineering students to Scrum. *Comput. Appl. Eng. Educ.* **2015**, *23*, 147–156. [CrossRef]
46. Fernandes, J.M.; Sousa, S.M. PlayScrum—A card game to learn the Scrum agile method. In Proceedings of the 2010 Second International Conference on Games and Virtual Worlds for Serious Applications, Braga, Portugal, 25–26 March 2010; pp. 52–59.
47. Marshburn, D.G.; Sieck, J.P. Don't break the build: Developing a Scrum retrospective game. In Proceedings of the 52nd Hawaii International Conference on System Sciences, Maui, HI, USA, 8–11 January 2019; pp. 6988–6996.
48. Von Wangenheim, C.G.; Savi, R.; Borgatto, A.F. SCRUMIA—An educational game for teaching Scrum in computing courses. *J. Syst. Softw.* **2013**, *86*, 2675–2687. [CrossRef]
49. Villavicencio, M.; Narvaez, E.; Izquierdo, E.; Pincay, J. Learning Scrum by doing real-life projects. In Proceedings of the 2017 IEEE Global Engineering Education Conference (EDUCON 2017), Athens, Greece, 25–28 April 2017; pp. 1450–1456.
50. May, J.; York, J.; Lending, D. Play Ball: Bringing Scrum into the classroom. *J. Inf. Syst. Educ.* **2016**, *27*, 87–92.

51. Schwaber, K.; Sutherland, J. Scrum Guide 2020. Available online: https://scrumguides.org/docs/scrumguide/v2020/2020-Scrum-Guide-US.pdf (accessed on 17 November 2023).
52. Agile Alliance Agile Alliance Web Portal. Available online: https://www.agilealliance.org (accessed on 17 November 2023).
53. Bishop, I.; Rizwan Abid, M. Survey of locomotion systems in virtual reality. In Proceedings of the 2nd International Conference on Information System and Data Mining, Lakeland, FL, USA, 9–11 April 2018; pp. 151–154.
54. Dumlu, B.N.; Demir, Y. Analyzing the user experience of virtual reality storytelling with visual and aural stimuli. In *Design, User Experience, and Usability. Design for Contemporary Interactive Environments, Proceedings of the 22nd HCI International Conference, HCII 2020, Copenhagen, Denmark, 19–24 July 2020*; Lecture Notes in Computer Science; Marcus, A., Rosenzweig, E., Eds.; Springer: Cham, Switzerland, 2020; Volume 12201.
55. Rangaswamy, S. Visual storytelling through lighting. In Proceedings of the Game Developers Conference, San Jose, CA, USA, 8–12 March 2000.
56. Cohen, J. *Statistical Power Analysis for the Behavioral Sciences*, 2nd ed.; Routledge: New York, NY, USA, 1988.
57. Caserman, P.; Hoffmann, K.; Müller, P.; Schaub, M.; Straßburg, K.; Wiemeyer, J.; Bruder, R.; Göbel, S. Quality criteria for serious games: Serious part, game part, and balance. *JMIR Serious Games* **2020**, *8*, e19037. [CrossRef]
58. Eppmann, R.; Bekk, M.; Klein, K. Gameful experience in gamification: Construction and validation of a gameful experience scale [GAMEX]. *J. Interact. Mark.* **2018**, *43*, 98–115. [CrossRef]
59. Brockmyer, J.H.; Fox, C.M.; Curtiss, K.A.; McBroom, E.; Burkhart, K.M.; Pidruzny, J.N. The development of the Game Engagement Questionnaire: A measure of engagement in video game-playing. *J. Exp. Soc. Psychol.* **2009**, *45*, 624–634. [CrossRef]
60. IJsselsteijn, W.A.; de Kort, Y.A.W.; Poels, K. *The Game Experience Questionnaire*; Technische Universiteit Eindhoven: Eindhoven, The Netherlands, 2013.
61. igroup.org—Project Consortium Igroup Presence Questionnaire (IPQ) Overview. Available online: https://www.igroup.org/pq/ipq (accessed on 17 November 2023).

virtual worlds

MDPI

Article

Adding a Web-Based Virtual Reality Classroom Experience to a Hybrid, Blended Course Modality

Laura Huisinga

Department of Art, Design and Art History, California State University Fresno Campus, CA 93740, USA; lhuisinga@csufresno.edu

Abstract: The blended classroom is a unique space for face-to-face (F2F) interaction and online learning. The blended classroom has three distinct interaction types: in-person synchronous, virtual synchronous, and virtual asynchronous; each of these modalities lends itself to different forms of extended reality. This case study looks at using a virtual reality (VR) classroom for an online synchronous weekly meetings for three upper-division or advanced (junior and senior level) higher education design classes at a university. The use of social web VR for a classroom can offer a collaborative, real-time environment that bridges the gap between virtual video conferences and gaming platforms. This paper examines how to use social web VR in a virtual classroom. Mixed methods were used to collect usability data at the end of the semester survey. The system usability scale (SUS) and several qualitative questions gathered student feedback. Overall, the students enjoyed using the VR classroom, but audio issues seemed to be the most significant pain point. While the overall response was positive, this study will address several areas for improvement from both the student and instructor perspectives. Social, web-based VR offers promising potential. Designing a human-centered virtual environment and considering all participants' total user experience is critical to a successful learning tool.

Keywords: virtual reality; blended learning classroom; social virtual reality; web-based virtual reality; virtual reality classroom; extended reality

Citation: Huisinga, L. Adding a Web-Based Virtual Reality Classroom Experience to a Hybrid, Blended Course Modality. *Virtual Worlds* **2023**, 2, 231–242. https://doi.org/10.3390/virtualworlds2030014

Academic Editor: Christos J. Bouras

Received: 28 January 2023
Revised: 18 May 2023
Accepted: 20 July 2023
Published: 1 August 2023

1. Introduction

Virtual reality (VR) is an advanced technology used across different sectors including medicine, aviation, art, and design [1,2]. Virtual reality can be used for training, therapy, exhibits, and gaming, yet it is not widely used in daily life. Virtual reality is not a new concept; the accessibility of VR technology has dramatically increased in the last few years. Social virtual worlds are increasingly embedded into e-commerce and e-learning [3]. In education, virtual reality technology is a way for teachers and students to create a simulated three-dimensional world [4].

Hardware like head-mounted displays (HMD) has become more cost-effective, yet it is not commonly owned by the masses like a smartphone. According to Pew Research, 85% of Americans own a smartphone. Web-based VR consists of 360-degree content that can be viewed and navigated using a web browser. In theory, any device capable of connecting to the internet could run a web-based VR experience. Web-based VR offers unique access across multiple devices, including phones, tablets, laptops, and head-mounted displays (HMDs). Leveraging existing devices increases digital equity and allows access to be scaled up quickly [5]. Web-based social VR is a subset of desktop-based VR and virtual worlds [6].

Unfortunately, there is often a digital divide issue in practice. While various devices like phones and tablets can, in theory, run web-based VR, many device variables can contribute to a negative user experience, such as older hardware and slow or inconsistent internet connection speeds. Ideally, access to head-mounted displays could give students additional immersion. However, the HMD should be an option used primarily for shorter meetings where movement and interaction in the space or with others is the primary objective; as noted in earlier studies, discomfort or VR sickness from long-term wear and difficulty with note taking while wearing an HMD are known issues [7–9]. In addition to the digital divide, digital skill gaps are increasingly an issue. There is a great need to establish projects addressing the digital skills needed for using social virtual environments or web-based VR higher education [10].

Social VR allows people to communicate in real time through avatars that can interact in a virtual world. Web-based social VR facilitates communication, collaboration, and interaction between people in a virtual world when meeting in real-life is too tricky, or inconvenient [11]. During the pandemic, many instructors sought alternatives to video conferencing to increase immersion and presence. Some turned to web-based virtual reality as a viable option. While research was already being conducted on distance learning using social virtual reality environments in education, the pandemic forced everyone to adopt distance learning, and some chose to explore the use of social virtual worlds. There was a significant rise in usage of this technology in multiple regions of the globe [12]. Current social VR platforms can provide an easy and affordable way for educators to utilize VR [13].

Several studies on Mozilla Hub web-based VR studies have been conducted since the pandemic [5,7,8,11,14]. Being unable to meet in person, especially for large events, made the virtual environment an exciting alternative. Conferences, expos, and festivals turned to VR to interact, collaborate, and meet up with people worldwide. One could even attend the annual Burning Man festival—where artists and makers gather to build Black Rock City, a participative temporary metropolis in the Nevada desert—in virtual reality in 2020.

Using avatars can create an enhanced sense of self for the learner since they can often customize and control the avatar that digitally represents them [10,15]. Some studies have even shown that the increased connection to the learner's avatar positively affected their engagement and ability to follow online discussions in the virtual world [16]. Social VR can be a successful tool in social learning spaces. [17] Some studies have shown that the VR learning environment can effectively ensure students' motivation and sociability in distance learning [18].

While there was an increase in the use and experimentation with virtual reality as a replacement for not being able to meet in person during a time of mandatory physical separation, previous studies on the use of virtual reality in education pre-COVID have shown how social virtual reality can be used as an educational tool to foster deep, meaningful learning [10]. Delivering course material via a virtual environment is beneficial to students [19]. Additionally, a literature review by Mystakidis et al., of studies before 2020 suggests, that social virtual reality Environments or SVREs "can provide authentic, simulated, cognitively challenging experiences in engaging, motivating environments for open-ended social and collaborative interactions and intentional, personalized Learning". This pre-pandemic literature review of social virtual reality environments or SVREs shows the promise of using virtual reality to facilitate deep, meaningful learning and foster engagement in a virtual setting across different disciplines through distance learning.

Social virtual reality environments can enhance distance education efficacy when used in combination with applying instructional methodologies such as situated learning, experiential learning, and game-based learning [20].

This case study looks at using a virtual reality (VR) classroom for an online synchronous weekly meeting for three upper-division advanced junior and senior-level design classes. During the height of the COVID-19 worldwide pandemic, all higher education institutions switched to a virtual teaching model. In many cases, this meant instructors provided class content in a learning management system (LMS) such as Canvas or Blackboard and then held classes over a video chat platform like Zoom or Microsoft Teams.

As institutions have navigated the process of bringing more instructors and students back to a face-to-face (F2F) campus environment, there have been various blended or hybrid learning options. A unique opportunity to research the use of web-based virtual reality for remote learning happened during the pandemic. New literature details the quick pivot to web-based virtual reality and what we have learned from relying solely on virtual reality as a point of interaction. Moving forward, educators can now look at how web-based virtual reality can fit into a blended learning environment. The blended classroom is a unique space for face-to-face (F2F) interaction and online learning. Blended learning has three distinct interaction types: in-person synchronous, virtual synchronous, and virtual asynchronous; each of these modalities lends itself to different forms of extended reality. Studies have also shown that when virtual environments are used as a supplement and incorporate traditional instruction strategies, they are more effective than autonomous learning experiences [21].

This work aims to look at how extended reality can pair with a blended classroom model. This study specifically looks at using a virtual reality (VR) classroom for an online synchronous weekly meeting for three upper-division design classes. The use of social web VR for a classroom can offer a collaborative real-time environment that bridges the gap between virtual video conferences and gaming platforms. The study is significant and relevant due to advances in extended reality web-based technology and the change in expected classroom modalities. A blended instruction model achieves greater flexibility for both instructors and students. This flexibility allows for quick pivots of classroom modality for any reason. In addition, it creates an equitable environment for students to continue receiving instruction even if they cannot attend F2F in-person classes for any reason.

2. Materials and Methods

Three advanced interactive multimedia classes in the Graphics Design Bachelor of Fine Arts (BFA) degree at California State University were used in this study, each class with a description is listed below.

GD142 User Experience and User Interface Design Course Description: An intermediate web design class for graphic designers. The class focuses on user experience design methods and practices to improve the usability and aesthetics of a user interface. Students will use user experience methods to engineer the whole experience surrounding a digital environment, emphasizing how data-driven research can improve the layout, hierarchy, typography, and color scheme of a user interface. Summary/outline of the course: Students will design website mock-ups and test functioning prototypes of their interfaces based on user experience methods. Through usability tests, they will refine their prototypes with multiple iterations to create finalized mock-ups ready for development. Similar to a style guide for a brand, they will create style guidelines to document the user interface systems they have created for their website.

GD157 Motiongraphics Course Description: Understand and implement animation principles for time-based media. Application of software to create visually integrated, concept-driven motion graphics and interactive web animations. Emphasis on research, including usability research and production of advanced time-based media projects.

GD159 Immersive Design Course Description: This course explores 3D digital modeling and its incorporation into augmented and virtual environments. Students will research and explore different ways to implement augmented and virtual reality. Summary/outline of the course: This course will be driven by research and experimental development of immersive technologies. Students will learn the basics of 3D modeling while researching how to implement them in different augmented and virtual environments. Time will also be spent considering the usability, UX (user experience) design, and UI (user interface) design of an augmented or virtual reality interface.

Mixed methods collected usability data at the end of the semester survey. In addition, the system usability scale (SUS) and several qualitative questions gathered feedback from the students. The classes are blended, hybrid class modalities meaning that on Mondays, students can join the instructor in the classroom face-to-face (F2F), join via Zoom or watch a recording asynchronously. On Wednesdays, students meet for check-in via Mozilla Hubs, a social web-based virtual reality platform. This is the text from the syllabus explaining the blended breakdown:

Group meetings will be held on Mondays to allow us to interact together. Most Mondays, there will be live face-to-face (F2F) meetings in person. Some Mondays will be held via a live Zoom meeting locations will be noted on the syllabus and on canvas. Attending the group meeting live is optional but highly recommended. You are responsible for reviewing the content and recordings of the meeting on canvas and asking questions if you cannot make the Monday F2F or Zoom meeting.

Weekly Check-ins will happen on Wednesdays. We will all join our virtual classroom in Mozilla Hubs for 30 min to have a progress check-in. The rest of class time will be work time. You have the option of signing up for an individual meeting with me during class time as well. Check-ins offer you time to ask questions or discuss anything class-related. You will include 1. What have you completed so far this week? 2. What do you plan to finish this week? 3. Any questions you have? 4. Screenshots or videos of any work you would like feedback on.

The same professor taught all three classes with different groups of students. During the check-in using Mozilla Hubs' web-based VR, the professor moderated a group discussion where each student took turns sharing their progress either using their microphone or typing in the chat. Visuals from students of their progress work were uploaded to a collaborative Google slide show and imported as a PDF before the meeting. There were approximately 15 students per class and attendance to the VR check-in fluctuated; 5–13 students would attend the VR check-in at a time. Mozilla Hubs was chosen for its ability to host the entire class, because it was free for the students to use, and because students could join from mobile, desktop, or HMD. At the end of the semester, students were given an option to participate in a post-activity survey asking a few qualitative questions on the system usability scale (SUS). This study meets the qualifications of an exempt Institutional Review Board (IRB) at the department-level review.

Qualitative questions included: How often did you attend the weekly Check-In in Mozilla Hubs? If you only attended a few times or never, Please explain if it was technology reasons or timing. What would have increased your desire to participate in the check-in? What did you like and not like about the VR classroom? What would improve your experience using the VR classroom?

The system usability scale (SUS) was worded as follows, using a 5-point Likert scale [strongly agree 1, 2, 3, 4, 5 strongly disagree].

1. I think that I would like to use this VR classroom frequently.
2. I found the VR classroom unnecessarily complex.
3. I thought the VR Classroom was easy to use.
4. I think that I would need the support of a technical person to be able to use this VR Classroom.
5. I found the various functions in this VR classroom were well integrated.
6. I thought there was too much inconsistency in this VR Classroom.
7. I would imagine that most people would learn to use this VR Classroom very quickly.
8. I found the VR classroom very cumbersome to use.
9. I felt very confident using the VR Classroom.
10. I needed to learn a lot of things before I could get going with this VR Classroom.

When reviewing the qualitative data, responses were run through voyant-tools.org to reveal additional correlations. Each response was read and coded based on key terms. The SUS was scored according to the SUS protocol. Each response is assigned a value for the SUS score calculation. The points breakdown for the responses are: Strongly Disagree—1 point, Disagree—2 points, Neutral—3 points, Agree—4 points, Strongly Agree—5 points. Then, tabulate the overall SUS score using the following framework:

- Add the total score for all odd-numbered questions and subtract 5 from the total to obtain (X).
- Add the total score for all even-numbered questions and subtract that total from 25 to obtain (Y).

- Add up the total score of the new values (X + Y) and multiply by 2.5.

The resulting score is the SUS score out of 100, with the average score being 68. Scoring above or below the average will give you immediate insight into the overall usability of the design solution [22,23].

3. Results

The results of the post-activity survey shed light on how students reacted to using Mozilla Hubs once a week for a full semester. While some students struggled with the modality because of technology, many also had issues that were unrelated to the modality and could have caused a drop in attendance/participation regardless of the modality. Several students appreciated the VR as an alternative to Zoom, while several students thought the check-in would have been simpler on Zoom, and one student would have preferred the whole class to be in-person F2F. Thirty-one out of thirty-five students opted to take the survey.

3.1. Findings from Qualitative Data

When asked, "how often did you attend the weekly check-in", four said a few times, nine said sometimes, one said never, five said most weeks, and twelve said almost every week. Nineteen people chose to answer: "If you only attended a few times or never, Please explain if it was technology reasons or timing. What would have increased your desire to participate in the check-in?" Twelve of those students attended sometimes/a few times/never, and seven attended most/every. After running the qualitative responses for this question through voyant-tools.org, the five most used words were work (6 uses), time (6 uses), timing (5 uses), technology (6 uses), and issues (6 uses). See Figure 1 for the collation of the most frequently used words.

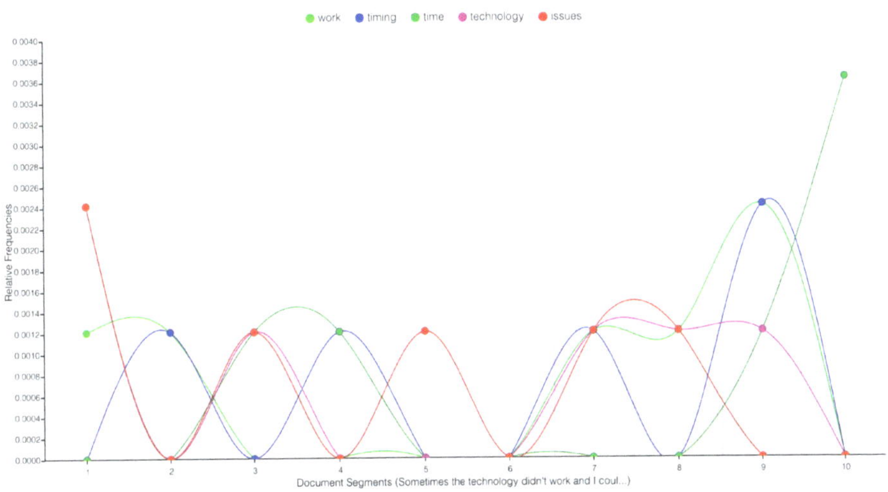

Figure 1. Correlation of trend words created with Voyant Tools for the qualitative questions, "Please explain if it was technology reasons or timing." and "What would have increased your desire to participate in the check-in?" [24].

After reviewing the context of each comment, seven of the students had technology issues that prevented them from attending more frequently. While seven other students had timing issues related to work schedules or personal/mental health, and time management issues. Five students fell outside the time/work category. One would have preferred in-person, two liked/loved using Hubs, and two stopped participating because they fell behind and "did not want to participate with nothing to share".

One student shared, "Mozilla Hubs was novel in the beginning, but it lost the human interaction that kept me engaged for most of the semester. Accessible, yes, but also isolating. Being able to see and hear the professor in-person and interact with my peers are a couple of reasons I enjoyed going to class." While two students who attended almost every time shared, "I loved the check-ins and how different it was to just Zoom. Would recommend more classes try this." and "[The] first time was confused but week after week I became familiar with it and like it".

Technology issues included having to reload the site multiple times, getting dropped from the room, audio/mic issues, lag, not working correctly on a cellphone, or not being able to enter the room:

"From the beginning, it was a bit buggy for me. For example, the audio would cut out sometimes or just lots of lag."; "Sometimes Mozilla Hubs does not comply with my phone. I would always get kicked out."; "I did encounter some technology issues when using Mozilla Hubs in which sometimes it would freeze so I would have to leave and come back in. And sometimes the sound would cut off, so it was hard to understand what people were saying."; "If it were easier to function on my phone, I would've been on every week".

When asked "What did you like and not like about the VR classroom?", students had more positive than negative responses.

After running the qualitative responses for this question through voyant-tools.org, the five most used words were liked (16 uses), like (14 uses), classroom (13 uses), vr (12 uses), and Zoom (8 uses). See Figure 2 for the correlation of trend words.

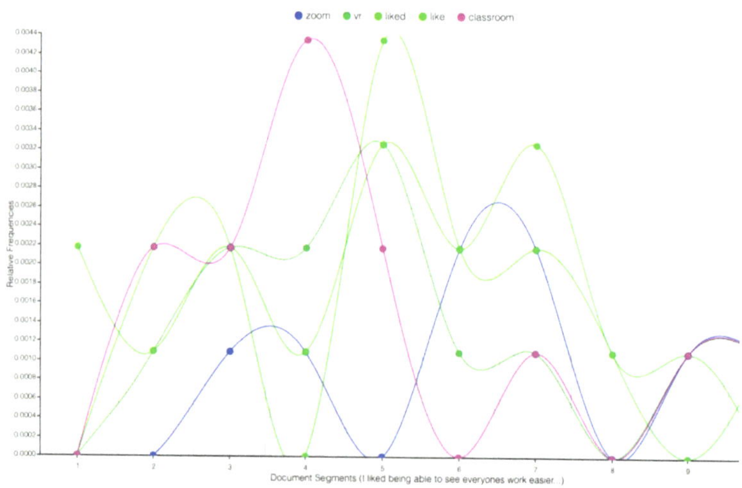

Figure 2. Correlation of trend words created with Voyant Tools for the qualitative question, "What did you like and not like about the VR classroom?" [25].

Some students liked the idea of the VR modality but disliked the technological issues they encountered: "I thought it was a different way of learning! It definitely kept me more engaged."; "I liked being able to see everyone's work easier, but the difficulties with the site and having to learn an entirely new program on top of the other ones we were learning was a lot."; "I liked that we got to share our progress without having to show our face and I disliked that the screen was small, so it was harder to see the presentations."; "I liked that it was a more interactive way to approach the classroom setting. The biggest issues I had with the VR classroom did not really have to do with the classroom itself, I've experienced a few technical issues on my end that made the VR classroom a little difficult".

Multiple students compared it to Zoom modalities:

"I like it because I learned new methods for education communication in technology not only Zoom class that we used to, but also it gives us the vibe we are in VR class room. I really do not have things that I do not like"; "I liked how we used something different and fun instead of just using Zoom, which does get boring from time to time."; "I liked that it was more interesting than the monotony of Zoom. I felt that audio was an issue for other students, though."; "I liked that it was a nice alternative to a Zoom meeting. I think being online in Zoom for two years gets very tiring, so personally, I like that this is a breath of fresh air."; "I liked the being able to see everyone virtually, and I did not dislike anything about it, but I do not think it offers anything that Zoom would not."; "I liked the idea of something knew other than Zoom but I think there may be better ways and software to accomplish this".

While some students commented on how they enjoyed that the VR modality reminded them of a video game, one student commented on how they disliked the game aspect. One student stated their preference for in-person F2F modality:

"I liked the fun factor that it adds. Each person being their own avatar and navigating a big open space. I loved it!"; "I liked how it was like playing a sort of video game but in a classroom"; "I liked that it was available without VR goggles, but I feel the experience would be better with VR goggles. Hopefully, with the amount of attention VR has been getting for use other than games will help bring more affordable options."; "I just did not really care for the video game format of the VR classroom. I like Zoom check-in better."; "I missed interacting with people and being in an actual physical environment that was meant for learning".

Students also commented on liking the flexibility the VR modality provided as well as it being a quick way to receive feedback and ask questions to acquire clarification as a group: "I loved the flexibility it offers to students who may not be able to attend physical class. I also really like the concept of it because I feel like it connects students who may have a fear of presenting, or who may struggle more in a typical classroom setting." Unfortunately, audio issues and the inability to see well were also problems: "Every time I joined the audio would start going static after just a few minutes in the VR classroom. I would have to close out the page and come back in for it work again, and then the problem would just continue repeating. I've tried fixing the audio settings in my devices, tried many different earbuds/mics, and several different devices like an IPad, phone, laptop, and had the same issue with all of them."; "I liked the space, but when we had to see something on the virtual board, it was hard to see."; "I like that the VR classroom made it easier to ask questions and receive feedback. It was hard to look at the screen with the slides as you needed to be at a certain angle".

These frustrations lowered students' feelings of engagement and reduced participation, especially among students joining with mobile devices. In future research, asking what device students joined on, what their internet speeds were, and if the connection was stable could verify if technological issues were related to the device type and/or poor internet connections. However, an even more interesting line of questions would look into the reason for device choice. Several students expressed the need to use mobile based on their work or athletic practice schedule conflicting with the class time. It is possible that even if students have access to higher-powered devices, they might still choose a lower-powered mobile device because of the location they join the class from. When asked what could improve their experience with the VR classroom, several mentioned phones. "I think if I used my laptop instead of my phone."; "If it was easier to use on cell phones,"; "I always got distracted and wanted to walk around. Additionally, It's not very mobile user friendly".

3.2. Findings from Quantitative System Usability Scale (SUS) Data

After calculating the SUS score for each student's response, the participants were almost equally divided above and below the average 68-point score for decent usability of the Mozilla Hubs web-based VR classroom experience. Fifteen scored it above 68, 13 scored it below 68, and three scored it at 67.5. The mean SUS score was 69.8. It should be noted that there may be a slight variance in the mental model of how students answered the SUS; some may have looked at it purely as evaluating the tool, while others may have viewed it through how it was used in class. For instance, one student who said they never attended the synchronous group check-in gave an SUS score of 85 based on interacting with the VR classroom asynchronously but not its performance during a synchronous meeting with multiple participants interacting since they did not attend group check-ins.

In response to the statement, "I think I would like to use this VR classroom frequently", thirty-one students (45%) strongly agreed/agreed, eight (25.8%) were neutral, and nine (29%) disagreed/strongly disagreed. When asked if they found the VR classroom unnecessarily complex, four (13%) strongly agreed/agreed, nine (29%) were neutral, and eighteen (58%) disagreed/strongly disagreed. Yet, twenty (64%) strongly agreed/agreed that the VR classroom was easy to use, with only four students (12.9%) neutral, and seven (22.6%) disagreed/strongly disagreed. When asked if they would need a technical support person to use the VR room, students strongly disagreed, with twenty-two (71%) strongly disagreeing and four (12.9%) disagreeing. Only three (9.7%) were neutral, and two agreed/strongly agreed; one each, representing 3.2%. Figures 3 and 4 show a cross-analysis of how the students answered multiple SUS questions overlayed with each other.

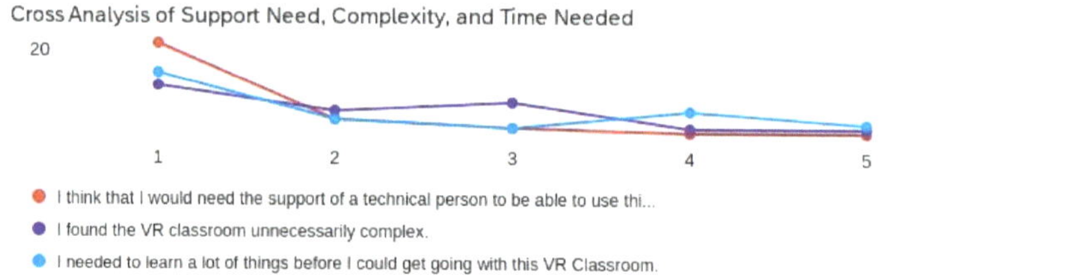

Figure 3. Cross Analysis of SUS questions showing the correlation between Support need, Perceived Complexity, and Time needed to learn the system. Numbers one-five correlate to student answers on a Likert scale.

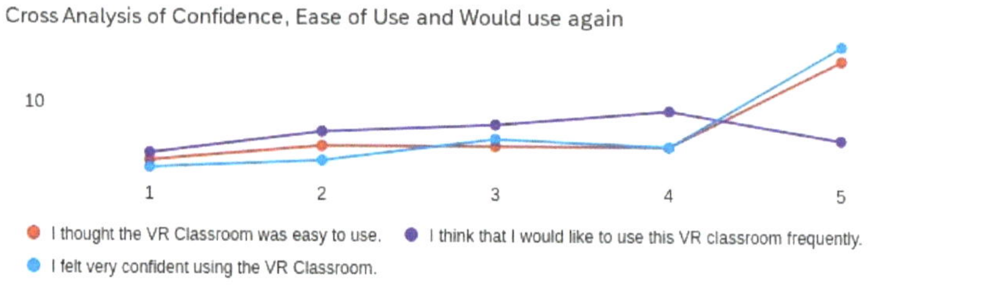

Figure 4. Cross Analysis of SUS questions showing the correlation between confidence, ease of use, and desire to use the system again. Numbers one-five correlate to student answers on a Likert scale.

While the students thought the classroom was easy to use and did not need technical support for the most part, they also were less sure that the functions of the VR classroom were well integrated, remaining largely neutral. While thirteen students (22%) agreed/strongly agreed that the various functions in the VR classroom were well integrated, the exact same amount was neutral (thirteen); only five (16%) disagreed, and none strongly disagreed. When asked if there was too much inconsistency in the VR classroom, students heavily disagreed, with seventeen students (56.7%) disagreeing/strongly disagreeing, eight feeling neutral (26.7%), and five (16.7%) agreeing/strongly agreeing. Students strongly agreed that most people would learn to use this VR classroom very quickly, with twenty-three students at 74% agreeing/strongly agreeing, only three (9.7%) feeling neutral, and five (16.2%) disagreeing/strongly disagreeing. When asked if they found the virtual reality classroom cumbersome to use, seven, or 22.6%, agreed/strongly agreed; seven (22.6%) were neutral, and seventeen (54.8%) disagreed/strongly disagreed. When asked if they were confident using the virtual reality classroom, twenty-two students (73.3%) agreed/strongly agreed, five (16.7%) were neutral, and three (10%) disagreed/strongly disagreed. The last SUS question stated, "I needed to learn a lot of things to get going with this VR Classroom". Nineteen students (61.3%) disagreed/strongly disagreed, two (6.5%) were neutral, and ten (32.3%) agreed/strongly agreed.

4. Discussion

Overall, the students enjoyed using the VR classroom. Still, audio issues seemed to be the most significant pain point mentioned by students. The audio issues seem to result from a lack of headphones, incorrect audio settings to use the headphones or not giving the browser permission to use the microphone/speaker. While the overall response was positive, there are several areas for improvement from both the student and instructor perspectives. Social, web-based VR offers promising potential for blended learning. Designing a human-centered virtual environment and considering all participants' total user experience is critical to a successful learning tool.

While seven out of thirty-one students cited technology issues including having to reload the room, audio/microphone issues, lag, and issues with using mobile devices, no one used or had access to head-mounted displays. While students can join a web-based VR experience from their phone, the immersion and usability of the interface on a small screen are very different from the immersive experience of an HMD, where the room responds naturally to head movement instead of trying to navigate on a small phone screen with your fingers. Future studies will need to look more closely at comparing students using HMD, Laptops, tablets, and phones, and additionally having students record their connectivity speed and if they have a stable connection. Similar audio issues and instances of participants being dropped from a Hubs VR room were also noted in a 2021 study by Eriksson, in the paper title, "Failure and Success in Using Mozilla Hubs for Online Teaching in a Movie Production Course". Erikson outlines two main audio issues mentioned by multiple students, including poor audio quality or crackling and issues with the spatial audio and distance from the speakers [8]. The survey for this study did not specifically ask about audio issues, so while many students mentioned them, they did not specify the root of the audio issues. However, despite telling students to use headphones with a microphone, students would frequently attend just using their computer microphone and speakers. When un-muted, the lack of headphones created considerable feedback. Students could also individually turn the volume up and down on the avatar who is speaking; however, many did not remember or know that they could do this. Students did not always state they were having audio issues while the problem was happening, but reported it after the fact, making troubleshooting difficult. Sometimes, audio issues were discussed during the class, and often solutions were found. For instance, about halfway through the semester, the instructor's right headphone would cause a static issue that only the other participants in the room could hear. This problem was solved by only using the left earbud for the rest of the semester.

Regarding the timing issues, either conflict with work, family obligations, mental health issues, or time management issues, which were not related specifically to the modality, may have affected attendance/participation regardless of class modality. Similar issues with disengagement and low attendance are discussed in McMurtrie's 2022 article titled, "A 'Stunning' Level of Student Disconnection", published in The Chronicle of Higher Education [26].

Many of the issues discussed by the student participants come back to frustrations involving audio and feelings of disconnection instead of immersion because of audio issues. Listed below are areas for improvement to create a better user experience with the Mozilla Hubs system:

1. Turn off positional audio during presentations and turn it back on for breaking into groups.

2. Have a very clearly defined use and reason for meeting in the VR space.
3. Removing unnecessary objects to reduce loading issues for mobile participants.
4. Take advantage of the media frames feature for screen-sharing presentations.
5. Using the objects menu to streamline the viewing of presentations from various points in the room.
6. Keep meetings short to avoid lag and the need to refresh the browser.
7. Having a separate viewing room for posted recordings or PDFs and an interaction room for meetings in order to limit load when joining as a group.

Additionally, make sure students have access to the tech they need to join web VR successfully. Access to a stable internet connection, quality headphones, with a microphone that works with their device. A device that can handle running web VR through its browser, ideally, access to head-mounted displays could give students additional immersion. Conducting multiple demonstrations and running in-person tests could also greatly improve the user experience for students. While a demonstration was led on how to use the Mozilla Hubs classroom, the students would have benefited from additional demonstrations and multiple test days when they all joined the VR classroom together while they were also physically present in the same room. Mystakidis (2021) discusses the importance of higher education in building up students' digital skills to better prepare them for VR technology.

In a blended hybrid learning environment, web-based VR supplements face-to-face (F2F) instruction, video conferencing, and the use of learning management systems like Canvas or Blackboard. VR is an additional tool to offer a flexible and diverse way of meeting that can increase presence and immersion in remote learning. Creating and using VR to teach requires careful planning to ensure the modality fits the activity and that the total user experience has been considered for the students.

5. Conclusions

Virtual reality (VR) is a technology that can be used to enhance classroom learning. It can be useful for teaching and learning in a blended environment. Virtual reality (VR) is an advanced technology used across different sectors. In education, virtual reality technology is a way for teachers and students to create a simulated three-dimensional world. Web-based social VR is a subset of desktop-based VR and virtual worlds. This work has looked at how extended reality can pair with a blended classroom model.

The main finding relates to the responses of students from three different upper-division design classes who met over Mozilla Hubs every Wednesday for a whole semester. Overall, the students enjoyed using the VR classroom, but audio issues seemed to be the most significant pain point. While the overall response was positive, this study identified several areas for improvement from both the student and instructor perspectives. Designing a human-centered virtual environment and considering all participants' total user experience is critical.

The results of the post-activity survey have shed light on how students responded to using Mozilla Hubs once a week for a full semester. This study shed light on the implications of the practical use of VR in a blended classroom. While some students struggled with the modality because of technology, many had issues that were unrelated to the modality and that could have caused a drop in attendance/participation regardless of the modality. At the same time, seven out of thirty-one students cited technology issues including having to reload the room, audio/microphone issues, lag, and issues with using mobile devices. Similar audio issues and instances of participants being dropped from a Mozilla Hubs VR room were noted in the study by Eriksson. Students did not always state that they were having audio issues while the problem was happening but reported it after the fact, making troubleshooting difficult. Virtual reality is not a new concept; the accessibility of VR technology has dramatically increased in the last few years. In education, virtual reality technology is a way for teachers and students to create a simulated three-dimensional world [4]. Hardware, like head-mounted displays (HMD), has become more cost-effective, yet it is not commonly owned by the masses like a smartphone. Any device capable of connecting to the internet could run a web-based VR experience. Web-based VR offers unique access across multiple devices, including phones, tablets, laptops, and head-mounted displays (HMDs).

This study was limited to only one semester and the hardware that the students already owned. By providing access to more robust hardware like hotspots, headphones with microphones, or even HMD, there could be an improvement in participation due to lower frustration levels. Additionally, more information should have been collected on the types of connections, hardware used, and audio issues students experienced.

To conclude, future research should look at web-based VR and how educators, designers, and developers can address digital equity issues to provide positive learning experiences for all students. Designing a human-centered virtual environment and considering all participants' total user experience is critical to the success of a learning tool. While students can join a web-based VR experience from their phone, it might not be the best option. The immersion and usability of the interface on a small screen are very different from the immersive experience of a head-mounted display (HMD), where the room responds naturally to head movement instead of trying to navigate on a tiny phone screen with your fingers. Creating and using VR to teach requires careful planning to ensure the modality fits the activity and that the total user experience has been considered for the students.

Funding: This research received no external funding.

Institutional Review Board Statement: This study was reviewed at the department level and noted as exempt, as it was conducted in the normal flow of a classroom setting, and students could opt in by providing feedback in the form of an optional post-activity survey. No identifying information was requested in the data. The study was conducted in accordance with the Declaration of Helsinki and approved as exempt by the Department Chair of Art, Design, and Art History at California State University—Fresno. Full Ethical review and approval were waived for this study As the study was conducted as a class activity in an established educational setting involving normal educational practices. Students were notified about the study before data collection and that their participation was voluntary, as per Section 3.4.4: Obligations of Investigators Regarding Informed Consent from the "Policy and Procedures for Research with Human Subjects" document at Fresno State.

Informed Consent Statement: Informed consent was obtained from all subjects involved in the study.

Data Availability Statement: Data available at https://voyant-tools.org/?corpus=de37481557034c9cfaa4f86f00d582a4&panels=cirrus,reader,trends,summary,contexts (accessed on 17 January 2023). And https://docs.google.com/spreadsheets/d/1tciZPjiiE6MYfWd3qeM6d52jHZQa65MOQSY0zhggFEE/edit?usp=sharing (accessed on 17 January 2023).

Conflicts of Interest: The authors declare no conflict of interest.

References

1. Azar, A.; Farahat, Z.; Benslimane, O.; Megdiche, K.; Ngote, N.; Samir, J. Implementation of a Virtual Reality Operating Room for Simulation Purposes in Medical Training. In Proceedings of the 2020 International Conference on Electrical and Information Technologies (ICEIT), Rabat, Morocco, 4–7 March 2020; IEEE: Piscataway, NJ, USA, 2020; pp. 1–6.
2. Roman, T.A.; Racek, J. Virtual reality as a pedagogical tool to design for social impact: A design case. *TechTrends* **2019**, *63*, 79–86. [CrossRef]
3. Jin, L.; Wen, Z.; Gough, N. Social virtual worlds for technology-enhanced learning on an augmented learning platform. *Learn. Media Technol.* **2010**, *35*, 139–153. [CrossRef]
4. Chang, X.; Zhang, D.; Jin, X. Application of virtual reality technology in distance learning. *Int. J. Emerg. Technol. Learn.* **2016**, *11*, 76. [CrossRef]
5. Williams, S.; Enatsky, R.; Gillcash, H.; Murphy, J.J.; Gračanin, D. Immersive technology in the public school classroom: When a class meets. In Proceedings of the 2021 7th International Conference of the Immersive Learning Research Network (iLRN), Eureka, CA, USA, 17 May–10 June 2021; IEEE: Piscataway, NJ, USA, 2021; pp. 1–8.
6. Pellas, N.; Mystakidis, S.; Christopoulos, A. A Systematic Literature Review on the User Experience Design for Game-Based Interventions via 3D Virtual Worlds in K-12 Education. *Multimodal Technol. Interact.* **2021**, *5*, 28. [CrossRef]
7. Canniff, K.; Cliburn, D.C. Teaching Virtual Reality in Virtual Reality. In Proceedings of the 2022 8th International Conference of the Immersive Learning Research Network (iLRN), Vienna, Austria, 30 May–4 June 2022; IEEE: Piscataway, NJ, USA, 2022; pp. 1–8.

8. Eriksson, T. Failure and success in using mozilla hubs for online teaching in a movie production course. In Proceedings of the 2021 7th International Conference of the Immersive Learning Research Network (iLRN), Eureka, CA, USA, 17 May–10 June 2021; IEEE: Piscataway, NJ, USA, 2021; pp. 1–8.
9. Yoshimura, A.; Borst, C.W. Evaluation and comparison of desktop viewing and headset viewing of remote lectures in vr with mozilla hubs. In Proceedings of the International Conference on Artificial Reality and Telexistence, and Eurographics Symposium on Virtual Environments (ICAT-EGVE), Virtual, 2–4 December 2020.
10. Mystakidis, S.; Berki, E.; Valtanen, J.P. Deep and meaningful e-learning with social virtual reality environments in higher education: A systematic literature review. *Appl. Sci.* **2021**, *11*, 2412. [CrossRef]
11. Huisinga, L. Virtual Exhibit Design: The UX of Student BFA Design Shows in Social VR. In *International Conference on Applied Human Factors and Ergonomics*; Springer: Cham, Switzerland, 2021; pp. 240–246.
12. Schwaiger, M. (Ed.) *Boosting Virtual Reality in Learning*; Focus Europe: Graz, Austria, 2020.
13. Genz, F.; Fuchs, N.; Kolb, D.; Müller, S.; Kranzlmüller, D. Evaluation of Proprietary Social VR Platforms for Use in Distance Learning. In Proceedings of the Augmented Reality, Virtual Reality, and Computer Graphics: 8th International Conference, AVR 2021, Virtual Event, 7–10 September 2021; Springer International Publishing: Berlin/Heidelberg, Germany, 2021; pp. 462–480.
14. Huisinga, L.A. User Experience of Social Web-Based Virtual Reality for the Hybrid and Blended Learning Classroom. *Hum. Side Serv. Eng.* **2022**, *62*, 55.
15. Schouten, A.P.; van den Hooff, B.; Feldberg, F. Virtual Team Work: Group Decision Making in 3D Virtual Environments. *Commun. Res.* **2016**, *43*, 180–210. [CrossRef]
16. Downey, S.; Mohler, J.; Morris, J.; Sanchez, R. Learner perceptions and recall of small group discussions within 2D and 3D collaborative environments. *Australas. J. Educ. Technol.* **2012**, *28*, 28. [CrossRef]
17. Scavarelli, A.; Arya, A.; Teather, R.J. Towards a framework on accessible and social VR in education. In Proceedings of the 2019 IEEE Conference on Virtual Reality and 3D User Interfaces (VR), Osaka, Japan, 23–27 March 2019; IEEE: Piscataway, NJ, USA, 2019; pp. 1148–1149.
18. Çoban, M.; GOKSU, İ. Using virtual reality learning environments to motivate and socialize undergraduates in distance learning. *Particip. Educ. Res.* **2022**, *9*, 199–218. [CrossRef]
19. Hodge, E.M.; Tabrizi MH, N.; Farwell, M.A.; Wuensch, K.L. Virtual reality classrooms: Strategies for creating a social presence. *Int. J. Soc. Sci.* **2008**, *2*, 105–109.
20. Mystakidis, S.; Berki, E.; Valtanen, J. Toward successfully integrating mini learning games into social virtual reality environments: Recommendations for improving open and distance learning. In *EDULEARN Proceedings*; IATED Academy: València, Spain, 2017.
21. Merchant, Z.; Goetz, E.T.; Cifuentes, L.; Keeney-Kennicutt, W.; Davis, T.J. Effectiveness of virtual reality-based instruction on students' learning outcomes in K-12 and higher education: A meta-analysis. *Comput. Educ.* **2014**, *70*, 29–40. [CrossRef]
22. Brooke, J. SUS-A quick and dirty usability scale. *Usability Eval. Ind.* **1996**, *189*, 4–7.
23. Smyk, A.; Herman, L.; Silveira, D.; Babich, N.; Kingston, C. The System Usability Scale & How It's Used in UX: Adobe XD Ideas. Available online: https://xd.adobe.com/ideas/process/user-testing/sus-system-usability-scale-ux/ (accessed on 20 December 2022).
24. Sinclair, S.; Rockwell, G. Trends. Voyant Tools. 2023. Available online: https://voyant-tools.org/?query=work&query=time&query=technology&query=issues&query=timing&mode=document&corpus=de37481557034c9cfaa4f86f00d582a4&view=Trends (accessed on 17 January 2023).
25. Sinclair, S.; Rockwell, G. Trends. Voyant Tools. 2023. Available online: https://voyant-tools.org/?query=liked&query=like&query=classroom&query=vr&query=zoom&mode=document&corpus=2b209a7e61dd11c16f6266fbc1749dba&view=Trends (accessed on 17 January 2023).
26. McMurtrie, B. A 'Stunning' Level of Student Disconnection. 2022. Available online: https://www.chronicle.com/article/a-stunning-level-of-student-disconnection (accessed on 17 January 2023).

virtual worlds

MDPI

Article

Physics-Based Watercraft Simulator in Virtual Reality

Kelly Ervin [1,*], Jonathan Boone [1], Karl Smink [1], Gaurav Savant [2], Keith Martin [2], Spicer Bak [2] and Shyla Clark [1]

[1] Information Technology Laboratory, U.S. Army Engineering Research and Development Center, Vicksburg, MS 39180, USA; jonathan.l.boone@erdc.dren.mil (J.B.); karl.a.smink@erdc.dren.mil (K.S.)
[2] Coastal and Hydraulics Laboratory, U.S. Army Engineering Research and Development Center, Vicksburg, MS 39180, USA; keith.martin@erdc.dren.mil (K.M.)
* Correspondence: kelly.b.ervin@erdc.dren.mil

Abstract: In this paper, watercraft and ship simulation is summarized, and the way that it can be extended through realistic physics is explored. A hydrodynamic, data-driven, immersive watercraft simulation experience is also introduced, using the Unreal Engine to visualize a Landing Craft Utility (LCU) operation and interaction with near-shore waves in virtual reality (VR). The VR application provides navigation scientists with a better understanding of how coastal waves impact landing operations and channel design. FUNWAVE data generated on the supercomputing resources at the U.S. Army Corps of Engineers (USACE) Engineering Research and Development Center (ERDC) are employed, and using these data, a graphical representation of the domain is created, including the vessel model and a customizable VR bridge to control the vessel within the virtual environment. Several dimension reduction methods are being devised to ensure that the FUNWAVE data can inform the model but keep the application running in real time at an acceptable frame rate for the VR headset. By importing millions of data points output from the FUNWAVE version 3.4 software into Unreal Engine, virtual vessels can be affected by physics-driven data.

Keywords: virtual reality; simulation; hydraulics; navigation; FUNWAVE; hydrodynamics; Unreal Engine; waves; Boussinesq; near-shore waves; physics engine; numerical models

Citation: Ervin, K.; Boone, J.; Smink, K.; Savant, G.; Martin, K.; Bak, S.; Clark, S. Physics-Based Watercraft Simulator in Virtual Reality. *Virtual Worlds* **2023**, 2, 422–438. https://doi.org/10.3390/virtualworlds2040024

Academic Editors: Anton Nijholt, Radu Comes, Dorin-Mircea Popovici, Calin Gheorghe Dan Neamtu and Jing-Jing Fang

Received: 11 April 2023
Revised: 22 August 2023
Accepted: 24 November 2023
Published: 14 December 2023

1. Introduction

Navigation channels are essential for the economy and national security. Ship pilots who traverse these channels can provide valuable feedback to the civil engineers who design them, and pilot-operated simulators are a popular means of gathering this feedback. Ship simulators can reproduce, imitate, or represent likely occurrences of real-world phenomena and have many applications such as informing risk-based decision making. One way to ensure that simulations are as accurate as possible is through numerical models of physical systems. Calculations of mathematical equations can offer a physics-based representation of common, natural phenomena such as fluid mechanics. In the case of vessel simulation, these natural forces can have important interactions with a ship, affecting its operation. To achieve our research objective of creating accurate simulations, it is imperative to focus on the intricate interactions of vessels with near-shore waves. Near-shore waves present unique challenges due to their complex behaviors influenced by coastal topography. As such, the selection of an appropriate hydrodynamic modeler becomes crucial for this task. Therefore, our research team has chosen to incorporate the hydrodynamic modeler FUNWAVE, renowned for its precision and reliability in capturing near-shore wave dynamics [1]. Many forces act upon a vessel, including waves, current, and wind. One of the most difficult kinds of waves to simulate is near-shore waves. For this application, our research team has incorporated the hydrodynamic modeler FUNWAVE as the most accurate data source for modeling near-shore waves.

Natural phenomena can be visualized using computer graphics applications, which are valuable in understanding and communicating the data. In the past, OpenGL was the powerful tool most often used for demonstrating this capability, but in recent years, video game engines have been leveraged for high-definition graphical renderings. To gain a market edge, game design companies have been at the forefront of graphics. These techniques have been proprietary and hidden until tools such as Unreal Engine and Unity provided amateur developers with similar capabilities. Communities of content creators can now share tools that make the process of visualization much easier. Scientists and engineers are using game design and visual effects techniques to create high-definition graphics simulations of physical systems. Advancements in visualization techniques have significantly impacted the field, particularly with the adoption of video game engines like Unreal Engine and Unity. These engines empower researchers, including both professionals and amateurs, to create visually stunning simulations. For our research, Unreal Engine proves to be an ideal choice, given its robust graphics rendering capabilities, which will be instrumental in enhancing the visualization of ship operations and near-shore wave dynamics. We have chosen this application because of the high quality of graphics capability with the software compared to other applications such as Unity. Unreal Engine utilizes a more advanced and sophisticated rendering pipeline, known as the Unreal Engine 4 (UE4) rendering system. It features cutting-edge graphical techniques such as physically based rendering (PBR) [2], high-quality global illumination through its precomputed radiance transfer (LPV) [3] or real-time ray tracing (DXR) [4], and cinematic-quality post-processing effects [5]. These features contribute to more visually stunning and realistic graphics in Unreal Engine compared to Unity. Beyond merely seeing a visualization, researchers can now be immersed in the data, thanks to virtual reality (VR). Smartphone technologies have led to a resurgence of VR hardware utilizing small and powerful graphics processing unit (GPU) chips and micro light-emitting diode (LED) screens. Game design tools such as Unreal Engine and Unity have also enabled the explosion of VR content created by independent developers. In academia, government, and private industry, developers are going beyond gaming with VR to produce immersive communication solutions. Data immersion can help stakeholders make better informed decisions based on an enhanced experience of the information.

In this study, we harness the potential of virtual reality to provide a transformative data immersion experience. By integrating Unreal Engine's cutting-edge graphics capabilities with VR technology (Table 1), our simulation will enable researchers and stakeholders to interact with the data in an immersive and comprehensive manner. The immersive nature of VR will foster a deeper understanding of the vessel behavior under various near-shore wave conditions, thereby contributing to enhanced decision making in coastal engineering, military operations, and navigational science.

Table 1. Hardware and software for virtual reality development.

PC Hardware Specs	VR Headsets	Software
Processor: Intel i9 Graphics Card: Nvidia GeForce RTX 3090	Valve Index	Unreal Engine 4.26
RAM: 64 GB Hard drive: 2TB SSD	HTC Vive Pro 2	FUNWAVE

2. Background

2.1. Ship Simulation

Ship simulation was developed to train mariners in areas such as safe vessel maneuvering techniques including avoiding collisions, which has been explored in previous studies [6]. While ship simulation was initially used for blue water navigation and deep-water harbors, the simulated environments have expanded to include the riverine and littoral environments. Its use promotes safe navigation in the world's sea lanes and navigation channels by allowing mariners to hone their skills in a zero-risk, laboratory environment [7]. In the 1980s and 1990s, the U.S. Army Corps of Engineers (USACE) Engineer Research and Development Center (ERDC) began using ship simulation in a unique way: the analysis of navigation channel design [8]. Throughout these studies, the ERDC has continually evolved its methods in support of safe and efficient channel design. The ERDC has applied ship simulation technology to design improvement projects in nearly every major U.S. port and commercially navigated waterway in the United States including Alaska, Hawaii, and Puerto Rico. Ship simulation has proven to be an invaluable tool in helping evaluate safety and economic issues for maritime development projects. Using local area expertise, field data, stakeholder input, and experience, the ERDC employs unique ship simulation methods to analyze channel and port design alternatives. Visualization is what makes simulation such a powerful training and analysis tool, giving the mariner a real-time view of the physical environment. The medium for these visual environments began with computer monitors and projectors and has advanced to high-resolution screens, projection systems, and LED domes.

Currently, the visualization software used for ship simulators is essentially the same as gaming and VR applications [9]. Many of the major companies such as Kongsberg Marine (Figure 1) and HR Wallingford (Figure 2) use Unity or Unreal Engine as the basis for their software due to the ability to create interactive experiences. In the past, game engines did not offer the ability to create functionality at the code level and only offered some asset importation and customization. This severely limited the ability to adjust physics parameters or extend any built-in physics. Physics-based simulations had to be developed without the use of game engines [10]. This research focused on Unreal Engine and its ability to create custom adaptations through coding in Unreal Blueprints or by utilizing plugins, which act as software libraries.

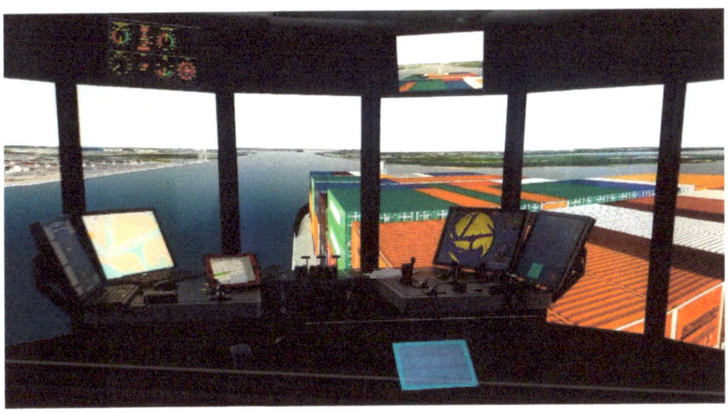

Figure 1. Kongsberg ship simulator at Engineering Research and Development Center.

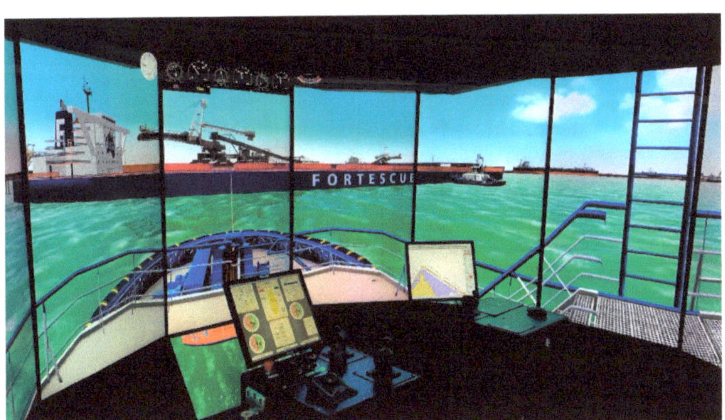

Figure 2. HR Wallingford ship simulator.

2.2. Virtual Reality Simulation in Gaming Engines

Virtual reality has been revolutionary in the field of ship and watercraft simulation by providing a more immersive and realistic training environment. The advancements of VR over the years have greatly enhanced the capabilities for these simulations, giving users the experience of realistic scenarios without the need to pilot a ship in the real world. The use of Unreal Engine, a powerful gaming engine known for its high-fidelity graphics and interactive capabilities, has played a crucial role in driving these advancements. The gaming engine's ability to render detailed environments and simulate complex physics has made it an ideal choice for watercraft and ship simulation.

The incorporation of VR allows for safer training scenarios and reduces the overall risk of accidents involved in training such as those that are common in the construction industry [11]. The realistic rendering of maritime environments enhances a pilot's preparedness in critical situations. The ability to model various vessels gives pilots a broad range of options for training that greatly increases their overall knowledge, and they can practice on various bridge types. VR is also very effective for remote learning [12]. Ship simulators can be very large, containing many parts that cannot be easily moved such as screens, consoles, and desktop computers. VR offers a more mobile solution, bringing the training to the student, and saving costs on travel.

2.3. Hydrodynamic Visualization

Watercraft simulation in a VR environment is currently limited by the lack of sophisticated near-shore wave models and the need for the better visualization of wave surfaces. Most traditional wave models, based on linear wave theory, fail to accurately capture nonlinear wave interactions, wave breaking, and near-shore dynamics [13]. These limitations lead to a lack of fidelity in simulating critical hydrodynamic phenomena, resulting in less reliable predictions of ship responses and behavior in realistic sea conditions. To remedy this, it is important to use wave modeling simulations with higher accuracy, which has been shown in previous studies [14]. Advancements in computer hardware, such as high-performance supercomputing, makes it possible to use numerical modeling, such as Navier–Stokes equations, to simulate the important factors affecting ships [15].

FUNWAVE is a fully nonlinear, shallow-to-intermediate water phase resolving, Boussinesq numerical wave model. It provides high-fidelity simulations for many coastal processes including near-shore waves, currents, wave breaking with run-up and overtopping, harbor resonance, infra-gravity waves, and vessel-generated waves. Many of its capabilities are only possible due to its ability to resolve the phases between different super-positioned wave frequencies. This high degree of accuracy, however, comes at the cost of the application being unable to run in real time. Researchers at the Coastal and Hydraulics Laboratory are utilizing an HPC to reduce the computational costs.

The most important components of an immersive and realistic simulated environment are physics calculations and visualization. This is especially true for maritime simulations where pilots sail in both deep water and near-shore (shallow water). Multiple wave types and conditions like spray, splashing, foam, and wakes are necessary to accurately render these different environments and create useful visuals. Pilots, for example, use breaking waves and foamy patches to navigate waters, especially in the near-shore. There are currently two main calculation methods for simulating deep-water ocean waves: parametric and statistical. The former uses mathematical equations to procedurally create simple, trochoidal Gerstner waves. This implementation is based on deep-water waves and is the method used in Unreal Engine's built-in water physics engine. The most formative example of a Gerstner-based wave simulation first appeared in the 1986 work of Fournier and Reeves [16]. Since then, oceanographers have moved beyond Gerstner waves and favor statistical models that generate "linear waves" or "gravity waves", which result in a more realistic representation of the open ocean's surface [17]. The statistical calculation method uses wave spectra data and Fast Fourier Transforms to statistically create a more realistic depiction of choppier waters. The individual waves themselves are still Gerstner waves, but they are superimposed in a way to create more complicated waveforms [18].

Simulating shallow water is more complex than simulating deep water. Oceanographers refer to these waves passing over a shallow bottom as "nonlinear waves" [17]. Unlike deep-water waves, which follow a sinusoidal shape, near-shore waves are sharp near the crest and flat near the trough. This change in shape results from the water depth and seabed terrain—not just wind and gravity. To simulate waves moving to the near-shore, a mathematical model of the seafloor topography is required. Previous work demonstrates that seafloor topography data and waveform data can be constructed simultaneously, making it possible to render near-shore waves in real time at a frame rate of 132 fps in OpenGL [19]. Perhaps more important than deep and shallow water rendering, in the context of ship simulation, is the rendering of visual context clues like breaking waves, spray, and foam. Extensive prior work has been conducted to realistically render breaking waves [16,20] and prove that very fast breaking wave behaviors are possible using OpenGL and NVIDIA Cg shading language [21]. Previous work has also shown how realistic ocean foam and spray can be achieved in real time using traditional texture-based methods [22]. More recent work has demonstrated improvements to these visualizations, including bubbles popping and clumping in natural patterns [23] and water spray as a two-continua for computer graphics wherein it does not appear to fall straight down [24].

In order to improve the near-shore wave physics of ship simulators, it is important to understand gaming physics engines. Programming logic combined with Newtonian equations offers the ability to simulate real-world physics-based events. These software packages are called "physics engines" for gaming and scientific simulation. Physics engines mainly deal with rigid body dynamics, soft body dynamics, collision response, and fluid dynamics. Physics-based particle systems for visual effects that simulate phenomena such as smoke, fog, dust, rain, snow, clouds, water, fire, and light offer enhanced virtual reality immersion [25]. In previous studies, physics engines have been compared, and some important factors have been identified [26]. Integrator performance determines numerical accuracy and is responsible for calculating a body's position given the forces acting upon it. Constraint stability, collision system, object representation, material properties, and the way objects are stacked were also evaluated [27].

Since our research is mostly focused on using Unreal Engine 4.26, we examined the Nvidia PhysX engine. The research did not evaluate Unreal Engine 5's new Chaos engine or Niagara Fluids but will be explored in a future work. For the PhysX system, three types of physics actors are static, dynamic, and kinematic. Static actors are immovable in the environment being used mostly for collision detection, dynamic actors are moveable bodies and act under the normal laws of physics, and finally, kinematic actors do not respond to outside forces and move under the user's control [28]. Several techniques have been evaluated with PhysX for water and fluid simulation including the forces acting upon particles [29].

Data sets have been visualized in different ways, from dashboards with real-time data [30] to VR applications using scatter plots on a 3D graph [31]. Many examples of 3D geospatial terrain data being ingested into virtual reality game engine simulations exist [32]. Other examples show how digital elevation models can be used to create 3D scenes for immersive geographical VR applications [33]. Data ingestion for simulations is not limited to terrain, and examples exist of how meteorological data can be imported to visualize real-time volumetric clouds using Python and Unreal Engine [34]. Researchers have gone beyond the earth and have even modeled real-time cosmological visualizations using Unreal Engine and galaxy image data [35]. Other rarer examples exist of actual simulators implemented such as a vehicle traffic simulator created in Unreal Engine [36]. DataTables are gameplay elements that Unreal Engine uses to store related data. They can be accessed using either C++ or Blueprints, the Unreal Engine visual scripting system. DataTables allow Unreal Engine to input and output data from comma-separated values (CSV) and JavaScript Object Notation (JSON) files [37].

3. Methods

The core of the methodology revolves around a prototype, Landing Craft Utility (LCU), which is piloted in virtual reality. Our unique approach was to ingest FUNWAVE output data into Unreal Engine and represent it in a fully immersive virtual reality simulator. This survey shows how a hybrid approach of virtual reality watercraft piloting, hydrodynamic models, high-definition water rendering, and data ingestion can lead to more advanced simulators in the future. Utilizing the information explained above, we have created a framework that integrates those pieces (Figure 3). We have chosen to use Unreal Engine over another application such as Unity due to its favorable graphics capabilities. Unreal Engine provides the common data environment for our numerical modeler, rigid body physics, realistic computer graphics, and virtual reality simulation. The application consists of a backend developed on Unreal Engine 4.26 and its native handling of physics using PhysX 3.3. The water plugin that was created by Epic Games has options for creating animated Gerstner waves and giving game actors buoyancy. Unreal Engine's water plugin does not have littoral or near-shore waves, which motivated this research. In order to enhance the realism of near-shore waves, we chose the FUNWAVE hydrodynamic numerical modeler as a source of data that could be ingested due to the high level of accuracy of the modeler.

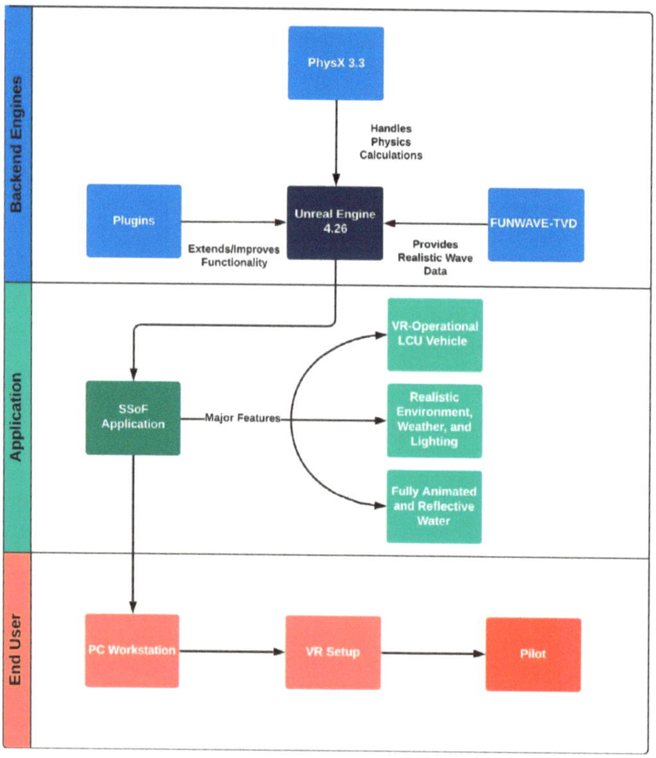

Figure 3. Diagram of current implementation framework.

3.1. *Unreal Engine Implementation*

Our development team utilized Unreal Engine 4.26 to simulate an ocean environment where the user can drive an LCU using a throttle for forward and backward motion and using a steering wheel to turn from left to right (Figure 4). Like previously implemented systems [38], the platform simulates real-time six-degrees-of-freedom ship motion (pitch, heave, roll, surge, sway, and yaw) under user interactions and environmental conditions, linear and angular velocity, user gaze direction, as well as control and lever angles taken from the bridge. The fully immersive virtual reality watercraft is buoyant and floats on the surface of the simulated water consisting primarily of Gerstner-type waves. Other auxiliary features include a horn that can be activated, emitting a realistic audio signature. The ship model was designed by ERDC CHL's Navigation branch. A menu system was included to give users a launch point and the ability to change options such as sound effects, music, and controller settings (Figure 5). A beach island scene was developed by the ITL team using Megascans library and a Combat Rubber Raiding Craft (CRRC) downloaded from Sketchfab.

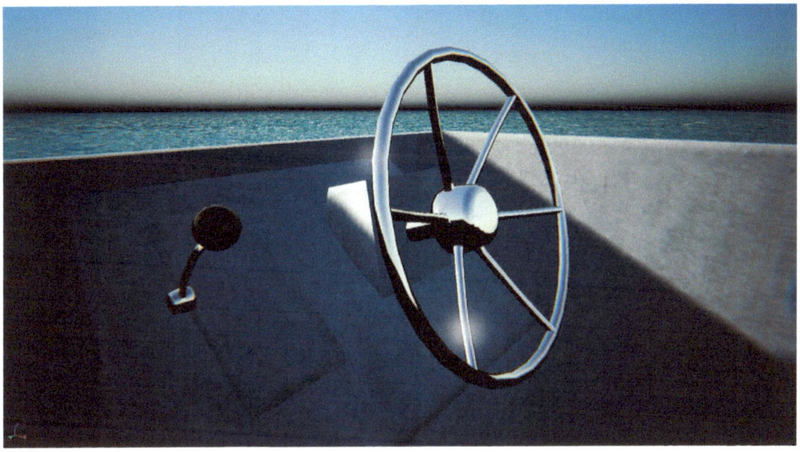

Figure 4. Steering and throttle modeled for Unreal Engine in Maya by the ITL team.

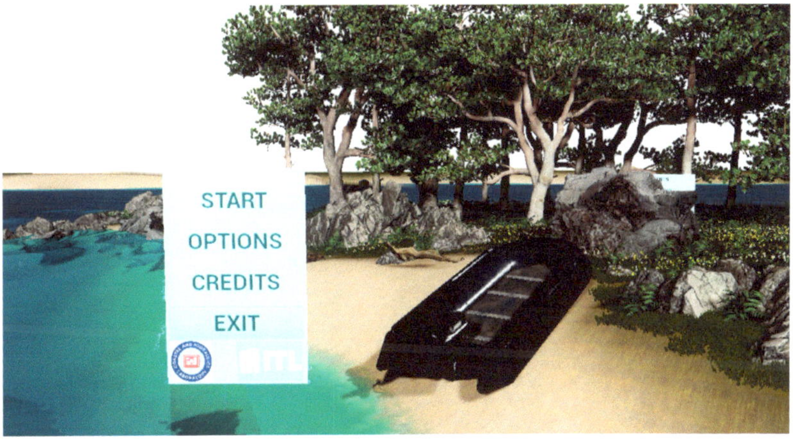

Figure 5. Beach environment main menu with default UE 4.26 water rendering.

3.2. Hydrodynamic Data Ingestion

Data from FUNWAVE are essential to integrate high-accuracy physics into a virtual simulation. Currently, there is no way to integrate a live Boussinesq model into a VR simulation at the level of accuracy in FUNWAVE; therefore, the developed capability relies on precomputed hydrodynamic data (Figure 6). Simulation data can be any phase-resolved nonlinear wave model, but for this project, we used FUNWAVE. The model output, packaged in binary files, comprise cross-shore velocities (u), alongshore velocities

(v), and water surface elevation (η). The data were unpacked from FUNWAVE's native format and converted to the CSV format to be ingestible by Unreal Engine's DataTables (Table 2). To unpack the binary file, our Python script (Figure 7), was used to convert the raw binary wave data into three columns of 7-point precision floating point numbers. Then, we transformed each float to 7-point precision before writing it as a string to the newly created CSV file.

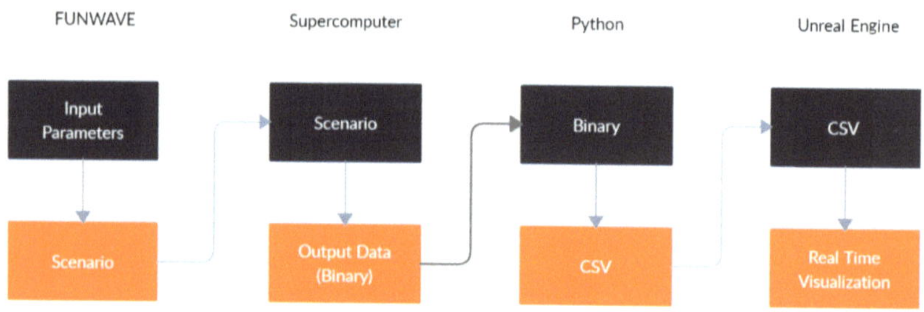

Figure 6. FUNWAVE to Unreal Engine workflow.

Table 2. Example of DataTable with FUNWAVE data with approx. 1 million rows.

u	v	η
0	0	1.001615
0.200694	0.001318	0.951349
0.380469	0.030034	0.914848
−0.33905	−0.01439	0.861739
0.217115	−0.06727	0.805298
0.342044	0.003659	0.761927
0.337063	0.004634	0.711583
0.344882	−0.00511	0.662127
0.352469	−0.06368	0.613077

```
import numpy as np
import csv

input_file = r'eta_00250'
float_file = r'eta_00250_float.csv'

with open(input_file) as f:
    floats = np.fromfile(f, dtype=float)
    with open(float_file, 'w') as s:
        for a in floats:
            a = "{:.7f}".format(a)
            s.write(str(a) + "\n")
```

Figure 7. Python code for reading in a binary file and converting it to CSV file.

FUNWAVE's data are output in a structured 2D grid. Data points are discretized along a user-entered resolution/value (every 1 m, 2 m, 0.5 m, etc.). For each discretized data point (here after referred to as a "cell"), there are 3 values that we had FUNWAVE calculate:

- U and V: Cross-shore and against-shore velocities (respectively);
- Eta: The spatio-temporal instantaneous water level oscillating around the still-water level; these values can be positive (peak) or negative (trough).

To render the simulation results of the littoral zone, a colored spatial grid was designed from the FUNWAVE data (Figure 8). Each colored cube represents one point in the FUNWAVE grid. Each cube represents a "u, v, eta" point, which will later be revised to be animated water in a future work. Red colored cubes represent the area where the ship is colliding with a FUNWAVE cell, illustrating how littoral waves affect the hydrodynamics of the ship, and vice versa. Data were accessed from each row in the DataTable, which consisted of three columns (u, v, eta) for each row. Each row represents a single time series point from FUNWAVE. Our Blueprint script iterated through the DataTable grabbed each row and assigned that to each cube.

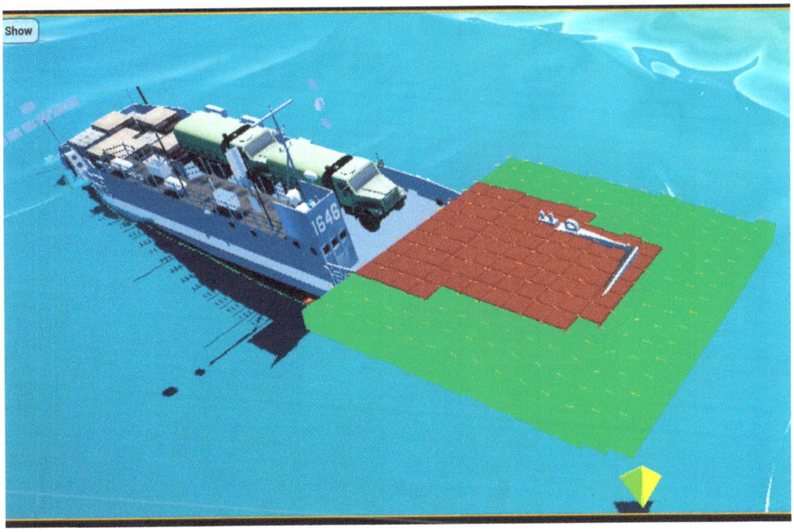

Figure 8. Spatial grid showing FUNWAVE data interacting with the ship.

The arrows on top of the cells indicate the direction in which they are pushing. The red cells are currently overlapping and pushing the ship, and as they come in and out, they will subscribe or unsubscribe themselves from the boat. The values can be adjusted on the side, such as the number of rows, columns, and the size of individual cells. These adjustments can be made prior to runtime, and the values are pulled from a DataTable generated from FUNWAVE that has the u, v, and eta columns, all stored in this data structure as floats.

The wave tile spawning construction script keeps an array of transforms, which are spots in 3D space (Figure 9). It loops through the DataTable and creates a square grid for those transforms (Figure 10). For each transform, it stores the three values from the DataTable in an array, loops over them by rows and columns, and sets those transforms equal to those values plus the offset from the starting location (Figure 11). The individual grid cells are represented by green blocks that turn red when they overlap. They possess a force vector, which tells the ship to keep track of them when they begin overlapping and to stop keeping track of them when they stop overlapping. The following figures are snippets of code written with Unreal Engine Blueprints.

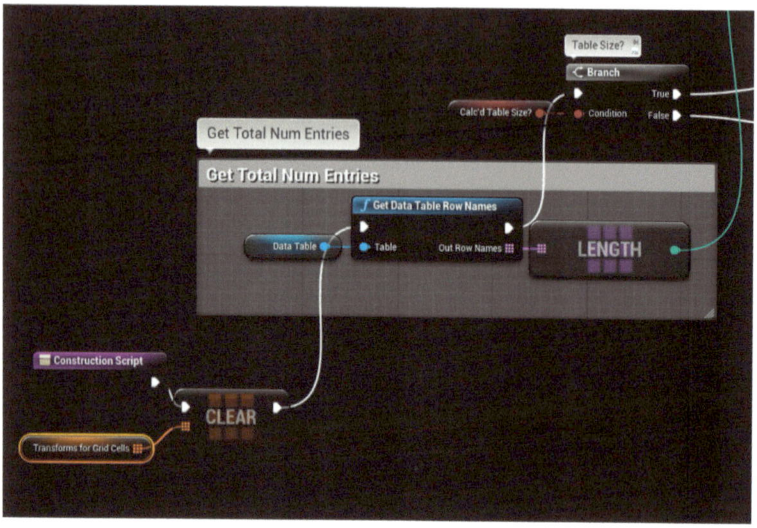

Figure 9. Blueprint snippet obtaining total number of entries.

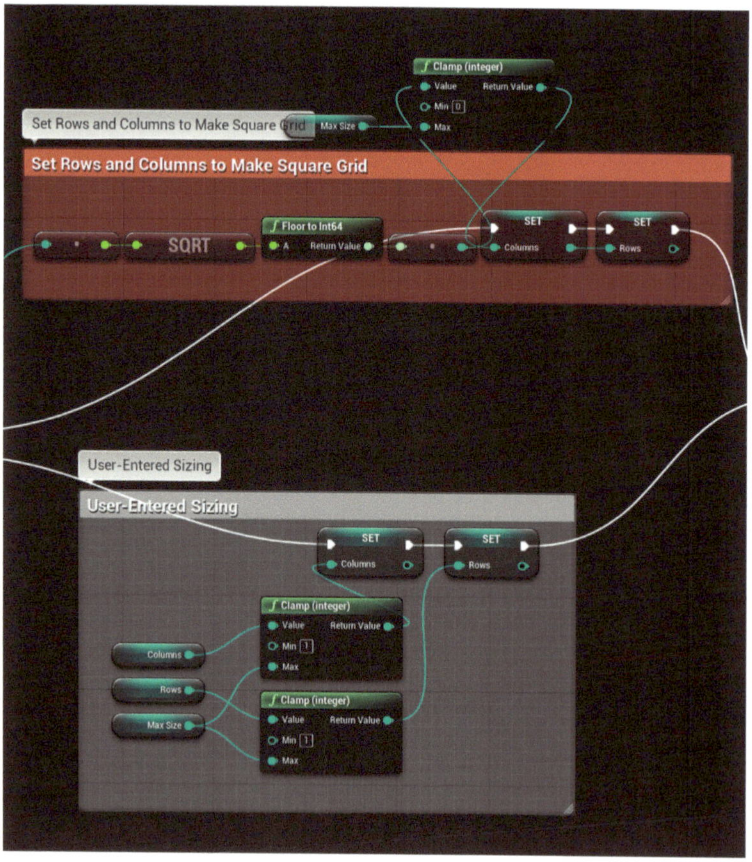

Figure 10. Blueprint snippet making a square grid and user-entered sizing.

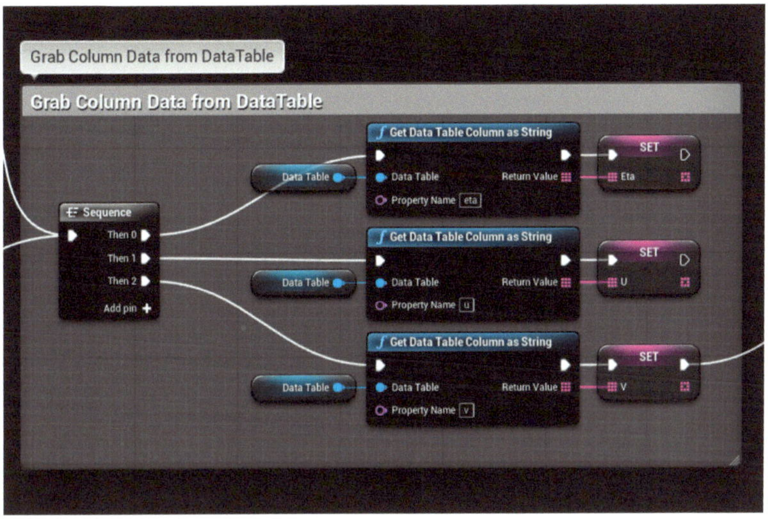

Figure 11. Blueprint script obtaining u, v, and eta values from the DataTable.

A Battleship-style board is used to illustrate the following example (Figure 12). The entire grid is too dense to load into memory at runtime, so we loaded a subset of those data, with a 1 cell radius around the vessel shown as highlighted areas. Because FUNWAVE's output is indexed, we did not have to loop over the entire grid to find and load the values for these cells. Instead, we took the known location of the vessel in 3D space (which Unreal provides as a "Transform"). We then obtained the Transform for the top left corner of the entire grid (red circle). The difference between the grid corner's location and the vessel's location, divided by the size of each grid cell in meters, tells us how many "cells" are along X the vessel (Figures 13 and 14).

$$(\text{ShipXLocation} - \text{GridCornerXLocation})/\text{CellSizeX} = \#\ \text{of Cells on X}$$

We used the same method to calculate how many cells away from the corner the ship is on Y.

$$(\text{ShipYLocation} - \text{GridCornerYLocation})/\text{CellSizeY} = \#\ \text{of Cells on Y}$$

The grid's maximum dimensions in X and Y are known. So, given an (X:Y) grid, we calculated the index (the yellow number) of the cell directly under the center of the vessel (the blue circle). In this example, the center of the ship is on G7 (rows in Battleship start at 1, not 0). If we replace "G", the column of that cell would also be 7 (on a Battleship board). The grid shown is 14 columns wide. So, each row is indexed as (0–13), (14–27), etc. See the yellow numbers (arrays in C++ start at 0, not 1). We know the center of the ship (blue circle) is on the 7th row of the grid, as well as the 7th column.

To calculate the index of this cell (the yellow number), we used the following formula:

$$\{[\text{ColumnWidth} * (\text{RowNum-1})] - 1\} + \text{ColumnNum}$$

$$\{[\text{ColumnWidth} * (\text{RowNum-1})] - 1\}$$

This portion accounts for all of the indexes of each "full" row above the target cell. It puts us on the correct "line"/row. We subtracted 1 from the RowNum so it did not count the row we were on as a full row (because we were not all the way to the right). We then subtracted 1 from the multiplied value to account for the fact that indexes in C++ arrays start at 0, and not 1. Rather than looping through the previous 90 cells and performing a calculation for each one to check if it was correct, we simply looked up the values for the cell at index 90. This changed the time complexity from O(n) to O(1), which is important due to FUNWAVE's grid being millions of cells in length. Our array lookup had a check based on the grid's dimensions to prevent wrapping (when the ship was at the grid's edge). In our code, this radius of loaded cells is dynamic. The user can enter how large of a radius they would like to load. This process enabled us to represent the ingested FUNWAVE data to our ability at this point.

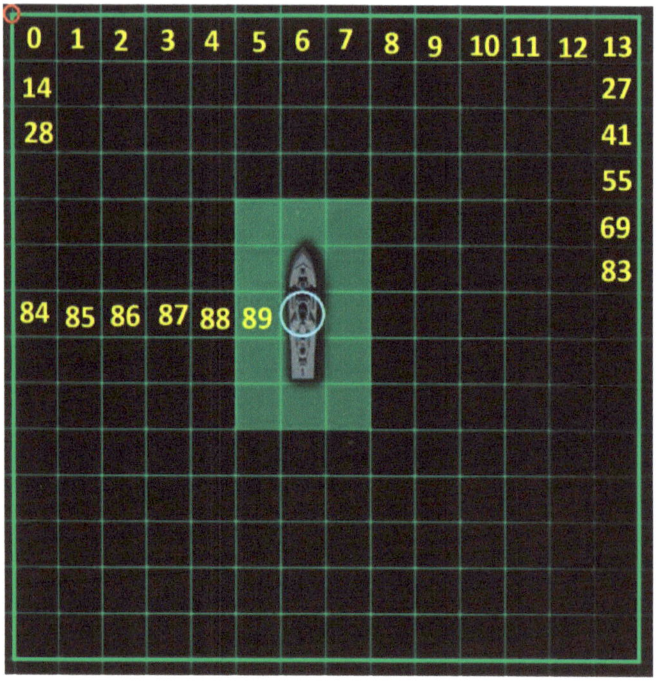

Figure 12. Battleship-style grid explaining radius of loaded cells.

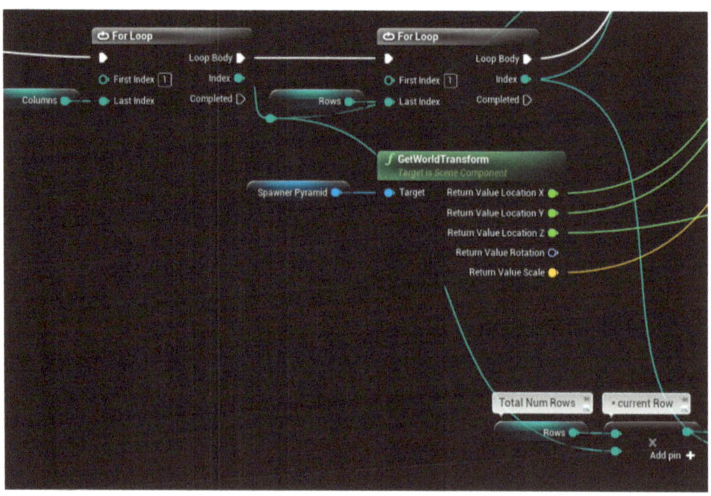

Figure 13. Blueprint snippet showing transform location.

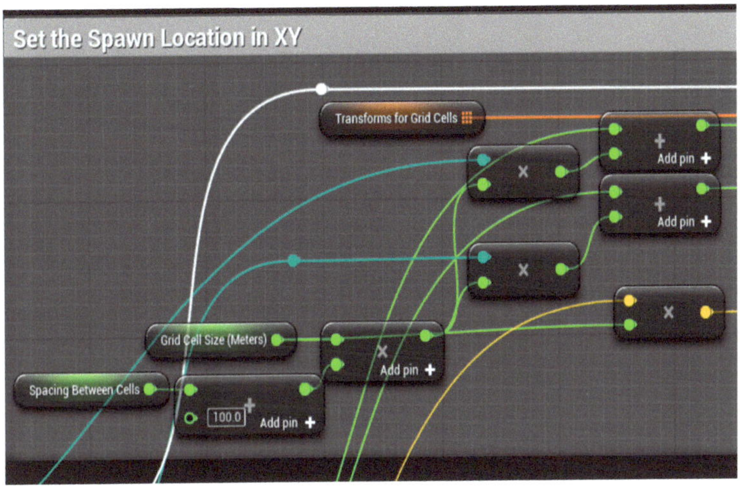

Figure 14. Blueprint snippet showing spawn location in XY.

Further exploration of data representation will allow us to render the grid in a more realistic way that represents water waves in a littoral zone. This is currently being studied and will be presented in a future work. The purpose of this technique was to show how the highly accurate FUNWAVE output could be ingested in an immersive environment. Reading the physics data is a crucial process toward combining these systems. Through the approach of hybridization, we outlined above that each data point could be integrated into the VR immersive system.

4. Results

The integration of FUNWAVE numerical modeling data was successfully integrated into a VR simulation, showing that highly accurate physics from numerical modeling can be incorporated. Although FUNWAVE data can be visualized via plotting, they have yet to be visualized in 3D, much less in virtual reality. Our final Unreal application shows our results of a hybrid methodology. In Figure 15, we can see the final visualization of our virtual watercraft simulation performing a beach landing. We also included the native FUNWAVE-generated results for comparison (Figure 16). These figures show that FUNWAVE's plot using Python can show more detail in the physics accuracy of the wave movements, but it lacks an immersive ability due to the nature of it being two-dimensional. A similar visualization can be rendered in 3D virtual reality in Unreal Engine, with integrated FUNWAVE data, greatly enhancing the physics accuracy of near-shore waves. Only a subset of the millions of data points was used due to being too computationally heavy, which resulted in lesser accuracy. Because FUNWAVE is run on a high-performance computer, this enables a high level of accuracy. We summarize the comparison in Table 3.

Table 3. Comparison between FUNWAVE visualization and Unreal Engine.

Application	Physics Accuracy	Visualization Capability
FUNWAVE	Higher (numerical modeler run on HPC)	Lower (only 2D plotting)
Unreal Engine	Lower (basic gaming physics engine)	Higher (fully immersive 3D VR)
Hybrid Approach	High accuracy of physics	High level of visual graphics and immersive virtual reality

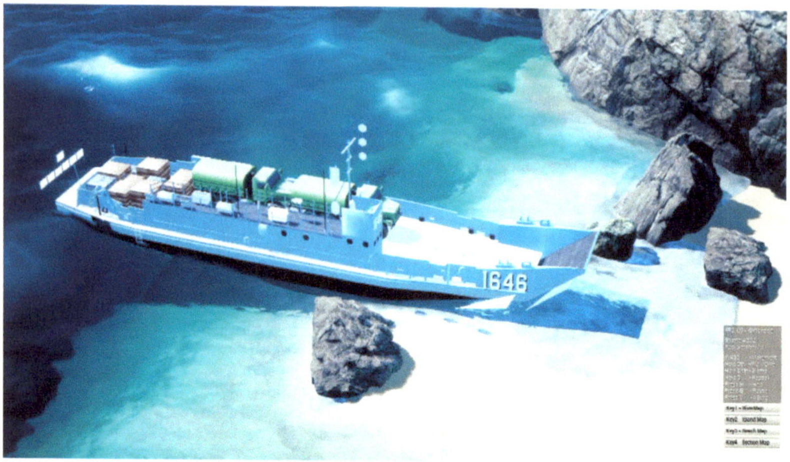

Figure 15. Fully immersive VR scene of LCU performing landing operation.

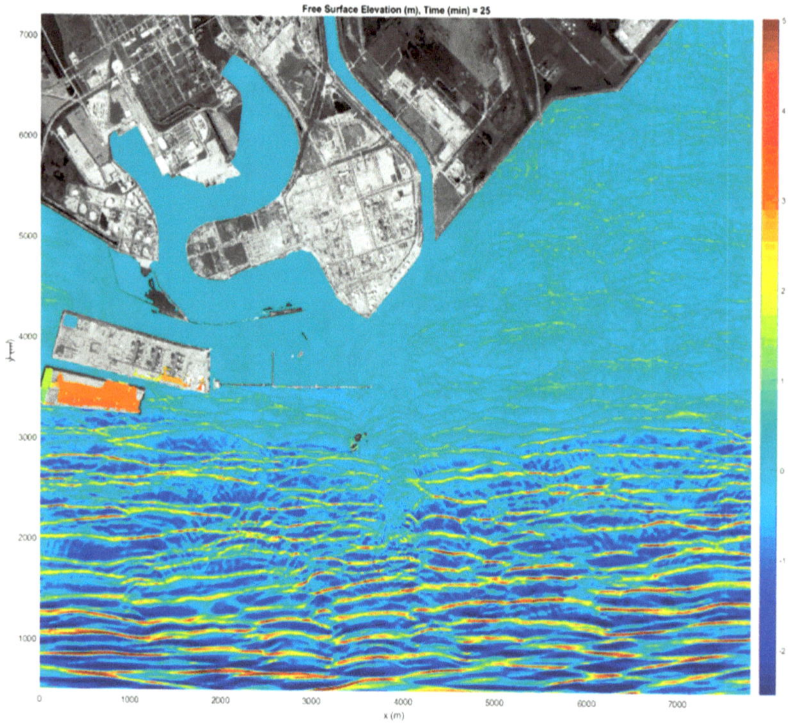

Figure 16. FUNWAVE plot using Python only available in 2D.

The hybrid prototype we developed demonstrates the ability to ingest physics-based output from computational modelers into a VR watercraft simulation running at 70 frames per second. We developed a framework to further explore this concept of physics data ingestion into VR development platforms for more immersive and scientifically accurate virtual experiences. Our current effort takes in FUNWAVE numerical output in the form of floating point numbers and ingests it into an Unreal Engine VR environment.

5. Discussion and Future Work

This project shows the potential of watercraft simulation advancement and the implications of adding valuable hydrodynamic numerical model data. By adding near-shore wave data through FUNWAVE simulation, LCU operators have a more accurate simulation that could potentially save soldiers' lives through more informed decisions relating to watercraft operation in littoral environments. Coupling our prototype with high-fidelity hydrodynamic numerical modeling within a VR environment provides a means to enhance ship survivability in operational deployments. Another direction could be for autonomous robotic ships that also operate in the littoral zones. Simulations for those systems could potentially save costs by providing a safer means of testing.

Future work should include upgrading to Unreal Engine 5 and should offer added functionality, better physics, and graphics capability. Reading in HDF5 and binary output directly into Unreal via C++ classes is currently being researched and could provide a faster ingestion method. A potential issue will be ingesting millions of numbers in parallel as opposed to a slow sequential reading function. Blueprints were primarily used for this project, but the use of C++ will be further explored for greater functionality. Additionally, this work focused on using FUNWAVE as a phase-resolved near-shore wave model, and the framework was built around the FUNWAVE HDF5 binary output. Celeris could provide a Unity implementation for highly accurate and immersive visualization [39]. There are a number of other phase-resolved wave models that can be used to generate the same spatial output (u, v, and eta, each as a function of time) including, but not limited to, SWASH [40], COULWAVE [41], and NHWAVE [42]. The framework can ingest these models with a simple conversion script between each of those native model outputs and the native HDF5 format can be used as an output from FUNWAVE.

6. Conclusions

The purpose of this research was to understand and integrate several systems toward an advanced watercraft simulator that is capable of physics-based water rendering. Hydrodynamic waves in VR have been limited to deep-water Gerstner waves and our application aims to incorporate near-shore wave models for more accuracy in wave rendering. In order to accomplish this, numerical modeler FUNWAVE data were ingested into Unreal Engine to supplement the native physics engine. The results show that this can be successfully achieved with the use of DataTables. Other methods are being explored, including reading in HDF5 and binary directly from output files without DataTables. Overall, the hybrid pieces of various data sources can come together for a comprehensive approach, creating a useful framework for further research in the field of game simulation using physics numerical models. This research will both accelerate development and facilitate the simulation, planning, and rehearsal of multi-domain operations by ensuring a seamless integration of sea- and land-based modeling and simulation tools to enable physics-based real-time accuracy and run-time efficiency.

Author Contributions: Conceptualization, G.S., K.M. and J.B.; methodology, K.E., K.S. and S.C.; software, K.S., K.E. and S.C.; validation, K.S., K.E., S.B. and S.C.; formal analysis K.S., K.E., S.B. and S.C.; investigation, G.S.; resources, G.S. and J.B.; data curation, K.S., K.E. and S.C.; writing—original draft preparation, K.E.; writing—review and editing, K.E., K.M., S.B. and S.C.; visualization, K.E. and K.S.; supervision, J.B.; project administration, G.S. and J.B.; funding acquisition, G.S. and J.B. All authors have read and agreed to the published version of the manuscript.

Funding: This research was funded by the U.S. Army Corps of Engineers, Engineering Research and Development Center Flex 4 Program and by the Coastal and Hydraulics Laboratory.

Institutional Review Board Statement: Not applicable.

Informed Consent Statement: Not applicable.

Data Availability Statement: The data presented in this study are available on request from the corresponding author. The data are not publicly available due to USACE ERDC security policy.

Acknowledgments: The authors would like to acknowledge the Engineering Research and Development Center, Coastal and Hydraulics Laboratory, and Information Technology Laboratory.

Conflicts of Interest: The authors declare no conflict of interest.

References

1. Shi, F.; Kirby, J.T.; Harris, J.C.; Geiman, J.D.; Grilli, S.T. A high-order adaptive time-stepping tvd solver for boussinesq modeling of breaking waves and coastal inundation. *Ocean Model.* **2012**, *43*, 36–51. [CrossRef]
2. Games, E. Rendering and Graphics, Physically Based, Unreal Engine 4 Documentation. Available online: https://docs.unrealengine.com/4.27/en-US/RenderingAndGraphics/Materials/PhysicallyBased/ (accessed on 1 August 2023).
3. Games, E. Building Worlds, Light Propagation Volumes, Unreal Engine 4 Documentation. Available online: https://docs.unrealengine.com/4.27/en-US/BuildingWorlds/LightingAndShadows/LightPropagationVolumes/ (accessed on 1 August 2023).
4. Games, E. Rendering and Graphics, Ray Tracing, Unreal Engine 4 Documentation. Available online: https://docs.unrealengine.com/4.27/en-US/RenderingAndGraphics/RayTracing/ (accessed on 1 August 2023).
5. Games, E. Rendering and Graphics, Post Process Effects, Unreal Engine 4 Documentation. Available online: https://docs.unrealengine.com/4.27/en-US/RenderingAndGraphics/PostProcessEffects/ (accessed on 1 August 2023).
6. Ni, S.; Liu, Z.; Cai, Y. Ship maneuverability-based simulation for ship navigation in collision situations. *J. Mar. Sci. Eng.* **2019**, *7*, 90. [CrossRef]
7. Fang, M.; Tsai, K.; Fang, C. A simplified simulation model of ship navigation for safety and collision avoidance in heavy traffic areas. *J. Navig.* **2018**, *71*, 837–860. [CrossRef]
8. Hewlett, J.C. *Ship Navigation Simulation Study, Houston-Galveston Navigation Channels, Texas. Report 1, Houston Ship Channel, Bay Segment*; U.S. Army Corps of Engineers: Washington, DC, USA; Waterways Experiment Station: Vicksburg, MS, USA, 1994.
9. Yin, J.; Ren, H.; Zhou, Y. The whole ship simulation training platform based on virtual reality. *IEEE Open J. Intell. Transp. Syst.* **2021**, *2*, 207–215. [CrossRef]
10. Lindberg, O.; Bingham, H.B.; Engsig-Karup, A.P.; Madsen, P.A. Towards real time simulation of ship-ship interaction. In Proceedings of the 27th International Workshop on Water Waves and Floating Bodies, Copenhagen, Denmark, 22–25 April 2012.
11. Lee, Y.S.; Rashidi, A.; Talei, A.; Beh, H.J.; Rashidi, S. A Comparison Study on the Learning Effectiveness of Construction Training Scenarios in a Virtual Reality Environment. *Virtual Worlds* **2023**, *2*, 36–52. [CrossRef]
12. Qi, J.; Tang, H.; Zhu, Z. Exploring an Affective and Responsive Virtual Environment to Improve Remote Learning. *Virtual Worlds* **2023**, *2*, 53–74. [CrossRef]
13. Ueng, S.; Lin, D.; Liu, C. A ship motion simulation system. *Virtual Real.* **2008**, *12*, 65–76. [CrossRef]
14. Chen, C.; Shiotani, S.; Sasa, K. Numerical ship navigation based on weather and ocean simulation. *Ocean. Eng.* **2013**, *69*, 44–53. [CrossRef]
15. Tai, T.C.; Carico, D. Simulation of dd-963 ship airwake by navier-stokes method. *J. Aircr.* **1995**, *32*, 1399–1401. [CrossRef]
16. Fournier, A.; Reeves, W.T. A simple model of ocean waves. In Proceedings of the 13th Annual Conference on Computer Graphics and Interactive Techniques, Philadelphia, PA, USA, 14–16 July 1986; pp. 75–84.
17. Tessendorf, J. Simulating ocean water. Simulating nature: Realistic and interactive techniques. *SIGGRAPH* **2001**, *1*, 5.
18. Zhang, W.; Zhang, J.; Zhang, T. Fast simulation method for ocean wave base on ocean wave spectrum and improved gerstner model with gpu. *J. Phys. Conf. Ser.* **2017**, *787*, 012027. [CrossRef]
19. Xu, J.; Gu, H.; Kang, F.; Yang, H.; Wang, S. Modeling and simulation of nearshore waves. *AsiaSim* **2012**, *323*, 358–364.
20. Mihalef, V.; Metaxas, D.; Sussman, M. Animation and control of breaking waves. In Proceedings of the 2004 ACM SIGGRAPH/Eurographics Symposium on Computer Animation, Grenoble, France, 27–29 August 2004; pp. 315–324.
21. Chen, J.; Yang, K.; Yuan, Y.; Wang, C. Visual simulation of breaking waves in shallow water. In Proceedings of the 2009 First International Workshop on Education Technology and Computer Science, Wuhan, China, 7–8 March 2009; IEEE: New York, NY, USA, 2009; Volume 2, pp. 246–249.
22. Takahashi, T.; Fujii, H.; Kunimatsu, A.; Hiwada, K.; Saito, T.; Tanaka, K.; Ueki, H. Realistic animation of fluid with splash and foam. In *Computer Graphics Forum*; Wiley Online Library: Hoboken, NJ, USA, 2003; Volume 22, pp. 391–400.
23. Yingst, M.; Alford, J.R.; Parberry, I. Very fast real-time ocean wave foam rendering using halftoning. In Proceedings of the 6th International North American Conference on Intelligent Games and Simulation (GAMEONNA); 2011; pp. 27–34. Available online: https://ianparberry.com/pubs/GAMEON-NA_GRAPH_04.pdf (accessed on 1 August 2023).
24. Nielsen, M.B.; Østerby, O. A two-continua approach to eulerian simulation of water spray. *ACM Trans. Graph. (TOG)* **2013**, *32*, 1–10. [CrossRef]
25. Wu, Y. A new exploration based on unreal engine4 particle effects of unreal engine in 3d animation scenes. *Int. J. Innov. Sci. Res. Technol.* **2021**, *6*, 691–696.
26. Hamano, T.; Onosato, M.; Tanaka, F. Performance comparison of physics engines to accelerate house-collapsing simulations. In Proceedings of the 2016 IEEE International Symposium on Safety, Security, and Rescue Robotics (SSRR), Lausanne, Switzerland, 23–27 October 2016; IEEE: New York, NY, USA, 2016; pp. 358–363.
27. Boeing, A.; Bräunl, T. Evaluation of real-time physics simulation systems. In Proceedings of the 5th International Conference on Computer Graphics and Interactive Techniques in Australia and Southeast Asia, Perth, Australia, 1–4 December 2007.

28. Hongpan, N.; Yong, G.; Zhongming, H. Application research of physx engine in virtual environment. In Proceedings of the 2010 International Conference on Audio, Language and Image Processing, Shanghai, China, 23–25 November 2010; IEEE: New York, NY, USA, 2010; pp. 587–591.
29. Wang, H.; Wan, J.; Zhang, F. Interaction of fluid simulation based on physx physics engine. In Proceedings of the 2015 4th International Conference on Sensors, Measurement and Intelligent Materials, Shenzhen, China, 27–28 December 2015; Atlantis Press: Dordrecht, The Netherlands, 2016; pp. 480–485.
30. Toasa, R.; Maximiano, M.; Reis, C.; Guevara, D. Data visualization techniques for real-time information—A custom and dynamic dashboard for analyzing surveys' results. In Proceedings of the 2018 13th Iberian Conference on Information Systems and Technologies (CISTI), Caceres, Spain, 13–16 June 2018; IEEE: New York, NY, USA, 2018; pp. 1–7.
31. Millais, P.; Jones, S.L.; Kelly, R. Exploring data in virtual reality: Comparisons with 2d data visualizations. In Proceedings of the Extended Abstracts of the 2018 CHI Conference on Human Factors in Computing Systems, Montreal, QC, Canada, 21–26 April 2018; pp. 1–6.
32. Stock, C.; Bishop, I.D.; O'Connor, A. Generating virtual environments by linking spatial data processing with a gaming engine. In Proceedings of the 6th International Conference for Information Technologies in Landscape Architecture, Dessau, Germany, 26 May 2005.
33. Keil, J.; Edler, D.; Schmitt, T.; Dickmann, F. Creating immersive virtual environments based on open geospatial data and game engines. *KN-J. Cartogr. Geogr. Inf.* **2021**, *71*, 53–65. [CrossRef]
34. Kenkenberg, A. Real-time Volumetric Cloud Visualization of Meteorological Simulation Data. Available online: https://gitlab2.cip.ifi.lmu.de/kenkenberg/cloud-thesis/-/tree/master (accessed on 1 February 2023).
35. Marsden, C.; Shankar, F. Using unreal engine to visualize a cosmological volume. *Universe* **2020**, *6*, 168. [CrossRef]
36. Prado, J.M. Using unreal engine as an engineering tool for traffic simulation and analysis. *Collect. Open Thesis Transp. Res.* **2020**, *2020*, 34.
37. Games, E. Data Driven Gameplay Elements, Making Interactive Experiences, Unreal Engine 4 Documentation. Available online: https://docs.unrealengine.com/4.26/en-US/InteractiveExperiences/DataDriven (accessed on 1 May 2021).
38. Sandurawan, D.; Kodikara, N.D.; Keppitiyagama, C.; Rosa, R. A six degrees of freedom ship simulation system for maritime education. *Int. J. Adv. ICT Emerg. Reg. (ICTer)* **2011**, *3*. [CrossRef]
39. Tavakkol, S.; Lynett, P. Celeris: A GPU-accelerated open source software with a Boussinesq-type wave solver for real-time interactive simulation and visualization. Comput. *Phys. Commun.* **2017**, *217*, 117–127. [CrossRef]
40. Marcel, Z.; Stelling, G.; Smit, P. SWASH: An operational public domain code for simulating wave fields and rapidly varied flows in coastal waters. *Coast. Eng.* **2011**, *58*, 992–1012.
41. Lynett, P.; Liu, P.L.F.; Sitanggang, K.I.; Kim, D.H. Modeling Wave Generation, Evolution, and Interaction with Depth Integrated, Dispersive Wave Equations COULWAVE Code Manual. Cornell University Long and Intermediate Wave Modeling Package v.2.0. 2002. Available online: https://www.semanticscholar.org/paper/Modeling-Wave-Generation-,-Evolution-,-and-with-,-v-Lynett-Liu/f07da390c4590b880607037be8d900538f42c992 (accessed on 1 February 2023).
42. Derakhti, M.O.; Kirby, J.T.; Shi, F.E.; Ma, G.A. *NHWAVE: Model Revisions and Tests of Wave Breaking in Shallow and Deep Water*; Research Report No. CACR-15-18; Center for Applied Coastal Research, Department of Civil and Environmental Engineering, University of Delaware: Newark, DE, USA, 2015.

virtual worlds

MDPI

Article

Field Trips and Their Effect on Student Learning: A Comparison of Knowledge Assessment for Physical versus Virtual Field Trips in a Construction Management Course

Amna Salman

McWhorter School of Building Science, Auburn University, Auburn, AL 36849, USA; azs0072@auburn.edu

Abstract: Teaching through field trips has been very effective in the architecture, engineering and construction (AEC) disciplines as it allows students to bridge the gap between theory and practice. However, it is not always feasible to take a large class on field trips due to time, safety, and cost limitations. To adequately prepare future professionals in the AEC industry, it is imperative that institutions adopt innovative methods of providing the field trip experience. One such approach is using virtual reality (VR) technology. Creating 3D VR construction environments and immersing students in that virtual world could provide an engaging and meaningful experience. Although researchers in AEC schools have developed and deployed many virtual field trips (VFTs) in education, little is known about their potential to provide the same knowledge base. For that reason, a VR app was created to teach students about the design and construction of steel structures, called the Steel Sculpture App (SSA). The SSA served as a VFT, and the location of the steel frame structure served as the actual field trip (AFT). The research was conducted in structure-related courses in the spring, summer, and fall of 2021 and the spring and fall of 2022 semesters. Each semester, students were split into groups, one being the control group and the other being the experimental group. The control groups learned through AFTs, whereas the experimental groups learned through VFTs. A knowledge test was administered at the end of each treatment to collect quantitative data on the students' performance, understanding, and knowledge retention. The results indicated that the students learning from VFTs scored higher than those learning from AFTs. The paper discusses student assessment results and student feedback about replacing AFTs with VFTs in times of need.

Keywords: virtual reality; construction education; pedagogical changes; steel structures; virtual field trips; learning assessments

Citation: Salman, A. Field Trips and Their Effect on Student Learning: A Comparison of Knowledge Assessment for Physical versus Virtual Field Trips in a Construction Management Course. *Virtual Worlds* **2023**, 2, 290–302. https://doi.org/10.3390/virtualworlds2030017

Academic Editors: Radu Comes, Dorin-Mircea Popovici, Calin Gheorghe Dan Neamtu and Jing-Jing Fang

Received: 8 August 2023
Revised: 1 September 2023
Accepted: 13 September 2023
Published: 18 September 2023
Corrected: 8 January 2025

1. Introduction

Given the pragmatic essence of the architecture, engineering, and construction (AEC) industry, it becomes crucial to delve into innovative teaching approaches to uphold elevated standards of education. In AEC education, educational field trips, often taking the form of site visits, play a pivotal role. These field trips offer participants a firsthand encounter with the topics or concepts discussed in the classroom. Nevertheless, organizing such field trips is not always practical due to constraints related to time, cost, and safety concerns [1]. It is crucial to find an alternative to having no field trips because the ability to visualize the built environment and learn the building construction processes is critical for students in the AEC disciplines [2]. For students lacking field experience, visualizing the construction processes and thus making informed decisions is difficult [3]. Creating 3D VR models and immersing students in the virtual world could provide an engaging and meaningful experience for all students in the AEC disciplines [4]. For this purpose, an interactive VR app was created for Oculus Quest, the "Steel Sculpture App" (SSA), to teach students about the design and construction of steel structures. Structural understanding is extremely important for all AEC students. However, teaching such skills in a traditional classroom setting becomes challenging.

The aim of the SSA app presented in this paper was to provide support to building science and architecture students, particularly in understanding onsite steel connections in a classroom-based education. This app was specifically created for structure-related courses in which students learn the design of steel, timber, and concrete structural members. The topic of steel connections was chosen because of its inherent complexity. In a steel building, connections play an important role, and many structural failures are attributed to connection failures [5]. The recent failure of the I-35W Bridge in Minneapolis in 2007 was due to the connection failure. The SSA is a self-explanatory interactive app that is also designed to cater to people with hearing impairments. In addition, for better understanding, the app shows the assembly and erection of steel members on a construction site. The app allows students to see modules again and again, pause, and exit at any time.

This interactive app could also bring an end to passive learners' attitudes, which are often found in traditional academic teaching settings [6]. Actual field trips, though helpful, require significant planning, funds, and time and still have many safety concerns. This paper explains the student learning assessment and student perspective of the VFT versus the AFT. The app served as the VFT, and the location of the actual steel structure served as the AFT. Controlled group and experimental group methods were used to analyze student learning assessments. After the learning assessment, all students were given a chance to experience both pedagogies to get their feedback.

2. Literature Review

The adoption of technology to effectively convey concepts to students is a common practice [6]. As technology advances, new means and methods are developed for integrating it effectively into teaching. When looking at mechanics and related courses, which are a vital part of understanding how a building carries loads, it is critical to clarify the concepts and details regarding the structural members using steel, timber, and concrete [1]. Such a task cannot be performed only within the boundaries of a classroom [7]. Visualization of these elements and their configuration is crucial for precise understanding and knowledge retention [7]. For this purpose, a field visit can enhance the concepts, where students can view these members being put together to form the structure rather than just reading them in a plan view [8]. The site visits, while educational, pose cost, safety, and time constraints. Visits are also dependent on the availability of the construction project during the structural phase [1].

VR was first used in the form of flight simulators, and it has come a long way since then [9]. As described by Merchant et al. [10], the aspect of being in a three-dimensional space, the ability to create and interact with three-dimensional objects, a digital representation of the learner in the form of an avatar, and the capability of communicating with other learners in the virtual world are all features of virtual reality. Virtual worlds are open-ended settings where users can design and develop their own objects, in contrast to the organized environments of simulations and games.

With immersive and interactive experiences in fields ranging from science and engineering to foreign languages and social sciences, virtual reality has long held promise as a tool to improve education [11]. As a cutting-edge teaching strategy that offers unique experiences to users, head-mounted VR-supported learning may influence students' self-efficacy in a specific area and further improve their future development [12]. Using VR modeling, you can better capture the audience's attention and immerse them to even change their attitude toward an issue such as environmental issues, and the model can be updated as new data is received [13]. In the medical industry, many surgical trainers use VR for educational purposes [14]. The use of VR for teaching anatomy was found to be more effective than traditional methods [15].

Virtual reality engages students in the learning process, particularly in lessons that require visualization and cannot be adequately addressed in conventional instruction [16]. For understanding concepts where spatial access is difficult, such as the world of atoms and molecules, VR has shown to improve the understanding of students, while making it much easier to teach [17]. On the other hand, students in a virtual reality learning environment have the potential to reach deeper levels of conceptual clarity, leading to knowledge retention, in a shorter amount of time, enabling students to focus on the learning scenario [18]. A 3D virtual environment was also shown to improve the cognitive skills of students with learning disabilities such as ADHD and dyslexia by allowing them to better visualize the material [19].

In addition, the concept of Industry 4.0 has an impact on the construction industry since structures are evolving into complex productions [20]. Construction management is integrating cutting-edge technologies like VR and augmented reality (AR) to improve efficiency and effectiveness in the construction process [21]. Therefore, it is important to equip students with the skills to use such technology in the classroom. According to Ververidis et al., virtual reality (VR) offers significant advantages in the realm of construction through its immersive visualization capabilities, enabling interactivity with the model, spatial awareness, and immediate real-time feedback [22].

While the architectural, engineering, and AEC industry would be transformed by integrating VR technologies and immersive collaboration among different stakeholders, it can be a valuable tool for improving students' capacity to recognize a range of building principles [23]. It is now possible to educate students by utilizing immersive digital environments that enable them to view and experiment with a 3D/4D full-scale virtual model of a construction project. A student's comprehension of complicated building projects can be considerably improved by this enhanced visual communication [2]. For example, for construction safety, VR is being used to develop simulations that give workers a first-person perspective of a construction process that has not yet begun, to spot potential issues before construction begins, and to train construction workers for potential hazards that may emerge on construction sites [24]. By using virtual reality technology, it has shown that most construction-related traffic incidents might be linked to workers who are easily distracted and are susceptible to boredom [25].

In order to teach the newer generation, which is fairly tech-savvy, the use of technology such as virtual reality (VR), augmented reality (AR), and mixed reality (MR) can provide ways to engage students in a social, collaborative, and active learning environment [4]. Kıral et al. [26] developed a V-SAFE app in which trainees are exposed to actual building risks in a secure virtual environment. Users become knowledgeable of the dangers they can encounter at work and experience the possible consequences of their own or other decisions [26]. In fact, virtual reality teaching is promoted for practical subjects like civil engineering and physics but not for theoretical subjects [27].

Recently, work has begun to see if VR technology can replace actual construction site visits [28]. This study used 360° panoramic photographs with modalities to enhance their experience through a focus on immersion, perception, and telepresence. For the modalities, iPads and VR headsets were used. Shahbaz et al., developed SimYA, which is an interactive 3D VR software where students can experience the basics of the construction process in a virtual environment and learn through trial and error as if they were at the construction site [29]. Özacar et al. conducted a complete building survey class in VR using tools like measuring tape, plumb, hose level, etc. The students and teachers were able to communicate using avatars using VRArchEducation [3].

It is evident that work is being performed to improve technology so that it can be used for teaching in the construction industry as well as education. To improve the learning experience and engagement of the newer generation, VR can be used, especially in courses where visualization is crucial. By providing an alternative to AFTs, a VFT can facilitate the instruction of important aspects of the construction site in a controlled and safe environment. Although a virtual trip may never completely replace or compare against AFTs, it can be helpful in times of need and can avoid time, cost, and safety concerns.

3. Research Methodology

This research study aimed to determine the validity of replacing VFTs with AFTs due to time, safety, and cost concerns in times of need. After an extensive literature review of VR in AEC academia and industry, a plan of approach was developed on how to compare a VFT with an AFT. For this purpose, the Steel Sculpture App (SSA) was developed in VR. The focus of this application was to create a virtual field trip and teach students about steel construction and connections in structure courses. The app was introduced in the Structures of Building-II course, where a major part of this course involved the design of steel, timber, and concrete structural members. Steel construction was selected due to its inherent complexity. The virtual trip explained seven basic connections of the steel structure, their uses, and a field example. The location of the steel sculpture served as the actual field trip, and the app served as the virtual field trip. The following objectives were established to investigate the efficacy of VFTs:

- To examine and assess student learning and understanding through VFT and AFT.
- To assess students' knowledge retention for VFT and AFT.
- To assess the challenges and student perspective of learning through VFT versus AFT.

To conduct this study, the following research hypothesis was developed.

Alternate Hypothesis: H_A: *Students who participated in AFT learn better than those who participated in VFT.*

Null Hypothesis: H_0: *There is no significant difference in student learning between the two ways of teaching.*

3.1. Research Design

To carry out this research, the action research method was chosen. Action research is a research philosophy and methodology that is commonly used in the social sciences. It seeks transformative change through the concurrent processes of action and research, which are linked by critical reflection involving the following steps:

- Diagnosis: finding problems.
- Action plan: how to approach the problem's solution.
- Action taking: application of the planned action.
- Evaluating: determination of the effects of the action.
- Specific learning: reflection on the action taken and recording the results.

The detailed action research road map is shown in Figure 1.

3.2. Steel Sculpture App (SSA) Development

After the 'Diagnosis' of the problem, 'Action Plan' was set to resolve the problem (Figure 1). The Steel Sculpture App (SSA) was developed, which served as VFT. For the development of the SSA, a sketch-up model of the steel sculpture was created (Figure 2, right). The location of the steel sculpture served as an AFT (Figure 2 left). This model was imported into Unity 3D (a virtual environment development software), where animations and voice-overs were added, and details were added for each connection type (Figure 3). The app developed in Unity 3D was then transferred to the Oculus Quest, where it was tested (Figure 4). The Oculus Quest can be seen in Figure 5.

3.3. Testing the SSA

The steps shown in Figure 6 were used to assess students' understanding of the SSA and knowledge retention of VFT versus AFT. For each semester, the students were separated into two groups, as detailed in Figure 6. One group was given a virtual tour using SSA, while the other was assigned a physical visit. In both trips, details regarding the model were taught to the students. A week after the trips, the students were evaluated through a quiz to determine their knowledge retention (Appendix A). In the next class period, students who had a VFT went on an AFT, and students who went on an AFT experienced the VFT. After both groups had gone through both trips, their feedback was collected. Both the feedback and the data from the quiz were then compiled and taken for analysis.

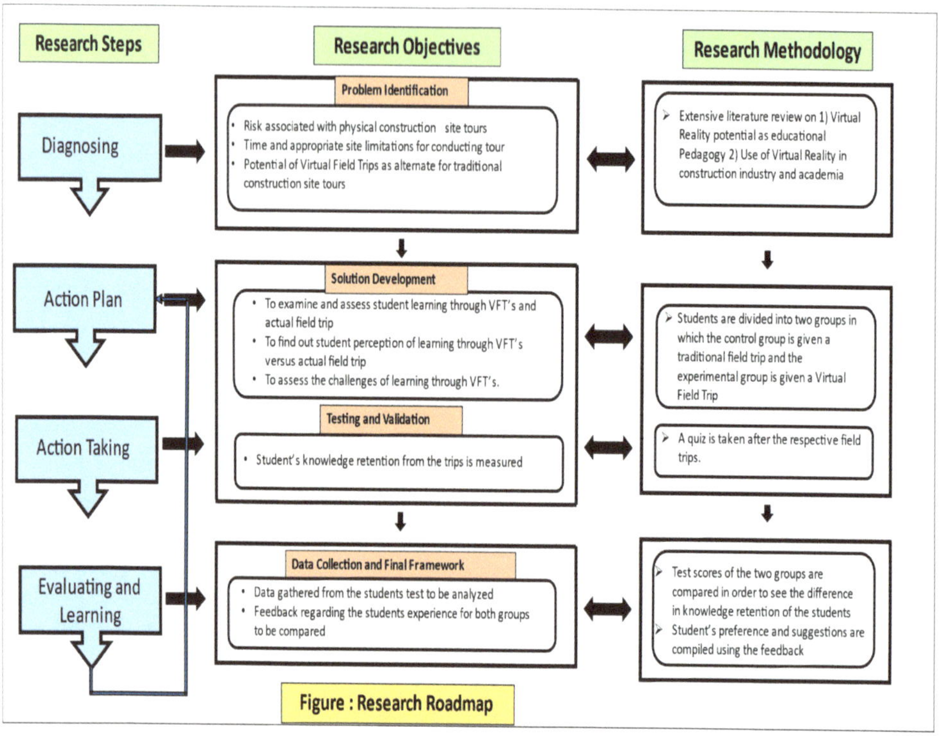

Figure 1. Research Design.

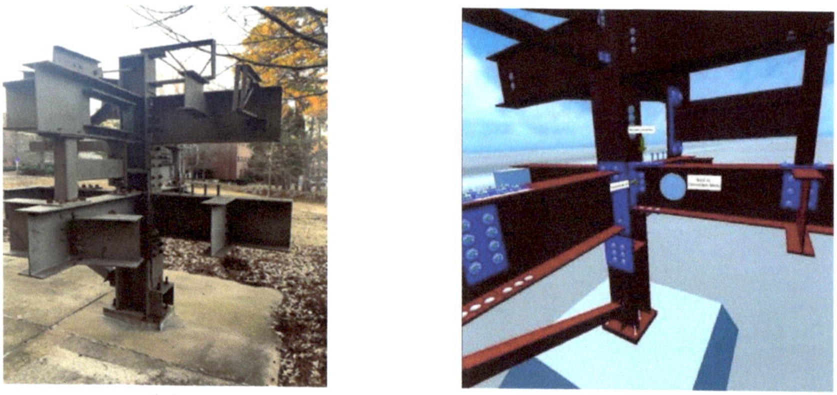

(a) (b)

Figure 2. Steel sculpture for AFT; (**a**) VS steel sculpture 3D model in Oculus (**b**).

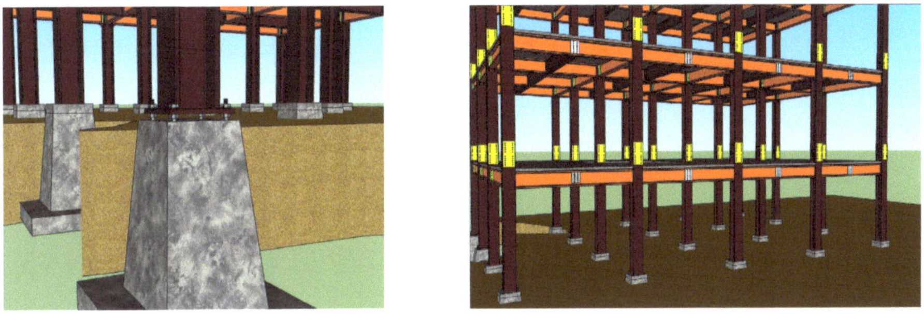

Figure 3. Images from the Steel Sculpture App.

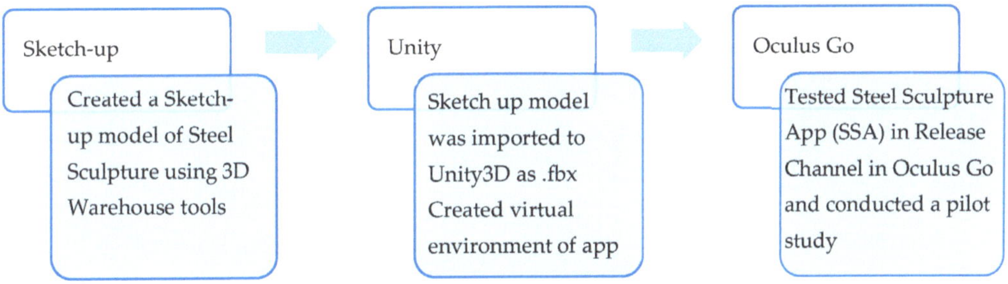

Figure 4. Development of SSA.

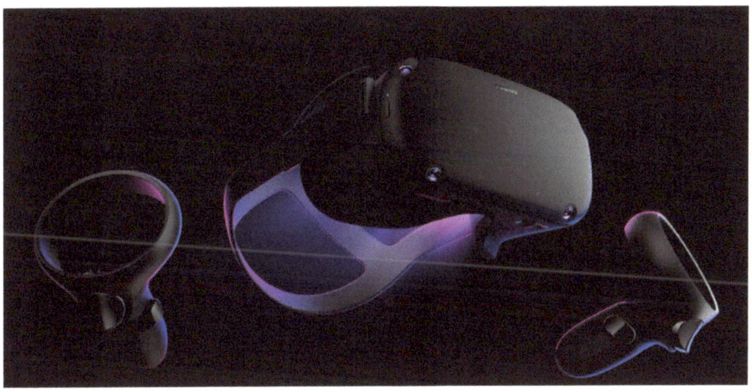

Figure 5. Oculus Quest.

3.4. Data Analysis

To evaluate the extent to which students retained knowledge from the two field trips, a quiz was administered one week after the trips occurred. Additionally, during the subsequent class period, students were exposed to both types of field trips to gauge their perceptions and feedback regarding each experience. To examine the data in detail, the student demographics and various tests used to analyze the data are given below.

3.5. Students' Demographic

To assess the effectiveness of the Steel Structure App (SSA), an experimental investigation of the VFT was carried out involving students from Auburn University's Architecture and Building Construction program. The study was conducted during the spring, summer, and fall of 2021 and the spring and fall of 2022. The study included a total of 182 students, of whom 94 were in the experimental group and 88 were in the controlled group. The results and analysis of the study incorporated feedback and assessments from 72 architecture students and 94 building science students.

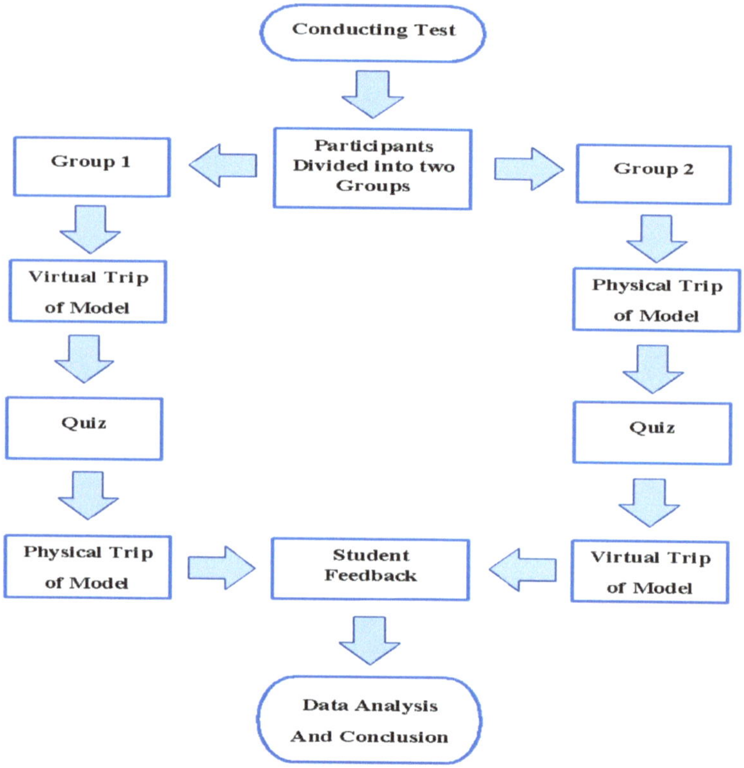

Figure 6. Flowchart for testing.

3.6. ANOVA Test (Analysis of Variance)

ANOVA is a statistical method employed to ascertain if there are significant differences in the means of two or more groups. It compares the means of various samples to assess the influence of one or more factors. ANOVA tests are commonly utilized to determine the significance of survey or experiment results. Essentially, they aid in making decisions regarding whether to accept the null hypothesis and reject the alternative hypothesis, or vice versa.

The null hypothesis in an ANOVA is valid when all the sample means are equal or do not have any significant difference. Thus, they can be considered part of a larger population. On the other hand, the alternate hypothesis is valid when at least one of the sample means is different from the rest of the sample means. This test is performed using MS Excel with a built-in plug-in. In simpler terms, if the p-value from the ANOVA test is < 0.05, then the alternate hypothesis is true. If the p-value is > 0.05, then the null hypothesis is true.

3.7. Mean and Standard Deviation

After determining if there was variance in the data, the mean score for the data was calculated. This was performed by taking the results of the students in the two groups and taking an average. This shows which of the two groups performed better in the test. The standard deviation was also calculated to see which of the two groups had more consistent data, i.e., less variance in their results. Both the mean and the standard deviation were then used to draw a conclusion.

3.8. Feedback

In terms of the feedback obtained from the students regarding both methods of tours, the data was collected on a Likert scale of 1–7, with "1" being strongly disagreed with and "7" being strongly agreed with. This data was then used to calculate the mean, mode, and standard deviation of the feedback statements. In addition, the weighted mean was also calculated for the statements.

4. Results and Discussion

To draw conclusions about the performance of the two groups, a quiz was administered one week after their respective tours. Upon analyzing the quiz results, it was observed that the experimental group, which underwent a virtual tour (group 1), achieved a higher mean/average score of 8.08 on the quiz. In contrast, the control group, which experienced a physical field trip (group 2), obtained a lower mean/average score of 7.39 (Table 1). These findings indicate that the performance of the experimental group was superior to that of the control group. Examining the standard deviations, the experimental group exhibited a standard deviation of 1.12, while the control group had a standard deviation of 1.27. As the standard deviation of the experimental group was lower than that of the control group, it can be inferred that there was less variation in the results of the experimental group.

Table 1. Student assessment results.

Groups	Count	Sum	Average	Standard Deviation	Variance
Group 1 (Virtual tour)	94	760	8.085106383	1.1232	1.261496225
Group 2 (Physical model visit)	88	651	7.397727273	1.2734	1.621603971

An ANOVA (Analysis of Variance) test was performed to find which of the hypotheses was true. By comparing the values gained from the ANOVA test, it was determined that group 1 had less variance in their scores, which shows that all students perceived roughly the same amount of information that was given to them during the virtual tour (Table 2). The F value is compared with the F-critical value to see if the test was significant. Since F > F-critical, the test is considered significant, and the null hypothesis can be rejected (Table 2). Also, to back up the results, the *p*-value was assessed. In this case, the *p*-value is <0.05, and the alternate hypothesis is true, meaning there is a difference in knowledge retention between students who took a VFT and those who took an AFT.

Student Feedback

To receive student perspectives about replacing AFT with VFT in times of need due to time, cost, and safety concerns, a survey was developed. Figure 7 shows the questions and student feedback from the survey. Table 3 shows the median, mode, SD, and weighted average of the results of the data received, where strongly agree = 7 and strongly disagree = 1.

Table 2. ANOVA test results.

Source of Variation	SS	df	MS	F	*p*-Value	F Crit
Between Groups	21.4749	1	21.4749	14.95939353	0.000153351	3.89364
Within Groups	258.399	180	1.43555			
Total	279.874	181				

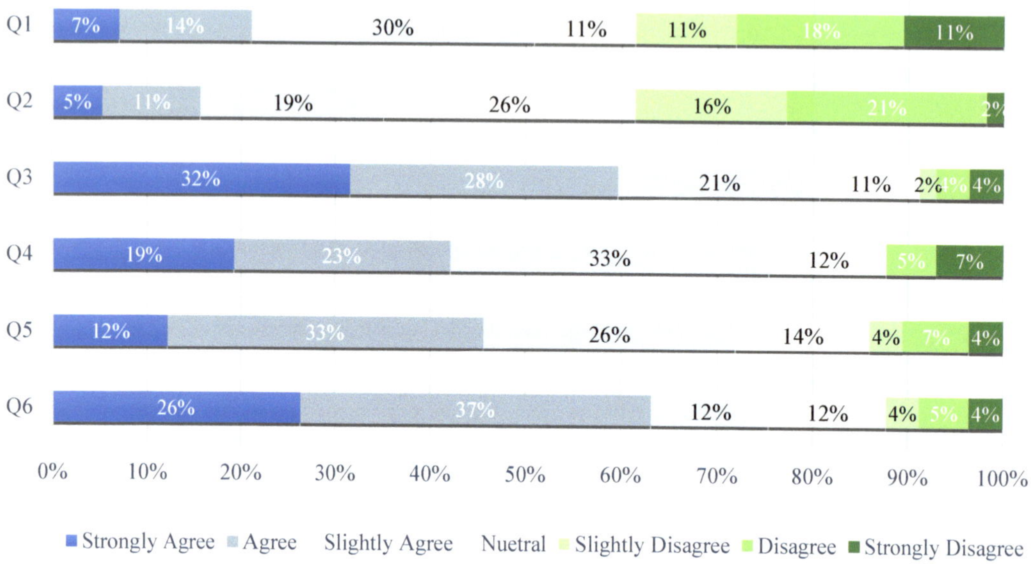

Figure 7. Student perception and feedback.

According to the survey results, 126 out of 168 students (75.4%) either slightly agree, agree, or strongly agree that virtual field trips (VFTs) can be used as an alternative to actual field trips (AFTs). The weighted average for this statement is 5.05, indicating that most of the students agree with this proposition (Table 3). However, it should be noted that there were a few students who were using the VR Oculus Quest headset for the first time, and it took longer for them to understand the subject matter (Q5: weighted average = 3.93). This suggests that there might be a learning curve associated with using virtual reality (VR) technology for educational purposes. Additionally, some students reported experiencing motion sickness during the VR experience (Table 3, Question 6, weighted average = 4.02). This highlights a potential drawback of VR technology, as certain individuals may be more susceptible to motion sickness when using VR headsets. Students also wanted to see more educational tools developed in VR (Q1, weighted average = 5.4).

In some open-ended questions, the students explained their likes and dislikes about the app. One student said, "I enjoyed how you were able to view the connections from multiple vantage points, as well as the aspect of if your instructor cannot plan a field trip, VR could be used as an alternate". Another student said, "that I could go back and hear the same thing again". Another student said, "I liked being able to see the structure from multiple angles, including from above; this is not possible in a real field trip". When asked about improvements in the app, a student said, "If there is a way to make it to where you don't get a headache, I think it would greatly improve my opinion about it". The students were also asked about what they did not like in the app, and one student said, "I did not like the voice changes, and the screen strained my eyes". These comments call for improvements in the technology to make it more comfortable for end users.

Overall, while the majority of students agreed that VFTs can serve as an alternative to AFTs, there were a few concerns related to the learning curve and potential discomfort associated with using VR technology. However, an informal discussion with the participants reached the conclusion that there are some experiences for which we must visit the actual site. Especially for freshmen and sophomores who have little field experience. However, for juniors and seniors, VR-based educational tools should be developed for conceptual clarity. These findings provide valuable insights into the students' experiences and perceptions regarding the use of VFTs in educational settings.

Table 3. Student perception and feedback.

Questions	N	Median	Mode	SD	Weighted Average
Q1: You want to see more educational tools developed in VR?	168	6	6	1.61	5.4
Q2: You enjoyed VFT without having to go out of classroom?	168	5	6	1.53	5.02
Q3: You believe we can sometimes use VFTs as an alternative to actual field trip?	168	5	5	1.66	5.05
Q4: Teaching a class of 30 students through the physical field trip will be challenging as some students may not be able to hear, some may be far away from the model to actually understand it well?	168	6	7	1.3	5.53
Q5: As a learner, it took longer to understand the subject matter in VR exercise than the physical field trip?	168	4	4	1.51	3.93
Q6: One of the reasons you did not enjoy VFTs is because you felt motion sickness during the VR experience?	168	5	5	1.8	4.02

5. Conclusions

In this study, student assessment and perception of virtual field trips (VFT) versus the actual field trip (AFT) were examined. A Steel Sculpture App (SSA) was created as the VFT, and the location of the actual steel sculpture model served as the AFT. The study was performed in the Structures of Building-II course, and students had no prior knowledge of steel connections or design. It was found that students not only learned better in VFTs but were also able to achieve conceptual clarity of the subject matter. During the AFT, students who were closer to the instructor were able to listen and see well, whereas those at a distance were either distracted, not able to listen, or could not see the connection properly. VFTs give students a chance to focus on subject matter very closely with visual demonstrations and applications. The actual field trips entail a lot of planning on the instructor's part. However, there are some experiences for which actual field trips are essential. Evidently, VFTs cannot provide the physical perception that one has in the field, such as touching soil, walking on muddy dirt, hearing sounds and smells, or climbing the stairs of a construction site. A well-designed VFT, involving proper visualization, real-time maps, sound, and video clips in a variety of formats, could, however, help students imagine what an actual site visit would be like. In targeting the learning objectives through a VFT, one must be realistic in its design, information presented, and voiceovers. The SSA created for this study is an Oculus Quest app that has been published for everyone to download from the Oculus library and incorporate into their curriculum. After the study, students proposed some improvements to the app, which are under process. In conclusion, VFTs offer a compelling alternative to actual field trips (AFTs) in construction education, considering the time, safety, and cost concerns involved. Using immersive technology, students can engage in realistic and interactive experiences that simulate real construction environments. Although students scored better with VFTs, they still expressed the belief that actual field trips are necessary, productive, and foundational. The students emphasized the importance of hands-on learning, as it allows students to physically engage with the construction site. While not advocating for replacing actual field trips entirely, students encouraged the development of better immersive educational apps, recognizing their potential to save in-class time. However, it was noted that having sufficient devices for all students in the class is crucial for effective implementation.

One of the primary advantages of VFTs is the time efficiency they provide. Traditional AFTs often require extensive planning, logistics, and travel time, which can be a significant constraint on the instructor. VFTs eliminate the need for physical travel, enabling students to explore multiple construction sites and scenarios within the convenience of the classroom. This allows for more frequent and varied learning experiences, enhancing students' exposure to different construction practices and projects.

Safety is another critical consideration in construction education, particularly when conducting site visits. Construction sites can present inherent risks, including heavy machinery, hazardous materials, and unstable structures. VFTs eliminate these safety concerns, ensuring a controlled and risk-free learning environment. Students can observe construction processes and safety protocols without exposure to actual hazards, reducing the potential for accidents or injuries.

Cost is often a limiting factor in organizing AFTs. Expenses related to transportation, accommodation, and site access can be substantial, making AFTs financially burdensome, especially for educational institutions with limited resources. VFTs offer a cost-effective alternative, as they require minimal additional expenses once the necessary VR equipment and software are in place. This affordability allows educational institutions to provide more opportunities for students to engage in experiential learning without straining their budgets.

However, it is important to acknowledge that VFTs may not completely replace AFTs in construction education and may only focus on one stage of the project. AFTs offer unique benefits, such as physical presence, tactile experiences, and real-time interactions with professionals on site. Therefore, a balanced approach that combines both VFTs and AFTs can provide a comprehensive learning experience, leveraging the advantages of each approach. As technology continues to advance, incorporating VFTs alongside AFTs can create a well-rounded and immersive learning environment for construction education, preparing students for the challenges of the industry while optimizing resources and ensuring their safety. VR is shaping up to be a powerful tool in teaching and is gradually becoming a part of classrooms. From this research, it is concluded that VFTs are directly linked to the students' knowledge retention and are responsible for a better understanding of the material. Thus, instructors can use VFTs in times of need due to time, safety, and cost limitations.

Funding: This research received no external funding.

Institutional Review Board Statement: In accordance with local legislation and institutional requirements, ethical review and approval were not required for the study of human participants. No personal information was collected.

Informed Consent Statement: Informed consent was obtained from all subjects involved in the study.

Data Availability Statement: The original contributions presented in the study are included in the article, further inquiries can be directed to the corresponding author.

Conflicts of Interest: The author declares no conflict of interest.

Appendix A

Virtual Steel Sculpture Quiz

Please answer the following questions from the best of your knowledge.

Question 1: Simple Connection are used to transmit _______________ forces

(a) Shear Forces (b) Bending Moment (c) Both Shear and Bending Moment (d) None of the above

Question 2: What is the purpose of moment connection?

(a) To transfer bending moments (b) To transfer bending moments and shear forces (c) To transfer only the dead loads (d) To transfer only the live loads

Question 3: In connecting beams to girders, when do we need to cop the beams?

(a) When beams and girders are of same depth (b) When beams and girders of same length (c) When beams have to connect with columns (d) None of the above

Question 4: The size of each member, plates and bolts is determined by the magnitude of load applied. (True/False)

Question 5: Which of the following connections do you recommend to use when a beam is too long to be transported in a single piece and has to be spliced i.e., transported in two pieces and joined at the jobsite?

Question 6: Which of the following connections is Shear Tab?

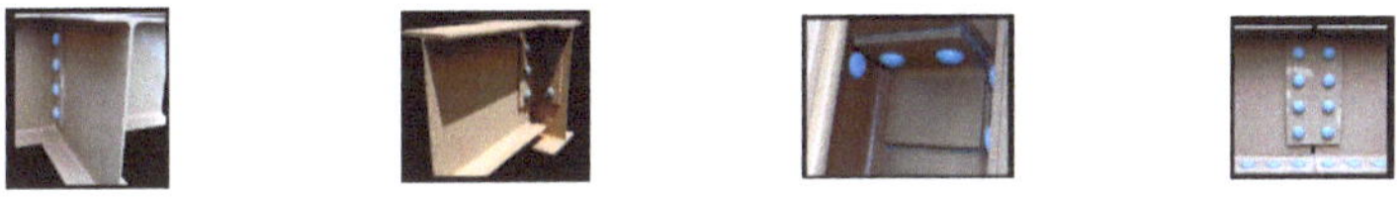

Question 7: Which of the following connection do you recommend to use when you have a concrete slab that is bonded to a beam and behaves as composite section?

Question 8: Which of the following connections do you recommend when you need a shear-moment connection between a girder and column?

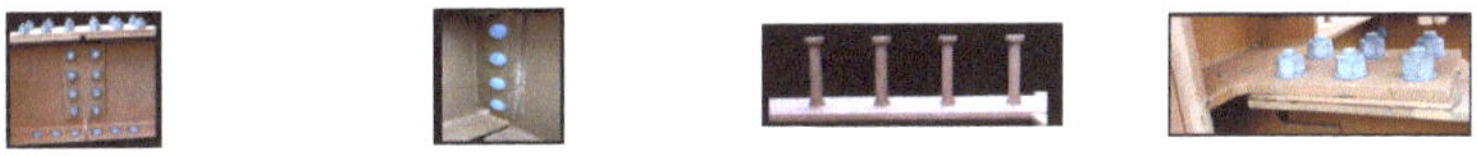

Question 9: Which of the following connections do you recommend when you need a shear-moment connection between a girder and column?

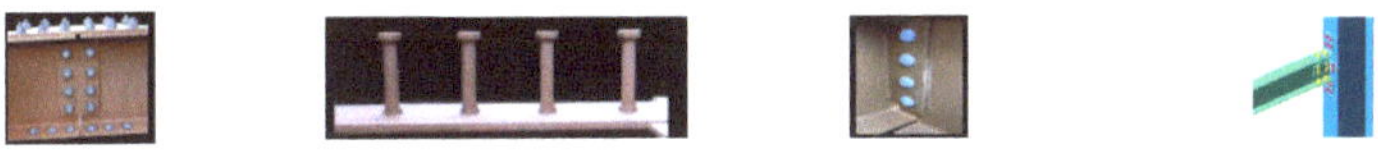

Question 10: Which of the following connection do you recommend when the column is too long to be transported in single piece and needs to be connected at the jobsite?

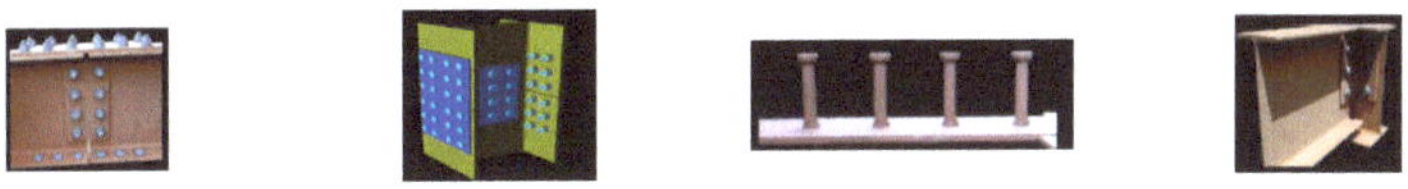

References

1. Kim, J. Comparing 360 Virtual Reality Learning Configurations for Construction Education. In *IOP Conference Series: Materials Science and Engineering*; IOP Publishing: Bristol, UK, 2022; Volume 1218, p. 012054.
2. Azhar, S.; Kim, J.; Salman, A. Implementing Virtual Reality and Mixed Reality Technologies in Construction Education: Students' Perceptions and Lessons Learned. In *ICERI2018 Proceedings*; IATED: Valencia, Spain, 2018; pp. 3720–3730.

3. Özacar, K.; Ortakcı, Y.; Küçükkara, M.Y. VRArchEducation: Redesigning Building Survey Process in Architectural Education Using Collaborative Virtual Reality. *Comput. Graph.* **2023**, *113*, 1–9. [CrossRef]
4. Azhar, S.; Han, D.; Dastider, S.G. Immersive VR Modules for Construction Safety Education of Generation Z Students. *EPiC Ser. Built Environ.* **2020**, *1*, 482–490.
5. Moaveni, S.; Chou, K. Teaching Steel Connections Using an Interactive Virtual Steel Sculpture. *J. STEM Educ.* **2015**, *16*, 61–68.
6. Amna Salman, M. Student Learning Assessment from a Virtual Field Trip. *EPiC Ser. Built Environ.* **2020**, *1*, 99–107.
7. Kisaumbi, A.M. External Factors and Adoption of New Technology in Education Support Organisations in Kenya: A Case of Cemastea. Ph.D. Thesis, Africa Nazarene University, Nairobi, Kenya, 2022.
8. Ullah, F.; Sepasgozar, S.; Tahmasebinia, F.; Sepasgozar, S.M.E.; Davis, S. Examining the Impact of Students' Attendance, Sketching, Visualization, and Tutors Experience on Students' Performance: A Case of Building Structures Course in Construction Management. *Constr. Econ. Build.* **2020**, *20*, 78–102. [CrossRef]
9. Sun, Y.; Albeaino, G.; Gheisari, M.; Eiris, R. Virtual Collaborative Spaces for Online Site Visits: A Plan-Reading Pilot Study. *EPiC Ser. Built Environ.* **2022**, *3*, 688–696.
10. Pantelidis, V.S. Reasons to Use Virtual Reality in Education and Training Courses and a Model to Determine When to Use Virtual Reality. *Themes Sci. Technol. Educ.* **2010**, *2*, 59–70.
11. Merchant, Z.; Goetz, E.T.; Cifuentes, L.; Keeney-Kennicutt, W.; Davis, T.J. Effectiveness of Virtual Reality-Based Instruction on Students' Learning Outcomes in K-12 and Higher Education: A Meta-Analysis. *Comput. Educ.* **2014**, *70*, 29–40. [CrossRef]
12. Boyles, B.D. *Virtual Reality and Augmented Reality in Education*; Center for Teaching Excellence, United States Military Academy: West Point, NY, USA, 2017.
13. Huang, W. Examining the Impact of Head-Mounted Display Virtual Reality on the Science Self-Efficacy of High Schoolers. *Interact. Learn. Environ.* **2019**, *30*, 100–112. [CrossRef]
14. Cho, Y.; Park, K.S. Designing Immersive Virtual Reality Simulation for Environmental Science Education. *Electronics* **2023**, *12*, 315. [CrossRef]
15. Haowen, J.; Vimalesvaran, S.; King Wang, J.; Boon, L.; Mogali, S.; Tudor Car, L. Virtual Reality in Medical Students' Education: A Scoping Review. *JMIR Med. Educ.* **2022**, *8*, e34860. [CrossRef] [PubMed]
16. Zhao, J.; Xu, X.; Jiang, H.; Ding, Y. The Effectiveness of Virtual Reality-Based Technology on Anatomy Teaching: A Meta-Analysis of Randomized Controlled Studies. *BMC Med. Educ.* **2020**, *20*, 127. [CrossRef]
17. Safikhani, S.; Keller, S.; Schweiger, G.; Pirker, J. Immersive Virtual Reality for Extending the Potential of Building Information Modeling in Architecture, Engineering, and Construction Sector: Systematic Review. *Int. J. Digit. Earth* **2022**, *15*, 503–526. [CrossRef]
18. Laricheva, E.N.; Ilikchyan, A. Exploring the Effect of Virtual Reality on Learning in General Chemistry Students with Low Visual-Spatial Skills. *J. Chem. Educ.* **2023**, *100*, 589–596. [CrossRef]
19. Hui, J.; Zhou, Y.; Oubibi, M.; Di, W.; Zhang, L.; Zhang, S. Research on Art Teaching Practice Supported by Virtual Reality (VR) Technology in the Primary Schools. *Sustainability* **2022**, *14*, 1246. [CrossRef]
20. Elfakki, A.O.; Sghaier, S.; Alotaibi, A.A. An Efficient System Based on Experimental Laboratory in 3D Virtual Environment for Students with Learning Disabilities. *Electronics* **2023**, *12*, 989. [CrossRef]
21. Das, P.; Perera, S.; Senaratne, S.; Osei-Kyei, R. Paving the Way for Industry 4.0 Maturity of Construction Enterprises: A State of the Art Review. *Eng. Constr. Archit. Manag.* **2022**. Available online: https://www.emerald.com/insight/content/doi/10.1108/ECAM-11-2021-1001/full/html (accessed on 1 September 2023).
22. Seyman Guray, T.; Kismet, B. VR and AR in Construction Management Research: Bibliometric and Descriptive Analyses. *Smart Sustain. Built Environ.* **2023**, *12*, 635–659. [CrossRef]
23. Ververidis, D.; Nikolopoulos, S.; Kompatsiaris, I. A Review of Collaborative Virtual Reality Systems for the Architecture, Engineering, and Construction Industry. *Architecture* **2022**, *2*, 476–496. [CrossRef]
24. Ghanem, S.Y. Implementing Virtual Reality-Building Information Modeling in the Construction Management Curriculum. *J. Inf. Technol. Constr.* **2022**, *27*, 48–69. [CrossRef]
25. Sacks, R.; Perlman, A.; Barak, R. Construction Safety Training Using Immersive Virtual Reality. *Constr. Manag. Econ.* **2013**, *31*, 1005–1017. [CrossRef]
26. Kim, N.; Yan, N.; Grégoire, L.; Anderson, B.A.; Ahn, C.R. Road Construction Workers' Boredom Susceptibility, Habituation to Warning Alarms, and Accident Proneness: Virtual Reality Experiment. *J. Constr. Eng. Manag.* **2023**, *149*, 04022175. [CrossRef]
27. Kiral, I.A.; Comu, S.; Kavaklioglu, C. *Enhancing the Construction Safety Training by Using Virtual Environment: V-SAFE*; University of British Columbia Library: Vancouver, BC, Canada, 2015.
28. An, D.; Deng, H.; Shen, C.; Xu, Y.; Zhong, L.; Deng, Y. Evaluation of Virtual Reality Application in Construction Teaching: A Comparative Study of Undergraduates. *Appl. Sci.* **2023**, *13*, 6170. [CrossRef]
29. Şahbaz, E. SimYA: A Virtual Reality–Based Construction Studio Simulator. *Int. J. Archit. Comput.* **2022**, *20*, 334–345. [CrossRef]

virtual worlds

MDPI

Article

Readers Theater in Desktop VR: A Pilot Study with Grade Nine Students

Linda Peschke [1,*], Anna Kiani [2,*], Ute Massler [2] and Wolfgang Müller [1]

1 Department of Media and Education Management, University of Education Weingarten, 88250 Weingarten, Germany; muellerw@ph-weingarten.de
2 English Department, University of Education Weingarten, 88250 Weingarten, Germany; massler@ph-weingarten.de
* Correspondence: linda.peschke@stud.ph-weingarten.de (L.P.); anna.kiani@stud.ph-weingarten.de (A.K.)

Abstract: Appropriate techniques for promoting reading fluency are difficult to implement in the classroom. There is little time to provide students with individualized feedback on reading aloud or to motivate them to do so. In this context, Virtual Reality (VR) can be beneficial for learning because it allows for individualized feedback and for increasing learner engagement. Studies that analyze established methods of language learning in VR at school are thus far lacking. Therefore, this pilot study is one of the first to analyze student acceptance of reading fluency training in desktop VR at a secondary school. The interview guide was developed in accordance with the Technology Acceptance Model. The desktop VR environment is web-based and provides individual and collaborative opportunities for training reading fluency, giving, and receiving feedback, and deepening content understanding of reading texts. To analyze the acceptance of the desktop VR environment, five guided interviews were conducted. The results reveal that despite various technical challenges within the VR environment, students not only accepted but also appreciated the reading fluency training in VR. The integration of established concepts of reading fluency training in foreign language classrooms has great potential as an additional value in addressing the challenges of face-to-face instruction.

Keywords: virtual reality; reading fluency training; language learning; acceptance; students; secondary school

Citation: Peschke, L.; Kiani, A.; Massler, U.; Müller, W. Readers Theater in Desktop VR: A Pilot Study with Grade Nine Students. *Virtual Worlds* **2023**, *2*, 267–289. https://doi.org/10.3390/virtualworlds2030016

Academic Editors: Radu Comes, Dorin-Mircea Popovici, Calin Gheorghe Dan Neamtu and Jing-Jing Fang

Received: 13 July 2023
Revised: 31 August 2023
Accepted: 4 September 2023
Published: 8 September 2023

1. Introduction

In the past, reading aloud was commonly employed in first language (L1) and second language (L2) learning to train reading fluency with reference to the skill of reading accurately, in a meaningful way, and with appropriate expression. Reading fluency training has gained popularity in L1 education after studies have made it evident that reading competence in L1 is closely linked to reading fluency [1]. While such research findings are limited, evidence suggests that reading fluency is also important for L2 learners [2,3].

Repeated reading of a text, assisted reading, and model reading have been proven to positively affect reading fluency [1]. However, these techniques require substantial amounts of time and resources. In addition, appropriate reading fluency instruction can hardly be met in school settings, as teachers already face a number of challenges such as the growing heterogeneity among their student bodies [4]. Subsequently, there is little to no time for each student to read aloud and receive sufficient feedback from the teacher. Additionally, motivating students to read aloud frequently proves difficult due to the perceived monotony of reading aloud activities [5]. Therefore, reading fluency training needs to be developed further by individualizing the learning process and student support, as well as making it more appealing. Moreover, training should reach beyond scholarly settings, giving students the chance to practice at home and allowing for "seamless learning" [6] (p. 98).

The overall objective of this project is, therefore, to evaluate student acceptance of a technology-based learning activity based on Virtual Reality (VR) and corresponding learning environments. The principle learning design draws from the Multilingual Readers' Theater (MELT), in which groups of students practice reading fluency using multilingual, dialogical texts until they are able to read them aloud fluently and expressively, and then perform them in plenum. The readers' theater (RT) is one of the reading-aloud methods that is able to achieve significant improvement in the area of reading fluency with regard to correct word recognition, reading speed, and prosody, while also significantly increasing young learners' motivation to read [7,8]. MELT and RT are based on cooperative role-playing, narrative approaches that provide an excellent starting point for research in the development of cooperative, VR-based methods for fostering foreign language learning.

The development of a digital system that is based on the previous approaches, MELT and RT, promises increased efficiency, easier structuring of the learning process, online collaboration, seamless learning at home and at school, and a more satisfying user experience for digital natives. Adding VR to MELT aims to provide students with a realistic and motivating learning experience that allows for flexible collaboration options. Using this backdrop, the specific objective of the project is to address the question: To what extent do students accept the use of MELT in the foreign language classroom in a VR environment? Furthermore, what are the specific internal (e.g., student motivation) and external factors (e.g., the design and features of the VR learning environment) that may influence student acceptance of VR applications in the foreign language classroom? Subsequently, what are the potential problems of VR application in MELT that need to be worked out? The research questions that guide this research are thus:

1. What internal and external factors influence a given student's intentions to use and accept VR in the context of MELT?
2. To what extent do students accept the performance of the reading fluency training phase of MELT in a VR application?
3. To what extent does VR have the potential to be used in foreign language classrooms to complement MELT?

This paper is organized as follows. First, related work is presented, with a specific focus on reading fluency and related technology-based approaches, such as the Technology Acceptance Model, and the application of VR in school-related learning scenarios in language learning. Second, the VR conception and design are described, followed by the study methodology. Third, the results are discussed; the research questions are addressed; and the conclusions are drawn. Lastly, the implications for the future design of VR applications in foreign language teaching are presented.

2. Related Work

2.1. Reading Fluency

Reading fluency (RF), a central factor in literacy, requires the mastery of accuracy, automaticity, and prosody [9]. Strategies that have a high potential for training RF are repeated reading and assisted reading [10]. Repeated reading of a text is used to strengthen automaticity in word recognition so that a reader's cognitive resources can be used for comprehension rather than the decoding of individual words [11]. Assisted reading refers to the "oral reading of a text while simultaneously listening to a fluent rendering of the same text" [12] (p. 514) which can be performed by a partner, a group choral reading, or an audio recording. Practicing assisted reading speeds up the learning progress, especially for text comprehension [12]. In combination with repeated reading, assisted repeated reading benefits reading speed, word recognition, as well as overall comprehension [13].

Even though RF is a central skill for educational, occupational, and societal success, it is rarely explicitly tackled in classroom settings, which is likely the result of method limitations. Most reading interventions require extensive amounts of time and human resources, both of which are scarce due to the growing heterogeneity of learner needs in the classroom, among other difficulties [4,14]. Further, weak readers are not able to improve their reading by practicing solely in school [15]. In addition, assisted and repeated reading require the monotonous task of reading the same text multiple times, which commonly lowers student motivation and prevents them from staying engaged for longer periods of time. These challenges cause the use of such interventions to fall short of their full potential [5].

2.2. Readers Theater

RT embeds repeated and assisted reading in a meaningful and motivational context because this method focuses on practicing a script that will eventually be performed in front of an audience [16]. "Readers Theatre, as well as other kinds of performance, gives students an authentic reason to engage in repeated reading of texts", Worthy and Prater [17] (p. 295) note. Moreso, this method focuses on meaning and comprehension instead of reading rate [16,17]. Rather than stereotypical theater, the use of props, costumes, and stage settings are rare in readers theater. Consequently, actors convey meaning by using appropriate intonation, rate, and accentuation [16,18]. Instead of text memorization, performers read from scripts. This shifts the purpose from memorization towards decoding words and adding them to the reader's visual vocabulary [19]. Additionally, readers can focus on precise and expressive oral reading, thus practicing prosody.

While traditional RT is constructed monolingually, its multilingual version allows practicing RF in several languages at the same time. MELT recognizes multilingualism in heterogeneous classrooms, allowing the inclusion of school language, foreign languages, and students' native tongues [19]. Furthermore, this method is able to provide a cooperative learning setting in which student heterogeneity is seen as a resource. In this setting, students with stronger reading skills support those with weaker skills by acting as reading models who also provide feedback [19]. Kutzelmann et al. [20] have created an eight-phase plan to guide teachers through the implementation of MELT in their classrooms (see Figure 1).

Teaching–Learning Process	*Social form*	*Approx. time*
1. Teacher introduces Multilingual Readers' Theatre	PL	15-20
2. Teacher reads book passages aloud	PL	5-10
3. Pupils read script scenes and are assigned roles	IW/GW	10-15
4. Pupils summarize content of their scenes	GW	15-25
5. Pupils introduce scenes and individual roles	PL	15-25
6. Pupils practice roles and provide mutual feedback	PW	20-45
7. General rehearsal and feedback	GW	20-45
8. Final performance	PL	25-45

Figure 1. Eight–phase MELT structure [20].

In addition to training RF in multiple languages, MELT has the potential to positively impact other areas of foreign language learning, such as listening comprehension, pronunciation, and vocabulary training [19]. The method further aims to promote social learning and reduce fear associated with speaking foreign languages simply because MELT's means of practice depends on group interaction. One study documents a high acceptance of this design on the part of the teachers and learners [19]. Teachers have also acknowledged its potential in terms of promoting RF, second language learning, and beyond. However, a comprehensive quantitative evaluation is still pending [19].

2.3. Digital Technologies and Reading Fluency Training

Digital approaches specifically targeted at the enhancement of RF used to be scarce. The Peabody Literacy Lab [21], a technology-based intervention for older school children, consists of a reading lab, a word lab, and a spelling lab. Instructions and feedback are provided by an animated tutor. Compared to a control group, the system was found to significantly foster auditory vocabulary, literal comprehension, inferential comprehension, and total reading comprehension.

Automatic speech recognition (ASR) was employed by Adams [22] and Mostow et al. [23]. In both cases, a Reading Assistant [22] or Reading Tutor [23] listens to a student reading aloud and provides feedback. Mostow's ASR provides feedback and gives supporting functions. Reading skills of students whose first language is English and also of students learning English as a second language [24] were improved in proof-of-concept studies. Adam's system additionally creates performance reports to assist teachers in monitoring student growth. In a 17-week study of grade 2–5 classrooms, she found that students using the Reading Assistant showed significantly greater gains in RF than students in the control group.

One study combined podcasting technology with traditional RT [25]. During a ten-week intervention, students practiced a new theater script each week that was then recorded and published online as podcasts. Results showed that publishing podcasts online not only increased the authenticity of the RT for the students, but also allowed them to self-evaluate, revise, and improve their reading performance.

Furthermore, RF training has also been enhanced with digital tools related to gamification [26,27]. For instance, GameLet implements meaningful digital media-based gamification mechanisms for the purpose of increasing pupil motivation in self-directed, individual, and cooperative learning in RF training [28].

Until recently, the few technology-based approaches used to complement classroom activities linked to RT assessments and feedback were limited to the evaluation of multiple-choice tests. More comprehensive approaches to automatic assessment, e.g., meaningful feedback, were largely lacking. However, in March 2023, Klett Publishing House launched the new reading tutor LaLeTu, which measures and promotes reading fluency with the help of AI [29]. According to information on the publisher's website, speech technology records and evaluates student reading samples in terms of reading speed, sentence stress, and reading errors. Allegedly, AI recognizes reading errors, long pauses, and incorrect intonations. It also has the capacity to recognize dialects and accents. With this technology, learners receive feedback while the teacher obtains an individualized analysis of reading performance. A playful reward system for reading motivation rounds off the offer. However, no studies have been published yet.

2.4. *VR and Learning*

For some time now, VR has been considered a strong contender in the world of learning technology. VR technologies are attributed to a high potential for generating added value in the context of learning applications. Studies have shown the positive effects of VR on learning [30]. The chances of improving teaching/learning processes through the use of VR are derived, among other things, from the high degree of immersion [31] that is achieved with these techniques, which can also address learners on an emotional level. The teaching/learning and the experienced environments merge, thus allowing learners to become immersed in the learning experience. At the same time, VR offers additional opportunities for interaction with the potential to improve individualization and flexibility of learning processes and strengthen cooperation between learners. Both aspects can be expected to provide strong arguments for initiating more successful and sustainable teaching/learning processes.

Although VR is still a relatively new technology in foreign language learning, it has been applied to this domain [32–34] mostly in the context of vocabulary learning and communicative processes training, which also fosters communicative skills. However, to our knowledge, applications at the school level that focus on training RF in a second language, do not exist. Nevertheless, two studies that used VR as a means to assess reading fluency have been carried out. In one recent study, Mirlaut et al. used VR glasses to assess beginner reading behavior and to measure their RF with the One-Minute Reading test [35]. While this study focused on native speakers, it showed that VR could be used as a legitimate tool for studying reading behavior in general terms [35]. As part of a master's thesis, the impact of reading in VR on a group of dyslexic student's reading fluency was explored [36]. The outcome of the study suggests that reading in VR may positively affect dyslexic readers, because it allows for the adjustment of fonts, text size, words per line, etc.

In general, applications of VR in school settings appear to be first and foremost linked to leveraging motivational aspects [37]. More comprehensive conceptualizations of learning scenarios linked to established methods in language learning at school and approaches for integrating classroom teaching with appropriate virtual learning methods appear to be missing thus far.

2.5. *Technology-Acceptance Model*

The perception of technologies can impact how these will be used in specific environments [38]. In this context, Davis et al. [39] developed the Technology-Acceptance Model (TAM) that was specifically designed to determine user acceptance of a specific type of technology—in this study: a VR application. According to Davis et al. [39], there are two key factors that could influence user attitudes and intentions to use a technology (see Figure 2): perceived ease of use and perceived usefulness. Perceived usefulness refers to whether users attribute added value to the technology, e.g., making training in reading fluency easier or more entertaining. Perceived ease of use is defined as the estimated effort that is required to use a specific technology. Since perceived ease of use and perceived usefulness are indicated as the most important factors influencing technology acceptance, they also play a central role in the context of this research.

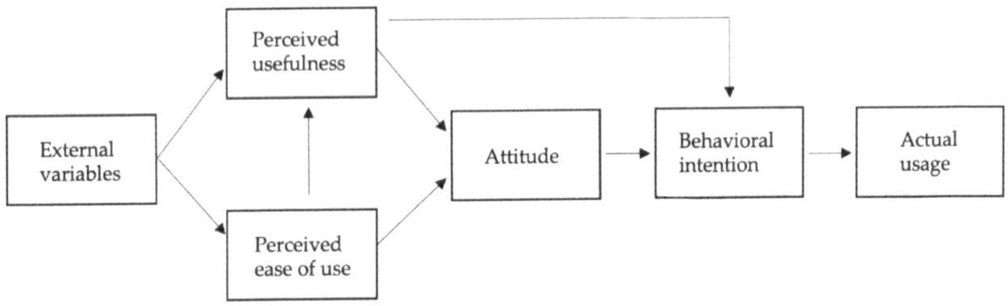

Figure 2. Technology-Acceptance Model (TAM) (our own illustration, based on Davis et al. [39]).

According to the model, the behavior of an individual is determined by their behavioral intention to use a specific technology. The behavioral intention to use a technology sheds light on a person's intentions to use it in the future [39]. Accordingly, users are more likely to accept applications that they find useful and are easier to use than those with little added value and complicated applications [40]. In the meantime, TAM has been used in a number of studies to examine attitudes towards new technologies [41]).

3. Concept and Design

3.1. *Learning Objectives*

The objectives behind the learning activities are, on the one hand, important for the development and promotion of good RF. On the other hand, these objectives were developed according to the general limitations and challenges of MELT, e.g., growing heterogeneity in classrooms [4], time restrictions for teacher feedback, and low motivation for reading aloud activities [28]. Therefore, with the implementation of MELT in a desktop VR school environment we hoped to develop the following: engaging, motivating reading tasks; personalized and intensified individual RF training and feedback options; and flexible collaboration opportunities for MELT in time and space. Based on these, the overarching learning objective for the desktop VR training session is for students to improve their RF by practicing reading scripts in a small group within the desktop VR environment. This is achieved by the following sub-learning objective in which students:

1. use the desktop VR environment to communicate and cooperate effectively with learning partners;

2. give and receive feedback on their performance of the text;
3. move through the desktop VR environment and interact appropriately with its features in order to improve their RF;
4. gain a deepened understanding of the story and its characters by interacting with props and images provided in the desktop VR environment.

3.2. Learning Scenario

Based on the learning objectives described in the previous chapter, the learning scenario of the desktop VR environment was developed.

3.2.1. Sub-Scenario of MELT Phases

For the implementation of the MELT concept in desktop VR, specific phases were chosen from the RF training concept. Based on the challenges of collaborative practice that occur in the classroom, e.g., limited spatial capacities at schools, certain phases of the collaborative RF training of MELT in particular were implemented in the desktop VR training phase and taken into account accordingly in the design of the desktop VR environment. This was conducted in an effort to address the challenges of traditional classroom instruction and to explore alternative design options for conducting MELT in VR. Thus, the focus was on the phase of collaborative RF training in various small groups of 3–4 students (n = 7). This correlated with phase 6 of the eight phases of MELT, as introduced by Kutzelmann et al. [20] (see Figure 1).

3.2.2. Desktop VR Concept (Implementation of MELT in Desktop VR)

To address the challenges of RF training in a classroom setting as described in the previous chapter, the desktop VR environment is based on the development of various virtual classroom types. For this purpose, a VR school environment was designed to consist of three large classrooms (see Figure 3a) and five small breakout rooms (see Figure 3b).

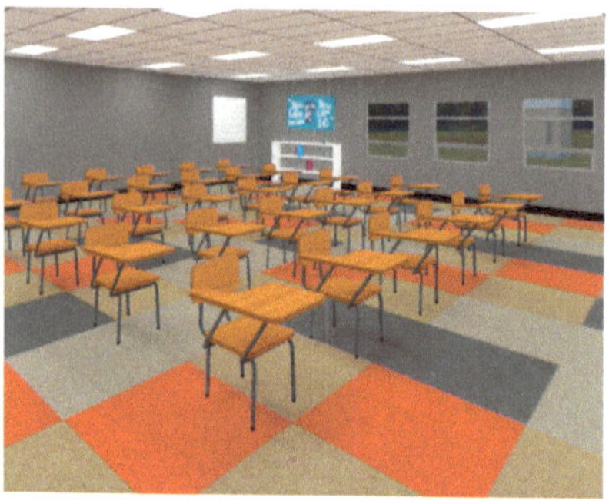

(a)

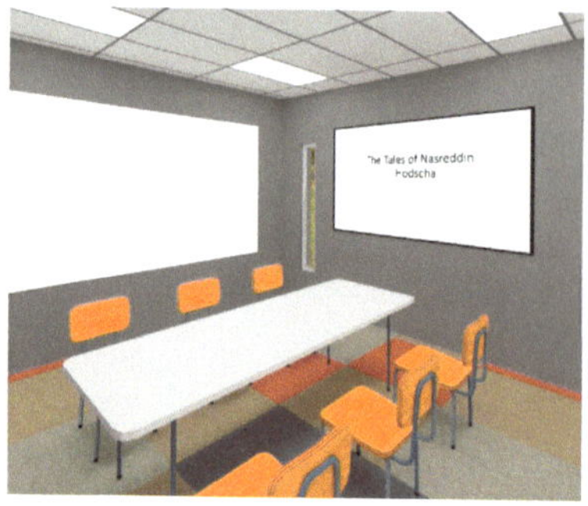

(b)

Figure 3. Available rooms in the desktop VR school environment: (**a**) Example for one of the three large classrooms; (**b**) Example for one of the five small breakout rooms.

In general, all of the eight VR rooms should be used for collaborative reading fluency training, i.e., MELT script out loud reading and giving others feedback. The collaborative reading training could take place both in tandem and in small groups (with three to four students per group). In addition, the VR school environment also provides ample space to conduct individual practice periods in which each student practices the MELT script on their own. However, since this was not the focus of this study project, this aspect will not be addressed.

In addition to the overarching goal of collaborative reading training, the learners were given additional tasks in two of the larger classrooms and the smaller group rooms.

The main purpose of the two larger classrooms was to create a space where the whole class, or in this case the study participants and the teacher, could come together for two different reasons. First, to acquire specific instructions from the teacher about the RF exercises that will be carried out, i.e., the task to be completed, time to complete the task, and group composition. Second, students should gather into their respective groups, determine reading roles, choose, and familiarize themselves with an individual avatar.

In the third large classroom, student groups present their scene to one another and receive feedback from the teacher and classmates. This means that both a final rehearsal and a performance of the MELT script are to be carried out in this classroom.

The small group work rooms were also designed to enable collaborative practice in small groups. Since these small rooms can only be entered via a link that opens a new browser window, these serve primarily for undisturbed reading training space. This degree of privacy should also be used by teachers to give groups individual feedback about their RF performance in an unthreatening atmosphere.

3.2.3. Desktop VR Design

For the development of the desktop VR learning environment, a VR school model was used that had already been made publicly available by the selected VR software, Hubs by Mozilla. This model already represented a school environment with a total of eight different classrooms. To adapt the model to the specific needs of conducting MELT in desktop VR, some modifications were made based on the one developed by Hubs. Some of the tables and chairs were removed from the large classrooms while a stage and partition wall were integrated, and avatars, shelves with props, and the MELT theater script were added. The links to both environments can be found in the supplementary materials.

The following describes how the individual rooms were designed, based on the tasks and functions that should take place in the individual rooms.

Practicing reading aloud cooperatively: In order to enable cooperative reading training in the rooms and to offer the students a wide range of cooperation opportunities, all rooms were equipped with chairs and tables analogous to real classrooms. However, these were arranged differently, making it possible to be used for different reading tasks. One of the large classrooms was furnished with free-standing chairs that had a foldable backrest, while the other one had various group tables. In both large classrooms, a free area without chairs and tables was set up for free use in the front area. A stage was integrated into the third large classroom for the purpose of conducting final rehearsals and reading performances with the entire class. Hence, the chairs in this room were arranged in rows staggered upwards, which are analogous to a lecture hall or theater hall, thus allowing all students to have a good view of the stage.

The five smaller classrooms, on the other hand, were set up identically. The reason here is to create a pleasant discussion atmosphere for feedback and at the same time offer space for collaborative practice in smaller student groups. Finally, a small meeting table with six chairs was integrated into all of the five small VR group rooms.

To support collaborative reading, the RT scripts were directly integrated as digital versions into all of the eight classrooms. On the one hand, the MELT scripts were first uploaded to each classroom in advance by the study instructors and pinned on the available media walls (see Figure 4a). Secondly, each student was given the option of viewing the RT scripts as cue cards (see Figure 4b) which they "carried" with them through the environment as they moved their avatars. This provided students with flexible and space-independent reading training.

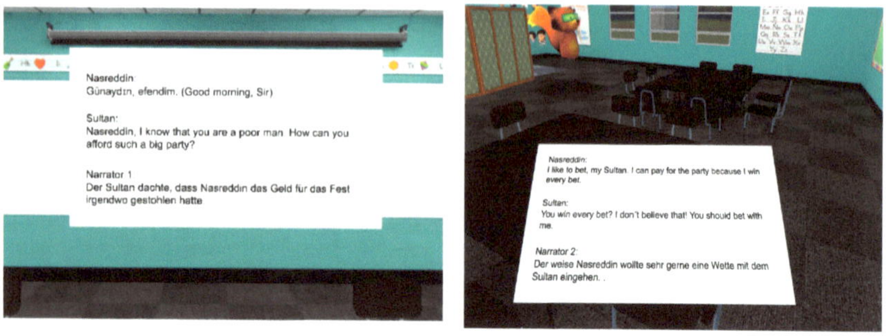

Figure 4. Versions of digital MELT scripts in the desktop VR environment: (**a**) Example of uploaded VR script on media wall; (**b**) Example of MELT script on individual cue cards.

In addition, audio zones were set up for all of the rooms so that students could hear only each other within the same room. The closer students placed their avatars towards each other, the louder their voices became. This provided enough space for individuals and groups to practice at the same time, which was designed with individual student needs in mind. Additionally, the feature allows for the receiving and giving of feedback in a private and non-threatening atmosphere.

Support further understanding of story and characters in the MELT script: To improve the overall prosodic composition of student reading, it is necessary to have a literary understanding of the MELT scripts [28]. For this reason, various props in the form of 3D objects (see Figure 5a) were integrated into the desktop VR environment in order to visualize central elements. Students could use these during cooperative reading sessions in order to highlight the content of their script, to give more expression to their own role, or the content of the readers' theater. Furthermore, posters were also integrated into the environment that illustrated central elements, characters, and contents of the RT (see Figure 5b).

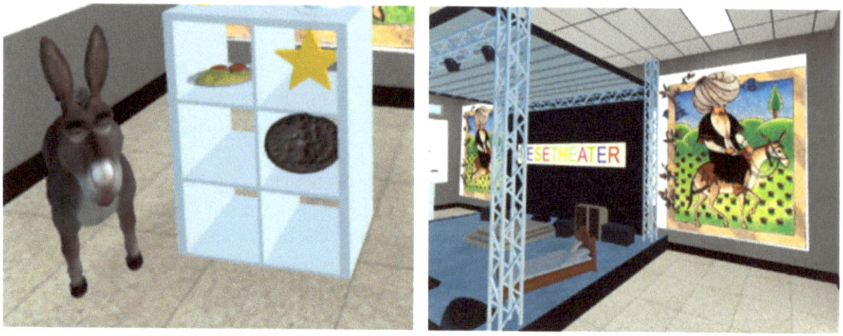

Figure 5. Elements supporting the further understanding of story and characters: (**a**) Example of a 3D object that appears in the MELT script; (**b**) Example of a poster that shows the main character of the MELT script.

To support engagement with their roles and characters, students were allowed to choose a personal avatar. In addition to an internal collection of avatars provided in Mozilla Hubs (see Figure 6a), additional and pre-designed avatars were provided directly in the desktop VR environment (see Figure 6b). These were specifically designed to reflect the roles and content of the underlying MELT scenario. In order to spatially delimit the choice of an avatar from the reading training area, the back of one of the large classrooms. A mirror wall was also integrated into this area, which should enable the students to look at the avatars and become familiar with them since the field of view of the students represents a first perspective.

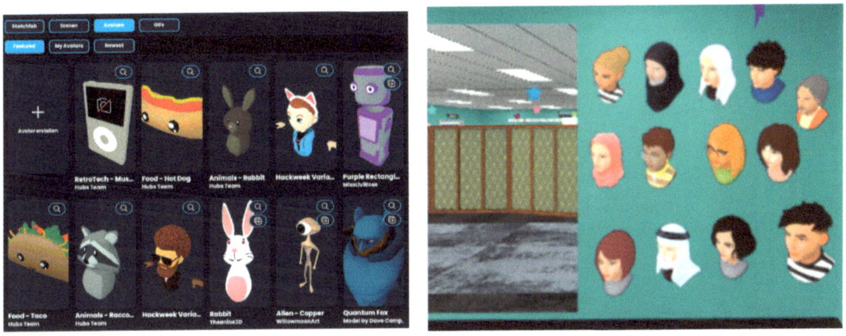

(**a**) (**b**)

Figure 6. Avatars supporting the further understanding of the characters: (**a**) Mozilla Hubs internal avatar collection; (**b**) Pre-designed avatars uploaded directly into the VR environment.

Asking for, giving, and receiving feedback: Due to the use of an avatar eliminating nonverbal behavior, such as e facial expressions and gestures, it is also important in VR that the students receive feedback on their expression and intonation while reading. To provide such feedback to each other, both auditory and visual options were made available in the desktop VR environment. Students could comment on how a classmate read aloud using two features that are provided in Mozilla Hubs. Students can either select an emoji from a dropdown menu or use a chat function. In addition, there was also the possibility of giving more detailed oral feedback. The smaller rooms were specifically designed for this purpose by offering a more private and unthreatening space than the large classrooms. This trains the perception of fluent reading and supports reading development.

Originally, the head of the study should have joined the VR environment by means of an iPad and avatar in order to coach students during the exercises (e.g., by giving feedback). However, this plan could not be realized due to technical problems.

3.2.4. Interaction Design

Since the students already use iPads in their everyday school life, this technology was selected for the study project in order not to overwhelm them with unfamiliar technology and VR software. In the following, the interaction design is described in relation to the use of the VR software on an iPad. The complete operation of the VR software was carried out using various tapping and swiping commands.

Avatar selection: By tapping once on the respective avatar, a button with the command "Choose an avatar" appears. By simply touching this button, the avatar could be selected and then automatically change its appearance.

Avatar navigation: The avatar could be moved forward by zooming in on the appropriate spot with two fingers. Backward movement is achieved by zooming out with two fingers. Swiping left or right rotated the avatar in those directions. Simultaneous movement and rotation could be performed using on-screen joysticks. With the help of these commands, one's own avatar could be moved through all rooms.

Seat avatar: To place the avatar on a chair, two fingers should tap simultaneously on the iPad screen and then select a chair.

Use of cue cards: Cue cards with the MELT text could be displayed by tapping the screen with two fingers and then selecting the magnifying glass icon. The entire MELT text was divided into different index card pages. Three roles were displayed on each index card page. After reading these, students need to manually switch to the next page of cue cards. This could be displayed by tapping the index card once. An arrow menu (left arrow (back one page) and right arrow (next page)) was then displayed, allowing students to navigate to the next cue card page by tapping on the desired arrow.

Prop usage: Props could be controlled by using a custom object menu that appears when tapping on an object. To rotate an object, the rotate icon is tapped while simultaneously specifying the direction by means of finger movement. Following the same principle, an object could be enlarged by holding the zoom-in icon and either moving the finger away from the object (zooming) or towards the object (zoom-out). While holding the object with a finger, it can be freely moved through the VR environment and shifted from one room to another.

4. Methodology

4.1. Study Design

The study was inspired by the idea of a design or feasibility study. The main purpose of the study was to conduct an initial assessment of applying MELT to the VR context. This evaluation could then serve as a basis for determining its potential applicability across different levels of the SAMR framework. It should be noted that while this study has predominantly addressed the substitution level and allowed for potential application at the augmentation level, it could also provide insights for further research, thus extending the implementation of MELT in desktop VR to the modification level and beyond.

The objective of this study was to investigate the acceptance and potential of MELT—a RF training format when performed by students in a desktop VR application. From this, design recommendations for future use of VR in the context of MELT should be derived. In this context, requirement surveys were conducted to analyze the challenges of traditional face-to-face instruction in foreign language classes, as well as the limitations of implementing MELT in the classroom. It was found that in implementing MELT in the classroom, and in particular, collaborative RF training in student groups, difficulties arose due to space limitations in schools and classrooms. For this reason, digital supplements are needed for flexible learning and facilitating the implementation of RF training, as well as collaborative RF practice. In particular, the study focused on testing collaborative RF training in various small groups (with three to four students each) (see Chapter 3.2).

The general approach was to ensure that the study design was as realistic as possible. It was therefore necessary to carry out the study design and collect data in a real school with real users, i.e., students and teachers. Moreover, the desktop VR study was carried out in the context of a MELT intervention in a real school. This means that the MELT concept was first explained to the students in the classroom. In this way, they became acquainted with and tried out all phases of MELT in a physical classroom setting. The collaborative RF training was the only phase carried out with a subset of the students in the VR environment. In addition, the study design relied on iPads, a technology that was already in use at the study school. The advantage was that the students were already familiar with this tool, thus making it easier for the students to participate in the study. Since the VR software was freely accessible via the Internet and did not have to be paid for separately, or installed on the iPads, it was possible to create highly realistic study conditions. As access to the environment is not location-bound, there is the possibility of including other schools, either nationally and/or internationally, in the training sessions, hence adding further potential for collaboration.

4.2. Subjects and Procedure

The study was conducted at a Secondary school in Ravensburg (Germany). Both the students and their parents were informed of the research project in advance. In order to participate in the interviews, a written declaration of consent was signed by both the parents and students. However, the students could independently decide whether to participate in the study or not.

The sample consisted of students (n = 28) in a bilingual English class in grade nine; the mean age was 14 years. Because the students had no prior experience with MELT, the study and data collection were preceded by two hours of classroom training (e.g., 90 min each) in order to introduce the students to the method. The two training sessions were, however, used solely for introductory reasons and were therefore not analyzed empirically. In total, the study consisted of two phases that built on each other (see Figure 7).

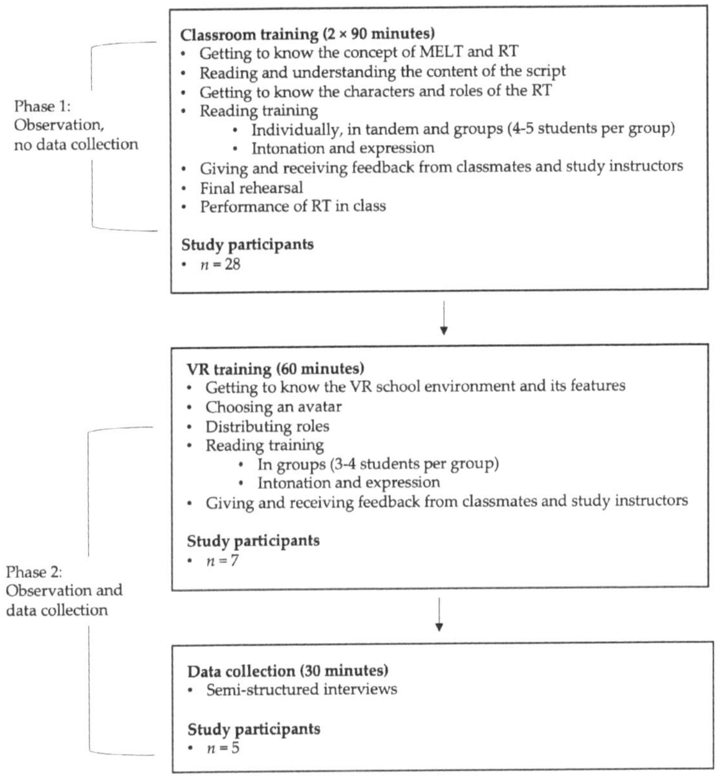

Figure 7. Study procedure (own illustration).

The study started with two synchronous classroom training sessions, based on the eight phases of MELT as introduced by Kutzelmann et al. [20]. Due to the limited time available, each phase was shortened to fit the timeframe of 90 min per session. The classroom training was conducted with the following learning objectives in mind:

1. Know the general concept of MELT;
2. Know and understand the story and characters in the MELT script (writing a table of consent);
3. Understand and learn the vocabulary used in the MELT script;
4. Practice reading the role aloud with others (e.g., intonation, emotions, etc.);
5. Give and receive feedback on group members' reading-aloud production.

The classroom training sessions took place in the students' classroom five and seven days before the VR study. All students attended these sessions during those two days. An overview of the contents addressed in classroom training can be found in Figure 7.

Following the classroom training sessions, those students who had completed the required declaration of consent (n = 7) participated in a synchronous desktop VR training session (60 min). First, as a group, all students were shown the desktop VR environment and its general functions (audio, chat, navigation, etc.) in the classroom (five minutes). However, the study itself took place in a different building where the school computer room was located. For this purpose, the students who were accompanied by the two study directors, changed buildings after the joint introduction in the classroom. There, the students were given the task of acquainting themselves independently with the VR environment by exploring its spaces and getting a feel for how to use and navigate it by means of an avatar (15 min). During the phase, each student was assigned an iPad (tablet).

After the self-exploration phase, students met in small groups to perform reading training, i.e., acting out or reading aloud one of the scenes of the MELT play. For the VR training session, only one phase of MELT was applied: the collaborative RF training. The previous phases (i.e., getting to know the play) had already been covered in the classroom training, at which time, they chose an appropriate avatar and met with their group which consisted of three to four students. The students were then given time to decide on which practice room to choose, and whether and how to integrate props into their reading training. Subsequent phases of MELT (such as the performance of the MELT script) could not be realized due to time constraints.

While students were engaging in the desktop VR activities, two study directors observed and noted their actions with guided, structured observation notes aimed at identifying aspects concerning RF, repetition, motivation, collaboration, and communication within the reading groups (see Chapter 5.2). After the activities were completed, some students ($n = 5$) were asked to provide additional qualitative feedback. One of the study directors conducted semi-structured interviews with five students that elicited the extent to which these students accepted the implementation of MELT in the desktop VR school environment and their reasons.

4.3. *Investigation Tools*

4.3.1. VR Software

There are various software applications that could be used to create VR environments for specific learning scenarios [42]. In the context of this study, we used the Mozilla Hubs platform [43], which features the creation and usage of virtual 3D rooms to facilitate various communication scenarios, in educational contexts. Mozilla Hubs is a web-based application that works on a browser and supports many devices. It can be used for a fully immersive experience with head-mounted displays, as well as for 2D web browser applications (e.g., desktop, laptop, smartphone, or tablet). The Mozilla Hubs rooms are private. Participants can enter a specific room by clicking on a web link generated by the room creator. The advantage of Mozilla Hubs is that it does not require further software installation. This particular ease of use was one of the reasons why we chose this application [44]. In addition, we selected Mozilla Hubs because of its free usage option for up to 10 users at a time, addressing concerns and risks of using VR in an educational context or class [45]. The restriction to 10 simultaneously active users did not represent a limitation in the context of the study, as training sessions with individual Reading Theatre Learning groups consisted of fewer students. It should be noted, however, that a regular implementation in class with possibly several parallel exercise groups therefore may require a modified solution with regard to the VR system to be used, but also possibly more comprehensive didactic measures that enable sufficient coaching of the different groups. Users are represented as avatars that they can choose from a large selection of pre-generated avatars. It is also possible for users to create an avatar with 3D modeling tools such as Blender. Further Mozilla Hubs features include display and media sharing (e.g., PDFs, images, videos, audios, 3D models, etc.), voice and text chat, and live reactions via emojis, among others.

4.3.2. Observation Notes

Observation notes were taken during the desktop VR training session by the two researchers who sat in the room with the participants. For a systematic recording of observations and subsequent comparability between the different observers, an observation protocol was developed with the following categories (see Appendix A): reading repetitions, reading of the RT script, design of the practice phases, communication within the groups, avatar and props, avatar movement and navigation, technique, and other notes/observations.

4.3.3. Construction Interview Questionnaire

In addition to the observation notes and to answer the research questions, additional, semi-structured interviews with the students were conducted that directly followed the desktop VR exercise phase. Overall, the interview guide was divided into four parts: (1) demographic information, (2) acceptance of the desktop VR RT (perceived ease of use and perceived usefulness), (3) effects of the desktop VR RT (joy, motivation, first impression) and (4) behavioral intention to use the desktop VR RT. The first part served to collect demographic information (1), consisting of a total of four questions about the students' media consumption (*"What technical devices do you own?"*, *"How and for what purpose do you use media in your everyday life/at school?"*) and previous experiences using VR applications (*"What has your experience with VR applications been like?"*).

Interview section two analyzed student acceptance of the VR school environment (2) and the implementation of the RT in this environment. While the questions were based on Davis et al. [39] original Technology Acceptance Model questionnaire, their content was adapted to the specific format of the RT in the VR school environment and translated into German. As postulated by Davis et al. [39], student acceptance was therefore divided into perceived ease of use and perceived usefulness. The six questions about perceived usefulness were primarily related to the practice phase, reading tasks, and or the use of an avatar during the performance of the RT in the VR environment (*"What did you like/dislike about the VR practice phase?"*, *"What did you like/dislike about the VR practice phase compared to face-to-face practice?"*, *"How did you feel about performing the reading practice tasks in VR?"*, *"What was easier/harder about performing the reading exercise in VR than in presence?"*, *"What did you find helpful/disruptive about the VR environment in order to complete the exercise?"*, *"How did you feel about being able to step into your role in the play with an avatar?"*).

The four questions on perceived ease of use focused primarily on the VR school environment and how students interact with it ("What did you like/dislike about the VR school environment?", "What did you like/dislike about the VR environment compared to face-to-face practice?", "How did you get along with the VR school environment?", "Were there any (technical) problems during the reading exercise in the VR school environment, if so—which ones?").

The third part of the questionnaire was related to what effects (3), e.g., general impression or joy, the implementation of the RT in the VR school environment had on the students (*"What was your first impression of the VR environment or practice phase?"*, *"How much did you enjoy today's practice period in VR compared to the practice period face-to-face?"*, *"Did you feel more like practicing the play in the VR environment than in presence? Why?"*).

The last interview section was to delve deeper into the reasons why students enjoyed using VR at school/in foreign language classes/in relation to RT, or not (4) in the future (*"What do you think are the advantages/disadvantages of performing a reader's theater in VR compared to being present?"*, *"Would you like to use more VR applications in school/foreign language class/in relation to RT in the future? And why?"*).

4.4. *Methodology of Data Evaluation*

4.4.1. Evaluation Procedure Observation Protocol

The observation protocol was completed individually by the two study directors following the desktop VR training session. Subsequently, the two observation protocols were compared in order to identify similarities or differences in the observations. The subsequent qualitative evaluation was carried out according to the previously discussed observation criteria.

4.4.2. Evaluation Procedure Interview Questionnaire

The interviews were subsequently evaluated by means of a qualitative content analysis in accordance with Mayring and Fenzl [46]. For this purpose, an iterative process was used to create a coding guide in the form of a category system with the following characteristics: main category, subcategory, definition of the category, and anchor example from the interview materials (see Table 1). The categories were formed both deductively along previous research findings and theories in the literature and inductively from the existing data material. The entire data material from the five interviews was analyzed with the help of this category system. Individual interview passages were assigned to the various categories in several iteration loops until a suitable category was found for all interview statements.

Table 1. Excerpt from the coding guide.

Main-Category	Sub-Category	Definition	Anchor Example
Effects of the VR RT	First impression of VR environment	In this category, study participants report on their first impression of the VR environment.	"I thought it was really good." (I. 1).
	Sense of fun and motivation	This category includes statements that relate to anything the study participants say about their motivation and enjoyment in using the VR environment or performing Reader's Theater in the VR environment.	"So it was even more fun." (I. 5).
Perceived Usefulness	Choice of an avatar	This category includes statements in which students comment on the choice and use of avatars in the VR environment.	"I just wanted it to fit my role a little bit. And because there were so many options to choose from, it was also good." (I. 3).
	Expression of emotions	This category includes statements related to the expression and perception of emotions when performing RT in VR.	"Disadvantage is just clear that you cannot hear these emotions and so good out." (I. 5).

5. Results

5.1. Description of the Sample

A total of n = 7 students participated in the desktop VR training session. Their behaviors were included in the observation protocols. Of these, four participants were female, and three participants were male. Only five of these students (four female and one male participant) participated in the interviews that are referred to in the following sample description. The average age at the time of the interviews was 14 years.

Use of technical devices in everyday life: With regards to the use of media in everyday life, it was found that participants use cell phones (n = 5), laptops (n = 3), tablets (e.g., family tablet) (n = 2), PC (n = 1) and TV (n = 1).

Use of technical devices in school: Three of the participants stated that they use their iPads at school.

Estimated duration of technical devices used per day: In terms of daily cell phone use, n = 2 students reported a daily duration of approximately two hours, n = 1 two to three hours, and n = 1 three hours. One student emphasized that her daily cell phone use had a fixed limit. In terms of daily iPad use at school, n = 2 students spoke of needing and using it for most of the school day. One study participant indicated that iPad use varied by subject, which approximated one to two hours per day. Overall, $n = 2$ of the students estimated their daily media use to be about three to four hours.

Previous experience with VR and VR environments: All participants ($n = 5$) reported having prior experience with various VR applications. While one student claimed never having been in a VR environment, 3 students named a school project that involved a VR art exhibit. One student talked about having used VR outside of school, two to three times at a friend's home. Finally, 2 students reported previous experience with VR glasses.

5.2. Observation Protocol

During the virtual reading training, the study participants were observed by the two study directors who used a guided, structured observation protocol with nine observation categories. The results are described below along these nine observation categories.

Reading repetitions: During the first reading of the RT scene in desktop VR, the students had trouble assigning the different RT roles and finding the appropriate page in the scripts while they read aloud in groups. As a result, the students would point out a missed cue, by saying "it's your turn". The second reading of the RT scene went smoothly.

Motivation to read: The students felt were motivated to read. It appears that they were more motivated during the desktop VR reading training than their classroom training. For instance, after the technical problems were solved, the students started to read the play on their own without being directly asked to do so by the study instructors. In presence, on the other hand, the students tended to occupy themselves with other things after a while. In addition, all students in a reading group had to take on a role unknown to them and read out unknown sentences. One student even had to take on two roles at the same time. The students had no inhibitions reading an unknown text and were motivated to read them. In addition, similar group dynamics with respect to reading motivation were evident in the desktop VR training as well as in the classroom training. For example, one student who motivated his group to read in presence also did so in VR. Reading motivation was also evident by the fact that the students did not take breaks during the reading training. After completing the first reading session, one group asked the study leader for the next reading task. In the physical classroom setting, the students did not ask the teacher for new tasks during the practice periods.

Reading Fluency: In terms of students' RF, no (positive/negative) differences were perceptible between the reading training in the desktop VR school environments and the classroom training sessions.

Communication & collaboration: At the beginning of the reading training in the presence, the students sat down next to each other and talked "in person" in order to distribute or discuss the division of the RT roles. This occurred above all when the first technical problems arose. After the technical problems were fixed, one reading group spread out on different floors in the hallway of the real school building while the other group spread out in a classroom to practice reading in presence.

Degree of distraction: During the reading training, most of the students were focused on their reading tasks and scripts. Only one student moved through the desktop VR environment with his avatar while his group members were reading, but then felt he had been caught by one of the study instructors.

Digital RT script: The study instructor first showed the students how to view and use the digital RT script in the desktop VR environment: i.e., how to keep clicking on the text shown on the media walls and how to view it on index card form. Even during the reading, some of the students needed help with setting and displaying the script. Nevertheless, all students voluntarily used the RT script available in the VR environment rather than their analog paper scripts.

Use of avatars and props: The study instructors observed that the students do not position their avatars in any special way while practicing reading. Instead, the avatars were randomly spread out in the room instead of being placed next to each other while reading.

This behavior resembles the RT reading practice in the presence where the students tend not to stand in any specific way, either. Even while reading per se, students did not move their avatars. With regard to the use of props during the reading training, students were observed to be aware of the props (e.g., by talking about them in their respective groups) but did not explicitly integrate them into the reading exercises.

Movement and navigation: The students intuitively and independently moved around and explored the environment and their features with their avatars immediately upon entering the desktop VR environment. This they were observed to do even without specific instruction from the study leader or an official warm-up phase that did not take place as planned due to technical problems. It was not apparent that the students had any inhibitions or fears about using the VR environment for reading practice.

Technical Equipment: The reading training start was delayed by audio problems in which the volume was too low so the students only partially heard themselves reading while their group members heard nothing at all. One student showed some frustration in this issue. In addition, Wi-Fi connection problems and the performance of the Internet in the school meant that students were forced to contend with re-accessing connectivity after being thrown out of the desktop VR environment. This problem meant an overall loss of reading practice time. In spite of this issue, the students remained motivated and patient while waiting for the technical problems to be resolved, or they searched for possible solutions themselves. Even though this took approx. 30 min, the students then became involved in the planned reading training which they carried out.

5.3. *Interview Results*

5.3.1. Student Acceptance of the Desktop VR RT

When analyzing interview results of the students' acceptance of participating in the virtual MELT, a distinction could be made between perceived usefulness and ease of use, as postulated by Davis et al. [39].

Perceived usefulness:

Choice of an avatar: Four of the five interviewees liked having the freedom to choose their own avatar. Two participants positively evaluated the variety of choices allotted to them. Various reasons were listed which were decisive for the choice of one's avatar. These were determined in accordance with the role in the RT play, personality, and the appearance of the avatar (e.g., *"what I find cool now"*, I. 4). In addition, one person said that the choice of avatar made it easier for her to identify with her reading role.

Reference to the RT play and use of props: For one student the use of props for the reader's theater play in the VR school environment was evaluated positively. Conversely, one student claimed not to have used any of the props in the desktop VR reading training.

Reference to the RT role: Contrasting results emerged with regards to the students' reading in the RT play on the desktop VR environment. One participant reported that she found it easier to gain entrance into her RT role in presence because she was able to draw more parallels to acting in a theater (e.g., voice changes), while another participant said it was easier for her to change into her role because of her avatar choice.

Spatial flexibility: Three of the study participants talked about how they liked the flexibility of the desktop VR environment which made it possible to read together without having to sit in the same room.

Level of variety: All five participants told us that they found conducting the MELT in a desktop VR environment to be very diversified in relation to their usual school day routine and that they liked this very much. One student went on to describe this aspect as follows: *"Because it's just something new and you don't do it every day..."* (I. 5).

Expression of emotions: With regard to the expression of emotions while reading the MELT script, differentiated results could be observed. Two students reported that it was more difficult for them to express their emotions and hear the emotions of other students when reading in VR than when reading in presence. The reason for this was the representation of oneself in the form of an avatar cannot show a facial expression. However, another student went on to say that there are no significant differences: *"I don't think it's a big difference. You can tell that other emotions are also shown whether you're standing opposite each other or there's another device in between."* (I. 3). In contrast, one student perceived emotions better when reading in the VR school environment than in presence.

Immersion: The statements by three students show that they experienced feelings of immersion during the reading training or in the desktop VR environment in general: *"It almost felt a bit like you were really in there"* (I. 1). Another student gave credence to the feeling of immersion as follows: *"It felt a little bit like being in school"* (I. 2).

Perceived ease of use:

Movement, navigation, and orientation: Two students stated that they could move freely and enter different rooms by means of their avatar in the desktop VR environment. Another participant reported needing time to learn how to navigate by avatar at the beginning of the reading training in the VR environment. However, he only needed three to five minutes to become accustomed to this function which worked well. One of the participants reported frequent navigation problems, in which her avatar became stuck to the environment furniture (e.g., a chair). This participant also referred to differences in the field of vision in the VR environment as compared to the real world, saying: *"You couldn't see exactly what you normally see, so you had to adjust to what you see a bit first"* (I. 5).

Degree of distraction: Four of the five participants stated that the VR environment did not distract them from the reading training and exercises. One student attributed this to her frequent use of an iPad at school. Another student justified this by saying that she focused mainly on the script and not the surroundings in the VR school environment while reading and practicing.

Digital RT script: Three of the participants perceived the presence of a digital theater script both on the media walls and in index card form positively. One of the participants explained as follows: *"It's not so boring with the paper at the front, but you can have it at the bottom, press on nicely"* (I. 2). Likewise, three of the study participants reported problems in using the digital theater script because one *"...always had to press on a cross at the top, so it wasn't so easy to see when it was your turn"* (I. 2).

Desktop VR school environment Design: Comments by four study participants concerning the design and structure of the VR environment were consistently positive. They found the virtual school building and the various classrooms to be realistic. The large number of classrooms surprised two of the study participants who said the school building and classrooms were a good representation of their real-life school. In addition, one of the interviewees commented specifically on the furnishings, which she claimed were *"...very colorful and um clearly arranged"* (I. 5).

Communication & collaboration: Communication and collaboration within one's group during the desktop VR reading training was described as difficult by two participants. They reported occasional difficulties with understanding the other group members which was mainly due to audio problems. Moreover, due to the use of the digital RT scripts, it was not always clearly recognizable whose turn it was to read next. The ability to hear and understand the other group members directly in the VR environment, as long as there were no audio problems, was found to be positive by two interviewees.

Degree of exercise/reading difficulty: Two students found the reading training in the desktop VR school environment to be more difficult than reading in presence. The reasons were as follows: technical problems, use of a digital script, and expression of emotions. One student, on the other hand, stated that she did not find the reading training in the VR environment more difficult than in the presence.

Technical problems: One of the participants said that it was difficult to hear the other group members at the beginning of the reading training. Towards the end of this phase, however, the volume problems could be solved, as she explained. With regard to audio-technical aspects, one study participant noted finding it "stupid" that most of the study participants did not have headphones with them. Two students also talked about how the time they were able to spend in the desktop VR environment was limited as a result of problems with the WIFI connection in the school building. These complications were evaluated differently by two students: One student said the technical problems were "*...not particularly bad now*" (I. 5), while the other felt it was "*...just a little bit stupid that it did not work out so perfectly then*" (I. 3).

5.3.2. Effects of the Desktop VR RT

The general impression of the Desktop VR environment (usefulness, ease of use, design) and the reading fluency training: Four of the five participants responded positively about their first impression of the VR environment and the reading exercises. They described it as: "*I thought it was really good*" (I. 2) or "*...it was cool*" (I. 3).

Sense of fun and motivation: Three of the five interviewees said they liked practicing the RT play more in VR than in presence. In addition, three interviewees also talked about how much more they enjoyed reading in the VR school environment than in the presence. One person, on the other hand, stated that she did not enjoy reading in VR any more or less than in presence. Moreover, she would prefer to use either format or a combination of both.

5.3.3. Behavioral Intent (Future Usage of Desktop VR RT)

Potential of RT in Desktop VR: All participants stated that they could imagine learning more in the future with VR applications because it is fun and offers variety. Of these, two of the interviewees specified that they would not want to use VR exclusively in class, but rather as a change from normal school lessons e.g., two to three times a month, or as a combination of both. As one participant put it: "*Well, I think it's best to have both together somehow*" (I. 3). In addition, one student said that he could imagine using VR, especially in English/foreign language classes, e.g., to learn and test vocabulary, engage in role plays, or read texts.

6. Discussion and Conclusions

Reading training formats that promote RF, e.g., repeated or assisted reading, are considered to be time-consuming. They often do not allow teachers to respond to the individual needs of students, nor give sufficient feedback. In addition, it is very difficult to motivate students as they sometimes find reading-aloud activities monotonous. Therefore, the overarching goal of this study was to determine the extent to which students accept the implementation of a specific phase of MELT in a VR environment for the purpose of cooperative reading fluency training. This may aid in increased efficiency, easier structuring of personal learning processes, individual feedback options, online collaboration, and a more satisfying and motivating user experience for the students.

In this section, we will now discuss how the learning objectives established in Chapter 3.1 could be implemented through the design of the VR environment and the didactic structure of the desktop VR training session. With regards to the sub-learning aim of providing opportunities for cooperative reading training, an important and surprising finding in this project is the overall positive response to the virtual RT, despite numerous technical difficulties at the beginning of the VR training session. In addition, the students indicated that they felt highly motivated and had more fun during the virtual RF training than during the face-to-face reading training (s. Chapter 5.3.2). However, two students explicitly stated that reading training in desktop VR was still more difficult for them than in presence, mainly due to technical challenges. Furthermore, the students perceived the presence of the digital MELT script as positive, even though they described its use as challenging and complicated (s. Chapter 5.3.1). In terms of testing the use of MELT and making student collaboration easier in VR, alternative possibilities should be created (e.g., the digital representation of the MELT script). In addition, the VR software that enables the reading text to be displayed and operated more easily should be tested.

Turning now to the second sub-learning objectives, (e.g., methods to encourage the giving of and receiving feedback), results showed that students did not use the chat and emoji features, even though they discovered them of their own accord. Due to the omission of non-verbal communication elements such as facial expressions or gestures, students are not able to interpret fellow readers reactions to their reading performance. In this context, it would be important to help students understand the relevance of giving and receiving verbal feedback about reading fluency as a means of support. In addition, various exercises should be integrated into the collaborative reading fluency training phases of VR. In this way, students can be instructed on not only how to give each other feedback, but also to encourage them to do so. For example, students could also be motivated to give feedback by means of a gamified approach, (e.g., a virtual badge award to the group that gave the most feedback).

Analysis of data concerning the third sub-learning objective that allows for movement and interaction within the desktop VR environment revealed that after initial difficulties and a short familiarization phase, most students were able to move their avatars around well. However, this feature distracted some of the students from the exercise task at hand, which then enticed them to continue exploring the VR environment and trying out the functions, (e.g., sitting on a chair, etc.). After a short introduction, they were also able to independently and intuitively use the other VR features (e.g., the digital MELT script). This ease of use is likely the result of their daily media use and, or prior VR experience (s. Chapter 5.2). However, it is unclear whether this ability improved their RF. This would require further experimental studies.

We now turn to the fourth sub-learning objective of gaining a better understanding of the story and its characters by means of interacting with props and images. Interview results showed that students very much liked how the design of the desktop VR environment was based on the content of the MELT script through the use of relevant props, even though they did not actively integrate them into their reading training. The free choice of an avatar was also described positively. However, only one student was able to benefit from the avatar that helped her identify in her role (s. Chapter 5.3.1). It is therefore recommended to integrate student input more into the design and development process of VR environments (e.g., avatar creation). This has the potential to promote learner discussion, as well as to support the process of understanding the MELT script content. In addition, there are a plethora of other features that could be integrated into a VR environment. For example, features that focus on practicing and improving RF are aimed at increasing student acceptance of VR or supporting students in giving and receiving feedback. Teachers and students would certainly benefit from functions similar to a recording studio that allow for uploading and recording audio files. In addition, an audio studio could also include a vocabulary pronunciation feature. Functions that support independent reading training could be integrated along with a comment function. Finally, integrating vocabulary lists would certainly add to the desktop VR environment learning experience.

Those factors associated with perceived usefulness, e.g., avatars, MELT content-specific environment design, and spatial flexibility of the VR environment, were perceived as useful and varied. However, a majority of the respondents found the expression and perception of emotions in the VR environment to be more challenging than in the presence (s. Chapter 5.3.1). To deal with this issue, students could benefit from instruction on and practicing the means to express emotions in the VR environment through intonation and voice pitch. In addition, when training in presence, one could create similar conditions for practicing the expression and perception of emotions as they occur in presence. For example, with closed eyes, students could listen to their classmate's expression of emotions with special emphasis on the emotions of their MELT character. An interesting paradox with regards to the perceived ease of use of the desktop VR environment emerged. Despite the difficulties with the digital script and various audio problems, students found these integrated features to be positive. It was not possible to carry out pre-tests under real study conditions within the scope of this study, due to limitations of time (i.e., hardware and software testing in advance with real study participants). For future studies, it is advisable that pre-tests are planned for and carried out in order to identify and eliminate technical problems early on. In this study, it was only possible to test the functionality of the hardware and software with one person in advance. Unfortunately, this was one of the study leaders. It would have been more advantageous to include a real number of study participants in this process. In addition, it is advisable to carry out the study with several study managers who can support participants in the event of technical difficulties.

In summary, an important and surprising result of this project revealed that despite numerous technical difficulties at the beginning of the desktop VR training session, the students' first impressions of the virtual RT were highly positive. Moreover, they indicated being highly motivated to engage in the activities and that they had had more fun as compared to face-to-face reading training (s. Chapter 5.3.2). In particular, due to the high levels of motivation and patience among the study participants, it can be concluded that they accepted the implementation of MELT in the desktop VR school environment. This aspect is consistent with previous research results and findings in the literature (see Chapter 2.4) [30]. This finding also suggests that with the above-mentioned improvements, the use of VR applications could potentially enable numerous design options, such as self-learning activities, personalized learning, and feedback, which are difficult to achieve in face-to-face settings. The results here provide evidence that supports the potential of the MELT reading fluency practice phase in a VR environment. Moreover, the findings suggest that the refinement and transfer of an established format for training reading fluency, such as in this project, creates additional added value that can, among other things, counter the limitations of the setting itself (e.g., the low motivation of the students to practice reading repeatedly).

In view of the limitations of this study, it must be stated that due to the time, financial, and personal resources available, an unrepresentative study was carried out. It should be noted that this study served as a pilot with a small sample size (n = 7). Moreover, we were unable to analyze speech patterns, nor the number of spoken words due to data privacy and technical constraints. Audio recordings were not permitted, thus preventing us from conducting an analysis of the aspects mentioned above. However, we do plan to address these dimensions in the future.

With regard to further research in this area, it is therefore essential to conduct a long-term study with a representative number of students in order to be able to draw more robust conclusions about their acceptance of the reading fluency practice phases of MELT in a VR application and RF development over a longer period of time. In addition, it is essential to test the various RF training phases and formats of a RT (e.g., individual, tandem, group) in order to assess how these affect student acceptance. It would also be exciting to explore the final performance of the MELT script in VR. In order to draw conclusions about the promotion of reading fluency in VR, an experimental study design would have to be carried out.

The above results can be considered a first evaluation of the acceptance of VR technologies in the context of reading fluency training at schools within the specific scenario of MELT. The next steps in this research will include a more comprehensive implementation of a VR-enhanced MELT scenario at schools and a more comprehensive evaluation over a longer time period, hence allowing for more informative insights on the possibilities and potentials for a permanent application of VR technologies in this context. Since the study results revealed the potential for the substitution and augmentation levels of the SAMR framework, further research will explore how modification of and even redefinition can be achieved by integrating MELT and VR technology. Corresponding research activities will also investigate the influence of specific VR technologies (e.g., VR glasses), as well as usability aspects and user experience in more detail.

Supplementary Materials: Original VR school environment link: https://hubs.mozilla.com/5JAX6Qa/ready-hidden-area (accessed on 1 September 2023); Customized VR school environment link: https://hubs.mozilla.com/link/EqYFJmf (accessed on 1 September 2023).

Author Contributions: Conceptualization, L.P.; Methodology, L.P., U.M. and W.M.; Evaluation, L.P. and A.K.; Writing, L.P., A.K., U.M. and W.M. All authors have read and agreed to the published version of the manuscript.

Funding: This research was partially funded by Baden-Wuerttemberg Ministry of Science, Research and Arts. Funding number: 31-7742.35/20.

Institutional Review Board Statement: Ethical review and approval was not required for the study on human participants in accordance with the local legislation and institutional requirements. The participants provided their written informed consent to participate in this study.

Informed Consent Statement: Informed consent was obtained from all subjects involved in the study.

Data Availability Statement: The data presented in this study are openly available in RADAR at https://doi.org/10.22000/1729 (accessed on 1 September 2023).

Conflicts of Interest: The authors declare no conflict of interest.

Appendix A

Main Category	Sub-Category	Observations
Turn Takings	Number	
	Smoothness/speaker overlaps	
	Repetitions	
	Missed cues	
Arrangement of practice phases	How often and how much is read/practiced?	
	How often are breaks taken?	
	Do students focus on practicing or are they otherwise engaged/distracted (with surroundings, etc.)	
	Do students finish before/after the given time?	
	Where do the students read their speaking text from?	
Avatar & Props	How do the students move/position their avatars in the environment? (Proxemics)	
	To what extend do the students use props/features of the environment?	
Technology	To what extend do (technical) issues arise? (audio-/image quality, WIFI problems, performance/speed of the tablet)	

Figure A1. Observation Protocol (Translated from German).

References

1. National Reading Panel. *Report of the National Reading Panel: Teaching Children to Read: An Evidence-Based Assessment of the Scientific Research Literature on Reading and Its Implications for Reading Instruction*; National Reading Panel: Bethesda, MD, USA, 2000.
2. Grabe, W. *Reading in a Second Language: Moving from Theory to Practice*; Cambridge University Press: New York, NY, USA, 2009.
3. Reynolds, D.; Goodwin, A. Supporting Students Reading Complex Texts: Evidence for Motivational Scaffolding. *ERA Open* **2016**, 2, 1–16. [CrossRef]

4. Jamshidifarsani, H.; Garbaya, S.; Lim, T.; Blazevic, P.; Ritchie, J.M. Technology-based reading intervention programs for elementary grades: An analytical review. *Comput. Educ.* **2019**, *128*, 427–451. [CrossRef]
5. Massler, U.; Gantikow, A.; Haake, S.; Müller, W.; Lopes, C. GameLet: Fostering Oral Reading Fluency with a Gamified, Media-Based Approach. In Proceedings of the European Conference on Games Based Learning; Southern Denmark, Denmark, 3–4 October 2019. [CrossRef]
6. Milrad, M.; Wong, L.-H.; Sharples, M.; Hwang, G.-J.; Looi, C.-K.; Ogata, H. Seamless Learning: An International Perspective on Next Generation Technology Enhanced Learning. In *Handbook of Mobile Learning*; Berge, Z.L., Muilenburg, L.Y., Eds.; Routledge: New York, NY, USA, 2013; pp. 95–108.
7. Mraz, M.; Nichols, W.; Caldwell, S.; Beisley, R.; Sargent, S.; Rupley, W. Improving oral reading fluency through readers theatre. *Read. Horiz.* **2013**, *52*, 163–180.
8. Tyler, B.-J.; Chard, D. Focus on Inclusion: Using Readers Theatre to foster fluency in struggling readers: A twist on the repeated reading strategy. *Read. Writ. Q.* **2000**, *16*, 163–168.
9. Rasinski, T. Reading Fluency Instruction: Moving Beyond Accuracy, Automaticity, and Prosody. *Read. Teach.* **2006**, *59*, 704–706. [CrossRef]
10. Ostovar-Namaghi, S.A.; Hosseini, S.M.; Norouzi, S. Reading Fluency Techniques from the Bottom-up: A Grounded Theory. *Int. J. Appl. Linguist. Engl. Lit.* **2015**, *4*, 29–35. [CrossRef]
11. Gorsuch, G.; Taguchi, E. Repeated reading for developing reading fluency and reading comprehension: The case of EFL learners in Vietnam. *System* **2008**, *36*, 253–278. [CrossRef]
12. Rasinski, T.; Hoffman, J. Oral reading in the school literacy curriculum. *Read. Res. Q.* **2003**, *38*, 510–522. [CrossRef]
13. Webb, S.; Chang, A.C.-S. Vocabulary Learning through Assisted and Unassisted Repeated Reading. *Can. Mod. Lang. Rev.* **2012**, *68*, 267–290. [CrossRef]
14. Vaughn, S.; Linan-Thompson, S.; Kouzekanani, K.; Pedrotty Bryant, D.; Dickson, S.; Blozis, S.A. Reading Instruction Grouping for Students with Reading Difficulties. *Remedial Spec. Educ.* **2003**, *24*, 301–315. [CrossRef]
15. Hußmann, A.; Wendt, H.; Bos, W.; Bremerich-Vos, A.; Kasper, D.; Lankes, E.M.; McElvany, N.; Stubbe, T.; Valentin, R. (Eds.) *IGLU 2016: Lesekompetenzen von Grundschulkindern in Deutschland im Internationalen Vergleich*; Waxman: Münster, Germany, 2017.
16. Young, C.; Rasinski, T. Implementing Readers Theatre as an Approach to Classroom Fluency Instruction. *Read. Teach.* **2009**, *63*, 4–13. [CrossRef]
17. Worthy, J.; Prater, K. "I thought about it all night": Readers Theatre for reading fluency and motivation. *Read. Teach.* **2002**, *56*, 294–297.
18. Drew, I.; Pedersen, R.R. Readers Theatre: A different approach to English for struggling readers. *Acta Didact. Nor.* **2010**, *4*, 1–18. [CrossRef]
19. Kutzelmann, S.; Massler, U.; Peter, K.; Götz, K.; Ilg, A. (Eds.) *Mehrsprachiges Lesetheater: Handbuch zu Theorie und Praxis*; Budrich: Leverkusen, Germany, 2017.
20. Kutzelmann, S.; Massler, U.; Peter, K. The Central Teaching and Learning Processes of Multilingual Readers' Theatre: A Guideline for the Classroom. Weingarten: Pädagogische Hochschule Weingarten. 2016. Available online: https://melt-multilingual-readers-theatre.eu/wp-content/uploads/2017/09/20170901_Kommentar_Englisch.pdf (accessed on 1 September 2023).
21. Hasselbring, T.S.; Goin, L.I. Literacy instruction for older struggling readers: What is the role of technology? *Read. Writ. Q.* **2004**, *20*, 123–144. [CrossRef]
22. Adams, M.J. The Promise of Automatic Speech Recognition for Fostering Literacy Growth in Children and Adults. In *International Handbook of Literacy and Technology*; McKenna, M.C., Labbo, L.D., Kieffer, R.D., Eds.; Lawrence Erlbaum Associates: Hillsdale, NJ, USA, 2006; pp. 109–128.
23. Mostow, J.; Aist, G.; Huang, C.; Junker, B. 4-Month Evaluation of a Learner-Controlled Reading Tutor That Listens. In *The Path of Speech Technologies in Computer Assisted Language Learning. From Research Toward Practice*, 1st ed.; Holland, M., Fisher, F.P., Eds.; Routledge: New York, NY, USA, 2007; pp. 201–219.
24. Mills-Tettey, G.A.; Mostow, J.; Dias, M.B.; Sweet, T.M.; Belousov, S.M.; Dias, M.F.; Gong, H. Improving Child Literacy in Africa: Experiments with an Automated Reading Tour. In Proceedings of the 3rd International Conference on Information and Communication Technologies and Development, Doha, Qatar, 17–19 April 2009; pp. 129–138. Available online: http://repository.cmu.edu/robotics/161 (accessed on 1 September 2023).
25. Vasinda, S.; McLeod, J. Extending Readers Theatre: A Powerful and Purposeful Match with Podcasting. *Read. Teach.* **2011**, *64*, 486–497. [CrossRef]
26. Kapp, K.M. *The Gamification of Learning and Instruction*; Pfeiffer/John Wiley & Sons: Hoboken, NJ, USA, 2012.
27. Deterding, S.; Dixon, D.; Khaled, R.; Nacke, L. From Game Design Elements to Gamefulness: Defining 'Gamification'. In Proceedings of the 15th International Academic MindTrek Conference: Envisioning Future Media Environments, Tampere, Finland, 28–30 September 2011; pp. 9–15.
28. Massler, U.; Müller, W.; Iurgel, I.; Haake, S.; Gantikow, A.; Hadzilacos, T. Meaningful, gamified training of reading fluency. *Front. Comput. Sci.* **2022**, *4*, 1–22. [CrossRef]
29. LaLeTu. Available online: https://www.laletu.de/home (accessed on 11 April 2023).
30. Luo, H.; Li, G.; Feng, Q.; Yang, Y.; Zuo, M. Virtual reality in K-12 and higher education: A systematic review of the literature from 2000 to 2019. *J. Comput. Assist. Learn.* **2021**, *37*, 887–901. [CrossRef]

31. Mestre, D. Immersion and Presence. 2023. Available online: https://www.researchgate.net/publication/239553303_Immersion_and_Presence (accessed on 1 September 2023).
32. Parmaxi, A. Virtual reality in language learning: A systematic review and implications for research and practice. *Interact. Learn. Environ.* **2023**, *31*, 172–184. [CrossRef]
33. Dhimolea, T.K.; Kaplan-Rakowski, R.; Lin, L. A systematic review of research on high-immersion virtual reality for language learning. *TechTrends* **2022**, *66*, 810–824. [CrossRef]
34. Symonenko, S.V.; Zaitseva, N.V.; Osadchyi, V.V.; Osadcha, K.P.; Shmeltser, E.O. Virtual reality in foreign language training at higher educational institutions. *CEUR-WS Org.* **2022**, *2547*, 37–49.
35. Mirlaut, J.; Albrand, J.-P.; Lassault, J.; Grainger, J.; Ziegler, J.C. Using Virtual Reality to Assess Reading Fluency in Children. *Front. Educ.* **2021**, *6*, 693355. [CrossRef]
36. Carrasco Orozco, M. Can Virtual Reality Improve Dyslexic English Students' Reading Fluency and Their Emotional Valence towards Reading? University of Oulu: Oulu, Finland, 2020.
37. Kavanagh, S.; Luxton-Reilly, A.; Wuensche, B.; Plimmer, B. A systematic review of virtual reality in education. *Themes Sci. Technol. Educ.* **2017**, *10*, 85–119.
38. Fussell, S.G.; Truong, D. Using virtual reality for dynamic learning: An extended technology acceptance model. *Virtual Real.* **2022**, *26*, 249–267. [CrossRef] [PubMed]
39. Davis, F.D.; Bagozzi, P.R.; Warshaw, P. User acceptance of computer technology: A comparison of two theoretical models. *Manag. Sci.* **1989**, *35*, 982–1003. [CrossRef]
40. Pletz, C.; Zinn, B. Technologieakzeptanz von virtuellen Lern- und Arbeitsumgebungen in technischen Domänen. *J. Tech. Educ.* **2018**, *6*, 86–105.
41. Aburbeian, A.M.; Owda, A.Y.; Owda, M. A Technology Acceptance Model Survey of the Metaverse Prospects. *AI* **2022**, *3*, 285–302. [CrossRef]
42. Liagkou, V.; Salmas, D.; Stylios, C. Realizing Virtual Reality Learning Environment for Industry 4.0. *Procedia CIRP* **2019**, *79*, 712–717. [CrossRef]
43. Mozilla Hubs. Available online: https://hubs.mozilla.com/ (accessed on 11 April 2023).
44. Le, D.A.; MacIntyre, B.; Outlaw, J. Enhancing the Experience of Virtual Conferences in Social Virtual Environments. In Proceedings of the IEEE Conference on Virtual Reality and 3D User Interfaces Abstracts and Workshops, Atlanta, GA, USA, 22–26 March 2020; pp. 485–494. [CrossRef]
45. Zender, R.; Buchner, J.; Schäfer, C.; Wiesche, D.; Kelly, K.; Tüshaus, L. Virtual Reality für Schüler_innen. Ein «Beipackzettel» für die Durchführung immersiver Lernszenarien im schulischen Kontext. *MedienPädagogik* **2022**, *47*, 26–52. [CrossRef]
46. Mayring, P.; Fenzl, T. Qualitative Inhaltsanalyse. In *Handbuch Methoden der Empirischen Sozialforschung*; Baur, N., Blasius, J., Eds.; Springer VS: Wiesbaden, Germany, 2019; pp. 633–648. [CrossRef]

virtual worlds

MDPI

Article

Piecewise: A Non-Isomorphic 3D Manipulation Technique that Factors Upper-Limb Ergonomics

Priya Kartick [1,†], Alvaro Uribe-Quevedo [1,*,†] and David Rojas [2,†]

1 Faculty of Business and IT, Ontario Tech University, 2000 Simcoe St. N, Oshawa, ON L1G 0C5, Canada
2 The Institute for Education Research, University of Toronto, 172 St. George St., Toronto, ON M5R 0A3, Canada
* Correspondence: alvaro.quevedo@ontariotechu.ca
† These authors contributed equally to this work.

Abstract: Virtual reality (VR) is gaining popularity as an educational, training, and healthcare tool due to its decreasing cost. Because of the high user variability in terms of ergonomics, 3D manipulation techniques (3DMTs) for 3D user interfaces (3DUIs) must be adjustable for comfort and usability, hence avoiding interactions that only function for the typical user. Given the role of the upper limb (i.e., arm, forearm, and hands) in interacting with virtual objects, research has led to the development of 3DMTs for facilitating isomorphic (i.e., an equal translation of controller movement) and non-isomorphic (i.e., adjusted controller visuals in VR) interactions. Although advances in 3DMTs have been proven to facilitate VR interactions, user variability has not been addressed in terms of ergonomics. This work introduces *Piecewise*, an upper-limb-customized non-isomorphic 3DMT for 3DUIs that accounts for user variability by incorporating upper-limb ergonomics and comfort range of motion. Our research investigates the effects of upper-limb ergonomics on time completion, skipped objects, percentage of reach, upper-body lean, engagement, and presence levels in comparison to common 3DMTs, such as normal (physical reach), object translation, and reach-bounded non-linear input amplification (RBNLIA). A 20-person within-subjects study revealed that upper-limb ergonomics influence the execution and perception of tasks in virtual reality. The proposed *Piecewise* approach ranked second behind the RBNLIA method, although all 3DMTs were evaluated as usable, engaging, and favorable in general. The implications of our research are significant because upper-limb ergonomics can affect VR performance for a broader range of users as the technology becomes widely available and adopted for accessibility and inclusive design, providing opportunities to provide additional customizations that can affect the VR user experience.

Keywords: 3D user interface; ergonomics; virtual reality; upper limb

Citation: Kartick, P.; Uribe-Quevedo, A.; Rojas, D. Piecewise: A Non-Isomorphic 3D Manipulation Technique that Factors Upper-Limb Ergonomics. *Virtual Worlds* **2023**, 2, 144–161. https://doi.org/10.3390/virtualworlds2020009

Academic Editors: Radu Comes, Dorin-Mircea Popovici, Calin Gheorghe Dan Neamtu and Jing-Jing Fang

Received: 15 February 2023
Revised: 10 April 2023
Accepted: 29 April 2023
Published: 17 May 2023

1. Introduction

Virtual reality (VR) is currently contributing to the development of psychomotor skills in education [1], training [2], and healthcare [3], among others, by allowing for immersion and exposure to scenarios that would otherwise be difficult or impossible to replicate in real life. However, despite the fact that recent breakthroughs in VR technology are mainly utilized in entertainment, one-size-fits-all solutions continue to be the norm, with advancements in comfort aimed at enhancing the user experience for more immersion and presence[4]. However, a lack of adequate ergonomics in virtual reality can have a negative effect on the user's immersion and presence [5], as well as causing motion sickness [6]. Several contributors to the poor impact on the user experience include an inadequate reach, height, and interpupillary distance, which are primarily the result of one-size-fits-all solutions.

Our research focuses on the upper limb since effective user interactions are essential for conducting real-world activities or tasks in virtual reality [7]. Upper-limb interactions are essential in virtual reality by allowing for reaching and gripping, which require a combination of movements resulting from the 27 degrees of freedom (DOFs) from the shoulder to the wrist, [8]. The 27 DOFs allow for the flexion and extension, abduction and adduction, and pronation and supination of the upper limb. Moving the upper limb within its range of motion should not result in tiredness and pain, which cause fatigue and/or discomfort. However, repetitive or prolonged physical activity, such as keeping arms in midair, may create weariness and elevate exertion levels, which may develop into musculoskeletal problems, such as the gorilla arm [4]. Three-dimensional manipulation techniques can minimize cognitive stress [1] and hazardous body movements linked with musculoskeletal illnesses [4] when combined with good ergonomics.

Research on 3DMTs, such as isomorphic (a mathematical term meaning "sameness") and non-isomorphic (i.e., "not the same") techniques for reaching, selecting, and grabbing objects in VR [9], is providing solutions for enhancing the VR user experience, such as *Erg-O*, a non-isomorphic 3DMT that remaps the position of VR objects [10]. Isomorphic and non-isomorphic 3DMTs are essential in VR applications, such as entertainment, education, healthcare, and training, to ensure that users can properly interact with the virtual environment. Object translation, commonly referred to as "distance grab," is a typical isomorphic 3DMT in which virtual objects are translated to the user's hand by stretching, expanding their reach. This 3DMT is included in various VR software development kits (SDKs) (e.g., Oculus, Steam VR, and the virtual reality toolkit (VRTK)) as it allows for interaction with objects out of physical reach. Although object translation improves reach, it can negatively impact immersion, presence, and embodiment as interactions no longer require arm movements matching those in VR. This scenario has sparked interest in the development of novel 3DMTs [11–13]. Rietzler et al. (2018) [5] examined the effects of virtual hand offsets on immersion and presence relative to the real hand location by examining the felt weight of virtual items in four tasks that allowed participants to interact with virtual objects. When portraying the weight of virtual objects, the study found that the offsets favor immersion and presence marginally.

Li, Cho, and Wartell (2018) compared the effects of offsets on four reaching conditions, focusing on efficiency, accuracy, and timely completion [14]. The four reaching conditions were: (i) no offset (physical reach), (ii) a fixed offset where the virtual hand would be translated one meter from the real hand position, (iii) a dynamic non-isomorphic linear offset that increased the virtual reach by adjusting the magnitude of the actual hand within different distances from the HMD, and (iv) a non-isomorphic quadratic gain reach approach (similar to the *GoGo* non-linear mapping technique [15]). The study enrolled 24 participants who used the Oculus Rift DK2 (discontinued), the Leap Motion, and the Razer Hydra (a discontinued computer desktop motion-sensing VR controller that uses magnetic tracking). The test subjects were instructed to grab a color-changing sphere at four different depth clusters. The results show that participants could only reach spheres in all four cluster depths when using non-isomorphic offsets, and the dynamic offset condition (iii) outperformed all other reach techniques. It is important to note that the Leap Motion remains a relevant 3DUI for dexterity used in human–computer interactions for graphical user interfaces, exergames, and educational applications [16]. Although the Oculus Rift DK2 and Razer Hydra are discontinued, the findings from Li, Cho, and Wartell remain fundamental for understanding the role of offsets in 3DMTs.

Another 3DMT that facilitates virtual object manipulation employs multi-object re-targeting with freehand movement, based on isomorphic visual-to-physical mapping, and an optimized computation for rendering the interactable objects with the least visual difference [10]. Re-targeting produces ease-of-use manipulations by remapping the targets to appear closer to the user, partitioning the physical and visual space with tetrahedrons. The study presented three layouts and three re-targeting strategies to 12 participants, who completed nine trials in total. The three layouts included one employing a a normal mode or physical reach mode, and two variations of the proposed *Erg-O* 3DMT for spacial consistent and ergonomics.

Murillo, Subramanian, and Plasencia [10] used re-targeting to facilitate VE manipulation by remapping the targets closer to the user. This approach allows for multi-object re-targeting with freehand movement, isomorphic visual-to-physical mapping, and an optimized computation for rendering interactable objects with the least visual discrepancy. Participants in the study were presented with three interaction layouts and three 3DMTs. The layouts consisted of (i) 15 spheres arranged in a 5×3 grid, (ii) 24 spheres distributed evenly within the participant's reach, and (iii) 24 spheres placed beyond the participant's reach. The 3DMTs included a normal mode (physical reach) and two variations of *Erg-O*, focusing on spatial consistency by leveraging visual dominance to keep VR elements close to the user rather than focusing on ergonomics to maintain objects within comfortable reach. Participants completed surveys regarding comfort and physical exertion. The study's findings indicate that spatially consistent remapping can reduce task execution times, whereas ergonomic configurations lead to the least amount of overstretching.

Wentzel, d'Eon, and Vogel [17] compared low and high non-linear input amplification techniques to create virtual offsets for *Erg-O* to better understand their role in comfort, physical motion path length, virtual motion path length, ease of reach, overstretching, body ownership, and sense of control. *Erg-O* was replicated, and ergonomics were calculated using the HTC Vive Pro HMD in conjunction with compatible HTC Vive trackers strapped to the participants' shoulders, elbows, and waist, as well as the Vive controllers and a Microsoft Kinect for body tracking. The study recruited 18 participants (9 of whom had moderate VR experience) and presented them with three different offset layouts: (i) no amplification, (ii) low amplification, and (iii) high amplification, in addition to three variations of *Erg-O*, including ergonomics, reach limits, and world fixation. The results demonstrate an increased comfort without reducing the task performance or body ownership when participants utilized the amplification layouts. Furthermore, physical path lengths decreased whereas virtual path lengths increased due to the offset created in the VE. No differences in time to completion were found, and comfort was determined by comparing the arm movement with comfortable ergonomic shoulder and elbow flexion and extension.

A follow-up study saw the recruitment of 18 participants (11 of whom had prior VR experience) who now experienced offset amplifications ranging from 0 percent to 45 percent at 5 percent increase intervals [17]. For this study, the HTC Vive trackers were removed in favor of body tracking using the Microsoft Kinect. At the same time, the VR headset was changed to the Oculus Rift S for a simplified setup, not requiring external tracking cameras for the headset. According to the second study, the offset's slope could not be less than one, and offsets that increase a user's arm reach by up to 30 percent are acceptable as long as the user maintains a sense of body ownership. Wentzel, d'Eon, and Vogel concluded that the participants' performance and time completion results were comparable to the *Erg-O* method. Nevertheless, their offset method is more easily reproducible in numerous VR and VE applications.

The evolution of 3DMTs toward providing manipulation techniques with a greater reach has led to the development of isomorphic and non-isomorphic solutions and their impacts on the overall user experience. According to the related works, offsets are crucial in extending the user's arm for interactions beyond their physical reach. For example, adding reach offsets can improve efficiency, accuracy, immersion, and task completion. Other approaches consider the upper limb's maximum reach to re-map targets closer to the user, but still out of physical reach, with positive effects on comfort, completion time, and physical effort. Finally, other methods employ linear amplifications to compensate for the user's reach in virtual reality, influencing comfort, embodiment, and task performance. While offsets and maximum reach provide manipulation techniques to improve the user experience, the related works do not integrate ergonomic ranges of motion as part of the 3DMT.

Ergonomic ranges of motion measure the impact of reach on the interactions [17]. In order to prevent overexertion or musculoskeletal disorders such as the gorilla arm [4], it is essential to keep movements within the ergonomic comfort range of movement. As the use of virtual reality (VR) continues to grow in popularity, one-size-fits-all ergonomics fail to account for user diversity. For instance, the COVID-19 pandemic increased VR adoption as a means of overcoming the limitations of traditional video calls in order to develop experiential learning and hands-on experiences [18], elderly care [19], and social connectedness [20], among others. By combining manipulation techniques for 3DUI principles and ergonomics, we intend to address one-size-fits-all reach in VR by factoring the upper-limb range of motion within a comfortable range.

In this paper, we present the development and evaluation of *Piecewise*, a non-isomorphic 3DMT for reaching and grabbing objects in VR that considers the ergonomics of the upper limb. We investigated the effects of accounting for upper-limb ergonomics on time to completion, task completion, percentage of reach, upper-body lean, engagement, and presence when compared to typical 3DMT methods, such as object translation (distance grab), reach-bounded non-linear input amplification (RBNLIA) [17], and the normal mode that relies on physically reaching for the objects in VR.

We hypothesize that *Piecewise*, a 3DMT in which the user is given an extended reach interaction customized to their upper-limb ergonomics to reposition the virtual hand in VR in comparison to normal (physical reach), object translation, and RBNLIA, will: (i) enable the execution of pick and place tasks in less time than other 3DMTs, (ii) reduce upper-body lean in comparison to the other 3DMTs, (iii) reduce the number of objects skipped in comparison to the other 3DMTs, (iv) maintain the percentage of reach within the comfort range of motion relative to other 3DMTs, and (v) provide a greater presence and immersion relative to other 3DMTs.

2. Materials and Methods

Our study consisted of a virtual scenario developed with the Unity game engine (2019.2.15f1) [21] and OpenVR [22]. Unity and OpenVR were chosen because, at the outset of the development process, they offered the tools required to support multiple VR headsets. Support for multiple VR headsets was required due to the restrictions imposed by the COVID-19 pandemic, which made collecting data online and remotely necessary. The study evaluated the effects on the engagement, presence, time, and task completion of four 3DMTs, including our proposed *Piecewise* method, which considers upper-limb ergonomics in comparison to object translation (distance grab), RBNLIA [17], and the normal mode, which rely on physically reaching for the objects in VR. In addition to performing the task in VR, the VR Questionnaire Toolkit [23] was utilized to house and display the Game Engagement Questionnaire (GEQ) [24] and the Presence Questionnaire (PQ) [25] in VR to minimize distractions and maintain the user's immersion and presence in VR.

2.1. Ergonomics

As depicted in Figure 1, human body movement includes flexion and extension in the sagittal or longitudinal plane, and abduction and adduction in the frontal or coronal plane. For comfort, these motions should remain within a specified range. According to Openshaw and Taylor [8], the optimal positioning for different types of tasks varies based on the activity, necessitating the need for ergonomic designs focusing on reducing fatigue and increasing comfort, which can influence productivity, reduce stress, and affect the quality of life.

The range of motion for comfort and safety is divided into four zones: (i) Zone 0, coded green for minimal stress on muscles and joints; (ii) Zone 1, coded yellow for minimal stress on muscles and joints; (iii) Zone 2, coded red for a greater strain on muscles and joints; and (iv) Zone 3 beyond the red zone for an extreme strain on muscles and joints that should be avoided. These zones indicate the optimal ranges for comfort, which is crucial for avoiding potential musculoskeletal disorders caused by repetitive movements, overexertion, and poor postures, such as the gorilla arm [4].

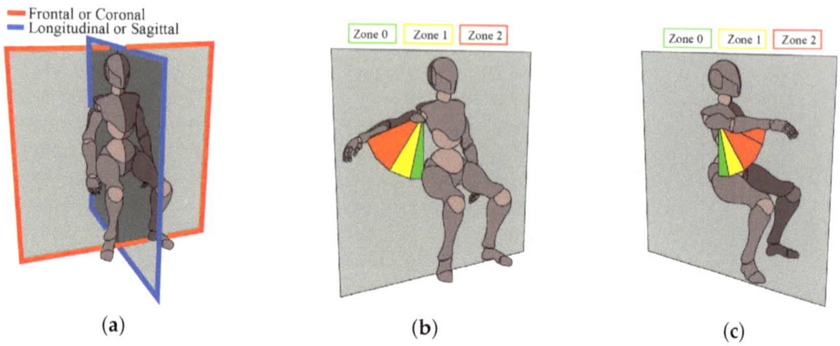

Figure 1. Ranges of motion showing outward and forward extension in the sagittal or longitudinal and frontal or coronal planes, respectively. (**a**) Frontal and longitudinal planes of motion. (**b**) Comfort zones for adduction and abduction movement. (**c**) Comfort zones for flexion and extension movement.

Piecewise, our proposed non-isomorphic 3DMT, is intended for reaching and grabbing objects in virtual reality. *Piecewise* takes upper-limb ergonomics into account through a calibration procedure that offsets the reach based on the range of motion to ensure that objects can be reached while remaining within the ergonomic comfort range (i.e., the green zone, Figure 1). The virtual scene requires the user to reach out and grab objects on a table's left and right sides from various distances. In order to compare our proposed *Piecewise* 3DMT, a management subsystem enables switching between three additional implemented manipulation methods, including object translation, RBNLIA, and a normal mode. A high-level overview of *Piecewise* is presented in Figure 2. An output data subsystem uses metrics that are recorded for calibration and performance metrics capture, such as task and time completion.

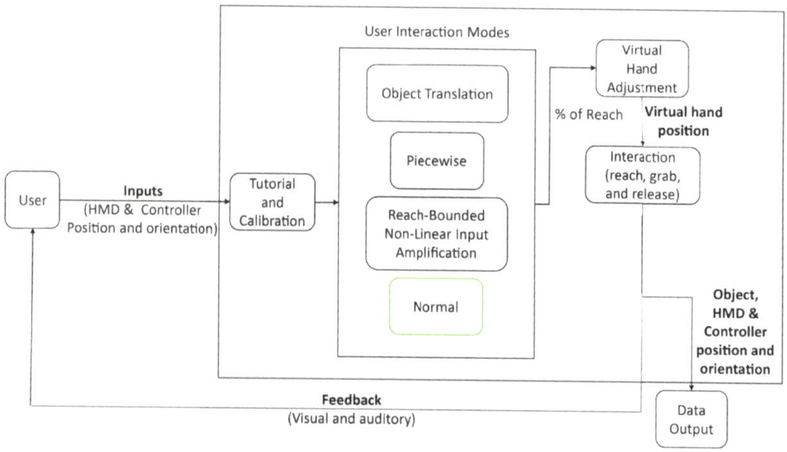

Figure 2. High-level overview of the proposed system and its components.

2.2. Calibration

Upper-limb calibration was used to capture user ergonomics, including their height when seated (referenced from the virtual floor calibration), the arms' length, and the virtual shoulders' location. A four-pose calibration consisting of: (i) arms up, (ii) arms forward, (iii) arms down, and (iv) arms outward allowed us to define both arms' length and virtual shoulder locations. The calibration poses are shown in Figure 3.

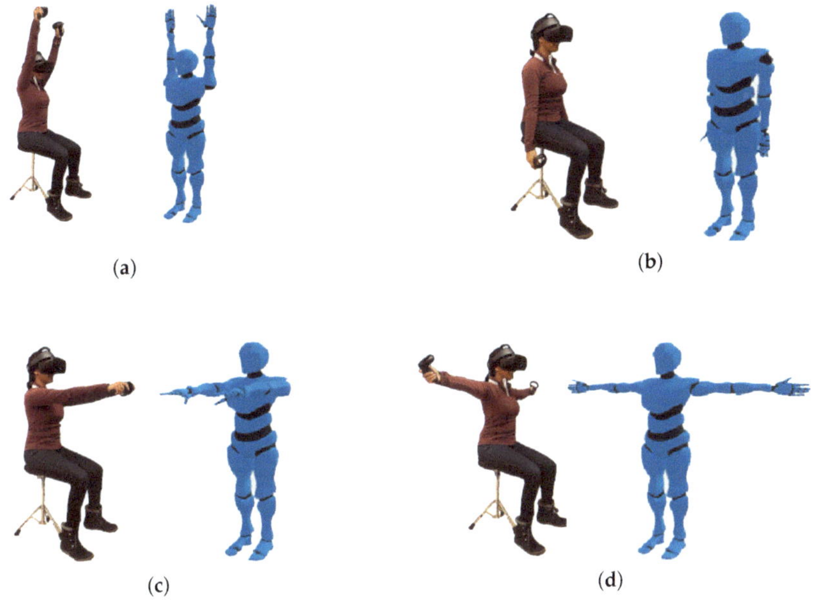

Figure 3. A virtual avatar models the calibration positions for the participant to imitate while seated throughout the upper-limb calibration process. (**a**) Step 1: Arms extended upward. (**b**) Step 2: Arms extended downward. (**c**) Step 3: Arms extended forward. (**d**) Step 4: Arms extended outward.

2.3. *Three-Dimensional Manipulation Techniques*

In addition to *Piecewise*, the following 3DMTs were added for our study: (i) the normal mode (physical reach), the object translation mode (also known as distance grab), and the RBNLIA mode [17]. The subsections that follow go over each 3DMT that was used.

2.3.1. Normal Mode

The normal mode is a universal, unaltered interaction method that relies on physical reach, as depicted in Figure 4a. This mode, which remains the most popular among VR installations and is easily accessible on a variety of SDKs, including OpenVR, SteamVR, and OpenXR, and it strongly depends on each user's upper-limb length and available VR area.

2.3.2. *Piecewise* Mode

The *Piecewise* mode, which factors in upper-limb calibration, extends the user's reach interaction by adding a scalar multiplier to the controller's location to reposition the virtual hand in VR. *Piecewise* was named after its multi-behavioral function, which is achieved by relocating the virtual hand in the VE using the forward vector based on the controller's local orientation (see Figure 4b). The visual modification is activated when the user's arms reach percentage hits 60% to maintain the range of motion within the comfort zone where a normal reach is performed. To reposition the controller, the scalar multiplier is doubled from a slope of 1 to a slope of 2 when the user's reach surpasses 60%. When the user's arm is fully extended, the maximum reach is adjusted by the scalar multiplier to be 140 percent. For instance, if the user's arms reach is 100 cm, the *Piecewise* mode's maximum reach is 140 cm. Nevertheless, the user will not experience an increase in reach until they cross 60% of their arm's reach; in this case, 60 cm.

2.3.3. Object Translation/Distance Grab Mode

The object translation mode (also known as distance grab) [26] is also readily available as a built-in interaction option in various VR SDKs, such as Oculus, SteamVR, OpenXR, and OpenVR. In the object translation mode, users can interact with far-off items by employing an extended invisible hand collider increase that secures objects to the virtual hand (Figure 4c). The distance grab is achieved by a constant range increasing the controller's local forward vector (see Figure 4). The maximum reach range in the object translation mode is 140 percent of the user's reach, with the arm's length being utilized to determine the 40% reach increase [17]. The additional range increase when interacting in the VE keeps a reach difference of 40% in centimeters (cm) from the user's actual maximum reach. The maximum reach possible with the object translation mode, for instance, is 140 cm if the user's arms reach is 100 cm. However, the user will always have an additional reach range of 40 cm added to their virtual hand position.

2.3.4. Reach-Bounded Non-Linear Input Amplification Mode

The RBNLIA mode leverages upper-limb ergonomics to expand the user's reach for virtual interactions (Figure 4d). RBNLIA is comparable to the Piecewise mode that we have proposed, with the primary difference being how the offset is determined. For example, RBNLIA exponentially increases the user's range so that, if the user's arms reach nears 100%, the exponential rise slows. The user interaction modification remains active throughout the mode and grants the user an additional 40 percent of reach. The virtual hand's size will expand exponentially from 0% to 60% based on the percentage of reach. As depicted in Figure 4d, an RBNLIA or slowing of the virtual hand will occur between 60 and 100 percent of the user's reach for fine motor interactions.

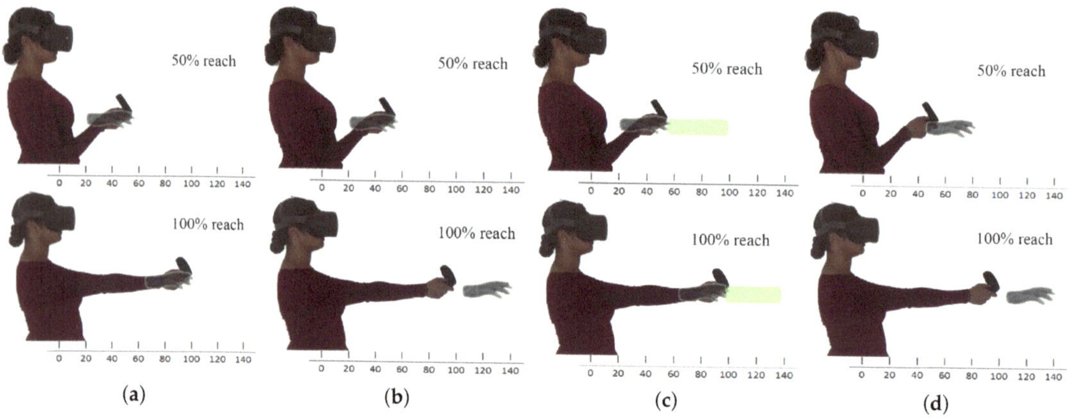

Figure 4. Percentage of reach comparison for the four user interaction modes, including normal, *Piecewise*, object translation, and RBNLIA. (**a**) Normal mode. (**b**) *Piecewise* mode. (**c**) Object translation mode. (**d**) Reach-bounded non-linear input amplification.

2.4. Study Design

A within-subjects study was conducted in which participants were exposed to all 3DMTs. A balanced Latin square was used to ensure that all participants access all conditions to minimize biases toward any interaction mode. Additionally, each condition was built into a separate executable file given to the participants who ran them as indicated by the study facilitator. The decision to provide the participants with the executables was made to minimize problems with larger files and errors when selecting the appropriate 3DMT. Due to the COVID-19 pandemic, the study was conducted online remotely, requiring participants to have access to a compatible desktop HMD and sufficient space for running the software in seated mode while having room to fully extend their arms forward, outward and upward as shown in Figure 3. The study software was compressed into an executable build and e-mailed to participants, along with additional documentation for running the study executable file, filling out the consent form, completing the surveys in VR after each manipulation technique, and finally uploading their data after the study was completed.

After the calibration (Figure 5a), the participants were immediately guided through the scene with a tutorial presenting the controller layout and interactions, with demonstrations given by a virtual avatar (Figure 5b). After completing the tutorial at the start of the study, the participants then proceeded to complete the pick-and-place task within the VE, employing the normal, *Piecewise*, RBNLIA, and object translation modes (Figure 5c). After completing each 3DUI mode, participants answered the questionnaires in VR, beginning with in-game GEQ and subsequently PQ (Figure 5d). The in-game GEQ survey captures each participant's experience with each 3DMT. The PQ questionnaire assesses the level of presence felt by the participants. However, the auditory, haptic, resolution, and interface quality subscales were omitted from the analysis because they were irrelevant to the current study. Figure 5 depicts a high-level summary of the study stages.

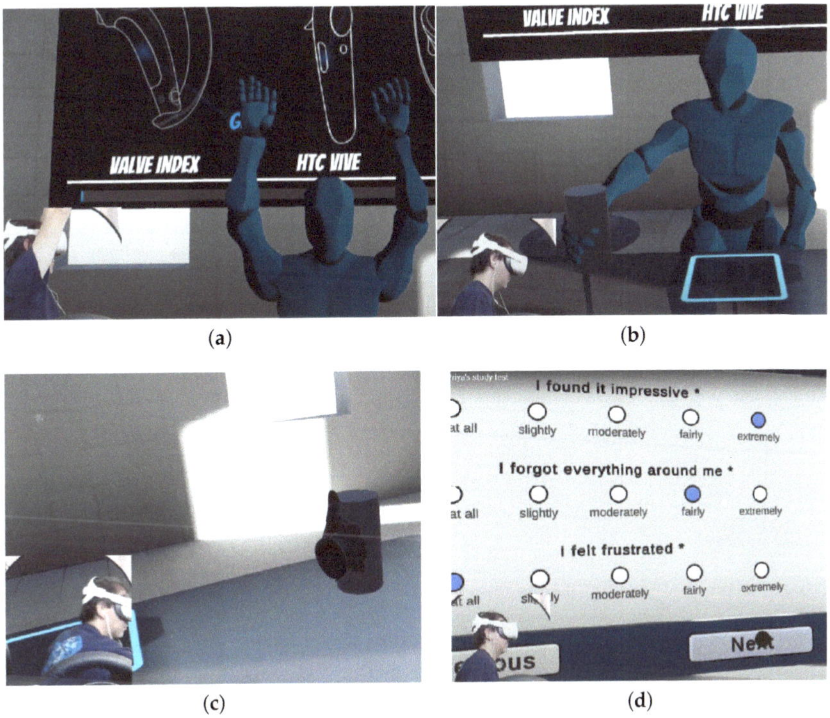

Figure 5. Step-by-step participant study journey. (**a**) Upper-limb calibration. (**b**) Tasks execution tutorial. (**c**) RBNLIA mode being used with a user reaching out to grab a cylinder. (**d**) Survey completion in VR where the * indicates mandatory questions.

2.5. Participants

The study recruited 20 individuals, 11 females and 9 males. Five percent of the participants were between the ages of 18 and 24, sixty-six percent were between the ages of 25 and 34, ten percent were between the ages of 35 and 54, and twenty percent were at least 55 years old. Seventeen individuals utilized the Meta Quest 1 HMD, whereas just three utilized the Meta Quest 2 HMD. A total of 75% of participants indicated no prior exposure to virtual reality, 15% reported using VR 1-5 times per month, 5% reported using VR 10–20 times per month, and 5% reported using VR 20+ times per month.

2.6. *VR Scene*

On a virtual table, the user is presented with a total of 12 virtual objects (cylinders) at varied distances within the ergonomic motion range reach, including Zone 0, Zone 1, and Zone 2 (see Figure 6). The objects on the left side of the virtual table are presented first, starting with Left object 1 (L1) and increasing to L6, followed by the objects on the right side, starting with Right object 1 (R1) and increasing to R6. The height of the virtual table was adjusted to 71 cm, which is the usual height for desks. In compliance with ergonomic requirements for the table height and comfortable range of motion [27], the table also contains the assistance, reply, and skip buttons, which were 38 cm from the user. The objects were equipped with interaction and tracking scripts to allow for interactions and timestamped metric monitoring. In order for the next object to appear, participants had to place the object in the Target area (T) in the bottom-center of the virtual table.

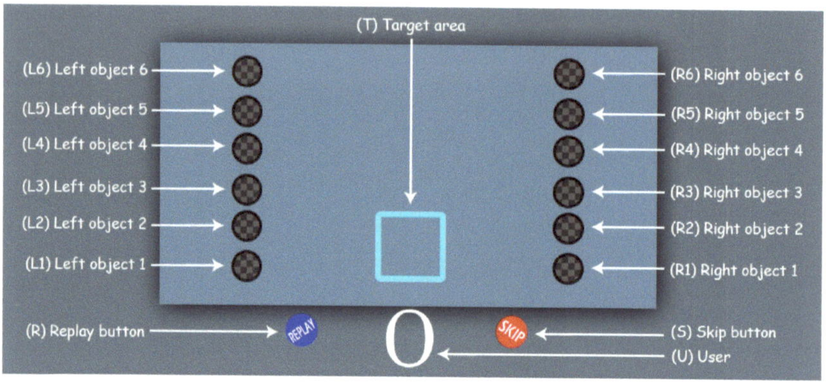

Figure 6. Objects, the user, and interactive buttons are presented on a virtual tabletop perspective.

Data Collection and Analysis

The data collected from the user study included the positions of the HMD and controllers, the position of the virtual hand, the start and end times to interact with an object and each mode, and the responses to the surveys asked in VR. Additionally, questions about their preferences toward any 3DMT and how exhausted they felt after completing the study were presented using a Google Form. Using the collected data, participant demographics and familiarity with VR were summarized, and the Statistical Package for the Social Sciences (SPSS) was used to analyze the collected data (i.e., time completion of each interaction mode, time completion of each object, percentage of arms reach, upper-body lean, and skipped objects). Using SPSS, the data were evaluated using the Shapiro–Wilk, Friedman, and Sign tests.

3. Results and Discussion

Our study's findings are organized into subsections based on time completion, skipped objects, percentage of reach, upper-body lean, engagement, and presence.

3.1. *Time Completion*

Time completion was utilized to determine how quickly a participant could interact with an object and how much time was spent in each interaction mode. The results indicate that the object translation mode had the shortest average time spent in the mode at 31 s (M = 2.756 s/object, SD = 2.422), followed by the normal mode at 33.52 s (M = 3.176 s/object, SD = 2.331), and then the two customized non-isomorphic interactions: RBNLIA mode at 37.28 s (M = 3.148 s/object, SD = 2.195), and *Piecewise* mode at 43.56 s (M = 3.728 s/object, SD = 3.797). A Shapiro–Wilk test found that the data set on time completion had not been normalized (see Tablereftab:TC swt), and a Friedman test revealed a statistically significant difference, $X^2(3) = 137.25, p \leq 0.001$ (see Table 1).

Table 1. Time completion Shapiro–Wilk results.

Shapiro–Wilk	N [1]	OT [2]	P [3]	F [4]
p-value	0.001	0.001	0.001	0.001

[1] Normal, [2] Object translation, [3] Piecewise, [4] RBNLIA.

A Bonferroni-adjusted non-parametric Sign test revealed a significant difference between all modes except for object translation and normal (see Table 2). The results disprove the hypothesis that customized non-isomorphic interactions will enable participants to complete tasks more quickly. The time spent in a mode was related to the number of objects that were skipped. In comparison to the *Piecewise* and RBNLIA modes, the normal and object translation modes had a larger average number of objects skipped (see Figure 7).

Table 2. Time completion Sign test results for the total time per mode.

Sign Test	P and N	OT and N	RBNLIA and N	OT and P	RBNLIA and P	RBNLIA and OT
p-value	0.001	0.239	0.001	0.001	0.001	0.001

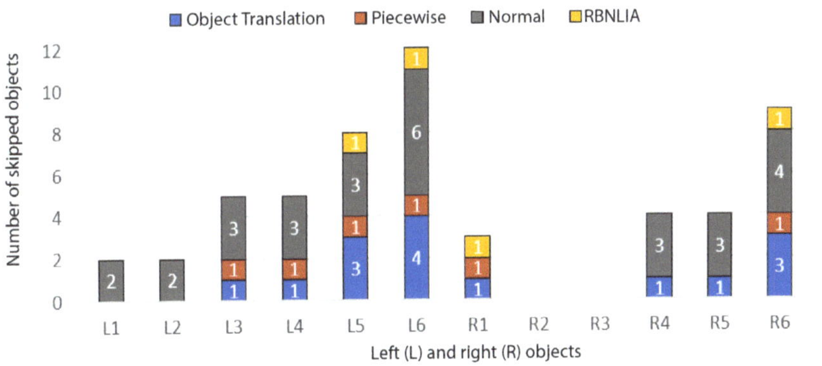

Figure 7. Number of skipped objects per 3DMT mode

3.2. Skipped Objects

Figure 7 presents the number of skipped objects per 3DMT, from the 48 objects (12 per mode): 29 objects were skipped in the normal mode, 15 objects were skipped in the object translation mode, 6 objects were skipped in the *Piecewise* mode, and 4 objects were skipped in the RBNLIA mode. The L6 object (the farthest object on the left) had the most skips (12), followed by the R6 object (the farthest object on the right), which was skipped 9 times (for the table layout distribution, see Figure 6). Curiously, some participants skipped over L1, L2, and R1 objects that were closest to them. Considering the motion data and participant input, we believe that this may have been caused by tracking errors and inadvertently pressing the skip button, an issue that will require future research.

The majority of skipped objects were encountered in the normal mode, as the farthest ones required participants to physically reach them, often leaning to extend their reach. The second most frequently skipped objects were met in the object translation mode, where collected motion data and participant input suggested that the virtual hand location made it difficult to aim at the objects. Unlike the normal and object translation modes, the participants skipped six objects when using *Piecewise*, and skipped four objects when using BRNLIA. Based on the number of skipped objects, *Piecewise* had a higher task completion than the normal and object translation modes.

3.3. *Percentage of Reach*

A Shapiro–Wilk analysis revealed that the data set for the percentage of reach did not have a normal distribution (see Table 3), and a Friedman test indicated that there were no statistically significant differences ($X^2(3) = 5.04$, $p = 0.168$). The average reach percentage per object, based on mode, showed that the reach percentages were all within the 90% range, but somewhat lower for objects positioned on the right side of the virtual table (see Table 4). Participants exhibited higher reach percentages when using the *Piecewise* and RBNLIA modes for objects on the left side of the virtual table, and when using the normal, object translation, and RBNLIA modes for objects on the right side.

Table 3. Percentage of reach Shapiro–Wilk significance results.

Shapiro–Wilk	N	OT	P	RBNLIA
p-value	0.001	0.001	0.001	0.001

The percentage of reach results is comparable across all DMT options (see Table 4). We believe that this is the case because the participants behaved as they would in real life, where extending the arm to reach objects is a more natural interaction than maintaining a reach percentage and leaning forward to correct for distance.

Table 4. Average percentage of reach of each object based on interaction mode.

Object	Normal	Distance	*Piecewise*	RBNLIA
L1	95.508%	96.176%	95.335%	93.625%
L2	95.703%	97.109%	97.132%	96.552%
L3	96.130%	95.398%	97.655%	98.246%
L4	96.519%	97.223%	98.541%	98.263%
L5	97.003%	96.752%	98.421%	97.698%
L6	96.824%	97.495%	98.394%	97.852%
R1	94.267%	92.687%	91.686%	90.999%
R2	96.890%	95.541%	93.585%	94.979%
R3	98.065%	97.333%	94.938%	96.933%
R4	97.804%	97.483%	94.947%	97.928%
R5	98.345%	98.112%	94.919%	98.802%
R6	99.035%	98.042%	94.977%	98.808%

3.4. *Upper-Body Lean*

A Shapiro–Wilk analysis indicated that the lean data set was not normalized (see Table 5), and a Friedman test revealed a statistically significant difference, $X^2(3) = 289.742$, $p \leq 0.001$. An additional analysis utilizing a non-parametric Sign test revealed statistically significant differences across all interaction types (see Table 6).

Table 5. Upper-body lean Shapiro–Wilk significance results.

Shapiro–Wilk	N	OT	P	RBNLIA
p-value	0.003	0.001	0.001	0.001

Table 6. Upper-body lean Sign test significance.

Sign Test	P and N	OT and N	RBNLIA and N	OT and P	RBNLIA and P	RBNLIA and OT
p-value	0.001	0.001	0.001	0.001	0.004	0.001

Figure 8 provides an overview of the average lean per object based on the interaction mode. The results indicated that the normal mode had the most upper-body lean

(M = 32.30 cm, SD = 17.998), followed by the object translation mode (M = 25.04 cm, SD = 17.948), RBNLIA mode (M = 16.10 cm, SD = 15.920), and *Piecewise* mode (M = 11.37 cm, SD = 15.236). The amount of leaning by participants using the normal mode was a result of extending their reach in the absence of any virtual visual manipulation or offsets. Interestingly, a similar behavior was present when using object translation, where leaning occured as an effort to increase reach and accuracy. Unlike the normal and object translation 3DMTs, *Piecewise* and RBNLIA both shifted the participant's virtual hand position in the virtual environment, which resulted in less leaning.

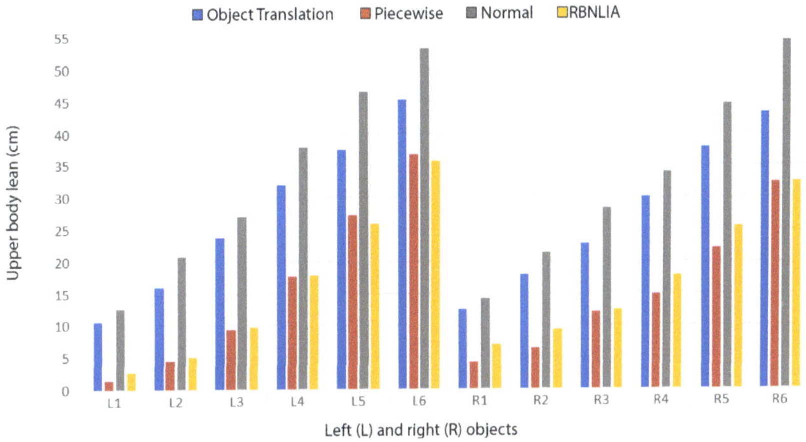

Figure 8. Upper-body lean average for each 3DMT mode.

3.5. Engagement

A Shapiro–Wilk test revealed that the data set was not normally distributed (see Table 7), and a Friedman test revealed significance in six of the seven GEQ categories: competence ($X^2(3) = 12.876$, p=.005), sensory ($X^2(3) = 94.320$, $p \leq 0.001$), flow ($X^2(3) = 7.826$, $p = 0.050$), tension ($X^2(3) = 70.541$, $p \leq 0.001$), challenge ($X^2(3) = 62.935$, $p \leq 0.001$), negative affect ($X^2(3) = 127.286$, $p \leq 0.001$), and positive affect ($X^2(3) = 40.271$, $p \leq 0.001$).

Table 7. In-game GEQ Shapiro–Wilk test.

Shapiro-Wilk	Chal [1]	Com [2]	Fl [3]	Neg [4]	Pos [5]	Sen [6]	Ten [7]
p-value	0.004	0.001	0.001	0.001	0.001	0.001	0.001

[1] Challenge, [2] Competence, [3] Flow, [4] Negative affect, [5] Positive affect, [6] Sensory, [7] Tension.

A non-parametric Sign test with a Bonferroni adjustment indicated statistically significant differences between the majority of modes in each GEQ category (see Table 8). The normal mode received the lowest scores for challenge, negative affect, and tension, indicating that this method of interaction was the least engaging. The *Piecewise* mode received the highest scores in the GEQ categories for flow, sensory, and immersion, while the RBNLIA mode received the lowest scores for negative affect and the highest scores for positive affect, and the object translation mode received the lowest scores for challenge and tension and the highest scores for competence.

The GEQ results (see Figure 9) indicate that non-isomorphic interactions were more engaging than isomorphic ones. The GEQ ratings corresponded to the degree of reach that was made available in each interaction style. The normal mode did not provide participants with enhanced reaching aids; as a result, the success rate of task completion was impaired, resulting in high scores in the categories of difficulty, negative affect, and tension. The *Piecewise* and RBNLIA modes both had a virtual offset and produced better engagement results. The participants' reach range increased the most in the object translation mode, and the findings reflect this.

Table 8. GEQ Sign test significance: P-Piecewise, N-Normal, OT-Object Translation, RBNLIA.

Sign Test	P and N	OT and N	FRBNLIA and N	OT and P	RBNLIA and P	RBNLIA and OT
Competence	0.076	0.002	0.001	0.001	0.0036	0.001
Sensory	0.001	0.019	0.001	0.001	1	0.001
Tension	0.001	0.001	0.001	0.001	0.156	1
Challenge	0.378	0.001	0.412	0.001	1	0.001
Negative	0.001	0.001	0.001	0.001	0.001	0.001
Positive	0.338	0.036	0.001	0.076	0.001	0.001

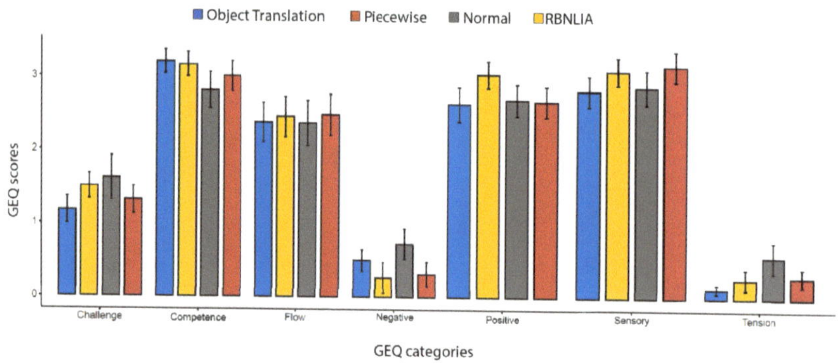

Figure 9. In-game GEQ results by category.

3.6. Presence

The Shapiro–Wilk test revealed that the data set was not normalized (see Table 9), and the Friedman test revealed a statistically significant relationship between the interaction modes in each of the PQ categories: control factors (CFs) ($X^2(3) = 94.242$, $p \leq 0.001$), sensory factors (SFs) ($X^2(3) = 36.000$, $p \leq 0.001$), distraction factors (DFs) ($X^2(3) = 38.571$, $p \leq 0.001$), realism factors (RFs) ($X^2(3) = 32.424$, $p \leq 0.001$), involvement/control (INV/C) ($X^2(3) = 65.217$, $p \leq 0.001$), and natural (NAT) ($X^2(3) = 33.288$, $p \leq 0.001$).

Table 9. PQ Shapiro–Wilk test.

Shapiro-Wilk	CF	SF	DF	RF	INV/C,	NAT
p-value	0.001	0.001	0.001	0.034	0.002	0.001

An additional analysis using a non-parametric Sign test with Bonferroni adjustment indicated significant differences between the majority of interaction modes within each PQ category (see Table 10).

Table 10. PQ Sign test significance.

Sign Test	P and N	OT and N	RBNLIA and N	OT and P	RBNLIA and P	RBNLIA and OT
CF	0.001	0.118	0.001	0.001	0.001	0.441
SF	0.378	0.097	0.001	1.000	0.097	0.001
DF	0.097	0.014	0.001	0.441	0.001	0.020
RF	0.14	0.118	0.001	0.441	1.000	0.001
INV/C	1.000	0.001	0.001	0.014	0.001	0.441
NAT	0.001	0.014	0.076	0.014	0.001	0.009

Figure 10 shows the PQ results, where the RBNLIA mode received the highest scores for all PQ categories, including CFs, SFs, DFs, RFs, INV/C, and NAT. The *Piecewise* mode yielded the second-most positive outcomes, after the object translation mode, while the normal mode yielded the least positive results. These results indicate that non-isomorphic 3DMTs that factor upper-limb VR had a higher presence level than those that do not. In spite of the visual manipulation of the virtual hand in the VE, participants believed that the RBNLIA mode produced the strongest level of presence. We believe that these results are the product of RBNLIA slowing the virtual hand's position utilizing a non-linear increase for finer motor control and interactions for all items within a 90% range.

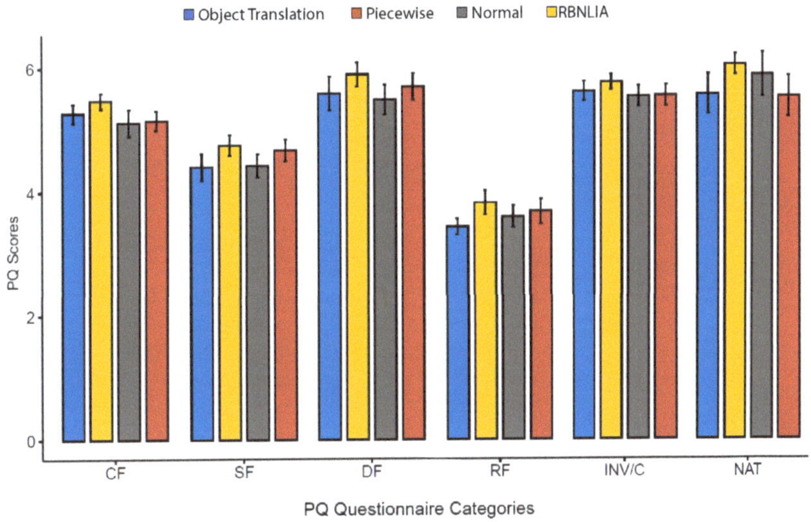

Figure 10. Presence results by category: CFs—control factors, SFs—sensory factors, DFs—distraction factors, RFs—realism factors, INV/C—involvement/control, NAT—natural.

3.7. *Preferred 3DMT and Perceived Fatigue*

After completing the GEQ and PQ surveys, the participants were asked to identify their preferred 3DMT. The object translation mode was preferred by 40% of participants, followed by RBNLIA with 32%, *Piecewise* with 12%, the normal mode with 8%, and, finally, no preference with 8%.

In addition, because the GEQ and PQ questionnaires were delivered in virtual reality, the participants were asked to report their level of fatigue upon completion of the study.The results indicate that 35% of participants reported "Feeling Great!", 20% reported "feeling good", 15% reported "feeling okay", 20% reported "feeling tired", and 10% reported feeling "Very Tired".

3.8. *Results Summary and Discussion by 3DMT*

3.8.1. Normal Mode

Participants missed a total of 29 objects in the normal mode, which was viewed as the most difficult 3DMT, increasing the challenge and anxiety, thus causing the highest tension and having the most negative impact on participants, affecting the overall engagement and presence (see Figure 9). Due to the physical reach nature of the normal mode, the participants found that it felt more natural than the object translation and *Piecewise* modes (see Figure 10). Additionally, 8% of the participants preferred the normal mode in terms of engagement. The normal mode produced the highest reach percentage per object and the greatest upper-body lean as a result of no offsets or upper-limb customizations.

3.8.2. Object Translation Mode

Forty percent of participants indicated object translation as their preferred interaction option. The participants spent the least amount of time in this mode, completed each object in the shortest amount of time, assessed it to be the least difficult, and experienced the least amount of tension (see Figure 9). In spite of having the quickest completion time, the object translation mode was deemed to be the least challenging, with 15 objects skipped. The time completion results indicated that the participants interacted with objects the quickest in this interaction mode; however, despite having the highest additional reach throughout the entirety of the interactions in the VE, there were nine and eleven more skips than in the *Piecewise* and RBNLIA modes, respectively. This non-isomorphic customized mode not only supplied the same maximum reach as the Piecewise and RBNLIA modes, but also included an increment to produce a greater interaction range from the participant's virtual hand. The large number of objects skipped in the object translation mode may have been influenced by the participant's inability to comprehend the extent of their interaction range. This may also be the result of the absence of a visual input, such as a laser beam or other visual help, to identify the complete reach range.

3.8.3. RBNLIA Mode

Participants using the RBNLIA mode skipped the fewest amount of objects: four. Despite having the second-longest completion time per object, 32% of participants self-reported RBNLIA mode as their preferred form of engagement. The design of the RBNLIA mode, which slows the offset rise, enables greater control for fine-motor interactions. The RBNLIA mode scores from the in-game GEQ suggest that participants felt the most positive effect and the least negative effect (see Figure 9), while the PQ results reveal that people felt the most present in the VE when interacting in this mode (see Figure 10).

3.8.4. Piecewise

The *Piecewise* 3DMT provided participants with up to 60% of their reach, followed by a virtual hand offset from 60% to 100% of the participant's reach. The *Piecewise* mode was self-reported as the most favored mode of interaction by 12% of participants, despite having the longest average completion time per object. We believe that the higher completion time is due to participants learning the technique and adjusting the reach based on their arm flexion and extension.

4. Conclusions

As VR continues to be adopted in non-entertainment scenarios such as education, training, and healthcare, users face usability difficulties due to a high user variability that hinders engagement, presence, and task execution. However, there have been advancements in providing VR customization in areas other than upper-limb ergonomics, such as setting the interpupillary distance, height calibration, adding tunneling vignettes for reducing motion sickness, and adjusting locomotion styles for ease of navigation. Therefore, it is essential to comprehend how upper-limb ergonomics influence presence, engagement, and task execution when integrated into a 3D manipulation technique.

This paper presented the development of a customized upper-limb 3DMT called *Piecewise* and compared it to existing isomorphic interactions, including normal and object translation (distance grab) modes, as well as RBNLIA, a non-isomorphic 3DMT for picking and placing objects set at various distances in front of the participants using both hands. Our research determined that the two 3DMTs that accounted for upper-limb ergonomics resulted in a greater presence and engagement, indicating that non-isomorphic techniques were more engaging than their isomorphic counterparts when immersing participants in the virtual environment. Despite having a greater number of omitted objects, isomorphic 3DMTs required less time to complete tasks than non-isomorphic modes according to our research. As a consequence of the number of skipped objects, non-isomorphic interactions permitted greater task completion with fewer skipped objects.

Following the analysis of the percentage of reach, both isomorphic and non-isomorphic 3DMTs produced comparable results. However, it is important to note that the participants had greater reach when using the *Piecewise* and RBNLIA modes for objects on the left side of the virtual table, and greater reach when using the normal, object translation, and RBNLIA modes for objects on the right side of the virtual table. Although the 3DMTs had no effect on the percentage of reach, the results of the upper-body lean revealed that the normal and object translation 3DMTs had a higher percentage than *Piecewise* and RBNLIA.

Our analysis of presence, engagement, time to completion, percentage of reach, and upper-body lean, as well as participant preferences, suggests that incorporating upper-limb ergonomics into a 3DMT has an effect on the performance of the task. Specifically, when compared to RBNLIA, our proposed *Piecewise* 3DMT ranked second in terms of preference, had the longest time to completion, the least amount of upper-body lean, the second highest rating in presence, and the most positive scores for flow, sensory, and imaginative immersion, while ranking behind RBNLIA's negative and positive affect. In terms of difficulty, tension, and proficiency, normal and object translation modes outperformed both non-isomorphic 3DMTs.

This paper contributes to 3DMTs by presenting the effects of factoring upper-limb ergonomics toward ensuring arm motion within the comfort zone when reaching and grasping objects in VR compared to a non-isomorphic (i.e., RBNLIA) and two isomorphic 3DMT models (i.e., normal and object translation). Our findings align with previous research on 3DMTs, further corroborating the importance of motion within ergonomics comfort. Furthermore, our results show how maintaining upper-limb movement with an ergonomic comfort range of motion can impact body posture and presence. Such findings are essential for advancing 3DMTs that can be used for accessible and inclusive immersive experiences. As VR becomes more widely adopted, eliminating one-size-fits-all barriers to immersive technologies is pertinent. Customizations tailored to each user will aid in performing duties and the experience of a greater presence and engagement.

Future Work

Future research will investigate the optimal combination of isomorphic and non-isomorphic 3DMTs for maximizing immersion, presence, and task success. Due to the cross-applications of 3DMT, additional use cases will be investigated in fields such as medicine, engineering, and inclusive design in order to study the effects on psychomotor skills development. Additional qualitative data will be collected from participants to better comprehend their perceptions of the provided amplification at various upper-limb flexion and extension ranges. Lastly, a larger study will be conducted to increase statistical power.

Author Contributions: Conceptualization, P.K., D.R. and A.U.-Q.; methodology, P.K., D.R. and A.U.-Q.; software, P.K.; validation, P.K., D.R. and A.U.-Q.; formal analysis, P.K., D.R. and A.U.-Q.; investigation, P.K., D.R. and A.U.-Q.; data curation, P.K.; writing—original draft preparation, P.K. and A.U.-Q.; writing—review and editing, P.K., D.R. and A.U.-Q.; supervision, A.U.-Q. and D.R.; project administration, A.U.-Q.; funding acquisition, A.U.-Q. All authors have read and agreed to the published version of the manuscript.

Funding: This research was funded by Natural Sciences and Engineering Research Council of Canada (NSERC) grant number RGPIN-2018-05917.

Institutional Review Board Statement: The study was conducted in accordance with the Declaration of Helsinki, and approved by the Institutional Review Board (or Ethics Committee) of Ontario Tech University [16652] on 7 March 2022.

Informed Consent Statement: Informed consent was obtained from all subjects involved in the study.

Data Availability Statement: The data are presented in aggregated format within this manuscript throughout the results section.

Acknowledgments: The authors would like to thank the support of the GAMER Lab at Ontario Tech University.

Conflicts of Interest: The authors declare no conflict of interest.

Abbreviations

The following abbreviations are used in this manuscript:

3DUI	3D User Interface
3DMT	3D Manipulation Technique
CFs	Control Factors
COVID-19	Coronavirus Disease of 2019
DFs	Distraction Factors
DK	Development Kit
DOFs	Degrees of Freedom
GEQ	Game Engagement Questionnaire
GUI	Graphical User Interface
HMD	Head-Mounted Display
INV/C	Involvement/Control
M	Mean
N	Normal
NAT	Natural
OT	Object Translation
P	Piecewise
PQ	Presence Questionnaire
RBNLIA	Reach-Bounded Non-Linear Input Amplification
RFs	Realism Factors
SD	Standard Deviation
SDK	Software Development Kit
SFs	Sensory Factors
VR	Virtual Reality
VRTK	Virtual Reality Toolkit

References

1. Chen, F.Q.; Leng, Y.F.; Ge, J.F.; Wang, D.W.; Li, C.; Chen, B.; Sun, Z.L. Effectiveness of virtual reality in nursing education: Meta-analysis. *J. Med. Internet Res.* **2020**, *22*, 1–13. [CrossRef] [PubMed]
2. King, D.; Tee, S.; Falconer, L.; Angell, C.; Holley, D.; Mills, A. Virtual health education: Scaling practice to transform student learning: Using virtual reality learning environments in healthcare education to bridge the theory/practice gap and improve patient safety. *Nurse Educ. Today* **2018**, *71*, 7–9. [CrossRef] [PubMed]
3. Monsky, W.L.; James, R.; Seslar, S.S. Virtual and Augmented Reality Applications in Medicine and Surgery-The Fantastic Voyage is here. *Anat. Physiol. Curr. Res.* **2019**, *9*, 1–6. [CrossRef]
4. Hansberger, J.T.; Peng, C.; Mathis, S.L.; Areyur Shanthakumar, V.; Meacham, S.C.; Cao, L.; Blakely, V.R. Dispelling the Gorilla Arm Syndrome: The Viability of Prolonged Gesture Interactions. In *Virtual, Augmented and Mixed Reality*; Lackey, S., Chen, J., Eds.; Springer International Publishing: Berlin/Heidelberg, Germany, 2017; pp. 505–520. [CrossRef]
5. Rietzler, M.; Geiselhart, F.; Gugenheimer, J.; Rukzio, E. Breaking the tracking: Enabling weight perception using perceivable tracking offsets. In Proceedings of the Conference on Human Factors in Computing Systems, Montreal, QC, Canada, 21–26 April 2018. [CrossRef]
6. Shafer, D.M.; Carbonara, C.P.; Korpi, M.F. Factors affecting enjoyment of virtual reality games: A comparison involving consumer-grade virtual reality technology. *Games Health J.* **2019**, *8*, 15–23. [CrossRef] [PubMed]
7. Flavián, C.; Ibáñez-Sánchez, S.; Orús, C. The impact of virtual, augmented and mixed reality technologies on the customer experience. *J. Bus. Res.* **2019**, *100*, 547–560. [CrossRef]
8. Openshaw, S.; Taylor, E. *Ergonomics and Design A Reference Guide*; Allsteel: Darby, PA, USA, 2006.
9. Coquand, T.; Danielsson, N.A. Isomorphism is equality. *Indag. Math.* **2013**, *24*, 1105–1120. [CrossRef]
10. Montano Murillo, R.A.; Subramanian, S.; Plasencia, D.M. *Erg-O*: Ergonomic optimization of immersive virtual environments. In Proceedings of the UIST 2017 30th Annual ACM Symposium on User Interface Software and Technology, Quebec City, QC, Canada, 22–25 October 2017; pp. 759–771. [CrossRef]
11. Hiramoto, K.; Hamamoto, K. Study on the Difference of Reaching Cognition between the Real and the Virtual Environment Using HMD and its Compensation. In Proceedings of the BMEiCON 2018 11th Biomedical Engineering International Conference, Chiang Mai, Thailand, 21–24 November 2018; pp. 8–12. [CrossRef]

12. Rothe, S.; Kegeles, B.; Allary, M.; Hußmann, H. The impact of camera height in cinematic virtual reality. In Proceedings of the ACM Symposium on Virtual Reality Software and Technology, VRST, Tokyo, Japan, 28 November–1 December 2018; pp. 9–10. [CrossRef]
13. Kim, J.S.; An, B.H.; Jeong, W.B.; Lee, S.W. Estimation of Interpupillary Distance Based on Eye Movements in Virtual Reality Devices. *IEEE Access* **2021**, *9*, 155576–155583. [CrossRef]
14. Li, J.; Cho, I.; Wartell, Z. Evaluation of cursor offset on 3D selection in VR. In Proceedings of the SUI 2018 Symposium on Spatial User Interaction, Berlin, Germany, 13–14 October 2018; pp. 120–129. [CrossRef]
15. Lisle, L.; Lu, F.; Davari, S.; Tahmid, I.A.; Giovannelli, A.; Llo, C.; Pavanatto, L.; Zhang, L.; Schlueter, L.; Bowman, D.A. Clean the Ocean: An Immersive VR Experience Proposing New Modifications to Go-Go and WiM Techniques. In Proceedings of the 2022 IEEE Conference on Virtual Reality and 3D User Interfaces Abstracts and Workshops (VRW), Christchurch, New Zealand, 12–16 March 2022; pp. 920–921.
16. Kintschner, N.R.; Liporace, T.L.; Blascovi-Assis, S.M.; Corrêa, A.G.D. The Use of Leap Motion in Manual Dexterity Testing by the Box and Blocks Test: A Review Study. In *Vision Sensors—Recent Advances*; Gallegos-Funes, D.F.J., Ed.; IntechOpen: Rijeka, Croatia, 2022; Chapter 5. [CrossRef]
17. Wentzel, J.; D'Eon, G.; Vogel, D. Improving Virtual Reality Ergonomics Through Reach-Bounded Non-Linear Input Amplification. In Proceedings of the Conference on Human Factors in Computing Systems, Honolulu, HI, USA, 25–30 April 2020; pp. 1–12. [CrossRef]
18. Alves, S.F.; Sivanathan, M.; Micallef, J.; Gino, B.; Mnaymneh, M.; Dubrowski, A.; Uribe-Quevedo, A. Cricothyroidotomy Simulator: A Makerspace and Augmented Reality Approach. In Proceedings of the 2022 IEEE Games, Entertainment, Media Conference (GEM), St. Michael, Bridgetown, Barbados, 27–30 November 2022; pp. 1–4.
19. Tabafunda, A.; Matthews, S.; Akhter, R.; Uribe-Quevedo, A.; Sun, W.; Horsburgh, S.; LaFontaine, C. Development of a non-immersive VR reminiscence therapy experience for patients with dementia. In Proceedings of the HCI International 2020–Late Breaking Posters: 22nd International Conference, HCII 2020, Copenhagen, Denmark, 19–24 July 2020; Proceedings, Part II; Springer: Berlin/Heidelberg, Germany, 2020; pp. 509–517.
20. Alves, S.F.; Uribe-Quevedo, A.; Chen, D.; Morris, J.; Radmard, S. Developing a VR simulator for robotics navigation and human robot interactions employing digital twins. In Proceedings of the 2022 IEEE Conference on Virtual Reality and 3D User Interfaces Abstracts and Workshops (VRW), Christchurch, New Zealand, 12–16 March 2022; pp. 121–125.
21. Unity3d. *Unity Real-Time Development Platform | 3D, 2D VR & AR Engine*; Unity Technologies: Seoul, Republic of Korea, 2020. Available online: https://unity.com/ (accessed on 1 March 2022).
22. Unity Technologies. Unity—Manual: OpenVR. Available online: https://docs.unity3d.com/Manual/VRDevices-OpenVR.html (accessed on 10 April 2023).
23. Feick, M.; Kleer, N.; Tang, A.; Krüger, A. The Virtual Reality Questionnaire Toolkit. In Proceedings of the UIST '20 Adjunct: 33rd Annual ACM Symposium on User Interface Software and Technology, Virtual, 20–23 October 2020. [CrossRef]
24. Law, E.L.C.; Brühlmann, F.; Mekler, E.D. Systematic review and validation of the game experience questionnaire (geq)-implications for citation and reporting practice. In Proceedings of the 2018 Annual Symposium on Computer-Human Interaction in Play, Melbourne, Australia, 28–31 October 2018; pp. 257–270.
25. Witmer, B.G.; Singer, M.J. Measuring Presence in Virtual Environments: A Presence Questionnaire. *ACM Comput. Surv.* **1998**, 7, 225–240. [CrossRef]
26. Facebook Technologies LLC. DistanceGrab Sample Scene. 2020. Available online: https://developer.oculus.com/documentation/unity/unity-sf-distancegrab/ (accessed on 1 February 2022).
27. Public Health Informatics Institute. Desk and Work Surface Height. In Health by Design. 2012. Available online: https://shop.healthydesign.com/Desk-and-work-surface-height.aspx (accessed on 1 May 2021).

sensors

MDPI

Review

In-Depth Review of Augmented Reality: Tracking Technologies, Development Tools, AR Displays, Collaborative AR, and Security Concerns

Toqeer Ali Syed [1], Muhammad Shoaib Siddiqui [1], Hurria Binte Abdullah [2], Salman Jan [3,4,*], Abdallah Namoun [1], Ali Alzahrani [1], Adnan Nadeem [1] and Ahmad B. Alkhodre [1]

1 Faculty of Computer and Information Systems, Islamic University of Madinah, Medina 42351, Saudi Arabia
2 School of Social Sciences and Humanities, National University of Science and Technology (NUST), Islamabad 44000, Pakistan
3 Malaysian Institute of Information Technology, Universiti Kuala Lumpur, Kuala Lumpur 50250, Malaysia
4 Department of Computer Science, Bacha Khan University Charsadda, Charsadda 24420, Pakistan
* Correspondence: salman.jan@unikl.edu.my

Abstract: Augmented reality (AR) has gained enormous popularity and acceptance in the past few years. AR is indeed a combination of different immersive experiences and solutions that serve as integrated components to assemble and accelerate the augmented reality phenomena as a workable and marvelous adaptive solution for many realms. These solutions of AR include tracking as a means for keeping track of the point of reference to make virtual objects visible in a real scene. Similarly, display technologies combine the virtual and real world with the user's eye. Authoring tools provide platforms to develop AR applications by providing access to low-level libraries. The libraries can thereafter interact with the hardware of tracking sensors, cameras, and other technologies. In addition to this, advances in distributed computing and collaborative augmented reality also need stable solutions. The various participants can collaborate in an AR setting. The authors of this research have explored many solutions in this regard and present a comprehensive review to aid in doing research and improving different business transformations. However, during the course of this study, we identified that there is a lack of security solutions in various areas of collaborative AR (CAR), specifically in the area of distributed trust management in CAR. This research study also proposed a trusted CAR architecture with a use-case of tourism that can be used as a model for researchers with an interest in making secure AR-based remote communication sessions.

Keywords: trusted augmented reality; augmented reality review; collaborative augmented reality; virtual reality review; display and tracking technology; display technologies in augmented reality

Citation: Syed, T.A.; Siddiqui, M.S.; Abdullah, H.B.; Jan, S.; Namoun, A.; Alzahrani, A.; Nadeem, A.; Alkhodre, A.B. In-Depth Review of Augmented Reality: Tracking Technologies, Development Tools, AR Displays, Collaborative AR, and Security Concerns. *Sensors* **2023**, *23*, 146. https://doi.org/10.3390/s23010146

Academic Editors: Calin Gheorghe Dan Neamtu, Radu Comes, Jing-Jing Fang and Dorin-Mircea Popovici

Received: 25 October 2022
Revised: 11 December 2022
Accepted: 13 December 2022
Published: 23 December 2022

1. Introduction

Augmented reality (AR) is one of the leading expanding immersive experiences of the 21st century. AR has brought a revolution in different realms including health and medicine, teaching and learning, tourism, designing, manufacturing, and other similar industries whose acceptance accelerated the growth of AR in an unprecedented manner [1–3]. According to a recent report in September 2022, the market size of AR and VR reached USD 27.6 billion in 2021, which is indeed estimated to reach USD 856.2 billion by the end of the year 2031 [4]. Big companies largely use AR-based technologies. For instance, Amazon, one of the leading online shopping websites, uses this technology to make it easier for customers to decide the type of furniture they want to buy. The rise in mobile phone technology also acted as an accelerator in popularizing AR. Earlier, mobile phones were not advanced and capable enough to run these applications due to their low graphics. Nowadays, however, smart devices are capable enough to easily run AR-based applications. A lot of research has been done on mobile-based AR. Lee et al. [5] developed a user-based design interface for educational purpose in mobile AR. To evaluate its conduct, fourth-grade elementary students were selected.

The adoption of AR in its various perspectives is backed up by a prolonged history. This paper presents an overview of the different integrated essential components that contribute to the working framework of AR, and the latest developments on these components are collected, analyzed, and presented, while the developments in the smart devices and the overall experience of the users have changed drastically [6]. The tracking technologies [7] are the building blocks of AR and establish a point of reference for movement and for creating an environment where the virtual and real objects are presented together. To achieve a real experience with augmented objects, several tracking technologies are presented which include techniques such as sensor-based [8], markerless, marker-based [9,10], and hybrid tracking technologies. Among these different technologies, hybrid tracking technologies are the most adaptive. As part of the framework constructed in this study, the simultaneous localization and mapping (SLAM) and inertial tracking technologies are combined. The SLAM technology collects points through cameras in real scenes while the point of reference is created using inertial tracking . The virtual objects are inserted on the relevant points of reference to create an augmented reality. Moreover, this paper analyzes and presents a detailed discussion on different tracking technologies according to their use in different realms i.e., in education, industries, and medical fields. Magnetic tracking is widely used in AR systems in medical, maintenance, and manufacturing. Moreover, vision-based tracking is mostly used in mobile phones and tablets because they have screen and camera, which makes them the best platform for AR. In addition, GPS tracking is useful in the fields of military, gaming, and tourism. These tracking technologies along with others are explained in detail in Section 3.

Once the points of reference are collected after tracking, then another important factor that requires significant accuracy is to determine at which particular point the virtual objects have to be mixed with the real environment. Here comes the role of display technologies that gives the users of augmented reality an environment where the real and virtual objects are displayed visually. Therefore, display technologies are one of the key components of AR. This research identifies state-of-the-art display technologies that help to provide a quality view of real and virtual objects. Augmented reality displays can be divided into various categories. All have the same task to show the merged image of real and virtual content to the user's eye. The authors have categorized the latest technologies of optical display after the advancements in holographic optical elements (HOEs). There are other categories of AR displays, such as video-based, eye multiplexed, and projected onto a physical surface. Optical see-through has two sub-categories, one is a free-space combiner and the other is a wave-guide combiner [11,12]. The thorough details of display technologies are presented in Section 4.

To develop these AR applications, different tools are used depending on the type of application used. For example, to develop a mobile-based AR application for Android or iOS, ARToolKit [13] is used. However, FLARToolKit [14] is used to create a web-based application using Flash. Moreover, there are various plug-ins available that can be integrated with Unity [15] to create AR applications. These development tools are reviewed in Section 6 of this paper. Figure 1 provides an overview of reviewed topics of augmented reality in this paper.

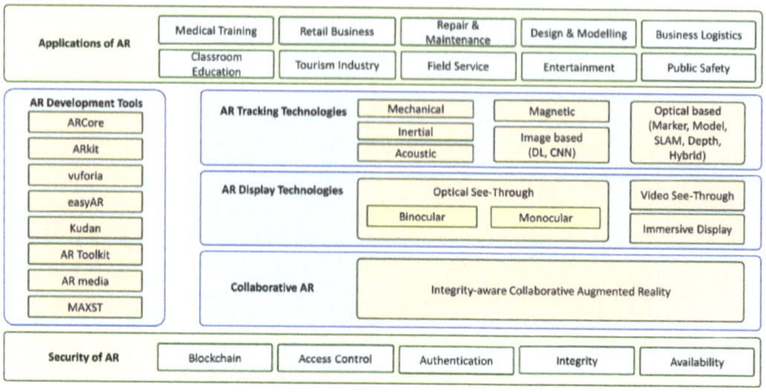

Figure 1. Overview of AR, VR, and collaborative AR applications, tools, and technologies.

After going through a critical review process of collaborative augmented reality, the research has identified that some security flaws and missing trust parameters need to be addressed to ensure a pristine environment is provided to the users. Hackers and intruders are always active to exploit different vulnerabilities in the systems and software, but the previous research conducted on collaborative augmented reality did not depict reasonable efforts made in this direction to make secure collaboration. To address the security flaws and to provide secure communication in collaborative augmented reality, this research considered it appropriate to come up with a security solution and framework that can limit danger and risks that may be posed in the form of internal and external attacks. To actualize the secure platform, this study came up with an architecture for presenting a secure collaborative AR in the tourism sector in Saudi Arabia as a case study. The focus of the case study is to provide an application that can guide tourists during their visit to any of the famous landmarks in the country. This study proposed a secure and trustful mobile application based on collaborative AR for tourists. In this application, the necessary information is rendered on screen and the user can hire a guide to provide more information in detail. A single guide can provide the services to a group of tourists visiting the same landmark. A blockchain network was used to secure the applications and protect the private data of the users [16,17]. For this purpose, we performed a thorough literature review for an optimized solution regarding security and tracking for which we studies the existing tracking technologies and listed them in this paper along with their limitations. In our use case, we used a GPS tracking system to track the user's movement and provide the necessary information about the visited landmark through the mobile application.

Observing the fact that AR operates in an integrated fashion that combines different technologies including tracking technologies, display technologies, AR tools, collaborative AR, and applications of AR has encouraged us to explore and present these conceptions and technologies in detail. To facilitate researchers on these different techniques, the authors have explored the research previously conducted and presented it in a Venn diagram, as shown in Figure 2. Interested investigators can choose their required area of research in AR. As can be seen in the diagram, most research has been done in the area of tracking technologies. This is further divided into different types of tracking solutions including fiducial tracking, video-based tracking, and inertial tracking. Some papers lie in several categories for, example some papers such as [18–20] fall in both the fiducial tracking and sensor categories. Similarly, computer vision and display devices have some common papers, and inertial tracking and video-based tracking also have some papers in common. In addition, display devices share common papers with computer vision, mobile AR, design guidelines, tool-kits, evaluation, AR tags, and security and privacy of AR. Furthermore, visualization has different papers in common with business, interior design, and human–robot communication. While education shares some paper with gaming, simulation, medicine, heritage, and manufacturing. In short, we have tried to summarize all papers and further elaborate in their sections for the convenience of the reader.

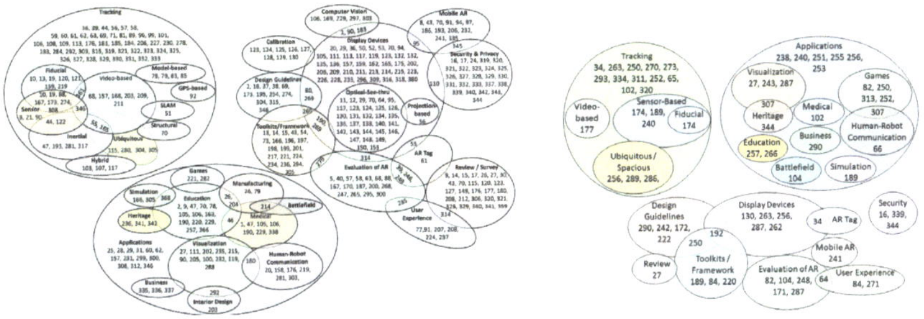

Papers related to Tracking, Display, Authoring Tools, Application, and security

Paper that Cover Collaborative Augmented Reality Only

Figure 2. Classification of reviewed papers with respect to tracking, display, authoring tools, application, Collaborative and security

Contribution: This research presents a comprehensive review of AR and its associated technologies. A review of state-of-the-art tracking and display technologies is presented followed by different essential components and tools that can be used to effectively create AR experiences. The study also presents the newly emerging technologies such as collaborative augmented reality and how different application interactions are carried out. During the review phase, the research identified that the AR-based solutions and particularly collaborative augmented reality solutions are vulnerable to external intrusion. It is identified that these solutions lack security and the interaction could be hijacked, manipulated, and sometimes exposed to potential threats. To address these concerns, this research felt the need to ensure that the communication has integrity; henceforth, the research utilizes the state-of-the-art blockchain infrastructure for the collaborating applications in AR. The paper further proposes complete secure framework wherein different applications working remotely have a real feeling of trust with each other [21].

Outline: This paper presents the overview of augmented reality and its applications in various realms in Section 2. In Section 3, tracking technologies are presented, while a detailed overview of the display technologies is provided in Section 4. Section 6 apprises readers on AR development tools. Section 7 highlights the collaborative research on augmented reality, while Section 8 interprets the AR interaction and input technologies. The paper presents the details of design guidelines and interface patterns in Section 9, while Section 10 discusses the security and trust issues in collaborative AR. Section 12 highlights future directions for research, while Section 13 concludes this research.

2. Augmented Reality Overview

People, for many years, have been using lenses, light sources, and mirrors to create illusions and virtual images in the real world [22–24]. However, Ivan Sutherland was the first person to truly generate the AR experience. Sketchpad, developed at MIT in 1963 by Ivan Sutherland, is the world's first interactive graphic application [25]. In Figure 3, we have given an overview of the development of AR technology from the beginning to 2022. Bottani et al. [26] reviews the AR literature published during the time period of 2006–2017. Moreover, Sereno et al. [27] use a systematic survey approach to detail the existing literature available on the intersection of computer-supported collaborative work and AR.

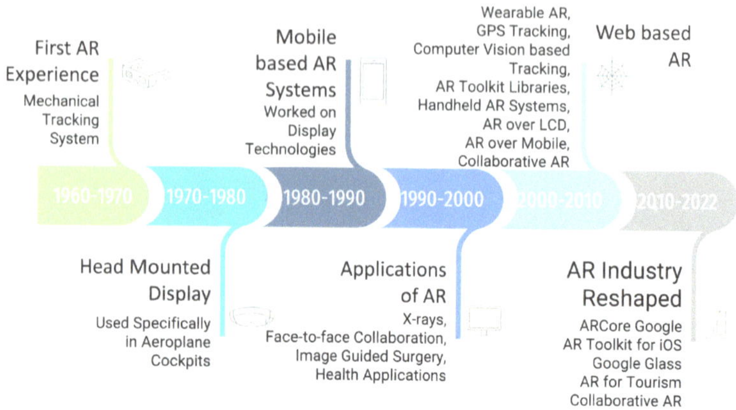

Figure 3. Augmented reality advancement over time for the last 60 years.

2.1. *Head-Mounted Display*

Ens et al. [28] review the existing work on design exploration for mixed-scale gestures where the Hololens AR display is used to interweave larger gestures with micro-gestures.

2.2. *AR Towards Applications*

ARToolKit tracking library [13] aimed to provide the computer vision tracking of a square marker in real-time which fixed two major problems, i.e., enabling interaction with real-world objects and secondly, the user's viewpoint tracking system. Researchers conducted studies to develop handheld AR systems. Hettig et al. [29] present a system called "Augmented Visualization Box" to asses surgical augmented reality visualizations in a virtual environment. Goh et al. [30] present details of the critical analysis of 3D interaction techniques in mobile AR. Kollatsch et al. [31] introduce a system that creates and introduces the production data and maintenance documentation into the AR maintenance apps for machine tools which aims to reduce the overall cost of necessary expertise and the planning process of AR technology. Bhattacharyya et al. [32] introduce a two-player mobile AR game known as Brick, where users can engage in synchronous collaboration while inhabiting the real-time and shared augmented environment. Kim et al. [33] suggest that this decade is marked by a tremendous technological boom particularly in rendering and evaluation research while display and calibration research has declined. Liu et al. [34] expand the information feedback channel from industrial robots to a human workforce for human–robot collaboration development.

2.3. *Augmented Reality for the Web*

Cortes et al. [35] introduce the new techniques of collaboratively authoring surfaces on the web using mobile AR. Qiao et al. [36] review the current implementations of mobile AR, enabling technologies of AR, state-of-art technology, approaches for potential web AR provisioning, and challenges that AR faces in a web-based system.

2.4. *AR Application Development*

The AR industry was tremendously increasing in 2015, extending from smartphones to websites with head-worn display systems such as Google Glass. In this regard, Agati et al. [18] propose design guidelines for the development of an AR manual assembly system which includes ergonomics, usability, corporate-related, and cognition.

AR for Tourism and Education: Shukri et al. [37] aim to introduce the design guidelines of mobile AR for tourism by proposing 11 principles for developing efficient AR design for tourism which reduces cognitive overload, provides learning ability, and helps explore the content while traveling in Malaysia. In addition to it, Fallahkhair et al. [38] introduce new guidelines to make AR technologies with enhanced user satisfaction, efficiency, and effectiveness in cultural and contextual learning using mobiles, thereby enhancing the tourism experience. Akccayir et al. [39] show that AR has the advantage of placing the virtual image on a real object in real time while pedagogical and technical issues should be addressed to make the technology more reliable. Salvia et al. [40] suggest that AR has a positive impact on learning but requires some advancements.

Sarkar et al. [41] present an AR app known as ScholAR. It introduces enhancing the learning skills of the students to inculcate conceptualizing and logical thinking among sevemth-grade students. Soleiman et al. [42] suggest that the use of AR improves abstract writing as compared to VR.

2.5. AR Security and Privacy

Hadar et al. [43] scrutinize security at all steps of AR application development and identify the need for new strategies for information security, privacy, and security, with a main goal to design and introduce capturing and mapping concerns. Moreover, in the industrial arena, Mukhametshin et al. [44] focus on developing sensor tag detection, tracking, and recognition for designing an AR client-side app for Siemen Company to monitor the equipment for remote facilities.

3. Tracking Technology of AR

Tracking technologies introduce the sensation of motion in the virtual and augmented reality world and perform a variety of tasks. Once a tracking system is rightly chosen and correctly installed, it allows a person to move within a virtual and augmented environment. It further allows us to interact with people and objects within augmented environments. The selection of tracking technology depends on the sort of environment, the sort of data, and the availability of required budgets. For AR technology to meet Azuma's definition of an augmented reality system, it must adhere to three main components:

1. it combines virtual and the real content;
2. it is interactive in real time;
3. is is registered in three dimensions.

The third condition of being "registered in three dimensions" alludes to the capability of an AR system to project the virtual content on physical surroundings in such a way that it seems to be part of the real world. The position and orientation (pose) of the viewer concerning some anchor in the real world must be identified and determined for registering the virtual content in the real environment. This anchor of the real world may be the dead-reckoning from inertial tracking, a defined location in space determined using GPS, or a physical object such as a paper image marker or magnetic tracker source. In short, the real-world anchor depends upon the applications and the technologies used. With respect to the type of technology used, there are two ways of registering the AR system in 3D:

- Determination of the position and orientation of the viewer relative to the real-world anchor: registration phase;
- Upgrading of viewer's pose with respect to previously known pose: tracking phase.

In this document, the word "tracking" would define both phases as common terminology. There are two main types of tracking techniques which are explained as follows (depicted in Figure 4).

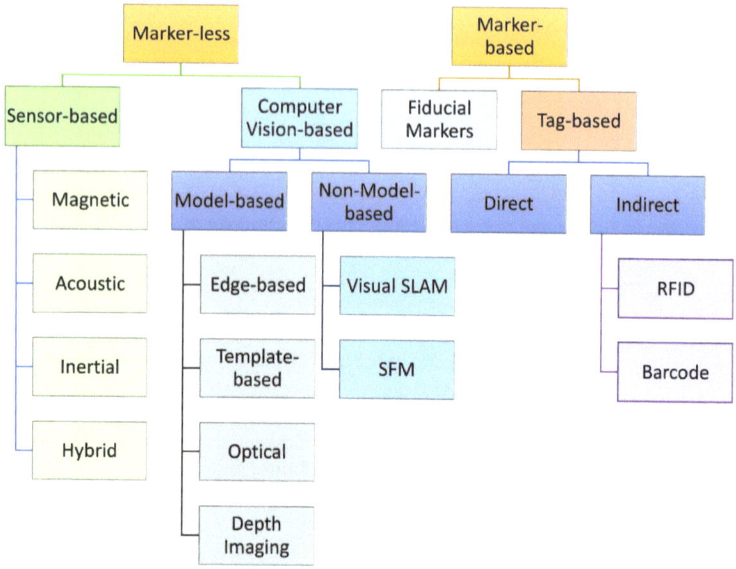

Figure 4. Categorization of augmented reality tracking techniques.

3.1. Markerless Tracking Techniques

Markerless tracking techniques further have two types, one is sensor based and another is vision based.

3.1.1. Sensor-Based Tracking

Magnetic Tracking Technology: This technology includes a tracking source and two sensors, one sensor for the head and another one for the hand. The tracking source creates an electromagnetic field in which the sensors are placed. The computer then calculates the orientation and position of the sensors based on the signal attenuation of the field. This gives the effect of allowing a full 360 range of motion. i.e., allowing us to look all the way around the 3D environment. It also allows us to move around all three degrees of freedom. The hand tracker has some control buttons that allow the user to navigate along the environment. It allows us to pick things up and understand the size and shape of the objects [45]. In Figure 5 we have tried to draw the tracking techniques to give a better understanding to the reader.

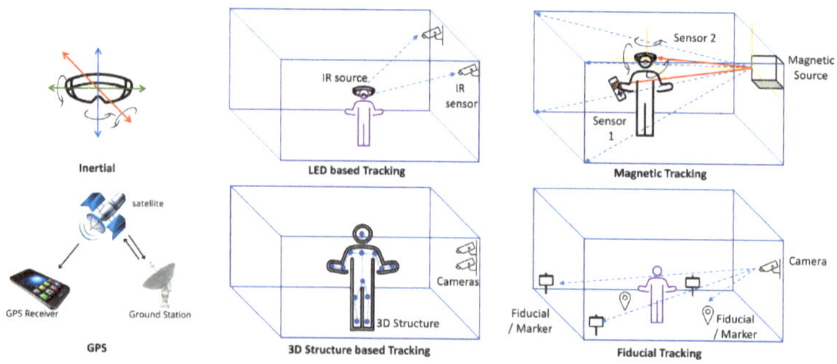

Figure 5. Augmented reality tracking techniques presentation.

Frikha et al. [46] introduce a new mutual occlusion problem handler. The problem of occlusion occurs when the real objects are in front of the virtual objects in the scene. The authors use a 3D positioning approach and surgical instrument tracking in an AR environment. The paradigm is introduced that is based on monocular image-based processing. The result of the experiment suggested that this approach is capable of handling mutual occlusion automatically in real-time.

One of the main issues with magnetic tracking is the limited positioning range [47]. Orientation and position can be determined by setting up the receiver to the viewer [48]. Receivers are small and light in weight and the magnetic trackers are indifferent to optical disturbances and occlusion; therefore, these have high update rates. However, the resolution magnetic field declines with the fourth power of the distance, and the strength of magnetic fields decline with the cube of the distance [49]. Therefore, the magnetic trackers have constrained working volume. Moreover, magnetic trackers are sensitive to environments around magnetic fields and the type of magnetic material used and are also susceptible to measurement jitter [50].

Magnetic tracking technology is widely used in the range of AR systems, with applications ranging from maintenance [51] to medicine [52] and manufacturing [53].

Inertial Tracking: Magnetometers, accelerometers, and gyroscopes are examples of inertial measurement units (IMU) used in inertial tracking to evaluate the velocity and orientation of the tracked object. An inertial tracking system is used to find the three rotational degrees of freedom relative to gravity. Moreover, the time period of the trackers' update and the inertial velocity can be determined by the change in the position of the tracker.

Advantages of Inertial Tracking: It does not require a line of sight and has no range limitations. It is not prone to optical, acoustic, magnetic, and RE interference sources. Furthermore, it provides motion measurement with high bandwidth. Moreover, it has negligible latency and can be processed as fast as one desires.

Disadvantages of Inertial Tracking: They are prone to drift of orientation and position over time, but their major impact is on the position measurement. The rationale behind this is that the position must be derived from the velocity measurements. The usage of a filter could help in resolving this issue. However, the issue could while focusing on this, the filter can decrease the responsiveness and the update rate of the tracker [54]. For the ultimate correction of this issue of the drift, the inertial sensor should be combined with any other kind of sensor. For instance, it could be combined with ultrasonic range measurement devices and optical trackers.

3.1.2. Vision-Based Tracking

Vision-based tracking is defined as tracking approaches that ascertain the camera pose by the use of data captured from optical sensors and as registration. The optical sensors can be divided into the following three categories:

- visible light tracking;
- 3D structure tracking;
- infrared tracking.

In recent times, vision-based tracking AR is becoming highly popular due to the improved computational power of consumer devices and the ubiquity of mobile devices, such as tablets and smartphones, thereby making them the best platform for AR technologies. Chakrabarty et al. [55] contribute to the development of autonomous tracking by integrating the CMT into IBVS, their impact on the rigid deformable targets in indoor settings, and finally the integration of the system into the Gazebo simulator. Vision-based tracking is demonstrated by the use of an effective object tracking algorithm [56] known as the clustering of static-adaptive correspondences for deformable object tracking (CMT). Gupta et al. [57] detail the comparative analysis between the different types of vision-based tracking systems.

Moreover, Krishna et al. [58] explore the use of electroencephalogram (EEG) signals in user authentication. User authentication is similar to facial recognition in mobile phones. Moreover, this is also evaluated by combining it with eye-tracking data. This research contributes to the development of a novel evaluation paradigm and a biometric authentication system for the integration of these systems. Furthermore, Dzsotjan et al. [59] delineate the usefulness of the eye-tracking data evaluated during the lectures in order to determine the learning gain of the user. Microsoft HoloLens2's designed Walk the Graph app was used to generate the data. Binary classification was performed on the basis of the kinematic graphs which users reported of their own movement.

Ranging from smartphones to laptops and even to wearable devices with suitable cameras located in them, visible light tracking is the most commonly used optical sensor. These cameras are particularly important because they can both make a video of the real environment and can also register the virtual content to it, and thereby can be used in video see-through AR systems.

Chen et al. [60] resolve the shortcomings of the deep learning lightning model (DAM) by combining the method of transferring a regular video to a 3D photo-realistic avatar and a high-quality 3D face tracking algorithm. The evaluation of the proposed system suggests its effectiveness in real-world scenarios when we have variability in expression, pose, and illumination. Furthermore, Rambach et al. [61] explore the details pipeline of 6DoF object tracking using scanned 3D images of the objects. The scope of research covers the initialization of frame-to-frame tracking, object registration, and implementation of these aspects to make the experience more efficient. Moreover, it resolves the challenges that we faced with occlusion, illumination changes, and fast motion.

3.1.3. Three-Dimensional Structure Tracking

Three-dimensional structure information has become very affordable because of the development of commercial sensors capable of accomplishing this task. It was begun after the development of Microsoft Kinect [62]. Syahidi et al. [63] introduce a 3D AR-based learning system for pre-school children. For determining the three-dimensional points in the scene, different types of sensors could be used. The most commonly used are the structured lights [64] or the time of flight [65]. These technologies work on the principle of depth analysis. In this, the real environment depth information is extracted by the mapping and the tracking [66]. The Kinect system [67], developed by Microsoft, is one of the widely used and well-developed approaches in Augmented Reality.

Rambach et al. [68] present the idea of augmented things: utilizing off-screen rendering of 3D objects, the realization of application architecture, universal 3D object tracking based on the high-quality scans of the objects, and a high degree of parallelization. Viyanon et al. [69] focus on the development of an AR app known as "AR Furniture" for providing the experience of visualizing the design and decoration to the customers. The customers fit the pieces of furniture in their rooms and were able to make a decision regarding their experience. Turkan et al. [70] introduce the new models for teaching structural analysis which has considerably improved the learning experience. The model integrates 3D visualization technology with mobile AR. Students can enjoy the different loading conditions by having the choice of switching loads, and feedback can be provided in the real-time by AR interface.

3.1.4. Infrared Tracking

The objects that emitted or reflected the light are some of the earliest vision-based tracking techniques used in AR technologies. Their high brightness compared to their surrounding environment made this tracking very easy [71,72]. The self-light emitting targets were also indifferent to the drastic illumination effects i.e., harsh shadows or poor ambient lighting. In addition, these targets could either be transfixed to the object being tracked and camera at the exterior of the object and was known as "outside-looking-in" [73]. Or it could be "inside-looking-out", external in the environment with camera attached to the target [74]. The inside-looking-out configuration, compared to the sensor of the inside-looking-out system, has greater resolution and higher accuracy of angular orientation. The inside-looking-out configuration is used in the development of several systems [20,75–77], typically with infrared LEDs mounted on the ceiling and a head-mounted display with a camera facing externally.

3.1.5. Model-Based Tracking

The three-dimensional tracking of real-world objects has been the subject of researchers' interest. It is not as popular as natural feature tracking or planner fiducials, however, a large amount of research has been done on it. In the past, tracking the three-dimensional model of the object was usually created by the hand. In this system, the lines, cylinders, spheres, circles, and other primitives were combined to identify the structure of objects [78]. Wuest et al. [79] focus on the development of the scalable and performance pipeline for creating a tracking solution. The structural information of the scene was extracted by using the edge filters. Additionally, for the determination of the pose, edge information and the primitives were matched [80].

In addition, Gao et al. [81] explore the tracking method to identify the different vertices of a convex polygon. This is done successfully as most of the markers are square. The coordinates of four vertices are used to determine the transformation matrix of the camera. Results of the experiment suggested that the algorithm was so robust to withstand fast motion and large ranges that make the tracking more accurate, stable, and real time.

The combination of edge-based tracking and natural feature tracking has the following advantages:

- It provides additional robustness [82].
- Enables spatial tracking and thereby is able to be operated in open environments [83].
- For variable and complex environments, greater robustness was required. Therefore, they introduced the concept of keyframes [84] in addition to the primitive model [85].

Figen et al. [86] demonstrate of a series of studies that were done at the university level in which participants were asked to make the mass volume of buildings. The first study demanded the solo work of a designer in which they had to work using two tools: MTUIs of the AR apps and analog tools. The second study developed the collaboration of the designers while using analog tools. The study has two goals: change in the behavior of the designer while using AR apps and affordances of different interfaces.

Developing and updating the real environment's map simultaneously had been the subject of interest in model-based tracking. This has a number of developments. First, simultaneous localization and map building (SLAM) was primarily done for robot navigation in unknown environments [87]. In augmented reality, [88,89], this technique was used for tracking the unknown environment in a drift-free manner. Second, parallel mapping and tracking [88] was developed especially for AR technology. In this, the mapping of environmental components and the camera tracks were identified as a separate function. It improved tracking accuracy and also overall performance. However, like SLAM, it did not have the capability to close large loops in the constrained environment and area (Figure 6).

Oskiper et al. [90] propose a simultaneous localization and mapping (SLAM) framework for sensor fusion, indexing, and feature matching in AR apps. It has a parallel mapping engine and error-state extended Kalman filter (EKF) for these purposes. Zhang et al.'s [91] Jaguar is a mobile tracking AR application with low latency and flexible object tracking. This paper discusses the design, execution, and evaluation of Jaguar. Jaguar enables a markerless tracking feature which is enabled through its client development on top of ARCoreest from Google. ARCore is also helpful for context awareness while estimating and recognizing the physical size and object capabilities, respectively.

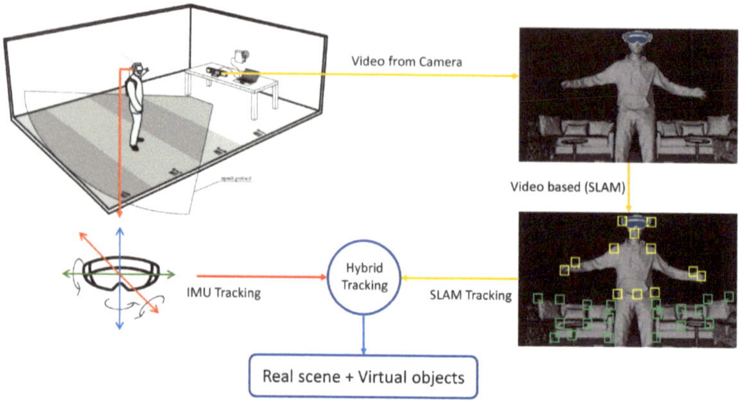

Figure 6. Hybrid tracking: inertial and SLAM combined and used in the latest mobile-based AR tracking.

3.1.6. Global Positioning System—GPS Tracking

This technology refers to the positioning of outdoor tracking with reference to the earth. The present accuracy of the GPS system is up to 3 m. However, improvements are available with the advancements in satellite technology and a few other developments. Real-time kinematic (RTS) is one example of them. It works by using the carrier of a GPS signal. The major benefit of it is that it has the ability to improve the accuracy level up to the centimeter level. Feiner's touring machine [92] was the first AR system that utilized GPS in its tracking system. It used the inclinometer/magnetometer and differential GPS positional tracking. The military, gaming [93,94], and the viewership of historical data [95] have applied GPS tracking for the AR experiences. As it only has the supporting positional tracking low accuracy, it could only be beneficial in the hybrid tracking systems or in the applications where the pose registration is not important. AR et al. [96] use the GPS-INS receiver to develop models for object motion having more precision. Ashutosh et al. [97] explore the hardware challenges of AR technology and also explore the two main components of hardware technology: battery performance and global positioning system (GPS). Table 1 provides a succinct categorization of the prominent tracking technologies in augmented reality. Example studies are referred to while highlighting the advantages and challenges of each type of tracking technology. Moreover, possible areas of application are suggested.

3.1.7. Miscellaneous Tracking

Yang et al. [98], in order to recognize the different forms of hatch covers having similar shapes, propose tracking and cover recognition methods. The results of the experiment suggest its real-time property and practicability, and tracking accuracy was enough to be implemented in the AR inspection environment. Kang et al. [99] propose a pupil tracker which consists of several features that make AR more robust: key point alignment, eye-nose detection, and infrared (NIR) led. NIR led turns on and off based on the illumination light. The limitation of this detector is that it cannot be applied in low-light conditions.

Table 1. Summary of tracking techniques and their related attributes.

No.	Tracking Technology	Category of Tracking Technique	Status of Technique, Used in Current Devices	Tools/Company Currently Using the Technology	Key Concepts	Advantages	Challenges	Example Application Areas	Example Studies
1	Magnetic	Marker-less/Sensor based	Yes	i. Edge Tracking/Pemo etc. ii. Most HMD/Most Recent Android Devices	Sensors are placedwithin an electromagnetic field	+360 degree motion +navigation around the environments +manipulationof objects	-limited positioning range -constrained working volume -highly sensitive to surrounding environments	Maintenance Medicine Manufacturing	[45–53]
2	Inertial	Marker-less/Sensor based	Yes	ARCore/Unity	Motion sensors (e.g., accelerometers and gyroscopes) are used to determine the velocity and orientation of objects	+high-bandwidth motion measurement +Negligible latency	-drift overtime impacting position measurement	Transport Sports	[54]
3	Optical	Marker-less/Vision based	Yes	i. Unity ii. Opti Track Used in conguction with Inertial sensors + Optical (Vision Based) sensors	Virtual content is added to real environments through cameras and optical sensors.Example approaches include visible light, 3D structure, and infrared tracking.	+Popular due to affordable consumer devices +Strong tracking algorithms +Applicationto real-world scenarios	-occlusion when objects are in close range	Education and Learning E-commerce Tourism	[100,101]
4	Model Based i. Edge-Based ii. Template-Based iii. Depth Imaging	Marker-less/Computer Vision-based	Yes	i. VisionLib ii. Unity iii. ViSP	A 3D model is visualized of real objects	+implicit knowledge of the 3D structure +empowersspatial tracking +robustness is achieved even in complex environments	-algorithms are required to track and predict movements -models need to be created using dedicated tools and libraries	Manufacturing Construction Entertainment	[78–86]
5	GPS	Marker-less/Sensor based	Yes	i. ARCore/ARKit ii. Unity/ARFoundation iii. Vuforia	GPS sensors are employed to track the price location of objects in the environment	+high tracking accuracy (up to cms)	-hardware requirements -objects should be modelled ahead	Gaming	[102–107]
6	Hybrid	Marker-less/Sensor based/Computer Vision	Yes	i. ARCore ii. ARKit	A mix of markerless technologies is used to overcome the challenges of a single-tracking technology	+improved tracking range and accuracy +higher degree of freedom +lower drift and jitter	-the need for multiple technologies (e.g., accelerators, sensors) so cost issues	Simulation Transport	[108–111]
7	SLAM	Marker-less/Computer Vision/Non-Model-based	Yes	i. WikiTude ii. Unity iii. ARCore	A map is created via a vision of the real environment to track the virtual object on it.	Can track unknown environments, Parallel mapping engine	Does not have the capability to close large loops in the constrained environment	Mobile based AR Tracking, Robot Navigation,	[112–114]
8	Structure from Motion (SFM)	Marker-Less/Computer Vision/Non-Model-Based	Yes	i. SLAM ii. Research Based	3D model reconstruction approach based on Multi View Stereo	Can be used for estimating the 3D structure of a scene from a series of 2D images	Shows limited reconstruction ability in vegetated environments	3-D scanning , augmented reality, and visual simultaneous localization and mapping (vSLAM)	[90]
9	Fiducial/Landmark	Marker-based /Fiducial	Yes	i. Solar/Unity ii. Uniducial/Unity	Tracking is made with reference to artificial landmarks (i.e., markers) added to the AR environment	+better accuracy is achieved +stable tracking with less cost	-the need for landmarks -requires image recognition (i.e., camera) -less flexible compared to marker-based	Marketing	[115–117]
10	QR Code based Tracking	Marker-Based/Tag-Based	Yes	Microsoft Hololense/Immersive Headsets/Unity	Tracking is made	+better accuracyis achieved +stable tracking with less cost	QR codes pose significant security risks.	Supply Chain Management	[115]

Moreover, Bach et al. [118] introduce an AR canvas for information visualization which is quite different from the traditional AR canvas. Therefore, dimensions and essential aspects for developing the visualization design for AR-canvas while enlisting the several limitations within the process. Zeng et al. [119] discuss the design and the implementation of FunPianoAR for creating a better AR piano learning experience. However, a number of discrepancies occurred with this system, and the initiation of a hybrid system is a more viable option. Rewkowski et al. [120] introduce a prototype system of AR to visualize the laparoscopic training task. This system is capable of tracking small objects and requires surgery training by using widely compatible and inexpensive borescopes.

3.1.8. Hybrid Tracking

Hybrid tracking systems were used to improve the following aspects of the tracking systems:

- Improving the accuracy of the tracking system.
- Coping with the weaknesses of the respective tracking methods.
- Adding more degrees of freedom.

Gorovyi et al. [108] detail the basic principles that make up an AR by proposing a hybrid visual tracking algorithm. The direct tracking techniques are incorporated with the optical flow technique to achieve precise and stable results. The results suggested that they both can be incorporated to make a hybrid system, and ensured its success in devices having limited hardware capabilities. Previously, magnetic tracking [109] or inertial trackers [110] were used in the tracking applications while using the vision-based tracking system. Isham et al. [111] use a game controller and hybrid tracking to identify and resolve the ultrasound image position in a 3D AR environment. This hybrid system was beneficial because of the following reasons:

- Low drift of vision-based tracking.
- Low jitter of vision-based tracking.
- They had a robust sensor with high update rates. These characteristics decreased the invalid pose computation and ensured the responsiveness of the graphical updates [121].
- They had more developed inertial and magnetic trackers which were capable of extending the range of tracking and did not require the line of sight. The above-mentioned benefits suggest that the utilization of the hybrid system is more beneficial than just using the inertial trackers.

In addition, Mao et al. [122] propose a new tracking system with a number of unique features. First, it accurately translates the relative distance into the absolute distance by locating the reference points at the new positions. Secondly, it embraces the separate receiver and sender. Thirdly, resolves the discrepancy in the sampling frequency between the sender and receiver. Finally, the frequency shift due to movement is highly considered in this system. Moreover, the combination of the IMU sensor and Doppler shift with the distributed frequency modulated continuous waveform (FMCW) helps in the continuous tracking of mobile due to multiple time interval developments. The evaluation of the system suggested that it can be applied to the existing hardware and has an accuracy to the millimeter level.

The GPS tracking system alone only provides the positional information and has low accuracy. So, GPS tracking systems are usually combined with vision-based tracking or inertial sensors. The intervention would help gain the full pose estimation of 6DoF [123]. Moreover, backup tracking systems have been developed as an alternative when the GPS fails [98,124]. The optical tracking systems [100] or the ultrasonic rangefinders [101] can be coupled with the inertial trackers for enhancing efficiency. As the differential measurement approach causes the problem of drift, these hybrid systems help resolve them. Furthermore, the use of gravity as a reference to the inertial sensor made them static and bound. The introduction of the hybrid system would make them operate in a simulator, vehicle, or in any other moving platform [125]. The introduction of accelerators, cameras, gyroscopes [126], global positioning systems [127], and wireless networking [128] in mobile phones such as tablets and smartphones also gives an opportunity for hybrid tracking. Furthermore, these devices have the capability of determining outdoor as well as indoor accurate poses [129].

3.2. Marker-Based Tracking

Fiducial Tracking: Artificial landmarks for aiding the tracking and registration that are added to the environment are known as fiducial. The complexity of fiducial tracking varies significantly depending upon the technology and the application used. Pieces of paper or small colored LEDs were used typically in the early systems, which had the ability to be detected using color matching and could be added to the environment [130]. If the position of fiducials is well-known and they are detected enough in the scene then the pose of the camera can be determined. The positioning of one fiducial on the basis of a well-known previous position and the introduction of additional fiducials gives an additional benefit that workplaces could dynamically extend [131]. A QR code-based fudicial/marker is also proposed by some researchers for marker-/tag-based tracking [115]. With the progression of work on the concept and complexity of the fiducials, additional features such as multi-rings were introduced for the detection of fiducials at much larger distances [116]. A minimum of four points of a known position is needed for determining for calculating the pose of the viewer [117]. In order to make sure that the four points are visible, the use of these simpler fiducials demanded more care and effort for placing them in the environment. Examples of such fiducials are ARToolkit and its successors, whose registration techniques are mostly planar fiducial. In the upcoming section, AR display technologies are discussed to fulfill all the conditions of Azuma's definition.

3.3. Summary

This section provides comprehensive details on tracking technologies that are broadly classified into markerless and marker-based approaches. Both types have many subtypes whose details, applications, pros, and cons are provided in a detailed fashion. The different categories of tracking technologies are presented in Figure 4, while the summary of tracking technologies is provided in Figure 7. Among the different tracking technologies, hybrid tracking technologies are the most adaptive. This study combined SLAM and inertial tracking technologies as part of the framework presented in the paper.

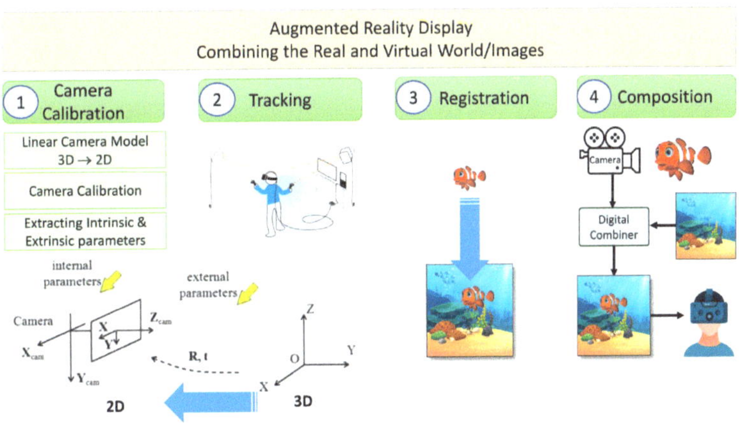

Figure 7. Steps for combining real and virtual content.

4. Augmented Reality Display Technology

For the combination of a real and the virtual world in such a way that they both look superimposed on each other, as in Azuma's definition, some technology is necessarily required to display them.

4.1. Combination of Real and the Virtual Images

Methods or procedures required for the merging of the virtual content in the physical world include camera calibration, tracking, registration, and composition as depicted in Figure 7.

4.2. Camera vs. Optical See Through Calibration

It is a procedure or an optical model in which the eye display geometry or parameters define the user's view. Or, in other words, it is a technique of complementing the dimensions and parameters of the physical and the virtual camera.

In AR, calibration can be used in two ways, one is camera calibration, and another is optical calibration. The camera calibration technique is used in video see-through (VST) displays. However, optical calibration is used in optical see-through (OST) displays. OST calibration can be further divided into three umbrellas of techniques. Initially, manual calibration techniques were used in OST. Secondly, semi-automatic calibration techniques were used, and thirdly, we have now automatic calibration techniques. Manual calibration requires a human operator to perform the calibration tasks. Semi-automatic calibration, such as simple SPAAM and display relative calibration (DRC), partially collect some parameters automatically, which usually needed to be done manually in earlier times by the user. Thirdly, the automatic OST calibration was proposed by Itoh et al. in 2014 with the model of interaction-free display calibration technique (INDICA) [132]. In video see through (VST), computer vision techniques such as cameras are used for the registration of real environments. However, in optical see through (OST), VST calibration techniques cannot be used as it is more complex because cameras are replaced by human eyes. Various calibration techniques were developed for OST. The author evaluates the registration accuracy of the automatic OST head-mounted display (HMD) calibration technique called recycled INDICA presented by Itoh and Klinker. In addition, two more calibration techniques called the single-point active alignment method (SPAAM) and degraded SPAAM were also evaluated. Multiple users were asked to perform two separate tasks to check the registration and the calibration accuracy of all three techniques can be thoroughly studied. Results show that the registration method of the recycled INDICA technique is more accurate in the vertical direction and showed the distance of virtual objects accurately. However, in the horizontal direction, the distance of virtual objects seemed closer than intended [133]. Furthermore, the results show that recycled INDICA is more accurate than any other common technique. In addition, this technique is also more accurate than the SPAAM technique. Although, different calibration techniques are used for OST and VST displays, as discussed in [133], they do not provide all the depth cues, which leads to interaction problems. Moreover, different HMDs have different tracking systems. Due to this, they are all calibrated with an external independent measuring system. In this regard, Ballestin et al. propose a registration framework for developing AR environments where all the real objects, including users, and virtual objects are registered in a common frame. The author also discusses the performance of both displays during interaction tasks. Different simple and complex tasks such as 3D blind reaching are performed using OST and VST HMDs to test their registration process and interaction of the users with both virtual and real environments. It helps to compare the two technologies. The results show that these technologies have issues, however, they can be used to perform different tasks [134].

Non-Geometric Calibration Method

Furthermore, these geometric calibrations lead to perceptual errors while converting from 3D to 2D [135]. To counter this problem, parallax-free video see-through HMDs were proposed; however, they were very difficult to create. In this regard, Cattari et al. in 2019 proposes a non-stereoscopic video see-through HMD for a close-up view. It mitigates perceptual errors by mitigating geometric calibration. Moreover, the authors also identify the problems of non-stereoscopic VST HMD. The aim is to propose a system that provides a view consistent with the real world [136,137]. Moreover, State et al. [138] focus on a VST HMD system that generates zero eye camera offset. While Bottechia et al. [139] present an orthoscope monocular VST HMD prototype.

4.3. Tracking Technologies

Some sort of technology is required to track the position and orientation of the object of interest which could either be a physical object or captured by a camera with reference to the coordinate plan (3D or 2D) of a tracking system. Several technologies ranging from computer vision techniques to 6DoF sensors are used for tracking the physical scenes.

4.4. Registration

Registration is defined as a process in which the coordinate frame used for manifesting the virtual content is complemented by the coordinate frame of the real-world scene. This would help in the accurate alignment of the virtual content and the physical scene.

4.5. Composition

Now, the accuracy of two important steps, i.e., the accurate calibration of the virtual camera and the correct registration of the virtual content relative to the physical world, signifies the right correspondence between the physical environment and the virtual scene which is generated on the basis of tracking updates. This process then leads to the composition of the virtual scene's image and can be done in two ways: Optically (or physically) or digitally. The physical or digital composition depends upon the configuration and dimensions of the system used in the augmented reality system.

4.6. Types of Augmented Reality Displays

The combination of virtual content in the real environment divides the AR displays into four major types, as depicted in Figure 8. All have the same job to show the merged image of real and virtual content to the user's eye. The authors have categorized the latest technologies of optical display after the advancements in holographic optical elements HOEs. There are other categories of AR display that arealso used, such as video-based, eye multiplexed, and projection onto a physical surface.

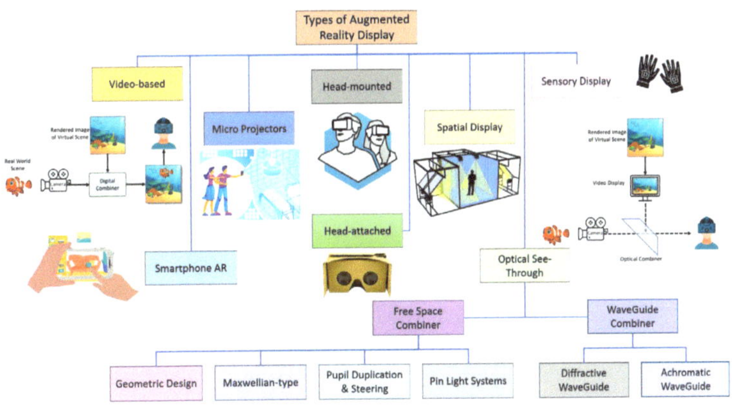

Figure 8. Types of augmented reality display technologies.

4.7. Optical See-Through AR Display

These kinds of displays use the optical system to merge the real scenes and virtual scene images. Examples of AR displays are head-up display HUD systems of advanced cars and cockpits of airplanes. These systems consist of the following components: beam splitters, which can be of two forms, combined prisms or half mirrors. Most beam splitters reflect the image from the video display. This reflected image is then integrated with a real-world view that can be visualized from the splitter. For half mirrors as a beam splitter, the working way is somewhat different: the real-world view is reflected on the mirror rather than the image of the video display. At the same time, the video display can also be viewed from the mirror. The transport projection system is semi-transparent optical technology used in optical display systems. Their semi-transparent property allows the viewer to witness the view at the back of the screen. Additionally, this system uses diffused light to manifest the exhibited image. Examples of semi-display optical systems are transparent projection film, transparent LCDs, etc. Optical combiners are used for the combination of virtual and real scene images. Optical see-through basically has two sub-categories, one is a free-space combiner and the other is a wave-guide combiner [140]. Additionally, now the advancement of technology has enabled technicians to make self-transparent displays. This self-transparent feature help in the miniaturization and simplification of the size and structure of the optical see-through displays.

4.7.1. Free-Space Combiners

Papers related to free space combiners are discussed here. Pulli et al. [11] introduce a second-generation immersive optical see-through AR system known as meta 2. It is based on an optical engine that uses the free-form visor to make a more immersive experience. Another traditional geometric display is ultra-fast high-resolution piezo linear actuators combined with Alvarez's lens to make a new varifocal optical see-through HMD. It uses a beamsplitter which acts as an optical combiner to merge the light paths of the real and virtual worlds [12]. Another type of free-space combiner is Maxwellian-type [112–114,141]. In [142], the author employs the random structure as a spatial light modulator for developing a light-field near-eye display based on random pinholes. The latest work in [143,144] introduces an Ini-based light field display using the multi-focal micro-lens to propose the extended depth of the field. To enhance the eyebox view there is another technique called puppil duplication steering[145–150]. In this regard, refs. [102,151] present the eyebox-expansion method for the holographic near-eye display and pupil-shifting holographic optical element (PSHOE) for the implementation. Additionally, the design architecture is discussed and the incorporation of the holographic optical element within the holographic display system is discussed. There is another recent technique similar to the Maxwellian view called pin-light systems. It increases the Maxwellian view with larger DoFs [103,104].

4.7.2. Wave-Guide Combiner

The waveguide combiner basically traps light into TIR as opposed to free-space, which lets the light propagate without restriction [104–106]. The waveguide combiner has two types, one is diffractive waveguides and another is achromatic waveguides [107,152–155].

4.8. Video-Based AR Displays

These displays execute the digital processes as their working principle [156]. To rephrase, the merging of the physical world video and the virtual images, in video display systems, is carried out by digital processing. The working of the video-based system depends upon the video camera system by which it fabricates the real-world video into digital. The rationale behind this system is that the composition of the physical world's video or scenario with the virtual content could be manifested digitally through the operation of a digital image processing technique [157]. Mostly, whenever the user has to watch the display, they have to look in the direction of the video display, and the camera is usually attached at the back of this display. So, the camera faces the physical world scene. These are known as "video see-through displays" because in them the real world is fabricated through the digitization (i.e., designing the digital illusion) of these video displays. Sometimes the design of the camera is done in such a way that it may show an upside-down image of an object, create the illusion of a virtual mirror, or site the image at a distant place.

4.9. Projection-Based AR Display

Real models [158] and walls [159] could be example of projection-based AR displays. All the other kinds of displays use the display image plan for the combination of the real and the virtual image. However, this display directly overlays the virtual scene image over the physical object. They work in the following manner:

- First, they track the user's viewpoint.
- Secondly, they track the physical object.
- Then, they impart the interactive augmentation [160].

Mostly, these displays have a projector attached to the wall or a ceiling. This intervention has an advantage as well as a disadvantage. The advantage is that this does not demand the user to wear something. The disadvantage is that it is static and restricts the display to only one location of projection. For resolving this problem and making the projectors mobile, a small-sized projector has been made that could be easily carried from one place to another [161]. More recently, with the advancement of technology, miniaturized projectors have also been developed. These could be held in the hand [162] or worn on the chest [163] or head [164].

4.10. Eye-Multiplexed Augmented Reality Display

In eye-multiplexed AR displays, the users are allowed to combine the views of the virtual and real scenes mentally in their minds [72]. Rephrased, these displays do not combine the image digitally; therefore, it requires less computational power [72]. The process is as follows. First, the virtual image gets registered to the physical environment. Second, the user will get to see the same rendered image as the physical scene because the virtual image is registered to the physical environment. The user has to mentally configure the images in their mind to combine the virtual and real scene images because the display does not composite the rendered and the physical image. For two reasons, the display should be kept near the viewer's eye: first, the display could appear as an inset into the real world, and second, the user would have to put less effort into mentally compositing the image.

The division of the displays on the basis of the position of the display between the real and virtual scenes is referred to as the "eye to world spectrum".

4.11. Head-Attached Display

Head-attached displays are in the form of glasses, helmets, or goggles. They vary in size from smaller to bigger. However, with the advancement of technology, they are becoming lighter to wear. They work by displaying the virtual image right in front of the user's eye. As a result, no other physical object can come between the virtual scene and the viewer's eye. Therefore, the third physical object cannot occlude them. In this regard, Koulieris et al. [165] summarized the work on immersive near-eye tracking technologies and displays. Results suggest various loopholes within the work on display technologies: user and environmental tracking and emergence–accommodation conflict. Moreover, it suggests that advancement in the optics technology and focus adjustable lens will improve future headset innovations and creation of a much more comfortable HMD experience. In addition to it, Minoufekr et al. [166] illustrate and examine the verification of CNC machining using Microsoft HoloLens. In addition, they also explore the performance of AR with machine simulation. Remote computers can easily pick up the machine models and load them onto the HoloLens as holograms. A simulation framework is employed that makes the machining process observed prior to the original process. Further, Franz et al. [88] introduce two sharing techniques i.e., over-the-shoulder AR and semantic linking for investigating the scenarios in which not every user is wearing HWD. Semantic linking portrays the virtual content's contextual information on some large display. The result of the experiment suggested that semantic linking and over-the-shoulder suggested communication between participants as compared to the baseline condition. Condino et al. [167] aim to explore two main aspects. First, to explore complex craniotomies to gauge the reliability of the AR-headsets [168]. Secondly, for non-invasive, fast, and completely automatic planning-to-patient registration, this paper determines the efficacy of patient-specific template-based methodology for this purpose.

4.12. Head-Mounted Displays

The most commonly used displays in AR research are head-mounted displays (HMDs). They are also known as face-mounted displays or near-eye displays. The user puts them on, and the display is represented right in front of their eyes. They are most commonly in the form of goggles. While using HMDs, optical and video see-through configurations are most commonly used. However, recently, head-mounted projectors are also explored to make them small enough to wear. Examples of smart glasses, Recon Jet, Google glass, etc., are still under investigation for their usage in head-mounted displays. Barz et al. [169] introduce a real-time AR system that augments the information obtained from the recently attended objects. This system is implemented by using head-mounted displays from the state-of-the-art Microsoft HoloLens [170]. This technology can be very helpful in the fields of education, medicine, and healthcare. Fedosov et al. [171] introduce a skill system, and an outdoor field study was conducted on the 12 snowboards and skiers. First, it develops a system that has a new technique to review and share personal content. Reuter et al. [172] introduce the coordinative concept, namely RescueGlass, for German Red Cross rescue dog units. This is made up of a corresponding smartphone app and a hands-free HMD (head-mounted display) [173]. This is evaluated to determine the field of emergency response and management. The initial design is presented for collaborative professional mobile tasks and is provided using smart glasses. However, the evaluation suggested a number of technical limitations in the research that could be covered in future investigations. Tobias et al. [174] explore the aspects such as ambiguity, depth cues, performed tasks, user interface, and perception for 2D and 3D visualization with the help of examples. Secondly, they categorize the head-mounted displays, introduce new concepts for collaboration tasks, and explain the concepts of big data visualization. The results of the study suggested that the use of collaboration and workspace decisions could be improved with the introduction of the AR workspace prototype. In addition, these displays have lenses that come between the virtual view and the user's eye just like microscopes and telescopes. So, the experiments are under investigation to develop a more direct way of viewing images such as the virtual retinal display developed in 1995 [175]. Andersson et al. [176] show that training, maintenance, process monitoring, and programming can be improved by integrating AR with human—robot interaction scenarios.

4.13. Body-Attached and Handheld Displays

Previously, the experimentation with handheld display devices was done by tethering the small LSDs to the computers [177,178]. However, advancements in technology have improved handheld devices in many ways. Most importantly, they have become so powerful to operate AR visuals. Many of them are now used in AR displays such as personal digital assistants [179], cell phones [180], tablet computers [181], and ultra-mobile PCs [182].

4.13.1. Smartphones and Computer tablets

In today's world, computer tablets and smartphones are powerful enough to run AR applications, because of the following properties: various sensors, cameras, and powerful graphic processors. For instance, Google Project Tango and ARCore have the most depth imaging sensors to carry out the AR experiences. Chan et al. [183] discuss the challenges faced while applying and investigating methodologies to enhance direct touch interaction on intangible displays. Jang et al. [184] aim to explore e-leisure due to enhancement in the use of mobile AR in outdoor environments. This paper uses three methods, namely markerless, marker-based, and sensorless to investigate the tracking of the human body. Results suggested that markerless tracking cannot be used to support the e-leisure on mobile AR. With the advancement of electronic computers, OLED panels and transparent LCDs have been developed. It is also said that in the future, building handheld optical see-through devices would be available. Moreover, Fang et al. [185] focus on two main aspects of mobile AR. First, a combination of the inertial sensor, 6DoF motion tracking based on sensor-fusion, and monocular camera for the realization of mobile AR in real-time. Secondly, to balance the latency and jitter phenomenon, an adaptive filter design is introduced. Furthermore, Irshad et al. [186] introduce an evaluation method to assess mobile AR apps. Additionally, Loizeau et al. [187] explore a way of implementing AR for maintenance workers in industrial settings.

4.13.2. Micro Projectors

Micro projectors are an example of a mobile phone-based AR display. Researchers are trying to investigate these devices that could be worn on the chest [188], shoulder [189], or wrist [190]. However, mostly they are handheld and look almost like handheld flash-lights [191].

4.13.3. Spatial Displays

Spatial displays are used to exhibit a larger display. Henceforth, these are used in the location where more users could get benefit from them i.e., public displays. Moreover, these displays are static, i.e., they are fixed at certain positions and can not be mobilized.

The common examples of spatial displays include those that create optical see-through displays through the use of optical beamers: half mirror workbench [192–195] and virtual showcases. Half mirrors are commonly used for the merging of haptic interfaces. They also enable closer virtual interaction. Virtual showcases may exhibit the virtual images on some solid or physical objects mentioned in [196–200]. Moreover, these could be combined with the other type of technologies to excavate further experiences. The use of volumetric 3D displays [201], autostereoscopic displays [202], and other three-dimensional displays could be researched to investigate further interesting findings.

4.13.4. Sensory Displays

In addition to visual displays, there are some sensors developed that work with other types of sensory information such as haptic or audio sensors. Audio augmentation is easier than video augmentation because the real world and the virtual sounds get naturally mixed up with each other. However, the most challenging part is to make the user think that the virtual sound is spatial. Multi-channel speaker systems and the use of stereo headphones with the head-related transfer function (HRTF) are being researched to cope with this challenge [203]. Digital sound projectors use the reverberation and the interference of sound by using a series of speakers [204]. Mic-throughand hear-through systems, developed by Lindeman [205,206,206], work effectively and are analogous to video and optical see-through displays. The feasibility test for this system was done by using a bone conduction headset. Other sensory experiences are also being researched. For example, the augmentation of the gustatory and olfactory senses. Olfactory and visual augmentation of a cookie-eating scene was developed by Narumi [207]. Table 2 gives the primary types of augmented reality display technologies and discusses their advantages and disadvantages.

Table 2. A Summary of Augmented Reality Display Technologies.

No.	Type	Technology Is Still Used or Obselete?	Technology Used in Devices/Software/Company	How Does It Work?	Advantages	Challenges	Practical Use Areas	Example Studies
1	Optical See-through	Yes	i. Microsoft's Hololens ii. Magic Leap One iii. Google Glass	Merges virtual and real scenes using optical systems through which users can see	+the real world can be viewed +achieves immersive augmented reality experiences	-system lags and calibration issues -reflections and limited field of view -occlusion may be challenging to achieve	Medicine Tourism Education	[11,102,112–114,140–151]
2	Video See-through	Yes	i. HTC Vive Headset ii. Handheld Devices with AR Library, such as, ARCore, ARKit	Combines a digital video of the physical world with virtual content using image processing	+enables a wide field of view +leveraging brightness of objects	-weak peripheral vision of the visuals -lags due to video rendering -disorientation	Advertisement Tourism	[156,157]
3	Projection based	Yes	Tile Five	Projects the virtual scene on a physical object (i.e., Wall or Ceiling) using a projector	+the user does not need to wear any equipment	-The projection is static -Projections are restricted to only one location	Entertainment	[158–164]
4	Eye multiplexed	Yes	Real Wear HMT-1	Integrates real scenes and virtual content in the mind of users	+requires less computational power	-Display must be close to the viewer's eyes		[72]
5	Head attached	Yes	SketchUp	Displays virtual images in front of the users' eyes using dedicatedequipment (e.g., helmets and glasses)	+does not block users' vision +enables user immersion and engagement	-Intrusive to wear -user and environment tracking could be challenging	Architecture Training	[88,165–168]
6	Head mounted	Yes	i. Avionic Displays ii. Solos iii. Beyeonics	Shows AR experiences in front of the users' eyes using HMDs	+VR world is compact in the smallest physical space +enables higher user focus on interaction with AR	-Must be worn, which could be disturbing -Lenses may impact the user experience	Education Medicine Healthcare	[208–213]
7	Body attached and handheld	Yes	Android iOS	Depicts AR visuals on regular handheld devices	+availability of affordable devices and apps +ubiquitous devices (e.g. smartphones) +ability to work with haptic and audio sensors	-interaction on tangible devices poses difficulty -visibility of handheld devices (e.g., brightness and contract)	Leisure	[177–182]

4.14. Summary

This section presented a comprehensive survey of AR display technologies. These displays not only focused on combing the virtual and real-world scenes of visual experience but also other ways of combining the sensory, olfactory, and gustatory senses are also under examination by researchers. Previously, head-mounted displays were most commonly in practice; however, now handheld devices and tablets or mobile-based experiences are widely used. These things may also change in the future depending on future research and low cost. The role of display technologies was elaborated first, thereafter, the process of combining the real and augmented contents and visualizing these to users was elaborated. The section elaborated thoroughly on where the optical see-through and video-based see-through are utilized along with details of devices. Video see-through (VST) is used in head-mounted displays and computer vision techniques such as cameras are used for registration of real environment, while in optical see-through (OST), VST calibration techniques cannot be used due to complexity, and cameras are replaced by human eyes. The optical see-through is a trendy approach as of now. The different calibration approaches are presented and analyzed and it is identified after analysis, the results show that recycled INDICA is more accurate than other common techniques presented in the paper. This section also presents video-based AR displays. Figure 8 present a classified representation of different display technologies pertaining to video-based, head-mounted, and sensory-based approaches. The functions and applications of various display technologies are provided in Table 2 Each of the display technologies presented has its applicability in various realms whose details are summarized in the same Table 2.

5. Walking and Distance Estimation in AR

The effectiveness of AR technologies depends on the perception of distance of users from both real and virtual objects [214,215]. Mikko et al. performed some experiments to judge depth using stereoscopic depth perception [216]. The perception can be changed if the objects are on the ground or off the ground. In this regard, Carlos et al. also proposed a comparison between the perception of distance of these objects on the ground and off the ground. The experiment was done where the participant perceived the distance from cubes on the ground and off the ground as well. The results showed that there is a difference between both perceptions. However, it was also shown that this perception depends on whether the vision is monocular or binocular [217]. Plenty of research has been done in outdoor navigation and indoor navigation areas with AR [214]. In this regard, Umair et al. present an indoor navigation system in which Google glass is used as a wearable head-mounted display. A pre-scanned 3D map is used to track an indoor environment. This navigation system is tested on both HMD and handheld devices such as smartphones. The results show that the HMD was more accurate than the handheld devices. Moreover, it is stated that the system needs more improvement [218].

6. AR Development Tool

In addition to the tracking and display devices, there are some other software tools required for creating an AR experience. As these are hardware devices, they require some software to create an AR experience. This section explores the tools and the software libraries. It will cover both the aspects of the commercially available tools and some that are research related. Different software applications require a separate AR development tool. A complete set of low-level software libraries, plug-ins, platforms, and standalones are presented in Figure 9 so they can be summarized for the reader.

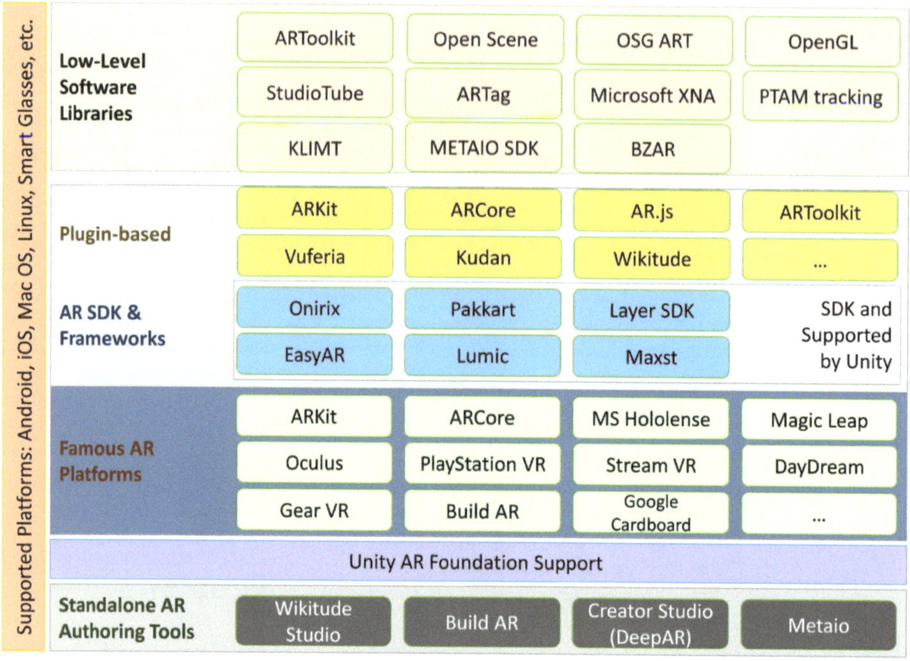

Figure 9. Stack of development libraries, plug-ins, platforms, and standalone authoring tools for augmented reality development.

In some tools, computer vision-based tracking (see Section 3.1.2) is preferred for creating an indoor experience, while others utilized sensors for creating an outdoor experience. The use of each tool would depend upon the type of platform (web or mobile) for which it is designed. Further in the document, the available AR tools are discussed, which consist of both novel tools and those that are widely known. Broadly, the following tools will be discussed:

- Low-level software development tools: needs high technological and programming skills.
- Rapid prototyping: provides a quick experience.
- Plug-ins that run on the existing applications.
- Standalone tools that are specifically designed for non-programmers.
- Next generation of AR developing tools.

6.1. Low-Level Software Libraries and Frameworks

Low-level software and frameworks make the functions of display and core tracking accessible for creating an AR experience. One of the most commonly used AR software libraries, as discussed in the previous section, is ARToolKit. ARToolKit is developed by Billing Hurst and Kato that has two versions [219]. It works on the principle of a fiducial marker-based registration system [220]. There are certain advances in the ARToolKit discussed related to the tracking in [213,221–224]. The first one is an open-source version that provides the marker-based tracking experience, while the second one provides natural tracking features and is a commercial version. It can be operated on Linux, Windows, and Mac OS desktops as it is written in the C language. It does not require complex graphics or built-in support for accomplishing its major function of providing a tracking experience, and it can operate simply by using low-level OpenGL-based rendering. ARToolKit requires some additional libraries such as osgART and OpenScene graph library so it can provide a complete AR experience to AR applications. OpenScene graph library is written in C language and operates as an open-source graph library. For graphic rendering, the OpenScene graph uses OpenGL. Similarly, the osgART library links the OpenScene graph and ARToolKit. It has advanced rendering techniques that help in developing the interacting AR application. OsgART library has a modular structure and can work with any other tracking library such as PTAM and BazAR, if ARtoolkit is not appropriate. BazAR is a workable tracking and geometric calibration library. Similarly, PTAM is a SLAM-based tracking library. It has a research-based and commercial license. All these libraries are available and workable to create a workable AR application. Goblin XNA [208] is another platform that has the components of interactions based on physics, video capture, a head-mounted AR display on which output is displayed, and a three-dimensional user interface. With Goblin XNA, existing XNA games could be easily modified [209]. Goblin XNA is available as a research and educational platform. Studierstube [210] is another AR system through which a complete AR application can be easily developed. It has tracking hardware, input devices, different types of displays, AR HMD, and desktops. Studierstube was specially developed to subsidize the collaborative applications [211,212]. Studierstube is a research-oriented library and is not available as commercial and workable easy-to-use software. Another commercially available SDK is Metaio SDK [225]. It consists of a variety of AR tracking technologies including image tracking, marker tracking, face tracking, external infrared tracking, and a three-dimensional object tracking. However, in May 2015, it was acquired by Apple and Metaio products and subscriptions are no longer available for purchase. Some of these libraries such as Studierstube and ARToolKit were initially not developed for PDAs. However, they have been re-developed for PDAs [226]. It added a few libraries in assistance such as open tracker, pocketknife for hardware abstraction, KLIMT as mobile rendering, and the formal libraries of communication (ACE) and screen graphs. All these libraries helped to develop a complete mobile-based AR collaborative experience [227,228]. Similarly, ARToolKit also incorporated the OpenScene graph library to provide a mobile-based AR experience. It worked with Android and iOS with a native development kit including some Java wrapping classes. Vuforia's Qualcomm low-level library also provided an AR experience for mobile devices. ARToolKit and Vuforia both can be installed as a plug-in in Unity which provides an easy-to-use application development for various platforms. There are a number of sensors and low-level vision and location-based libraries such as Metaio SDK and Droid which were developed for outdoor AR experience. In addition to these low-level libraries, the Hit Lab NZ Outdoor AR library provided high-level abstraction for outdoor AR experience [229]. Furthermore, there is a famous mobile-based location AR tool that is called Hoppala-Augmentation. The geotags given by this tool can be browsed by any of the AR browsers including Layar, Junaio, and Wikitude [230].

6.2. ARTag

ARTag is designed to resolve the limitations of ARToolkit. This system was developed to resolve a number of issues:

- Resolving inaccurate pattern matching by preventing the false positive matches.
- Enhancing the functioning in the presence of the imbalanced lightening conditions.
- Making the occlusion more invariant.

However, ARTag is no longer actively under development and supported by the NRC Lab. A commercial license is not available.

6.3. Wikitude Studio

This is also a web-based authoring tool for creating mobile-based AR applications. It allows the utilization of computer vision-based technology for the registration of the real world. Several types of media such as animation and 3D models can be used for creating an AR scene. One of the important features of Wikitude is that the developed mobile AR content can be uploaded not only on the Wikitude AR browser app but also on a custom mobile app [231]. Wikitude's commercial plug-in is also available in Unity to enhance the AR experience for developers.

6.4. Standalone AR Tools

Standalone AR tools are mainly designed to enable non-programmer users to create an AR experience. A person the basic computer knowledge can build and use them. The reason lies in the fact that most AR authoring tools are developed on a graphical user interface. It is known as a standalone because it does not require any additional software for its operation. The most common and major functions of standalone are animation, adding interactive behaviors, and construction. The earliest examples of the standalone tools are AMIRE [232] and CATOMIR [233]. However, AMIRE and CATOMIR have no support available and are not maintained by the development team.

BuildAR

This standalone AR authoring tool has the advantage of quickly adding to the development of the AR experience. BuildAR has important characteristics. This allows the user to add video, 3D models, sound, text, and images. It has both arbitrary images and the square marker for which it provides computer vision-based tracking. They use the format of proprietary file format for saving the content developed by the user. BuildAR viewer software can be downloaded for free and it helps in viewing the file. However, BuildAR has no support available and the exe file is not available on their website.

Limitation: It does not support adding new interactive features. However, Choi et al. [234] have provided a solution to this constraint. They have added the desktop authoring tool that helps in adding new interactive experiences.

6.5. Rapid Prototyping/Development Tools

In order to cope with the limitation of low-level libraries, another more fast and more rapid AR application development tool is required. The major idea behind the development of rapid prototyping was that it rapidly shows the user the prototype before executing the hard exercise of developing the application. In the following paragraphs, a number of different tools are explained for developing rapid prototyping. For the creation of multimedia content, Adobe Flashis one of the most famous tools. It was developed on desktop and web platforms. Moreover, the web desktop and mobile experiences can be prototyped by it. Flash developers can use the FLARManager, FLARToolKit, or any other plug-ins for the development of AR experience. Porting the version of ARToolKit over the flash on the web creates the AR experience. Its process is so fast that just by writing a few lines, the developer can:

- Activate their camera.
- The AR markers could be viewed in a camera.
- The virtual content could be overlaid and loaded on the tracked image.

FLARToolkit is the best platform for creating AR prototyping because it has made it very easy for being operated by anyone. Anyone who has a camera and flash-enabled web browser can easily develop the AR experience. Alternatives to Flash: According to the website of Adobe, it no longer supports Flash Player after 31 December 2020 and blocked Flash content from running in Flash Player beginning 12 January 2021. Adobe strongly recommends all users immediately uninstall Flash Player to help protect their systems. However, some AR plug-ins could be used as an alternative to Flash-based AR applications. For instance, Microsoft Silverlight has the SLARToolKit. HTML5 is also recently used by researchers for creating web-based AR experiences. The major benefit of using HTML5 is that the interference of the third-party plug-in is not required. For instance, the AR natural feature tracking is implemented on WebGL, HTML5, and JavaScript. This was developed by Oberhofer and was viewable on mobile web browsers and desktops. Additionally, the normal HTML, with few web component technologies, has been used by Ahn [235] to develop a complete mobile AR framework.

6.6. Plug-ins to Existing Developer Tools

For the creation of AR experiences, the software libraries require tremendous programming techniques. So, plug-ins could be used as an alternative. Plug-ins are devices that could be plugged into the existing software packages. The AR functionality is added to the software packages that to the existing two-dimensional or three-dimensional content authoring tools. If the user already knows the procedure of using authoring tools that are supported by plug-ins, then AR plug-ins for the non-AR authoring tools are useful. These tools are aimed at:

- AR tracking and visualization functions for the existing authoring tools.
- It depends on the content authoring function supplied by the main authoring tool.

There are certain tools available as plug-ins and standalone through which AR applications can be built comparatively simply. These are commercial and some of them are freely available. As discussed earlier, Vuforia can be installed as a plug-in in Unity [236] and also has a free version. However, with complete support of tools certain amount needs to be paid. Similarly, ARtoolkit is available standalone and a plug-in for Unity is available. It is freely available for various platforms such as Android, iOS, Linux, and Windows. Moreover, ARCore and ARKit are also available for Android and iOS, respectively, and can work with Unity and Unreal authoring tools as a plug-in. ARCore is available and free for developers. MAXST and Wikitude also can work in integration with Unity, though they have a licensing price for the commercial version of the software. MAXST had a free version as well. All these tools, the abovementioned libraries, and standalone tools are depicted in Figure 9. Cinema 4D, Maya, Trimble SketchUp 3D modeling software, 3Ds Max, and many others were created by a number of plug-ins that acted as authoring tools for three-dimensional content. While 3D animation and modeling tools are not capable of providing interactive features, it is very productive in creating three-dimensional scenes. SketchUp can utilize the AR plug-in by creating a model for the content creators. This model is then viewable in the AR scene provided by a free AR media player. The interactive three-dimensional graphic authoring tools are also available for the creation of highly interactive AR experiences, for instance, Wizard [237], Quest3D [238], and Unity [236]. All of these authoring tools have their own specific field of operation; however, Unity can be utilized to create a variety of experiences. The following are examples that justify the use of Unity over different solutions available:

- The AR plug-in of the Vuforia tracking library can be used with Unity 3D. This integration will help Vuforia in the creation of AR applications for the android or iOS platform.
- Similarly, the ARToolkit for Unity also provides marker-based experiences. It provides both image and marker-based AR visualization and tracking.

In such integrations, the highly interactive experiences are created by the normal Unity3D scripting interface and visual programming. Limitations of AR plug-ins: The following are the limitations accrued with the AR plug-in:

- The need for proprietary software could arise for the content produced by the authoring tool. The design provided by the authoring tools could restrict the user's interactive and interface designs.
- Moreover, the authoring tools can also restrict the configurations of hardware or software within a certain limit.

Moreover, Nebeling et al. [239] reviewed the issues with the authoring tools of AR/VR. The survey of the tools has identified three key issues. To make up for those limitations, new tools are introduced for supporting the gesture-based interaction and rapid prototyping of the AR/VR content. Moreover, this is done without having technical knowledge of programming, gesture recognition, and 3D modeling. Mladenov et al. [240] review the existing SDKs and aim to find the most efficient SDK for the AR applications used in industrial environments. The paper reveals that currently available SDKs are very helpful for users to create AR applications with the parameters of their choice in industrial settings.

6.7. Summary

This section presents a detailed survey of different software and tools required for creating an AR experience. The section outlines hardware devices used in AR technology and various software to create an AR experience. It further elaborates on the software libraries required and covers bother the aspects of the commercially available tools. Table 3 provides a stack of software libraries, plug-ins, supported platforms, and standalone authoring tools. The figure also presents details of whether the mentioned tools are active or inactive. As an example, BazAR is used in tracking and geometric calibration. It is an open-source library for Linux or windows available under research-based GPL and can be used for research to detect an object via camera, calibrate it, and initiate tracking to put a basic virtual image on it; however, this library is not active at the present. Commercially used AR tools such as plug-ins have the limitations of only working efficiently in the 2D GUI and become problematic when used for 3D content. The advancement of technology may bring about a change in the authoring tools by making them capable of being operated for 3D and developing more active AR interfaces.

Table 3. A summary of development and authoring tools for augmented reality application development.

Authoring Tool	AR Component	Features	Research Based or Commercial	Active/Not	Used in/by Software/Tool	Platform Supported
OpenScene	Graph Library	-OpenScene is a graph library -Can be linked with OpenGL and osgART	Researched/Commercial	Active	ARToolKit	GNULinux/Windows/OSX
PTAM	SLAM Tracking Library	OpenSource/Available Under GPL	Research-Based	Can be used for research and open source. However, for productionARCore/ARKit implementation of SLAMis available/Not Active	Standalone	Linux/OSX
BazAR	Tracking and Geometric Calibration	OpenSource/Available Under GPL	Research-Based	Can beused for research to detectan object via camera, calibrate it and initiatetracking to put a basicvirtual image onit/Not Active	Standalone	Linux/Windows
Goblin XNA	-Platform for Mobile-based AR -Marker Based tracking with ARTag	Free Windows Platform	Research/Education Based	Can beused forresearch and educationpurposes, to generate 3Dand track the object/NotActive	Standalone	Windows
Studierstube	Open Tracker	-Open Source/Free -Have Builtin Hardware Tracking -Used for Collaborative AR	Research/Education Based	Can beused forresearch and educationpurposes to test varioustracking and AR apps/NotActive	Standalone	Linux
Metaio SDK	Image, Marker, Face, infrared, and 3D object Tracking	-Support Localization -Tracking	The source code can be provided after proper owner's approval on their website	Active	Standalone	Andoird/iOS
ARTag	-Maker-Based (Fiducial) Tracking	Tracking Library that support AR application development	No support available	Not Active	Standalone	Windows
WikiTude Studio	-SLAM -Image Tracking -Calibration Manager -Geo AR -Inertial	It is an SDK that can help to build an AR app without any other tools needed for Android, iOS, Windows, and Linux.	Commercial	Active	Native API, JavaScript API, Unity Plugin, Cordova Plugin, Flutter Plugin,	Windows, Linux, iOS, Android
BuildAR	Marker based tracking	-Standalone easy to create new AR applications. -	Free	Not Active	Standalone	Windows

Table 3. *Cont.*

Authoring Tool	AR Component	Features	Research Based or Commercial	Active/Not	Used in/by Software/Tool	Platform Supported
AMIRE and CATOMIR	Standalone ARTools		No support availble	Active		
ARCore	SLAM + Inertial forTracking and understanding the environment Integrated Display	ARCore support Motion tracking with SLAM and Inertial, Depth Understanding, Light Estemation,	Free	Active	Android, Android NDK, Unity(AR Foundation), iOS, Unreal, Web	Android, iOS
MS HoloLense	-Vision Based Tracking -OST Display -VST Display	Is an augmented reality headset for running AR apps	Commercial	Active	Unity, Unreal, Vuforia	Windows 10
ARKit	-Motion Tracking -Camera Scene Capture -Advanced Scene Processing	With ARKit one can create a complete AR application. It has tracking, display and development environment to develop AR app.	Commercial for application development	Active	Plugin Available for Unity	iOS
Vuforia	Supports -Marker less (vision-based) and -Marker based tracking (Fiducial) -Calibration Library	-A complete SDK for AR application development. -Supports many languages for AR development for API - C++, Java, Net	Free and Commercial both versions are available.	Active	-Standalone Native development -Plugin available for Unity	iOS, Android
ARToolKit	-Tracking Library Supports both -Video See Through(VST) -Optical See Through(OST) -ARTag variant of ARToolKit supports Marker based(Fiducial)	-C and C++ Language Support for AR -JARToolKit for Java Support -A Modified Marker Base -ARToolKitPlus	Free and Commercial both are available.	Active	-Standalone -Unity plugin is also available for Integration with Unity libraries	Linux, Windows, McOS X
DeepAR (Creator Studio)	Embdded Tracking, VST Display	Standalone easy to create AR applications for non-programmers	Commercial	Active	DeepAR SDK Web SDK	Windows, iOS, Android,

7. Collaborative Research on Augmented Reality

In general, collaboration in augmented reality is the interaction of multiple users with virtual objects in the real environment. This interaction is regardless of the users' location, i.e., they can participate remotely or have the same location. In this regard, we have two types of collaborative AR: co-located collaborative AR and remote collaborative AR. We mention it further in Figure 10.

7.1. Co-Located Collaborative AR

In this type of collaborative AR, the users interact with the virtual content rendered in the real environment while sharing the same place. The participant are not remote in such case. In this regard, Wells et al. [241] aim to determine the impact on the co-located group activities by varying the complexity of AR models using mobile AR. The paper also discusses different styles of collaborative AR such as:

- hlActive Discussion: A face-to-face discussion including all participants.
- Single Shared view: The participants focus on a single device.
- Disjoint and Shared View: Two to three participants focus on a single device.
- Disjoint and Distributed View: One to two people focus on their devices while the others are discussing.
- Distributed View: Participants focus on their devices with no discussion.
- Distributive View with Discussion: Participants focus on their devices while discussing in the group.

In this paper, the author did not contribute to the technology of co-located collaborative AR, but rather performed analysis on the effectiveness of different collaborative AR.

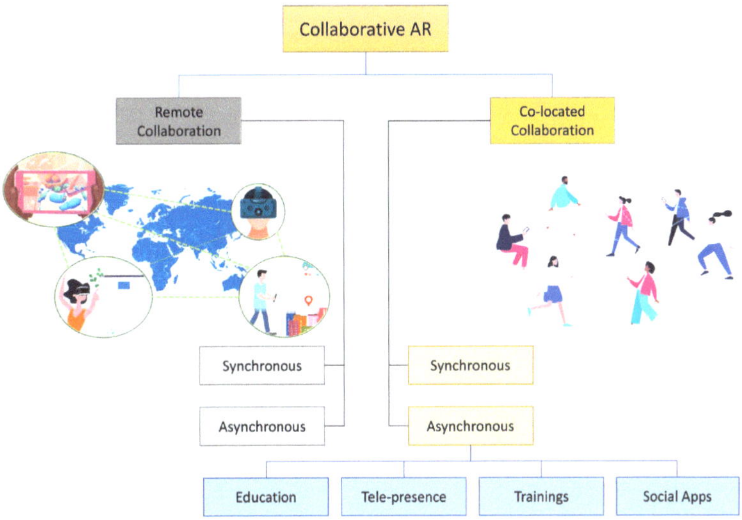

Figure 10. Collaborative augmented reality research domains.

Grandi et al. [242] target the development of design approaches for synchronous collaboration to resolve complex manipulation tasks. For this, purpose fundamental concepts of design interface, human collaboration, and manipulation are discussed. This research the spiral model of research methodology which involves the development, planning, analysis, and evaluation. In addition, Dong et al. [243] introduce "ARVita", a system where multiple users can interact with virtual simulations of engineering processes by wearing a head-mounted display. This system uses a co-located AR technique where the users are sitting around a table.

7.1.1. Applications of Co-located Collaborative AR

Kim et al. [244] propose a PDIE model to make a STEAM educational class while incorporating AR technology into the system. Furthermore, the "Aurasma" application is used to promote AR in education. In addition, Kanzanidis et al. [245] focus on teaching mobile programming using synchronous co-located collaborative AR mobile applications in which students are distributed in groups. The result showed that the students were satisfied with this learning methodology. Moreover, Chang et al. [246] explore the use of a mobile AR (MAR) application to teach interior design activities to students. The results identified that the students who were exposed to MAR showed more effectiveness in learning than those who were taught traditionally. Lastly, Sarkar et al. [247] discuss three aspects of synchronous co-located collaboration-based problem-solving: first, students' perspectives on AR learning activities, either in dyads or individually are determined; second, the approach adopted by students while problem-solving is determined; third, the students' motivation for using ScholAR is determined. Statistical results suggested that 90.4% students preferred the collaborative AR experience, i.e., in dyads. Meanwhile, motivation level and usability scores were higher for individual experiences. Grandi et al. [248] introduce the design for the collaborative manipulation of AR objects using mobile AR. This approach has two main features. It provides a shared medium for collaboration and manipulation of 3D objects as well as provides precise control of DoF transformations. Moreover, strategies are presented to make this system more efficient for users in pairs. Akccayir et al. [249] explore the impact of AR on the laboratory work of university students and their attitudes toward laboratories. This study used the quasi-experimental design with 76 participants—first year students aged 18–20 years. Both qualitative and quantitative methods were used for the analyses of data. A five-week implementation of the experiment proved that the use of AR in the laboratory significantly improved the laboratory skills of the students. However, some teachers and students also discussed some of the negative impacts of other aspects of AR. Rekimoto et al. [250] propose a collaborative AR system called TransVision. In this system, two or more users use a see-through display to look at the virtual objects rendered in a real environment using synchronous co-located collaborative AR. Oda et al. [251] propose a technique for avoiding interference for hand-held synchronous co-located collaborative AR. This study is based on first-person two-player shooting AR games. Benko et al. [87] present a collaborative augmented reality and mixed reality system called "VITA" or "Visual Interaction Tool For Archaeology". They have an off-site visualization system that allows multiple users to interact with a virtual archaeological object. Franz et al. [88] present a system of collaborative AR for museums in which multiple users can interact in a shared environment. Huynh et al. [252] introduce art of defense (AoD), a co-located augmented reality board game that combines handheld devices with physical game pieces to create a unique experience of a merged physical and virtual game. Nilsson et al. [253] focus on a multi-user collaborative AR application as a tool for supporting collaboration between different organizations such as rescue services, police, and military organizations in a critical situation.

7.1.2. Asynchronous Co-Located Collaborative AR

Tseng et al. [254] present an asynchronous annotation system for collaborative augmented reality. This system can attribute virtual annotations with the real world due to a number of distinguishing capabilities, i.e., playing back, placing, and organizing. Extra context information is preserved by the recording of the perspective of the annotator. Furthermore, Kashara et al. [255] introduce "Second Surface", an asynchronous co-located collaborative AR system. It allows the users to render images, text, or drawings in a real environment. These objects are stored in the data server and can be accessed later on.

7.2. Remote Collaborative AR

In this type of collaborative AR, all the users have different environments. They can interact with virtual objects remotely from any location. A number of studies have been done in this regard. Billinghurst et al. [256] introduce a wearable collaborative augmented reality system called "WearCom" to communicate with multiple remote people. Stafford et al. [257] present God-like interaction techniques for collaboration between outdoor AR and indoor tabletop users. This paper also describes a series of applications for collaboration. Gauglitz et al. [258] focus on a touchscreen interface for creating annotations in a collaborative AR environment. Moreover, this interface is also capable of virtually navigating a scene reconstructed live in 3D. Boonbrahm et al. [259] aim to develop a design model for remote collaboration. The research introduces the multiple marker technique to develop a very stable system that allows users from different locations to collaborate which also improves the accuracy. Li et al. [260] suggest the viewing of a collaborative exhibit has been considerably improved by introducing the distance-driven user interface (DUI). Poretski et al. [261] describe the behavioral challenges faced in interaction with virtual objects during remote collaborative AR. An experiment was performed to study users' interaction with shared virtual objects in AR. Clergeaud et al. [262] tackle the limitations of collaboration in aerospace industrial designs. In addition, the authors propose prototype designs to address these limitations. Oda et al. [263] present the GARDEN (gesturing in an augmented reality depth-mapped environment) technique for 3D referencing in a collaborative augmented reality environment. The result shows that this technique is more accurate than the other comparisons. Muller et al. [85] investigate the influence of shared virtual landmarks (SVLs) on communication behavior and user experience. The results show that enhancement in user experience when SVLs were provided. Mahmood et al. [264] present a remote collaborative system for co-presence and sharing information using mixed reality. The results show improvements in user collaborative analysis experience.

7.2.1. Applications of Remote Collaborative AR

Munoz et al. [265] present a system called GLUEPS-AR to help teachers in learning situations by integrating AR and web technologies i.e., Web 2.0 tools and virtual learning environments (VLEs) [266]. Bin et al. [267] propose a system to enhance the learning experience of the students using collaborative mobile augmented reality learning application (CoMARLA). The application was used to teach ICT to students. The results showed improvement in the learning of the students using CoMARLA. Dunleavy et al. [268] explore the benefits and drawbacks of collaborative augmented reality simulations in learning. Moreover, a collaborative AR system was proposed for computers independent of location, i.e., indoor or outdoor. Maimone et al. [269] introduce a telepresence system with real-time 3D capture for remote users to improve communication using depth cameras. Moreover, it also discusses the limitations of previous telepresence systems. Gauglitz et al. [270] present an annotation-based remote collaboration AR system for mobiles. In this system, the remote user can explore the scene regardless of the local user's camera position. Moreover, they can also communicate through annotations visible on the screen. Guo et al. [271] introduce an app, known as Block, that enables the users to collaborate irrespective of their geographic position, i.e., they can be either co-located or remote. Moreover, they can collaborate either asynchronously or synchronously. This app allows users to create structures that persist in the real environment. The result of the study suggested that people preferred synchronous and collocated collaboration, particularly one that was not restricted by time and space. Zhang et al. [272] propose a collaborative augmented reality for socialization app (CARS). This app improves the user's perception of the quality of the experience. CARS benefits the user, application, and system on various levels. It reduces the use of computer resources, end-to-end latency, and networking. Results of the experiment suggest that CARS acts more efficiently for users of cloud-based AR applications. Moreover, on mobile phones, it reduces the latency level by up to 40%. Grandi et al. [242] propose an edge-assisted system, known as CollabAR, which combines both collaboration image recognition and distortion tolerance. Collaboration image recognition enhances recognition accuracy by exploiting the "spatial-temporal" correlation. The result of the experiment suggested that this system has significantly decreased the end-to-end system latency up to 17.8 ms for a smartphone. Additionally, recognition accuracy for images with stronger distortions was found to be 96%.

7.2.2. Synchronous Remote Collaborative AR

Lien et al. [273] present a system called "Pixel-Point Volume Segmentation" in collaborative AR. This system is used for object references. Moreover, one user can locate the objects with the help of circles drawn on the screen by other users in a collaborative environment. Huang et al. [274] focus on sharing hand gestures and sketches between a local user and a remote user by using collaborative AR. The system is named "Handsin-Touch". Ou et al. [275] present the DOVE (drawing over video environment) system, which integrates live-video and gestures in collaborative AR. This system is designed to perform remote physical tasks in a collaborative environment. Datcu et al. [276] present the creation and evaluation of the handheld AR system. This is done particularly to investigate the remote forensic and co-located and to support team-situational awareness. Three experienced investigators evaluated this system in two steps. First, it was investigated with one remote and one local investigator. Secondly, with one remote and two local investigators. Results of the study suggest the use of this technology resolves the limitation of HMDs. Tait et al. [277] propose the AR-based remote collaboration that supports view independence. The main aim of the system was to enable the remote user to help the local user with object placement. The remote user uses a 3D reconstruction of the environment to independently find the local user's scene. Moreover, a remote user can also place the virtual cues in the scene visible to the local user. The major advantage of this system is that it allows the remote user to have an independent scene in the shared task space. Fang et al. [278] focus on enhancing the 3D feel of immersive interaction by reducing communication barriers. WebRTC, a real-time video communication framework, is developed to enable the operator site's first-hand view of the remote user. Node.js and WebSocket, virtual canvas-based whiteboards, are developed which are usable in different aspects of life. Mora et al. [279] explain the CroMAR system. The authors aim to help the users in crowd management who are deployed in a planned outdoor event. CroMAR allows the users to share viewpoints via email, and geo-localized tags allow the users to visualize the outdoor environment and rate these tags. Adcock et al. [280] present three remote spacial augmented reality systems "Composite Wedge", "Vector Box", and "Eyelight" for off-surface 3D viewpoints visualization. In this system, the physical world environment of a remote user can be seen by the local user. Lincoln et al. [281] focus on a system of robotic avatars of humans in a synchronous remote collaborative environment. It uses cameras and projectors to render a humanoid animatronic model which can be seen by multiple users. This system is called "Animatronic Shader Lamps Avatars". Komiyama et al. [282] present a synchronous remote collaborative AR system. It can transition between first person and third person view during collaboration. Moreover, the local user can observe the environment of the remote user. Lehment et al. [283] present an automatically aligned videoconferencing AR system. In this system, the remote user is rendered and aligned on the display of the local user. This alignment is done automatically regarding the local user's real environment without modifying it. Oda et al. [284] present a remote collaborative system for guidance in a collaborative environment. In this system, the remote expert can guide a local user with the help of both AR and VR. The remote expert can create virtual replicas of real objects to guide a local user. Piumsomboon et al. [285] introduce an adaptive avatar system in mixed reality (MR) called "Mini Me" between a remote user using VR and a local user using AR technology. The results show that it improves the overall experience of MR and social presence. Piumsomboon et al. [286] present "CoVAR", a collaboration consisting of both AR and VR technologies. A local user can share their environment with a remote VR user. It supports gestures, head, and eye gaze to improve the collaboration experience. Teo et al. [287] present a system that captures a 360 panorama video of one user and shares it with the other remote user in a mixed reality collaboration. In this system, the users communicate through hand gestures and visual annotation. Thanyadit et al. [288] introduce a system where the instructor can observe students in a virtual environment. The system is called "ObserVAR" and uses augmented reality to observe students' gazes in a virtual environment. Results show that this system is more improved and flexible in several scenarios. Sodhi et al. [289] present a synchronous remote collaborative system called "BeThere" to explore 3D gestures and spatial input. This system enables a remote user to perform virtual interaction in the local user's real environment. Ong et al. [290] propose a collaborative system in which 3D objects can be seen by all the users in a collaborative environment. Moreover, the changes made to these objects are also observed by the users. Butz et al. [84] present EMMIE (environment management for multi-user information environments) in a collaborative augmented reality environment in which virtual objects can be manipulated by the users. In addition, this manipulation is visible to each user of this system.

7.2.3. Asynchronous Remote Collaborative AR

Irlitti et al. [291] explore the challenges faced during the use of asynchronous collaborative AR. Moreover, the author further discusses how to enhance communication while using asynchronous collaborative AR. Quasi-systems do not fulfill Azuma's [292] definition of AR technology. However, they are very good at executing certain aspects of AR as other full AR devices are doing. For instance, mixed-space collaborative work in a virtual theater [268]. This system explained that if someone wants two groups to pay attention to each other, a common spatial frame of reference should be created to have a better experience of social presence. In the spatially aware educational system, students were using location-aware smartphones to resolve riddles. This was very useful in the educational system because it supported both engagement and social presence [245,265,269]. However, this system did not align the 3D virtual content in the virtual space. Therefore, it was not a true AR system. In order to capture a remote 3D scene, Fuchs and Maimone [293] developed an algorithm. They also developed a proof of concept for teleconferencing. For capturing images, RGB-D cameras were used. The remote scene was displayed on the 3D stereoscopic screen. These systems were not fully AR, but they still exhibited a very good immersion. Akussah et al. [294] focus on developing a marker-based collaborative augmented reality app for learning mathematics. First, the system focuses on individual experience and later on expands it to collaborative AR.

7.3. Summary

This section provides comprehensive details on collaborative augmented reality which is broadly classified into co-located collaborative AR, where participants collaborate with each other in geographically the same location, and remote collaboration. The applications of both approaches are presented as well. Co-located collaborative AR is mostly adopted in learning realms for sharing information, for example, in museums. On the other hand, in remote collaborative AR the remote user can explore the scene regardless of the local user's camera position. The applications of this technology are mostly found in education.

8. AR Interaction and Input Technologies

The interaction and input technologies are detailed in this section. There are a number of input methods that are utilized in AR technologies. First, multimode and 3D interfaces such as speech, gesture and handheld wands. Second, the mouse, and keyboard traditional two-dimensional user interfaces (UI). The type of interaction task needed for the interface defines which input method would be utilized in the application. A variety of interfaces have been developed: three-dimensional user interfaces, tangible user interfaces, multimedia interfaces, natural user interfaces, and information browsers.

8.1. AR Information Browsers

Wikitude and Navicam are one of the most popular examples of AR information browsers. The only problem with AR browsers is that they cannot provide direct interaction with the virtual objects.

8.2. Three-Dimensional User Interfaces

A three-dimensional user interface uses the controllers for providing the interaction with virtual content. By using the traditional 3D user interface techniques, we can directly interact with the three-dimensional object in the virtual space. There are a number of 3D user interface interaction techniques as follows: **3D motion tracking sensors** are one of the most commonly used devices for AR interaction. The motion tracking sensors allow the following functions: tracking the parts of the user's body and allow pointing as well as the manipulation of the virtual objects [295]. Haptic devices are also used for interacting with AR environments [296–298]. They mainly used as 3D pointing devices. In addition, they provide tactile and forces feedback. This will create the illusion of a physical object existing in the real world. Thereby, it helps in complementing the virtual experience. They are used in training, entertainment, and design-related AR applications.

8.3. Tangible User Interface

The tangible user interface is one of the main concepts of human–computer interface technology research. In this, the physical object is used for interaction [299]. It bridges the gap between the physical and the virtual object [300]. Chessa et al. incorporated grasping behavior in a virtual reality systems [301], while Han et al. presented and evaluated hand interaction techniques using tactile feedback (haptics) and physical grasping by mapping a real object with virtual objects [302].

8.4. Natural User Interfaces in AR

Recently, more accurate gesture and motion-based interactions for AR and VR applications have become extensively available due to the commercialization of depth cameras such as Microsoft Kinect and technical advances. Bare-hand interaction with a virtual object was made possible by the introduction of a depth camera. It provided physical interaction by tracking the dexterous hand motion. For instance, the physical objects and the user's hands were recognized by the use of Kinect Camera, designed by the Microsoft HoloDesk [299]. The virtual objects were shown on the optical see-through AR workbench. It also allowed the users to interact with the virtual objects presented on the AR workbench. The user-defined gestures have been categorized into sets by the Piumsomboon [300]. This set can be utilized in AR applications for accomplishing different tasks. In addition, some of the mobile-based depth-sensing cameras are also under investigation. For instance, the SoftKinetic and Myo gesture armband controller. SodtKinetic is aimed at developing hand gesture interaction in mobile phones and wearable devices more accurately, while the Myo gesture armband controller is a biometric sensor that provides interaction in wearable and mobile environments.

8.5. Multimodal Interaction in AR

In addition to speech and gesture recognition, there are other types of voice recognition are being investigated. For example, the whistle-recognition system was developed by Lindeman [303] in mobile AR games. In this, the user had to whistle the right length and pitch to intimidate the virtual creatures in the game. Summary: The common input techniques and input methods have been examined in this section. These included simple information browsers and complex AR interfaces. The simple ones have very little support for the interaction and virtual content, while the complex interfaces were able to recognize even the speech and gesture inputs. A wide range of input methods are available for the AR interface; however, they are needed to be designed carefully. The following section delineates the research into the interface pattern, design, and guideline for AR experiences.

9. Design Guidelines and Interface Pattern

The previous section detailed the wide range of different AR input and interaction technologies; however, more rigorous research is required to design the AR experience. This section explores the interface patterns and design guidelines to develop an AR experience.

The development of new interfaces goes through four main steps. First, the prototype is demonstrated. Second, interaction techniques are adopted from the other interface metaphors. Third, new interface metaphors are developed that are appropriate to the medium. Finally, the formal theoretical models are developed for modeling the interaction of users. In this regard, Wang et al. [304] employ user-centered AR instruction (UcAI) in procedural tasks. Thirty participants were selected for the experiment while having both the control and experiment groups. The result of the experiment suggested that introduction of UcAI increased the user's spatial cognitive ability, particularly in the high-precision operational task. This research has the potential of guiding advanced AR instruction designs to perform tasks of high cognitive complexity. For instance, WIMP (windows, icons, menus, and pointers) is a very well-known desktop metaphor. In development, it has gone through all of these stages. There are methods developed that are used to predict the time taken by the mouse will select an icon of a given size. These are known as formal theoretical models. Fitts law [305] is among those models that help in determining the pointing times in the user interfaces. There are also a number of virtual reality interfaces available that are at the third stage with reference to the techniques available. For example, the manipulation and selection in immersive virtual worlds can be done by using the go-go interaction method [306]. On the other hand, as evident in the previous section, AR interfaces have barely surpassed the first two stages. Similarly, a number of AR interaction methods and technologies are available; however, by and large, they are only the extensions or versions of the existing 3D and 2D techniques present in mobiles, laptops, or AR interfaces. For instance, mobile phone experiences such as the gesture application and the touch screen input are added to AR. Therefore, there is a dire need to develop AR-specific interaction techniques and interface metaphors [307]. A deeper analysis and study of AR interfaces will help in the development of the appropriate metaphor interfaces. AR interfaces are unique in the sense that they need to develop close interaction between the real and the virtual worlds. A researcher, MacIntyre, has argued that the definition and the fusion of the virtual and real worlds are required for creating an AR design [308]. The primary goal of this is to depict the physical objects and user input onto the computer-generated graphics. This is done by using a suitable interaction interface. As a result, an AR design should have three components:

- The physical object.
- The virtual image to be developed.
- An interface to create an interaction between the physical world and the virtual objects.

Use of *design patterns* could be an alternative technique to develop the AR interface design. These design patterns are most commonly used in the fields of computer science and design interface. Alexander has defined the use of design patterns in the following words: "Each pattern describes a problem that occurs over and over again in our environment, and then describes the core of the solution to that problem in such a way that you can use this solution a million times over, without ever doing it the same way twice" [309,310]. The pattern language approach could be used to enhance AR development, as suggested by Reicher [311]. This idea has evolved from the earlier research works of MacWilliam [312]. This approach has two main functionalities. First, it is more focused on the software engineering aspect. Secondly, it suggests ways to develop complex AR systems by combining different modules of design patterns. So, they describe each pattern by the number of its aspects such as name, motivation, goal, description, consequences, known project usage, and general usability. One of the most notable examples of it is the DWARF framework [313]. DWARF is a component-based AR framework that is developed through the design pattern approach. In contrast to the pattern language approach, the user experience of design in the AR handheld device could be used for developing designs. This was described by Xu and the main concern was pre-patterns. Pre-patterns are the components that bridge the gap between the game design and the interaction design. For determining the method of using of design patterns,seamful design could be used. This suggests that the designer should integrate the AR handheld game design and the technology in such a way that they should blend into each other. Some users need more attention for designing effective AR experiences; therefore, the designing of special needs is another intervention to resolve this discrepancy. For instance, as pointed out by Rand and MacIntyre [314], in designing an AR system for the age group of 6–9, the developmental stages of the children should be accounted for in it. The research has also suggested that a powerful educational experience could be created through the use of AR. In addition to this development, it was also stated that the developmental stages of the students should be considered [315,316]. However, there is no extensive research that suggests the development of AR experiences for children [317]. Radu, in his paper, has determined the key four areas that should be considered while designing AR for children: attention, motor, special, logic, and memory abilities [318].

10. Security, Trust, and Collaborative AR

Security is very important in augmented reality, especially in collaborative augmented reality. While using collaborative AR applications, the data are exposed to external attacks, which increases concerns about security relating to AR technologies. Moreover, if the users who share the same virtual collaborative environments are unknown to each other, it also elevates these issues. In [319], the basic premise of the research is that the developed abstraction device not only improves the privacy but also the performance of the AR apps, which lays the groundwork for the development of future OS support for AR apps. The results suggested that the prototype enables secure offloading of heavyweight, incurs negligible overhead, and improves the overall performance of the app. In [320], the authors aim to resolve security and privacy challenges in multi-user AR applications. They have introduced an AR-sharing module along with systematized designs and representative case studies for functionality and security. This module is implemented as a prototype known as ArShare for the HoloLens. Finally, it also lays the foundation for the development of fully fledged and secure multi-user AR interaction. In [321], the authors used AR smart glasses to detail the "security and safety" aspect of AR applications as a case study. In the experiment, cloud-based architecture is linked to the oil extractor in combination with Vuzix Blade smart glasses. For security purposes, this app sends real-time signals if a dangerous situation arrives. In [322], deep learning is used to make the adaptive policies for generating the visual output in AR devices. Simulations are used that automatically detect the situation and generate policies and protect the system against disastrous malicious content. In [323], the authors discussed the case study of challenges faced by VR and AR in the field of security and privacy. The results showed that the attack reached the target of distance 1.5 m with 90 percent accuracy when using a four-digit password. In [324], the authors provide details and goals for developing security. They discuss the challenges faced in the development of edge computing architecture which also includes the discussion regarding reducing security risks. The main idea of the paper is to detail the design of security measures for both AR and non-AR devices. In [325], the authors presented that the handling of multi-user outputs and handling of data are demonstrated are the two main obstacles in achieving security and privacy of AR devices. It further provides new opportunities that can significantly improve the security and privacy realm of AR. In [326], the authors introduce the authentication tool for ensuring security and privacy in AR environments. For these purposes, the graphical user password is fused with the AR environments. A doodle password is created by the touch-gesture-recognition on a mobile phone, and then doodles are matched in real-time size. Additionally, doodles are matched with the AR environment. In [327], the authors discussed the immersive nature of augmented reality engenders significant threats in the realm of security and privacy. They further explore the aspects of securing buggy AR output. In [328], the authors employ the case study of an Android app, "Google Translator", to detect and avoid variant privacy leaks. In addition, this research proposes the foundational framework to detect unnecessary privacy leaks. In [329], the authors discuss the AR security-related issues on the web. The security related vulnerabilities are identified and then engineering guidelines are proposed to make AR implementation secure. In [330], the past ten years of research work of the author, starting from 2011, in the field of augmented reality is presented. The main idea of the paper is to figure out the potential problems and to predict the future for the next ten years. It also explains the systematization for future work and focuses on evaluating AR security research. In [331], the authors presented various AR-related security issues and identified managing the virtual content in the real space as a challenge in making AR spaces secure for single and multi-users. The authors in [332] believe that there is a dire need of cybersecurity risks in the AR world. The introduction of systemized and universal policy modules for the AR architecture is a viable solution for mitigating security risks in AR. In [333], the authors discuss the challenge of enabling the different AR apps to augment the user's world experience simultaneously, pointing out the conflicts between the AR applications.

11. Summary

In this paper, the authors have reviewed the literature extensively in terms of tracking and displays technology, AR, and collaborative AR, as can be seen in Figure 10. It has been observed that collaborative AR has further two classifications i.e., co-located AR and remote collaboration [334]. Each of these collocated and remote collaborations has two further types i.e., synchronous and asynchronous. In remote collaborative AR, there are a number of use cases wherein it has been observed that *trust management* is too important a factor to consider because there are unknown parties that participate in remote activities to interact with each other and as such, they are unknown to each other as well [21,335–338]. There has been a lack of trust and security concerns during this remote collaboration. There are more chances of intrusion and vulnerabilities that can be possibly exploited [331,339,340]. One such collaboration is from the tourism sector, which has boosted the economy, especially in the pandemic era when physical interactors were not allowed [341]. To address these concerns, this research felt the need to ensure that the communication has integrity and for this purpose, the research utilized state-of-the-art blockchain infrastructure for collaborative applications in AR. The paper has proposed a complete secure framework wherein different applications working remotely are having a real feeling of trust in each other [17,342,343]. The participants within the collaborative AR subscribed to a trusted environment to further make interaction with each other in a secure fashion while their communication was protected through state-of-the-art blockchain infrastructure [338,344]. A model of such an application is shown in Figure 11.

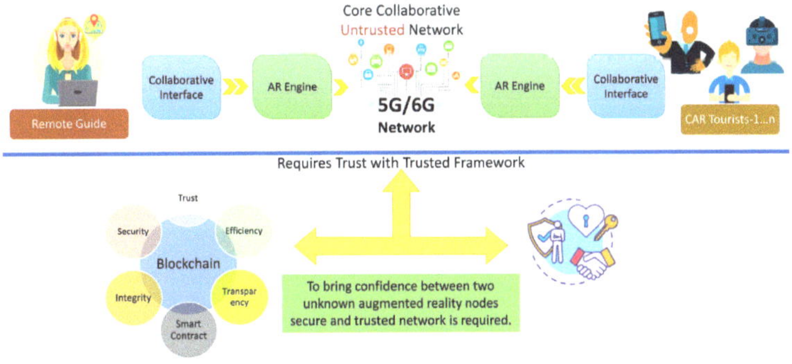

Figure 11. A model of blockchain-based trusted and secured collaborative AR system.

Figure 12 demonstrates the initiation of the AR App in step 1, while in step 2 of Figure 12, the blockchain is initiated to record transactions related to sign-up, record audio calls, proceed with payment/subscription, etc. In step 3, when the transaction is established, AR is initiated, which enables the visitor to receive guidance from the travel guide. The app creates a map of the real environment. The created map and the vision provide a SLAM, i.e., SLAM provides an overall vision and details of different objects in the real world. Inertial tracking controls the movement and direction in the augmented reality application. The virtual objects are then placed after identifying vision and tracking. In a collaborative environment, the guides are provided with an option of annotation so they can circle a particular object or spot different locations and landmarks or point to different incidents [16].

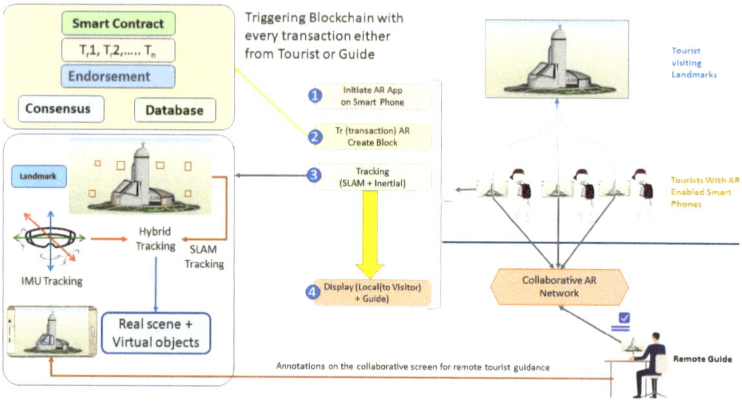

Figure 12. Sharing of the real-time environment of CAR tourist app for multiple users [16].

12. Directions for Research

The commercialization efforts of companies have made AR a mainstream field. However, for the technology to reach its full potential, the number of research areas should be expanded. Azuma has explained the three major obstacles in the way of AR: interface limitation, technological limitations, and the issue of social acceptance. In order to overcome these barriers, the two major models are developed: first, Roger's innovation diffusion theory [345] and the technology acceptance model (developed by Martinez) [346]. Roger has explained the following major restriction towards the adoption of this technology: limited computational power of AR technology, social acceptance, no AR standards, tracking inaccuracy, and overloading of information. The main research trends in display technology, user interface, and tracking were identified by Zho by evaluating ten years of ISMAR papers. The research has been conducted in a wide number of areas except for social acceptance. This section aims at exploring future opportunities and ongoing research in the field of AR, particularly in the four key areas: display, tracking, interaction, and social acceptance. Moreover, there are a number of other topics including evaluation techniques, visualization methods, applications, authoring and content-creating tools, rendering methods, and some other areas.

13. Conclusions

This document has detailed a number of research papers that address certain problems of AR. For instance, AR tracking techniques are detailed in Section 3. Display technologies, such as VST and OST, and its related calibration techniques in Section 4, authoring tools in Section 6, collaborative AR in Section 7, AR interaction in Section 8, and design guidelines in Section 9. Finally, promising security and trust-related papers are discussed in the final section. We presented the problem statement and a short solution to the problem is provided. These aspects should be covered in future research and the most pertinent among these are the hybrid AR interfaces, social acceptance, etc. The speed of research is significantly increasing, and AR technology is going to dramatically impact our lives in the next 20 years.

Author Contributions: Conceptualization of the paper is done by T.A.S. Sections Organization, is mostly written by T.A.S. and S.J.; The protype implementation is done by the development team, however, the administration and coordination is performed by A.A., A.N. (Abdullah Namoun) and A.B.A.; Validation is done by A.A. and A.N. (Adnan Nadeem); Formal Analysis is done by T.A.S. and S.J.; Investigation, T.A.S.; Resources and Data Curation, is done by A.N. (Adnan Nadeem); Writing—Original Draft Preparation, is done by T.A.S. and S.J., Writing—Review & Editing is carried out by H.B.A.; Visualization is mostly done by T.A.S. and M.S.S.; Supervision, is done by T.A.S.; Project Administration, is done by A.A.; Funding Acquisition, T.A.S. All authors have read and agreed to the published version of the manuscript.

Funding: This project is funded by the Deputyship For Research and Innovation, Ministry of Education, Kingdom of Saudi Arabia, under project No (20/17), titled Digital Transformation of Madinah Landmarks using Augmented Reality.

Acknowledgments: Thanks to the Deanship of Research, Islamic University of Madinah. We would like to extend special thanks to our other team members (Anas and his development team at 360Folio, Ali Ullah and Sajjad Hussain Khan) who participated in the development, writeup, and finding of historical data. Ali Ullah has a great ability to understand difficult topics in AR, such as calibration and tracking.

Conflicts of Interest: The authors declare no conflict of interest.

References

1. Berciu, A.G.; Dulf, E.H.; Stefan, I.A. Flexible Augmented Reality-Based Health Solution for Medication Weight Establishment. *Processes* **2022**, *10*, 219. [CrossRef]
2. Sırakaya, M.; Alsancak Sırakaya, D. Augmented reality in STEM education: A systematic review. *Interact. Learn. Environ.* **2022**, *30*, 1556–1569. [CrossRef]
3. Chouchene, A.; Ventura Carvalho, A.; Charrua-Santos, F.; Barhoumi, W. Augmented Reality-Based Framework Supporting Visual Inspection for Automotive Industry. *Appl. Syst. Innov.* **2022**, *5*, 48. [CrossRef]
4. Augmented Reality and Virtual Reality Market. 2022, Available online: https://www.marketsandmarkets.com/Market-Reports/augmented-reality-virtual-reality-market-1185.html?gclid=CjwKCAjwtKmaBhBMEiwAyINuwNi_hv87XEg2rZqpBVQGtOr1gL8mNrLbRsYaSZmNYOXF4Za63Bhb4xoChZkQAvD_BwE (accessed on 16 October 2022).
5. Lee, W.H.; Lee, H.K. The usability attributes and evaluation measurements of mobile media AR (augmented reality). *Cogent Arts Humanit.* **2016**, *3*, 1241171. [CrossRef]
6. Mourtzis, D.; Angelopoulos, J.; Panopoulos, N. Challenges and Opportunities for Integrating Augmented Reality and Computational Fluid Dynamics Modeling under the Framework of Industry 4.0. *Procedia CIRP* **2022**, *106*, 215–220. [CrossRef]
7. Carter, D. Immersive Employee Experiences in the Metaverse: Virtual Work Environments, Augmented Analytics Tools, and Sensory and Tracking Technologies. *Psychosociological Issues Hum. Resour. Manag.* **2022**, *10*, 35–49.
8. Zhang, Z.; Wen, F.; Sun, Z.; Guo, X.; He, T.; Lee, C. Artificial Intelligence-Enabled Sensing Technologies in the 5G/Internet of Things Era: From Virtual Reality/Augmented Reality to the Digital Twin. *Adv. Intell. Syst.* **2022**, *2022*, 2100228. [CrossRef]
9. Yu, J.; Denham, A.R.; Searight, E. A systematic review of augmented reality game-based Learning in STEM education. *Educ. Technol. Res. Dev.* **2022**, *70*, 1169–1194.
10. Moro, M.; Marchesi, G.; Hesse, F.; Odone, F.; Casadio, M. Markerless vs. Marker-Based Gait Analysis: A Proof of Concept Study. *Sensors* **2022**, *22*, 2011. [CrossRef]
11. Pulli, K. 11–2: Invited Paper: Meta 2: Immersive Optical-See-Through Augmented Reality. In *SID Symposium Digest of Technical Papers*; Wiley Online Library: Hoboken, NJ, USA, 2017; Volume 48, pp. 132–133.
12. Wilson, A.; Hua, H. Design and demonstration of a vari-focal optical see-through head-mounted display using freeform Alvarez lenses. *Opt. Express* **2019**, *27*, 15627–15637. [CrossRef]
13. Khan, D.; Ullah, S.; Yan, D.M.; Rabbi, I.; Richard, P.; Hoang, T.; Billinghurst, M.; Zhang, X. Robust tracking through the design of high quality fiducial markers: an optimization tool for ARToolKit. *IEEE Access* **2018**, *6*, 22421–22433. [CrossRef]
14. Ramadar, P. NS Flartoolkit Flash Augmented Reality Alt Actionscript, Journal=Buku AR Online Solo. 2014. Available online: https://artoolworks.com/products/open-source-software/flartoolkit-2.html (accessed on 16 October 2022).
15. Linowes, J.; Babilinski, K. *Augmented Reality for Developers: Build Practical Augmented Reality Applications with Unity, ARCore, ARKit, and Vuforia*; Packt Publishing Ltd.: Birmingham, UK, 2017.
16. Syed, T.A.; Jan, S.; Siddiqui, M.S.; Alzahrani, A.; Nadeem, A.; Ali, A.; Ullah, A. CAR-Tourist: An Integrity-Preserved Collaborative Augmented Reality Framework-Tourism as a Use-Case. *Appl. Sci.* **2022**, *12*, 12022. [CrossRef]
17. Syed, T.A.; Alzahrani, A.; Jan, S.; Siddiqui, M.S.; Nadeem, A.; Alghamdi, T. A comparative analysis of blockchain architecture and its applications: Problems and recommendations. *IEEE Access* **2019**, *7*, 176838–176869. [CrossRef]

18. Agati, S.S.; Bauer, R.D.; Hounsell, M.d.S.; Paterno, A.S. Augmented reality for manual assembly in industry 4.0: Gathering guidelines. In Proceedings of the 2020 22nd Symposium on Virtual and Augmented Reality (SVR), Porto de Galinhas, Brazil, 7–10 November 2020; pp. 179–188.
19. Brooker, J. The polytechnic ghost: Pepper's ghost, metempsychosis and the magic lantern at the Royal Polytechnic Institution. *Early Pop. Vis. Cult.* **2007**, *5*, 189–206. [CrossRef]
20. Drascic, D.; Grodski, J.J.; Milgram, P.; Ruffo, K.; Wong, P.; Zhai, S. ARGOS: A display system for augmenting reality. In Proceedings of the INTERACT'93 and CHI'93 Conference on Human Factors in Computing Systems, Amsterdam, The Netherlands, 24–29 April 1993; p. 521.
21. Abdeen, M.; Jan, S.; Khan, S.; Ali, T. Employing Takaful Islamic Banking Through State of The Art Blockchain: A Case Study. *Int. J. Adv. Comput. Sci. Appl.* **2019**, *10*, 648–654. [CrossRef]
22. Kerber, R. Advanced tactic targeted grocer. *The Boston Globe*. 2008. Available online: https://seclists.org/isn/2008/Mar/126 (accessed on 20 October 2022).
23. Mansfield-Devine, S. Interview: BYOD and the enterprise network. *Comput. Fraud Secur.* **2012**, *2012*, 14–17. [CrossRef]
24. Nofer, M.; Gomber, P.; Hinz, O.; Schiereck, D. Blockchain. *Bus. Inf. Syst. Eng.* **2017**, *59*, 183–187. [CrossRef]
25. Behzadan, A.H.; Aziz, Z.; Anumba, C.J.; Kamat, V.R. Ubiquitous location tracking for context-specific information delivery on construction sites. *Autom. Constr.* **2008**, *17*, 737–748. [CrossRef]
26. Bottani, E.; Vignali, G. Augmented reality technology in the manufacturing industry: A review of the last decade. *IISE Trans.* **2019**, *51*, 284–310. [CrossRef]
27. Sereno, M.; Wang, X.; Besançon, L.; McGuffin, M.J.; Isenberg, T. Collaborative work in augmented reality: A survey. *IEEE Trans. Vis. Comput. Graph.* **2020**, *28*, 2530–2549. [CrossRef]
28. Ens, B.; Quigley, A.; Yeo, H.S.; Irani, P.; Piumsomboon, T.; Billinghurst, M. Counterpoint: Exploring mixed-scale gesture interaction for AR applications. In Proceedings of the Extended Abstracts of the 2018 CHI Conference on Human Factors in Computing Systems, Montreal, QC, Canada, 21–26 April 2018; pp. 1–6.
29. Hettig, J.; Engelhardt, S.; Hansen, C.; Mistelbauer, G. AR in VR: Assessing surgical augmented reality visualizations in a steerable virtual reality environment. *Int. J. Comput. Assist. Radiol. Surg.* **2018**, *13*, 1717–1725. [CrossRef] [PubMed]
30. Goh, E.S.; Sunar, M.S.; Ismail, A.W. 3D object manipulation techniques in handheld mobile augmented reality interface: A review. *IEEE Access* **2019**, *7*, 40581–40601. [CrossRef]
31. Kollatsch, C.; Klimant, P. Efficient integration process of production data into Augmented Reality based maintenance of machine tools. *Prod. Eng.* **2021**, *15*, 311–319. [CrossRef]
32. Bhattacharyya, P.; Nath, R.; Jo, Y.; Jadhav, K.; Hammer, J. Brick: Toward a model for designing synchronous colocated augmented reality games. In Proceedings of the 2019 CHI Conference on Human Factors in Computing Systems, Glasgow, UK 4–9 May 2019; pp. 1–9.
33. Kim, K.; Billinghurst, M.; Bruder, G.; Duh, H.B.L.; Welch, G.F. Revisiting trends in augmented reality research: A review of the 2nd decade of ISMAR (2008–2017). *IEEE Trans. Vis. Comput. Graph.* **2018**, *24*, 2947–2962. [CrossRef]
34. Liu, H.; Wang, L. An AR-based worker support system for human-robot collaboration. *Procedia Manuf.* **2017**, *11*, 22–30. [CrossRef]
35. Cortés-Dávalos, A.; Mendoza, S. Collaborative Web Authoring of 3D Surfaces Using Augmented Reality on Mobile Devices. In Proceedings of the 2016 IEEE/WIC/ACM International Conference on Web Intelligence (WI), Omaha, NE, USA, 13–16 October 2016; pp. 640–643.
36. Qiao, X.; Ren, P.; Dustdar, S.; Liu, L.; Ma, H.; Chen, J. Web AR: A promising future for mobile augmented reality—State of the art, challenges, and insights. *Proc. IEEE* **2019**, *107*, 651–666. [CrossRef]
37. Shukri, S.A.A.; Arshad, H.; Abidin, R.Z. The design guidelines of mobile augmented reality for tourism in Malaysia. In *AIP Conference Proceedings*; AIP Publishing LLC: Melville, NY, USA, 2017; Volume 1891, p. 020026.
38. Fallahkhair, S.; Brito, C.A. Design Guidelines for Development of Augmented Reality Application with Mobile and Wearable Technologies for Contextual Learning. *Braz. J. Technol. Commun. Cogn. Sci.* **2019**, *7*, 1–16.
39. Akçayır, M.; Akçayır, G. Advantages and challenges associated with augmented reality for education: A systematic review of the literature. *Educ. Res. Rev.* **2017**, *20*, 1–11. [CrossRef]
40. da Silva, M.M.; Teixeira, J.M.X.; Cavalcante, P.S.; Teichrieb, V. Perspectives on how to evaluate augmented reality technology tools for education: A systematic review. *J. Braz. Comput. Soc.* **2019**, *25*, 1–18. [CrossRef]
41. Sarkar, P.; Pillai, J.S.; Gupta, A. ScholAR: A collaborative learning experience for rural schools using Augmented Reality application. In Proceedings of the 2018 IEEE Tenth International Conference on Technology for Education (T4E), Chennai, India, 10–13 December 2018; pp. 8–15.
42. Soleimani, H.; Jalilifar, A.; Rouhi, A.; Rahmanian, M. Augmented Reality and Virtual Reality Scaffoldings in Improving the Abstract Genre Structure in a Collaborative Learning Environment: A CALL Study. *J. Engl. Lang. Teach. Learn.* **2019**, *11*, 327–356.
43. Hadar, E. Toward Development Tools for Augmented Reality Applications—A Practitioner Perspective. In *Workshop on Enterprise and Organizational Modeling and Simulation*; Springer: Berlin/Heidelberg, Germany, 2018; pp. 91–104.
44. Mukhametshin, S.; Makhmutova, A.; Anikin, I. Sensor tag detection, tracking and recognition for AR application. In Proceedings of the 2019 International Conference on Industrial Engineering, Applications and Manufacturing (ICIEAM), Tokyo, Japan, 12–15 April 2019; pp. 1–5.

45. Santoni, F.; De Angelis, A.; Moschitta, A.; Carbone, P. MagIK: A Hand-Tracking Magnetic Positioning System Based on a Kinematic Model of the Hand. *IEEE Trans. Instrum. Meas.* **2021**, *70*, 1–13. [CrossRef]
46. Frikha, R.; Ejbali, R.; Zaied, M. Handling occlusion in augmented reality surgical training based instrument tracking. In Proceedings of the 2016 IEEE/ACS 13th International Conference of Computer Systems and Applications (AICCSA), Agadir, Morocco, 29 November–2 December 2016; pp. 1–5.
47. Wang, M.; Shi, Q.; Song, S.; Meng, M.Q.H. A novel magnetic tracking approach for intrabody objects. *IEEE Sensors J.* **2020**, *20*, 4976–4984. [CrossRef]
48. Davis, F.D.; Bagozzi, R.P.; Warshaw, P.R. User acceptance of computer technology: A comparison of two theoretical models. *Manag. Sci.* **1989**, *35*, 982–1003. [CrossRef]
49. Davison, A.J.; Reid, I.D.; Molton, N.D.; Stasse, O. MonoSLAM: Real-time single camera SLAM. *IEEE Trans. Pattern Anal. Mach. Intell.* **2007**, *29*, 1052–1067. [CrossRef] [PubMed]
50. De Smet, J. The Smart Contact Lens: From an Artificial Iris to a Contact Lens Display. Ph.D. Thesis, Ghent University, Ghent, Belgium, 2014.
51. Dissanayake, M.G.; Newman, P.; Clark, S.; Durrant-Whyte, H.F.; Csorba, M. A solution to the simultaneous localization and map building (SLAM) problem. *IEEE Trans. Robot. Autom.* **2001**, *17*, 229–241. [CrossRef]
52. Dodgson, N.A. Autostereoscopic 3D displays. *Computer* **2005**, *38*, 31–36. [CrossRef]
53. De Smet, J.; Avci, A.; Joshi, P.; Schaubroeck, D.; Cuypers, D.; De Smet, H. Progress toward a liquid crystal contact lens display. *J. Soc. Inf. Disp.* **2013**, *21*, 399–406. [CrossRef]
54. Heidemann, G.; Bax, I.; Bekel, H. Multimodal interaction in an augmented reality scenario. In Proceedings of the 6th International Conference on Multimodal Interfaces, State College, PA, USA, 13–15 October 2004; pp. 53–60.
55. Chakrabarty, A.; Morris, R.; Bouyssounouse, X.; Hunt, R. Autonomous indoor object tracking with the Parrot AR. Drone. In Proceedings of the 2016 International Conference on Unmanned Aircraft Systems (ICUAS), Arlington, VA, USA, 7–10 June 2016; pp. 25–30.
56. Buttner, S.; Sand, O.; Rocker, C. Exploring design opportunities for intelligent worker assistance: A new approach using projetion-based AR and a novel hand-tracking algorithm. In Proceedings of the European Conference on Ambient Intelligence, Malaga, Spain, 26–28 April 2017; Springer: Berlin/Heidelberg, Germany, 2017; pp. 33–45.
57. Gupta, S.; Chaudhary, R.; Gupta, S.; Kaur, A.; Mantri, A. A survey on tracking techniques in augmented reality based application. In Proceedings of the 2019 Fifth International Conference on Image Information Processing (ICIIP), Shimla, India, 15–17 November 2019; pp. 215–220.
58. Krishna, V.; Ding, Y.; Xu, A.; Höllerer, T. Multimodal biometric authentication for VR/AR using EEG and eye tracking. In Proceedings of the Adjunct of the 2019 International Conference on Multimodal Interaction, Suzhou, China, 14–18 October 2019; pp. 1–5.
59. Dzsotjan, D.; Ludwig-Petsch, K.; Mukhametov, S.; Ishimaru, S.; Kuechemann, S.; Kuhn, J. The Predictive Power of Eye-Tracking Data in an Interactive AR Learning Environment. In Proceedings of the Adjunct Proceedings of the 2021 ACM International Joint Conference on Pervasive and Ubiquitous Computing and Proceedings of the 2021 ACM International Symposium on Wearable Computers, Virtual, 21–26 September 2021; pp. 467–471.
60. Chen, L.; Cao, C.; De la Torre, F.; Saragih, J.; Xu, C.; Sheikh, Y. High-fidelity Face Tracking for AR/VR via Deep Lighting Adaptation. In Proceedings of the IEEE/CVF Conference on Computer Vision and Pattern Recognition, Nashville, TN, USA, 20–25 June 2021 pp. 13059–13069.
61. Rambach, J.; Pagani, A.; Schneider, M.; Artemenko, O.; Stricker, D. 6DoF object tracking based on 3D scans for augmented reality remote live support. *Computers* **2018**, *7*, 6. [CrossRef]
62. Ha, T.; Billinghurst, M.; Woo, W. An interactive 3D movement path manipulation method in an augmented reality environment. *Interact. Comput.* **2012**, *24*, 10–24. [CrossRef]
63. Syahidi, A.A.; Tolle, H.; Supianto, A.A.; Arai, K. AR-Child: Analysis, Evaluation, and Effect of Using Augmented Reality as a Learning Media for Preschool Children. In Proceedings of the 2019 5th International Conference on Computing Engineering and Design (ICCED), Purwokerto, Indonesia, 5–6 August 2019; pp. 1–6.
64. Wang, X.; Dunston, P.S. User perspectives on mixed reality tabletop visualization for face-to-face collaborative design review. *Autom. Constr.* **2008**, *17*, 399–412. [CrossRef]
65. Wang, X.; Dunston, P.S. Comparative effectiveness of mixed reality-based virtual environments in collaborative design. *IEEE Trans. Syst. Man Cybern. Part C* **2011**, *41*, 284–296. [CrossRef]
66. Hauptmann, A.G. Speech and gestures for graphic image manipulation. In Proceedings of the SIGCHI Conference on Human Factors in Computing Systems, Austin, TX, USA, 30 April–4 June 1989; pp. 241–245.
67. Heath, C.; Luff, P. Disembodied conduct: Communication through video in a multi-media office environment. In Proceedings of the SIGCHI Conference on Human Factors in Computing Systems, New Orleans, LA, USA, 27 April–2 May 1991; pp. 99–103.
68. Rambach, J.; Pagani, A.; Stricker, D. [poster] Augmented things: Enhancing AR applications leveraging the internet of things and universal 3D object tracking. In Proceedings of the 2017 IEEE International Symposium on Mixed and Augmented Reality (ISMAR-Adjunct), Nantes, France, 9–13 October 2017; pp. 103–108.

69. Viyanon, W.; Songsuittipong, T.; Piyapaisarn, P.; Sudchid, S. AR furniture: Integrating augmented reality technology to enhance interior design using marker and markerless tracking. In Proceedings of the 2nd International Conference on Intelligent Information Processing, Bangkok Thailand, 17–18 July 2017; pp. 1–7.
70. Turkan, Y.; Radkowski, R.; Karabulut-Ilgu, A.; Behzadan, A.H.; Chen, A. Mobile augmented reality for teaching structural analysis. *Adv. Eng. Inform.* **2017**, *34*, 90–100. [CrossRef]
71. Dorfmüller, K. Robust tracking for augmented reality using retroreflective markers. *Comput. Graph.* **1999**, *23*, 795–800. [CrossRef]
72. Danielsson, O.; Holm, M.; Syberfeldt, A. Augmented reality smart glasses for operators in production: Survey of relevant categories for supporting operators. *Procedia CIRP* **2020**, *93*, 1298–1303. [CrossRef]
73. Dörner, R.; Geiger, C.; Haller, M.; Paelke, V. Authoring mixed reality—A component and framework-based approach. In *Entertainment Computing*; Springer: Berlin/Heidelberg, Germany, 2003; pp. 405–413.
74. Drascic, D.; Milgram, P. Positioning accuracy of a virtual stereographic pointer in a real stereoscopic video world. In Proceedings of the Stereoscopic Displays and Applications II, San Jose, CA, USA, 25–27 February 1991; Volume 1457, pp. 302–313.
75. Drascic, D.; Milgram, P. Perceptual issues in augmented reality. In Proceedings of the Stereoscopic Displays and Virtual Reality Systems III. International Society for Optics and Photonics, San Jose, CA, USA, 30 January–2 February 1996; Volume 2653, pp. 123–134.
76. Dünser, A. Supporting low ability readers with interactive augmented reality. *Annu. Rev. Cybertherapy Telemed.* **2008**, *6*, 39–46.
77. Dünser, A.; Hornecker, E. Lessons from an AR book study. In Proceedings of the 1st International Conference on Tangible and Embedded Interaction, Baton Rouge, LA, USA, 15–17 February 2007; pp. 179–182.
78. Gibson, L.; Hanson, V.L. Digital motherhood: How does technology help new mothers? In Proceedings of the SIGCHI Conference on Human Factors in Computing Systems, Paris, France, 27 April–2 May 2013; pp. 313–322.
79. Wuest, H.; Engekle, T.; Wientapper, F.; Schmitt, F.; Keil, J. From CAD to 3D Tracking—Enhancing & Scaling Model-Based Tracking for Industrial Appliances. In Proceedings of the 2016 IEEE International Symposium on Mixed and Augmented Reality (ISMAR-Adjunct), Merida, Mexico, 19–23 September 2016; pp. 346–347.
80. LaViola, J.J. A discussion of cybersickness in virtual environments. *ACM SIGCHI Bull.* **2000**, *32*, 47–56. [CrossRef]
81. Gao, Y.F.; Wang, H.Y.; Bian, X.N. Marker tracking for video-based augmented reality. In Proceedings of the 2016 International Conference on Machine Learning and Cybernetics (ICMLC), Jeju Island, Republic of Korea, 10–13 July 2016; Volume 2, pp. 928–932.
82. Szalavári, Z.; Eckstein, E.; Gervautz, M. Collaborative gaming in augmented reality. In Proceedings of the ACM Symposium on Virtual Reality Software and Technology, Taipei, Taiwan, 2–5 November 1998; pp. 195–204.
83. Dolata, M.; Agotai, D.; Schubiger, S.; Schwabe, G. Pen-and-paper rituals in service interaction: Combining high-touch and high-tech in financial advisory encounters. *Proc. ACM Hum.-Comput. Interact.* **2019**, *3*, 1–24. [CrossRef]
84. Butz, A.; Hollerer, T.; Feiner, S.; MacIntyre, B.; Beshers, C. Enveloping users and computers in a collaborative 3D augmented reality. In Proceedings of the 2nd IEEE and ACM International Workshop on Augmented Reality (IWAR'99), San Francisco, CA, USA, 20–21 October 1999; pp. 35–44.
85. Müller, J.; Rädle, R.; Reiterer, H. Remote collaboration with mixed reality displays: How shared virtual landmarks facilitate spatial referencing. In Proceedings of the 2017 CHI Conference on Human Factors in Computing Systems, Denver, CO, USA, 6–11 May 2017; pp. 6481–6486.
86. Gül, L.F. Studying gesture-based interaction on a mobile augmented reality application for co-design activity. *J. Multimodal User Interfaces* **2018**, *12*, 109–124. [CrossRef]
87. Benko, H.; Ishak, E.W.; Feiner, S. Collaborative mixed reality visualization of an archaeological excavation. In Proceedings of the Third IEEE and ACM International Symposium on Mixed and Augmented Reality, Arlington, VA, USA, 5 November 2004; pp. 132–140.
88. Franz, J.; Alnusayri, M.; Malloch, J.; Reilly, D. A comparative evaluation of techniques for sharing AR experiences in museums. *Proc. ACM Hum.-Comput. Interact.* **2019**, *3*, 1–20. [CrossRef]
89. An, Z.; Xu, X.; Yang, J.; Liu, Y.; Yan, Y. Research of the three-dimensional tracking and registration method based on multiobjective constraints in an AR system. *Appl. Opt.* **2018**, *57*, 9625–9634. [CrossRef]
90. Oskiper, T.; Samarasekera, S.; Kumar, R. [POSTER] CamSLAM: Vision Aided Inertial Tracking and Mapping Framework for Large Scale AR Applications. In Proceedings of the 2017 IEEE International Symposium on Mixed and Augmented Reality (ISMAR-Adjunct), Nantes, France, 9–13 October 2017; pp. 216–217.
91. Zhang, W.; Han, B.; Hui, P. Jaguar: Low latency mobile augmented reality with flexible tracking. In Proceedings of the 26th ACM International Conference on Multimedia, Seoul, Republic of Korea, 22–26 October 2018; pp. 355–363.
92. Tokusho, Y.; Feiner, S. Prototyping an outdoor mobile augmented reality street view application. In *ISMAR Workshop on Outdoor Mixed and Augmented Reality*; Citeseer: Princeton, NJ, USA, 2009; Volume 2.
93. Henrysson, A.; Ollila, M. UMAR: Ubiquitous mobile augmented reality. In Proceedings of the 3rd International Conference on Mobile and Ubiquitous Multimedia, College Park, MD, USA, 27–29 October 2004; pp. 41–45.
94. Henrysson, A.; Ollila, M.; Billinghurst, M. Mobile phone based AR scene assembly. In Proceedings of the 4th International Conference on Mobile and Ubiquitous Multimedia, Christchurch, New Zealand, 8–10 December 2005; pp. 95–102.
95. Hilliges, O.; Kim, D.; Izadi, S.; Weiss, M.; Wilson, A. HoloDesk: Direct 3d interactions with a situated see-through display. In Proceedings of the SIGCHI Conference on Human Factors in Computing Systems, Austin, TX, USA, 5–10 May 2012; pp. 2421–2430.

96. Ar, Y.; Ünal, M.; Sert, S.Y.; Bostanci, E.; Kanwal, N.; Güzel, M.S. Evolutionary Fuzzy Adaptive Motion Models for User Tracking in Augmented Reality Applications. In Proceedings of the 2018 2nd International Symposium on Multidisciplinary Studies and Innovative Technologies (ISMSIT), Ankara, Turkey, 19–21 October 2018; pp. 1–6.
97. Ashutosh, K. Hardware Performance Analysis of Mobile-Based Augmented Reality Systems. In Proceedings of the 2020 International Conference on Computational Performance Evaluation (ComPE), Shillong, India, 2–4 July 2020; pp. 671–675.
98. Yang, X.; Fan, X.; Wang, J.; Yin, X.; Qiu, S. Edge-based cover recognition and tracking method for an AR-aided aircraft inspection system. *Int. J. Adv. Manuf. Technol.* **2020**, *111*, 3505–3518. [CrossRef]
99. Kang, D.; Heo, J.; Kang, B.; Nam, D. Pupil detection and tracking for AR 3D under various circumstances. *Electron. Imaging* **2019**, *2019*, 55-1–55-5. [CrossRef]
100. Hu, X.; Hua, H. Design of an optical see-through multi-focal-plane stereoscopic 3d display using freeform prisms. In *Frontiers in Optics*; Optical Society of America: Washington, DC, USA, 2012; p. FTh1F–2.
101. Hourcade, J.P. *Interaction Design and Children*; Now Publishers Inc.: Delft, The Netherland, 2008.
102. Kang, D.; Ma, L. Real-Time Eye Tracking for Bare and Sunglasses-Wearing Faces for Augmented Reality 3D Head-Up Displays. *IEEE Access* **2021**, *9*, 125508–125522. [CrossRef]
103. Jeong, J.; Lee, C.K.; Lee, B.; Lee, S.; Moon, S.; Sung, G.; Lee, H.S.; Lee, B. Holographically printed freeform mirror array for augmented reality near-eye display. *IEEE Photonics Technol. Lett.* **2020**, *32*, 991–994. [CrossRef]
104. Park, S.g. Augmented and mixed reality optical see-through combiners based on plastic optics. *Inf. Disp.* **2021**, *37*, 6–11. [CrossRef]
105. Lee, Y.H.; Zhan, T.; Wu, S.T. Prospects and challenges in augmented reality displays. *Virtual Real. Intell. Hardw.* **2019**, *1*, 10–20. [CrossRef]
106. Jang, C.; Mercier, O.; Bang, K.; Li, G.; Zhao, Y.; Lanman, D. Design and fabrication of freeform holographic optical elements. *ACM Trans. Graph. (TOG)* **2020**, *39*, 1–15. [CrossRef]
107. Yu, C.; Peng, Y.; Zhao, Q.; Li, H.; Liu, X. Highly efficient waveguide display with space-variant volume holographic gratings. *Appl. Opt.* **2017**, *56*, 9390–9397. [CrossRef]
108. Gorovyi, I.M.; Sharapov, D.S. Advanced image tracking approach for augmented reality applications. In Proceedings of the 2017 Signal Processing Symposium (SPSympo), Auckland, New Zealand, 27–30 November 2017; pp. 1–5.
109. Hix, D.; Gabbard, J.L.; Swan, J.E.; Livingston, M.A.; Hollerer, T.H.; Julier, S.J.; Baillot, Y.; Brown, D. A cost-effective usability evaluation progression for novel interactive systems. In Proceedings of the 37th Annual Hawaii International Conference on System Sciences, Big Island, HI, USA, 5–8 January 2004.
110. Hodges, S.; Williams, L.; Berry, E.; Izadi, S.; Srinivasan, J.; Butler, A.; Smyth, G.; Kapur, N.; Wood, K. SenseCam: A retrospective memory aid. In Proceedings of the International Conference on Ubiquitous Computing, Seoul, Republic of Korea, 21–24 September 2008; Springer: Berlin/Heidelberg, Germany, 2006; pp. 177–193.
111. Isham, M.I.M.; Mohamed, F.; Siang, C.V.; Yusoff, Y.A.; Abd Aziz, A.A.; Dewi, D.E.O. A framework of ultrasounds image slice positioning and orientation in 3D augmented reality environment using hybrid tracking method. In Proceedings of the 2018 IEEE Conference on Big Data and Analytics (ICBDA), Seattle, WA, USA, 10–13 December 2018; pp. 105–110.
112. Park, J.H.; Kim, S.B. Optical see-through holographic near-eye-display with eyebox steering and depth of field control. *Opt. Express* **2018**, *26*, 27076–27088. [CrossRef]
113. Chakravarthula, P.; Peng, Y.; Kollin, J.; Fuchs, H.; Heide, F. Wirtinger holography for near-eye displays. *ACM Trans. Graph. (TOG)* **2019**, *38*, 1–13. [CrossRef]
114. Peng, Y.; Choi, S.; Padmanaban, N.; Wetzstein, G. Neural holography with camera-in-the-loop training. *ACM Trans. Graph. (TOG)* **2020**, *39*, 1–14. [CrossRef]
115. Ruan, W.; Yao, L.; Sheng, Q.Z.; Falkner, N.J.; Li, X. Tagtrack: Device-free localization and tracking using passive rfid tags. In Proceedings of the 11th International Conference on Mobile and Ubiquitous Systems: Computing, Networking and Services, London, UK, 2–5 December 2014; pp. 80–89.
116. Ellis, S.R.; Menges, B.M. Studies of the Localization of Virtual Objects in the Near Visual Field. In *Fundamentals of Wearable Computers and Augmented Reality*, 1st ed.; CRC Press: Boca Raton, FL, USA, 2001.
117. Evennou, F.; Marx, F. Advanced integration of WiFi and inertial navigation systems for indoor mobile positioning. *EURASIP J. Adv. Signal Process.* **2006**, *2006*, 1–11. [CrossRef]
118. Bach, B.; Sicat, R.; Pfister, H.; Quigley, A. Drawing into the AR-CANVAS: Designing embedded visualizations for augmented reality. In *Workshop on Immersive Analytics*; IEEE Vis: Piscataway, NJ, USA, 2017.
119. Zeng, H.; He, X.; Pan, H. FunPianoAR: A novel AR application for piano learning considering paired play based on multi-marker tracking. *J. Phys. Conf. Ser.* **2019**, *1229*, 012072. [CrossRef]
120. Rewkowski, N.; State, A.; Fuchs, H. Small Marker Tracking with Low-Cost, Unsynchronized, Movable Consumer Cameras For Augmented Reality Surgical Training. In Proceedings of the 2020 IEEE International Symposium on Mixed and Augmented Reality Adjunct (ISMAR-Adjunct), Recife, Brazil, 9–13 November 2020; pp. 90–95.
121. Hoffman, H.G. Physically touching virtual objects using tactile augmentation enhances the realism of virtual environments. In Proceedings of the IEEE 1998 Virtual Reality Annual International Symposium (Cat. No. 98CB36180), Atlanta, GA, USA, 14–18 March 1998; pp. 59–63.

122. Mao, W.; He, J.; Qiu, L. Cat: High-precision acoustic motion tracking. In Proceedings of the 22nd Annual International Conference on Mobile Computing and Networking, New York, NY, USA, 3–7 October 2016; pp. 69–81.
123. Höllerer, T.; Wither, J.; DiVerdi, S. "Anywhere augmentation": Towards mobile augmented reality in unprepared environments. In *Location Based Services and TeleCartography*; Springer: Berlin/Heidelberg, Germany, 2007; pp. 393–416.
124. Hong, J. Considering privacy issues in the context of Google glass. *Commun. ACM* **2013**, *56*, 10–11. [CrossRef]
125. Hua, H.; Brown, L.D.; Gao, C.; Ahuja, N. A new collaborative infrastructure: SCAPE. In Proceedings of the IEEE Virtual Reality, 2003. Proceedings, Los Angeles, CA, USA, 22–26 March 2003; IEEE: Piscataway, NJ, USA, 2003; pp. 171–179.
126. Huang, Y.; Weng, D.; Liu, Y.; Wang, Y. Key issues of wide-area tracking system for multi-user augmented reality adventure game. In Proceedings of the 2009 Fifth International Conference on Image and Graphics, Xi'an, China, 20–23 September 2009; pp. 646–651.
127. Huber, M.; Pustka, D.; Keitler, P.; Echtler, F.; Klinker, G. A system architecture for ubiquitous tracking environments. In Proceedings of the 2007 6th IEEE and ACM International Symposium on Mixed and Augmented Reality, Nara, Japan, 13–16 November 2007; pp. 211–214.
128. Hugues, O.; Fuchs, P.; Nannipieri, O. New augmented reality taxonomy: Technologies and features of augmented environment. In *Handbook of Augmented Reality*; Springer: Berlin/Heidelberg, Germany, 2011; pp. 47–63.
129. Inami, M.; Kawakami, N.; Sekiguchi, D.; Yanagida, Y.; Maeda, T.; Tachi, S. Visuo-haptic display using head-mounted projector. In Proceedings of the Proceedings IEEE Virtual Reality 2000 (Cat. No. 00CB37048), New Brunswick, NJ, USA, 18–22 March 2000; IEEE: Piscataway, NJ, USA, 2000; pp. 233–240.
130. Ekman, P.; Friesen, W.V. *The Repertoire of Nonverbal Behavior: Categories, Origins, Usage, and Coding*; De Gruyter Mouton: Berlin, Germany, 2010.
131. Ellis, S.R.; Menges, B.M. Judgments of the distance to nearby virtual objects: Interaction of viewing conditions and accommodative demand. *Presence Teleoperators Virtual Environ.* **1997**, *6*, 452–460. [CrossRef]
132. Grubert, J.; Itoh, Y.; Moser, K.; Swan, J.E. A survey of calibration methods for optical see-through head-mounted displays. *IEEE Trans. Vis. Comput. Graph.* **2017**, *24*, 2649–2662. [CrossRef] [PubMed]
133. Moser, K.; Itoh, Y.; Oshima, K.; Swan, J.E.; Klinker, G.; Sandor, C. Subjective evaluation of a semi-automatic optical see-through head-mounted display calibration technique. *IEEE Trans. Vis. Comput. Graph.* **2015**, *21*, 491–500. [CrossRef] [PubMed]
134. Ballestin, G.; Chessa, M.; Solari, F. A registration framework for the comparison of video and optical see-through devices in interactive augmented reality. *IEEE Access* **2021**, *9*, 64828–64843. [CrossRef]
135. Cattari, N.; Cutolo, F.; D'amato, R.; Fontana, U.; Ferrari, V. Toed-in vs parallel displays in video see-through head-mounted displays for close-up view. *IEEE Access* **2019**, *7*, 159698–159711. [CrossRef]
136. Banks, M.S.; Read, J.C.; Allison, R.S.; Watt, S.J. Stereoscopy and the human visual system. *SMPTE Motion Imaging J.* **2012**, *121*, 24–43. [CrossRef]
137. Cutolo, F.; Fontana, U.; Ferrari, V. Perspective preserving solution for quasi-orthoscopic video see-through HMDs. *Technologies* **2018**, *6*, 9. [CrossRef]
138. State, A.; Keller, K.P.; Fuchs, H. Simulation-based design and rapid prototyping of a parallax-free, orthoscopic video see-through head-mounted display. In Proceedings of the Fourth IEEE and ACM International Symposium on Mixed and Augmented Reality (ISMAR'05), Vienna, Austria, 5–8 October 2005; pp. 28–31.
139. Bottecchia, S.; Cieutat, J.M.; Merlo, C.; Jessel, J.P. A new AR interaction paradigm for collaborative teleassistance system: The POA. *Int. J. Interact. Des. Manuf. (IJIDeM)* **2009**, *3*, 35–40. [CrossRef]
140. Xiong, J.; Hsiang, E.L.; He, Z.; Zhan, T.; Wu, S.T. Augmented reality and virtual reality displays: Emerging technologies and future perspectives. *Light. Sci. Appl.* **2021**, *10*, 1–30. [CrossRef]
141. Do, H.; Kim, Y.M.; Min, S.W. Focus-free head-mounted display based on Maxwellian view using retroreflector film. *Appl. Opt.* **2019**, *58*, 2882–2889. [CrossRef]
142. Song, W.; Cheng, Q.; Surman, P.; Liu, Y.; Zheng, Y.; Lin, Z.; Wang, Y. Design of a light-field near-eye display using random pinholes. *Opt. Express* **2019**, *27*, 23763–23774. [CrossRef] [PubMed]
143. Wang, X.; Hua, H. Depth-enhanced head-mounted light field displays based on integral imaging. *Opt. Lett.* **2021**, *46*, 985–988. [CrossRef] [PubMed]
144. Huang, H.; Hua, H. High-performance integral-imaging-based light field augmented reality display using freeform optics. *Opt. Express* **2018**, *26*, 17578–17590. [CrossRef]
145. Kim, S.B.; Park, J.H. Optical see-through Maxwellian near-to-eye display with an enlarged eyebox. *Opt. Lett.* **2018**, *43*, 767–770. [CrossRef]
146. Shrestha, P.K.; Pryn, M.J.; Jia, J.; Chen, J.S.; Fructuoso, H.N.; Boev, A.; Zhang, Q.; Chu, D. Accommodation-free head mounted display with comfortable 3D perception and an enlarged eye-box. *Research* **2019**, *2019*, 9273723. [CrossRef]
147. Lin, T.; Zhan, T.; Zou, J.; Fan, F.; Wu, S.T. Maxwellian near-eye display with an expanded eyebox. *Opt. Express* **2020**, *28*, 38616–38625. [CrossRef]
148. Jo, Y.; Yoo, C.; Bang, K.; Lee, B.; Lee, B. Eye-box extended retinal projection type near-eye display with multiple independent viewpoints. *Appl. Opt.* **2021**, *60*, A268–A276. [CrossRef] [PubMed]
149. Xiong, J.; Li, Y.; Li, K.; Wu, S.T. Aberration-free pupil steerable Maxwellian display for augmented reality with cholesteric liquid crystal holographic lenses. *Opt. Lett.* **2021**, *46*, 1760–1763. [CrossRef] [PubMed]

150. Ratnam, K.; Konrad, R.; Lanman, D.; Zannoli, M. Retinal image quality in near-eye pupil-steered systems. *Opt. Express* **2019**, *27*, 38289–38311. [CrossRef] [PubMed]
151. Jang, C.; Bang, K.; Li, G.; Lee, B. Holographic near-eye display with expanded eye-box. *ACM Trans. Graph. (TOG)* **2018**, *37*, 1–14. [CrossRef]
152. Shi, X.; Liu, J.; Xiao, J.; Han, J. Design of a compact waveguide eyeglass with high efficiency by joining freeform surfaces and volume holographic gratings. *JOSA A* **2021**, *38*, A19–A26. [CrossRef]
153. Weng, Y.; Zhang, Y.; Cui, J.; Liu, A.; Shen, Z.; Li, X.; Wang, B. Liquid-crystal-based polarization volume grating applied for full-color waveguide displays. *Opt. Lett.* **2018**, *43*, 5773–5776. [CrossRef]
154. Lee, Y.H.; Tan, G.; Yin, K.; Zhan, T.; Wu, S.T. Compact see-through near-eye display with depth adaption. *J. Soc. Inf. Disp.* **2018**, *26*, 64–70. [CrossRef]
155. Yoo, C.; Bang, K.; Chae, M.; Lee, B. Extended-viewing-angle waveguide near-eye display with a polarization-dependent steering combiner. *Opt. Lett.* **2020**, *45*, 2870–2873. [CrossRef]
156. Ghasemi, S.; Otsuki, M.; Milgram, P.; Chellali, R. Use of random dot patterns in achieving x-ray vision for near-field applications of stereoscopic video-based augmented reality displays. *Presence* **2017**, *26*, 42–65. [CrossRef]
157. Gabbard, J.L.; Fitch, G.M.; Kim, H. Behind the glass: Driver challenges and opportunities for AR automotive applications. *Proc. IEEE* **2014**, *102*, 124–136. [CrossRef]
158. Kansaku, K.; Hata, N.; Takano, K. My thoughts through a robot's eyes: An augmented reality-brain–machine interface. *Neurosci. Res.* **2010**, *66*, 219–222. [CrossRef] [PubMed]
159. Kato, H.; Billinghurst, M. Marker tracking and hmd calibration for a video-based augmented reality conferencing system. In Proceedings of the Proceedings 2nd IEEE and ACM International Workshop on Augmented Reality (IWAR'99), San Francisco, CA, USA, 20–21 October 1999; pp. 85–94.
160. Azuma, R. Tracking requirements for augmented reality. *Commun. ACM* **1993**, *36*, 50–51. [CrossRef]
161. Kato, H.; Billinghurst, M.; Poupyrev, I.; Imamoto, K.; Tachibana, K. Virtual object manipulation on a table-top AR environment. In Proceedings of the Proceedings IEEE and ACM International Symposium on Augmented Reality (ISAR 2000), Munich, Germany, 5–6 October 2000; pp. 111–119.
162. Ke, Y.; Sukthankar, R. PCA-SIFT: A more distinctive representation for local image descriptors. In Proceedings of the 2004 IEEE Computer Society Conference on Computer Vision and Pattern Recognition (CVPR 2004), Washington, DC, USA, 27 June–2 July 2004; Volume 2.
163. Kerawalla, L.; Luckin, R.; Seljeflot, S.; Woolard, A. "Making it real": Exploring the potential of augmented reality for teaching primary school science. *Virtual Real.* **2006**, *10*, 163–174. [CrossRef]
164. Kijima, R.; Ojika, T. Transition between virtual environment and workstation environment with projective head mounted display. In Proceedings of the Proceedings of IEEE 1997 Annual International Symposium on Virtual Reality, Albuquerque, NM, USA, 1–5 March 1997; pp. 130–137.
165. Koulieris, G.A.; Akşit, K.; Stengel, M.; Mantiuk, R.K.; Mania, K.; Richardt, C. Near-eye display and tracking technologies for virtual and augmented reality. In *Computer Graphics Forum*; Wiley Online Library: Hoboken, NJ, USA, 2019; Volume 38, pp. 493–519.
166. Minoufekr, M.; Schug, P.; Zenker, P.; Plapper, P.W. Modelling of CNC Machine Tools for Augmented Reality Assistance Applications using Microsoft Hololens. In Proceedings of the ICINCO (2), Prague, Czech Republic, 29–31 July 2019; pp. 627–636.
167. Condino, S.; Montemurro, N.; Cattari, N.; D'Amato, R.; Thomale, U.; Ferrari, V.; Cutolo, F. Evaluation of a Wearable AR Platform for Guiding Complex Craniotomies in Neurosurgery. *Ann. Biomed. Eng.* **2021**, *49*, 2590–2605. [CrossRef] [PubMed]
168. Milanović, V.; Kasturi, A.; Yang, J.; Hu, F. A fast single-pixel laser imager for VR/AR headset tracking. In Proceedings of the MOEMS and Miniaturized Systems XVI, San Francisco, CA, USA, 30 January–1 February 2017; International Society for Optics and Photonics: San Diego, CA, USA, 2017; Volume 10116, p. 101160E.
169. Barz, M.; Kapp, S.; Kuhn, J.; Sonntag, D. Automatic Recognition and Augmentation of Attended Objects in Real-time using Eye Tracking and a Head-mounted Display. In Proceedings of the ACM Symposium on Eye Tracking Research and Applications, Stuttgart Germany, 25–29 May 2021; pp. 1–4.
170. Evans, G.; Miller, J.; Pena, M.I.; MacAllister, A.; Winer, E. Evaluating the Microsoft HoloLens through an augmented reality assembly application. In *Degraded Environments: Sensing, Processing, and Display*; SPIE: Philadelphia, PA, USA, 2017; Volume 10197, p. 101970V.
171. Fedosov, A.; Niforatos, E.; Elhart, I.; Schneider, T.; Anisimov, D.; Langheinrich, M. Design and evaluation of a wearable AR system for sharing personalized content on ski resort maps. In Proceedings of the 15th International Conference on Mobile and Ubiquitous Multimedia, Rovaniemi, Finland, 12–15 December 2016; pp. 141–152.
172. Reuter, C.; Ludwig, T.; Mischur, P. RescueGlass: Collaborative Applications involving Head-Mounted Displays for Red Cross Rescue Dog Units. *Comput. Support. Coop. Work (CSCW)* **2019**, *28*, 209–246. [CrossRef]
173. Medin, R. Gesture-Driven Interaction in Head-Mounted Display AR: Guidelines for Design within the Context of the Order Picking Process in Logistic Warehouses. 2018. Available online: http://www.diva-portal.se/smash/get/diva2:1483645/FULLTEXT01.pdf (accessed on 16 October 2022).
174. Tobias, D. Data Visualisation using Augmented Reality with a Focus set on Head Mounted Displays and Collaborative Tasks. In Proceedings of the International Symposium on NDT in Aerospace, Dresden, Germany, 24–26 October 2018; Volume 10, pp. 1–9.

175. Kim, S.; Suh, Y.; Lee, Y.; Woo, W. Toward ubiquitous VR: When VR meets ubiComp. In Proceedings of the 4th International Symposium on Ubiquitous VR, 2006; pp. 1–4. Available online: http://icserv.gist.ac.kr/mis/publications/data/2006/ISUVR2006_SKim.pdf (accessed on 20 October 2022).
176. Andersson, N.; Argyrou, A.; Nägele, F.; Ubis, F.; Campos, U.E.; De Zarate, M.O.; Wilterdink, R. AR-enhanced human-robot-interaction-methodologies, algorithms, tools. *Procedia CIRP* **2016**, *44*, 193–198. [CrossRef]
177. Kiyokawa, K.; Takemura, H.; Yokoya, N. A collaboration support technique by integrating a shared virtual reality and a shared augmented reality. In Proceedings of the IEEE SMC'99 Conference Proceedings, 1999 IEEE International Conference on Systems, Man, and Cybernetics (Cat. No. 99CH37028), Tokyo, Japan, 12–15 October 1999; Volume 6, pp. 48–53.
178. Kiyokawa, K.; Takemura, H.; Yokoya, N. SeamlessDesign for 3D object creation. *IEEE Multimed.* **2000**, *7*, 22–33. [CrossRef]
179. Klein, G.; Drummond, T. Sensor fusion and occlusion refinement for tablet-based AR. In Proceedings of the Third IEEE and ACM International Symposium on Mixed and Augmented Reality, Arlington, VA, USA, 5 November 2004; pp. 38–47.
180. Klein, G.; Murray, D.W. Simulating low-cost cameras for augmented reality compositing. *IEEE Trans. Vis. Comput. Graph.* **2009**, *16*, 369–380. [CrossRef]
181. Klein, G.; Murray, D. Parallel tracking and mapping for small AR workspaces. In Proceedings of the 2007 6th IEEE and ACM International Symposium on Mixed and Augmented Reality, Nara, Japan, 13–16 November 2007; pp. 225–234.
182. Kiyokawa, K.; Kurata, Y.; Ohno, H. An optical see-through display for mutual occlusion with a real-time stereovision system. *Comput. Graph.* **2001**, *25*, 765–779. [CrossRef]
183. Chan, L.W.; Kao, H.S.; Chen, M.Y.; Lee, M.S.; Hsu, J.; Hung, Y.P. Touching the void: Direct-touch interaction for intangible displays. In Proceedings of the SIGCHI Conference on Human Factors in Computing Systems, Atlanta, GA, USA, 10–15 April 2010; pp. 2625–2634.
184. Jang, S.W.; Ko, J.; Lee, H.J.; Kim, Y.S. A Study on Tracking and Augmentation in Mobile AR for e-Leisure. *Mob. Inf. Syst.* **2018**, *2018*, 4265352 . [CrossRef]
185. Fang, W.; Zheng, L.; Deng, H.; Zhang, H. Real-time motion tracking for mobile augmented/virtual reality using adaptive visual-inertial fusion. *Sensors* **2017**, *17*, 1037. [CrossRef] [PubMed]
186. Irshad, S.; Awang, D.R.B. A UX Oriented Evaluation approach for Mobile Augmented Reality Applications. In Proceedings of the 16th International Conference on Advances in Mobile Computing and Multimedia, Yogyakarta, Indonesia, 19–21 November 2018; pp. 108–112.
187. Loizeau, Q.; Danglade, F.; Ababsa, F.; Merienne, F. Methodology for the Field Evaluation of the Impact of Augmented Reality Tools for Maintenance Workers in the Aeronautic Industry. *Front. Virtual Real.* **2021**, *1*, 41. [CrossRef]
188. Kraut, R.E.; Miller, M.D.; Siegel, J. Collaboration in performance of physical tasks: Effects on outcomes and communication. In Proceedings of the 1996 ACM Conference on Computer Supported Cooperative Work, Boston, MA, USA, 16–20 November 1996; pp. 57–66.
189. Krum, D.M.; Suma, E.A.; Bolas, M. Augmented reality using personal projection and retroreflection. *Pers. Ubiquitous Comput.* **2012**, *16*, 17–26. [CrossRef]
190. Kutter, O.; Aichert, A.; Bichlmeier, C.; Traub, J.; Heining, S.; Ockert, B.; Euler, E.; Navab, N. Real-time volume rendering for high quality visualization in augmented reality. In *International Workshop on Augmented Environments for Medical Imaging Including Augmented Reality in Computer-Aided Surgery (AMI-ARCS 2008)*; Citeseer: New York, NY, USA, 2008; pp. 104–113.
191. Kolsch, M.; Bane, R.; Hollerer, T.; Turk, M. Multimodal interaction with a wearable augmented reality system. *IEEE Comput. Graph. Appl.* **2006**, *26*, 62–71. [CrossRef]
192. Kuzuoka, H. Spatial workspace collaboration: A SharedView video support system for remote collaboration capability. In Proceedings of the SIGCHI Conference on Human Factors in Computing Systems, Monterey, CA, USA, 3–7 May 1992; pp. 533–540.
193. Lang, P.; Kusej, A.; Pinz, A.; Brasseur, G. Inertial tracking for mobile augmented reality. In Proceedings of the IMTC/2002. Proceedings of the 19th IEEE Instrumentation and Measurement Technology Conference (IEEE Cat. No. 00CH37276), Anchorage, AK, USA, 21–23 May 2002; Volume 2, pp. 1583–1587.
194. LaViola, J. Whole-Hand and Speech Input in Virtual Environments. CS-99-15. Master's Thesis, Department of Computer Science, Brown University, Providence, RI, USA, 1999, *Unpublished*.
195. Lee, G.A.; Kim, G.J.; Billinghurst, M. Interaction design for tangible augmented reality applications. In *Emerging Technologies of Augmented Reality: Interfaces and Design*; IGI Global: Hershey, PA, USA, 2007; pp. 261–282.
196. Lee, G.A.; Billinghurst, M. A component based framework for mobile outdoor ar applications. In Proceedings of the 12th ACM SIGGRAPH International Conference on Virtual-Reality Continuum and Its Applications in Industry, Hong Kong, China, 17–19 November 2013; pp. 207–210.
197. Lee, G.A.; Kim, G.J.; Park, C.M. Modeling virtual object behavior within virtual environment. In Proceedings of the ACM Symposium on Virtual Reality Software and Technology, Hong Kong, China, 11–13 November 2002; pp. 41–48.
198. Lee, G.A.; Billinghurst, M.; Kim, G.J. Occlusion based interaction methods for tangible augmented reality environments. In Proceedings of the 2004 ACM SIGGRAPH International Conference on Virtual Reality Continuum and Its Applications in Industry, Singapore, 16–18 June 2004; pp. 419–426.
199. Lee, G.A.; Nelles, C.; Billinghurst, M.; Kim, G.J. Immersive authoring of tangible augmented reality applications. In Proceedings of the Third IEEE and ACM International Symposium on Mixed and Augmented Reality, Arlington, VA, USA, 2–5 November 2004; pp. 172–181.

200. Santos, M.E.C.; Taketomi, T.; Yamamoto, G.; Rodrigo, M.M.T.; Sandor, C.; Kato, H.; et al. Augmented reality as multimedia: The case for situated vocabulary learning. *Res. Pract. Technol. Enhanc. Learn.* **2016**, *11*, 1–23. [CrossRef]
201. Lee, G.A.; Kim, G.J.; Billinghurst, M. Immersive authoring: What you experience is what you get (wyxiwyg). *Commun. ACM* **2005**, *48*, 76–81. [CrossRef]
202. Lee, G.A.; Yang, U.; Son, W. Layered multiple displays for immersive and interactive digital contents. In Proceedings of the International Conference on Entertainment Computing, Cambridge, UK, 20–22 September 2006; Springer: Berlin/Heidelberg, Germany, 2006; pp. 123–134.
203. Lee, G.A.; Kang, H.; Son, W. Mirage: A touch screen based mixed reality interface for space planning applications. In Proceedings of the 2008 IEEE Virtual Reality Conference, Reno, NV, USA, 8–12 March 2008; pp. 273–274.
204. Lee, G.A.; Yang, U.; Son, W.; Kim, Y.; Jo, D.; Kim, K.H.; Choi, J.S. Virtual reality content-based training for spray painting tasks in the shipbuilding industry. *ETRI J.* **2010**, *32*, 695–703. [CrossRef]
205. Lee, G.A.; Dünser, A.; Kim, S.; Billinghurst, M. CityViewAR: A mobile outdoor AR application for city visualization. In Proceedings of the 2012 IEEE International Symposium on Mixed and Augmented Reality-Arts, Media, and Humanities (ISMAR-AMH), Altanta, GA, USA, 5–8 November 2012; pp. 57–64.
206. Lee, G.A.; Dünser, A.; Nassani, A.; Billinghurst, M. AntarcticAR: An outdoor AR experience of a virtual tour to Antarctica. In Proceedings of the 2013 IEEE International Symposium on Mixed and Augmented Reality-Arts, Media, and Humanities (ISMAR-AMH), Adelaide, Australia, 1–4 October 2013; pp. 29–38.
207. Lee, J.Y.; Rhee, G.W.; Seo, D.W. Hand gesture-based tangible interactions for manipulating virtual objects in a mixed reality environment. *Int. J. Adv. Manuf. Technol.* **2010**, *51*, 1069–1082. [CrossRef]
208. Köse, H.; Güner-Yildiz, N. Augmented reality (AR) as a learning material in special needs education. *Educ. Inf. Technol.* **2021**, *26*, 1921–1936. [CrossRef]
209. Oda, O.; Lister, L.J.; White, S.; Feiner, S. Developing an augmented reality racing game. In Proceedings of the 2nd International Conference on Intelligent Technologies for interactive enterTAINment, Cancun Mexico, 8–10 January 2008.
210. Schmalstieg, D.; Fuhrmann, A.; Hesina, G.; Szalavári, Z.; Encarnaçao, L.M.; Gervautz, M.; Purgathofer, W. The studierstube augmented reality project. *Presence Teleoperators Virtual Environ.* **2002**, *11*, 33–54. [CrossRef]
211. Taehee Lee, T.; Handy, A. Markerless inspection of augmented reality objects using fingertip tracking. In Proceedings of the IEEE International Symposium on Wearable Computers, Boston, MA, USA, 11–13 October 2007.
212. Lenhardt, A.; Ritter, H. An augmented-reality based brain-computer interface for robot control. In Proceedings of the International Conference on Neural Information Processing, Sydney, NSW, Australia, 22–25 November 2010; Springer: Berlin/Heidelberg, Germany, 2010; pp. 58–65.
213. Fiala, M. Artag revision 1, a fiducial marker system using digital techniques. *Natl. Res. Counc. Publ.* **2004**, *47419*, 1–47.
214. Renner, R.S.; Velichkovsky, B.M.; Helmert, J.R. The perception of egocentric distances in virtual environments-a review. *ACM Comput. Surv. (CSUR)* **2013**, *46*, 1–40. [CrossRef]
215. Creem-Regehr, S.H.; Stefanucci, J.K.; Thompson, W.B.; Nash, N.; McCardell, M. Egocentric distance perception in the oculus rift (dk2). In Proceedings of the ACM SIGGRAPH Symposium on Applied Perception, Tübingen, Germany, 13–14 September 2015; pp. 47–50.
216. Kytö, M.; Mäkinen, A.; Tossavainen, T.; Oittinen, P.T. Stereoscopic depth perception in video see-through augmented reality within action space. *J. Electron. Imaging* **2014**, *23*, 011006. [CrossRef]
217. Rosales, C.S.; Pointon, G.; Adams, H.; Stefanucci, J.; Creem-Regehr, S.; Thompson, W.B.; Bodenheimer, B. Distance judgments to on-and off-ground objects in augmented reality. In Proceedings of the 2019 IEEE Conference on Virtual Reality and 3D User Interfaces (VR), Osaka, Japan, 23–27 March 2019; pp. 237–243.
218. Rehman, U.; Cao, S. Augmented-reality-based indoor navigation: A comparative analysis of handheld devices versus google glass. *IEEE Trans. Hum.-Mach. Syst.* **2016**, *47*, 140–151. [CrossRef]
219. Fischler, M.A.; Bolles, R.C. Random sample consensus: A paradigm for model fitting with applications to image analysis and automated cartography. *Commun. ACM* **1981**, *24*, 381–395. [CrossRef]
220. Favalora, G.E. Volumetric 3D displays and application infrastructure. *Computer* **2005**, *38*, 37–44. [CrossRef]
221. Feiner, S.; MacIntyre, B.; Haupt, M.; Solomon, E. Windows on the world: 2D windows for 3D augmented reality. In Proceedings of the 6th Annual ACM Symposium on User Interface Software and Technology, Atlanta, GA, USA, 3–5 November 1993; pp. 145–155.
222. Feiner, S.; MacIntyre, B.; Seligmann, D. Knowledge-based augmented reality. *Commun. ACM* **1993**, *36*, 53–62. [CrossRef]
223. Feiner, S.; MacIntyre, B.; Höllerer, T.; Webster, A. A touring machine: Prototyping 3D mobile augmented reality systems for exploring the urban environment. *Pers. Technol.* **1997**, *1*, 208–217. [CrossRef]
224. Fergason, J.L. Optical System for a Head Mounted Display Using a Retro-Reflector and Method of Displaying an Image. U.S. Patent 5,621,572, 15 April 1997.
225. Amin, D.; Govilkar, S. Comparative study of augmented reality SDKs. *Int. J. Comput. Sci. Appl.* **2015**, *5*, 11–26.
226. Fisher, R.W. Head-Mounted Projection Display System Featuring Beam Splitter and Method of Making Same. U.S. Patent 5,572,229, 5 November 1996.
227. Lepetit, V.; Fua, P. Keypoint recognition using randomized trees. *IEEE Trans. Pattern Anal. Mach. Intell.* **2006**, *28*, 1465–1479. [CrossRef]

228. Leutenegger, S.; Chli, M.; Siegwart, R.Y. BRISK: Binary robust invariant scalable keypoints. In Proceedings of the 2011 International Conference on Computer Vision, Barcelona, Spain, 6–13 November 2011; pp. 2548–2555.
229. Leventon, M.E. A Registration, Tracking, and Visualization System for Image-Guided Surgery. Ph.D. Thesis, Massachusetts Institute of Technology, Cambridge, MA, USA, 1997.
230. Kyza, E.A.; Georgiou, Y. Digital tools for enriching informal inquiry-based mobile learning: the design of the TraceReaders location-based augmented reality learning platform. In Proceedings of the 3rd Asia-Europe Symposium on Simulation & Serious Gaming, Zhuhai, China, 3–4 December 2016; pp. 195–198.
231. Carmigniani, J.; Furht, B.; Anisetti, M.; Ceravolo, P.; Damiani, E.; Ivkovic, M. Augmented reality technologies, systems and applications. *Multimed. Tools Appl.* **2011**, *51*, 341–377. [CrossRef]
232. Lindeman, R.W.; Lee, G.; Beattie, L.; Gamper, H.; Pathinarupothi, R.; Akhilesh, A. GeoBoids: A mobile AR application for exergaming. In Proceedings of the 2012 IEEE International Symposium on Mixed and Augmented Reality-Arts, Media, and Humanities (ISMAR-AMH), Altanta, GA, USA, 5–8 November 2012; pp. 93–94.
233. Lingley, A.R.; Ali, M.; Liao, Y.; Mirjalili, R.; Klonner, M.; Sopanen, M.; Suihkonen, S.; Shen, T.; Otis, B.; Lipsanen, H.; et al. A single-pixel wireless contact lens display. *J. Micromechan. Microeng.* **2011**, *21*, 125014. [CrossRef]
234. Choi, J.; Kim, Y.; Lee, M.; Kim, G.J.; Nam, Y.; Kwon, Y. k-MART: Authoring tool for mixed reality contents. In Proceedings of the 2010 IEEE International Symposium on Mixed and Augmented Reality, Seoul, Republic of Korea, 13–16 October 2010; pp. 219–220.
235. Lindeman, R.W.; Sibert, J.L.; Hahn, J.K. Towards usable VR: An empirical study of user interfaces for immersive virtual environments. In Proceedings of the SIGCHI Conference on Human Factors in Computing Systems, Pittsburgh, PA, USA, 15–20 May 1999; pp. 64–71.
236. Chong, U.; Alimardanov, S. Audio augmented reality using unity for marine tourism. In Proceedings of the International Conference on Intelligent Human Computer Interaction, Kent, OH, USA, 20–22 December 2021; Springer: Berlin/Heidelberg, Germany, 2021; pp. 303–311.
237. Konopka, B.; Hönemann, K.; Brandt, P.; Wiesche, M. WizARd: A No-Code Tool for Business Process Guidance through the Use of Augmented Reality. 2022. Available online: https://ceur-ws.org/Vol-3216/paper_258.pdf (accessed on 16 October 2022).
238. Zhao, S.; Wang, L.; Song, J. P-2.8: Research on multi-user interaction design in augmented reality. In *SID Symposium Digest of Technical Papers*; Wiley Online Library: Hoboken, NJ, USA, 2022; Volume 53, pp. 651–654.
239. Nebeling, M.; Speicher, M. The trouble with augmented reality/virtual reality authoring tools. In Proceedings of the 2018 IEEE International Symposium on Mixed and Augmented Reality Adjunct (ISMAR-Adjunct), Munich, Germany, 16–20 October 2018; pp. 333–337.
240. Mladenov, B.; Damiani, L.; Giribone, P.; Revetria, R. A short review of the SDKs and wearable devices to be used for ar application for industrial working environment. In Proceedings of the World Congress on Engineering and Computer Science, San Francisco, CA, USA, 23–25 October 2018; Volume 1, pp. 23–25.
241. Wells, T.; Houben, S. Collabar–investigating the mediating role of mobile ar interfaces on co-located group collaboration. In Proceedings of the 2020 CHI Conference on Human Factors in Computing Systems, Honolulu, HI, USA, 25–30 April 2020; pp. 1–13.
242. Grandi, J.G. Design of collaborative 3D user interfaces for virtual and augmented reality. In Proceedings of the 2017 IEEE Virtual Reality (VR), Venice, Italy, 21–25 May 2017; pp. 419–420.
243. Dong, S.; Behzadan, A.H.; Chen, F.; Kamat, V.R. Collaborative visualization of engineering processes using tabletop augmented reality. *Adv. Eng. Softw.* **2013**, *55*, 45–55. [CrossRef]
244. Kim, J.O.; Kim, J. Augmented Reality Tools for Integrative Science and Arts STEAM Education. *Int. J. Pure Appl. Math.* **2018**, *118*.
245. Kazanidis, I.; Tsinakos, A.; Lytridis, C. Teaching mobile programming using augmented reality and collaborative game based learning. In Proceedings of the Interactive Mobile Communication, Technologies and Learning, Thessalonikē, Greece, 29 November–1 December 2017; Springer: Berlin/Heidelberg, Germany, 2017; pp. 850–859.
246. Chang, Y.S.; Hu, K.J.; Chiang, C.W.; Lugmayr, A. Applying Mobile Augmented Reality (AR) to teach Interior Design students in layout plans: Evaluation of learning effectiveness based on the ARCS Model of learning motivation theory. *Sensors* **2020**, *20*, 105. [CrossRef]
247. Sarkar, P.; Kadam, K.; Pillai, J.S. Collaborative approaches to problem-solving on lines and angles using augmented reality. In Proceedings of the 2019 IEEE Tenth International Conference on Technology for Education (T4E), Goa, India, 9–11 December 2019; pp. 193–200.
248. Grandi, J.G.; Debarba, H.G.; Bemdt, I.; Nedel, L.; Maciel, A. Design and assessment of a collaborative 3D interaction technique for handheld augmented reality. In Proceedings of the 2018 IEEE Conference on Virtual Reality and 3D User Interfaces (VR), Reutlingen, Germany, 22 March 2018; pp. 49–56.
249. Akçayır, M.; Akçayır, G.; Pektaş, H.M.; Ocak, M.A. Augmented reality in science laboratories: The effects of augmented reality on university students' laboratory skills and attitudes toward science laboratories. *Comput. Hum. Behav.* **2016**, *57*, 334–342. [CrossRef]
250. Rekimoto, J. Transvision: A hand-held augmented reality system for collaborative design. In Proceeding of International Conference on Virtual Systems and Multimedia, Gifu, Japan, 18–20 September 1996; Volume 96, pp. 18–20.
251. Oda, O.; Feiner, S. Interference avoidance in multi-user hand-held augmented reality. In Proceedings of the 2009 8th IEEE International Symposium on Mixed and Augmented Reality, Orlando, FL, USA, 19–22 October 2009; pp. 13–22.

252. Huynh, D.N.T.; Raveendran, K.; Xu, Y.; Spreen, K.; MacIntyre, B. Art of defense: A collaborative handheld augmented reality board game. In Proceedings of the 2009 ACM SIGGRAPH Symposium on Video Games, New Orleans, LA, USA, 4–6 August 2009; pp. 135–142.
253. Nilsson, S.; Johansson, B.; Jonsson, A. Using AR to support cross-organisational collaboration in dynamic tasks. In Proceedings of the 2009 8th IEEE International Symposium on Mixed and Augmented Reality, Orlando, FL, USA, 19–22 October 2009; pp. 3–12.
254. Tseng, P.Y.; Haraldsson, H.; Belongie, S. Annotate All! A Perspective Preserved Asynchronous Annotation System for Collaborative Augmented Reality. 2019. Available online: https://static1.squarespace.com/static/5c3f69e1cc8fedbc039ea739/t/5d0294ab169b78000195c0f1/1560450226075/32_Annotate_all__A_Perspective_Preserved_Asynchronous__Annotation_System_for_Collaborative_Augmented_Reality.pdf (accessed on 16 October 2022).
255. Kasahara, S.; Heun, V.; Lee, A.S.; Ishii, H. Second surface: Multi-user spatial collaboration system based on augmented reality. In Proceedings of the SIGGRAPH Asia 2012 Emerging Technologies, Singapore, 28 November–1 December 2012; pp. 1–4.
256. Billinghurst, M.; Bowskill, J.; Morphett, J. WearCom: A wearable communication space. In Proceedings of the CVE, Manchester, UK, 17–19 June 1998; Volume 98, pp. 123–130.
257. Stafford, A.; Piekarski, W.; Thomas, B.H. Implementation of god-like interaction techniques for supporting collaboration between outdoor AR and indoor tabletop users. In Proceedings of the 2006 IEEE/ACM International Symposium on Mixed and Augmented Reality, Santa Barbard, CA, USA, 22–25 October 2006; pp. 165–172.
258. Gauglitz, S.; Nuernberger, B.; Turk, M.; Höllerer, T. In touch with the remote world: Remote collaboration with augmented reality drawings and virtual navigation. In Proceedings of the 20th ACM Symposium on Virtual Reality Software and Technology, Edinburgh, UK, 11–13 November 2014; pp. 197–205.
259. Boonbrahm, P.; Kaewrat, C.; Boonbrahm, S. Effective Collaborative Design of Large Virtual 3D Model using Multiple AR Markers. *Procedia Manuf.* **2020**, *42*, 387–392. [CrossRef]
260. Li, X.; Chen, W.; Wu, Y. Distance-driven user interface for collaborative exhibit viewing in augmented reality museum. In Proceedings of the The Adjunct Publication of the 32nd Annual ACM Symposium on User Interface Software and Technology, New Orleans, LA, USA, 20–23 October 2019; pp. 42–43.
261. Poretski, L.; Lanir, J.; Arazy, O. Normative tensions in shared augmented reality. *Proc. ACM Hum.-Comput. Interact.* **2018**, *2*, 1–22. [CrossRef]
262. Clergeaud, D.; Roo, J.S.; Hachet, M.; Guitton, P. Towards seamless interaction between physical and virtual locations for asymmetric collaboration. In Proceedings of the 23rd ACM Symposium on Virtual Reality Software and Technology, Gothenburg, Sweden, 8–10 November 2017; pp. 1–4.
263. Oda, O.; Feiner, S. 3D referencing techniques for physical objects in shared augmented reality. In Proceedings of the 2012 IEEE International Symposium on Mixed and Augmented Reality (ISMAR), Atlanta, GA, USA, 5–8 November 2012; pp. 207–215.
264. Mahmood, T.; Fulmer, W.; Mungoli, N.; Huang, J.; Lu, A. Improving information sharing and collaborative analysis for remote geospatial visualization using mixed reality. In Proceedings of the 2019 IEEE International Symposium on Mixed and Augmented Reality (ISMAR), Beijing, China, 10–18 October 2019; pp. 236–247.
265. Munoz-Cristóbal, J.A.; Gallego-Lema, V.; Arribas-Cubero, H.F.; Asensio-Pérez, J.I.; Martínez-Monés, A. Game of Blazons: Helping teachers conduct learning situations that integrate web tools and multiple types of augmented reality. *IEEE Trans. Learn. Technol.* **2018**, *11*, 506–519. [CrossRef]
266. Muñoz-Cristóbal, J.A.; Prieto, L.P.; Asensio-Pérez, J.I.; Jorrín-Abellán, I.M.; Martínez-Monés, A.; Dimitriadis, Y. GLUEPS-AR: A system for the orchestration of learning situations across spaces using augmented reality. In Proceedings of the European Conference on Technology Enhanced Learning, Paphos, Cyprus, 17–21 September 2013; Springer: Berlin/Heidelberg, Germany, 2013; pp. 565–568.
267. bin Hanafi, H.F.; Said, C.S.; Ariffin, A.H.; Zainuddin, N.A.; Samsuddin, K. Using a collaborative Mobile Augmented Reality learning application (CoMARLA) to improve Improve Student Learning. In *IOP Conference Series: Materials Science and Engineering*; IOP Publishing: Bristol, UK, 2016; Volume 160, p. 012111.
268. Dunleavy, M.; Dede, C.; Mitchell, R. Affordances and limitations of immersive participatory augmented reality simulations for teaching and learning. *J. Sci. Educ. Technol.* **2009**, *18*, 7–22. [CrossRef]
269. Maimone, A.; Fuchs, H. Encumbrance-free telepresence system with real-time 3D capture and display using commodity depth cameras. In Proceedings of the 2011 10th IEEE International Symposium on Mixed and Augmented Reality, Basel, Switzerland, 26–29 October 2011; pp. 137–146.
270. Gauglitz, S.; Nuernberger, B.; Turk, M.; Höllerer, T. World-stabilized annotations and virtual scene navigation for remote collaboration. In Proceedings of the 27th Annual ACM Symposium on User Interface Software and Technology, Honolulu, HI, USA, 5–8 October 2014; pp. 449–459.
271. Guo, A.; Canberk, I.; Murphy, H.; Monroy-Hernández, A.; Vaish, R. Blocks: Collaborative and persistent augmented reality experiences. *Proc. ACM Interact. Mobile Wearable Ubiquitous Technol.* **2019**, *3*, 83. [CrossRef]
272. Zhang, W.; Han, B.; Hui, P.; Gopalakrishnan, V.; Zavesky, E.; Qian, F. CARS: Collaborative augmented reality for socialization. In Proceedings of the 19th International Workshop on Mobile Computing Systems & Applications, Tempe, AZ, USA, 12–13 February 2018; pp. 25–30.

273. Lien, K.C.; Nuernberger, B.; Höllerer, T.; Turk, M. PPV: Pixel-point-volume segmentation for object referencing in collaborative augmented reality. In Proceedings of the 2016 IEEE International Symposium on Mixed and Augmented Reality (ISMAR), Merida, Mexico, 19–23 September 2016; pp. 77–83.
274. Huang, W.; Billinghurst, M.; Alem, L.; Kim, S. HandsInTouch: Sharing gestures in remote collaboration. In Proceedings of the 30th Australian Conference on Computer-Human Interaction, Melbourne, Australia, 4–7 December 2018; pp. 396–400.
275. Ou, J.; Fussell, S.R.; Chen, X.; Setlock, L.D.; Yang, J. Gestural communication over video stream: Supporting multimodal interaction for remote collaborative physical tasks. In Proceedings of the 5th International Conference on Multimodal Interfaces, Vancouver, BC, Canada, 5–7 November 2003; pp. 242–249.
276. Datcu, D.; Lukosch, S.G.; Lukosch, H.K. Handheld augmented reality for distributed collaborative crime scene investigation. In Proceedings of the 19th International Conference on Supporting Group Work, Sanibel Island, FL, USA, 13–16 November 2016; pp. 267–276.
277. Tait, M.; Billinghurst, M. The effect of view independence in a collaborative AR system. *Comput. Support. Coop. Work (CSCW)* **2015**, *24*, 563–589. [CrossRef]
278. Fang, D.; Xu, H.; Yang, X.; Bian, M. An augmented reality-based method for remote collaborative real-time assistance: From a system perspective. *Mob. Netw. Appl.* **2020**, *25*, 412–425. [CrossRef]
279. Mora, S.; Boron, A.; Divitini, M. CroMAR: Mobile augmented reality for supporting reflection on crowd management. *Int. J. Mob. Hum. Comput. Interact. (IJMHCI)* **2012**, *4*, 88–101. [CrossRef]
280. Adcock, M.; Feng, D.; Thomas, B. Visualization of off-surface 3D viewpoint locations in spatial augmented reality. In Proceedings of the 1st Symposium on Spatial User Interaction, Los Angeles, CA, USA, 20–21 July 2013; pp. 1–8.
281. Lincoln, P.; Welch, G.; Nashel, A.; Ilie, A.; State, A.; Fuchs, H. Animatronic shader lamps avatars. In Proceedings of the 2009 8th IEEE International Symposium on Mixed and Augmented Reality, Orlando, FL, USA, 19–22 October 2009; pp. 27–33.
282. Komiyama, R.; Miyaki, T.; Rekimoto, J. JackIn space: Designing a seamless transition between first and third person view for effective telepresence collaborations. In Proceedings of the 8th Augmented Human International Conference, Silicon Valley, CA, USA, 16–18 March 2017; pp. 1–9.
283. Lehment, N.H.; Merget, D.; Rigoll, G. Creating automatically aligned consensus realities for AR videoconferencing. In Proceedings of the 2014 IEEE International Symposium on Mixed and Augmented Reality (ISMAR), Munich, Germany, 10–12 September 2014; pp. 201–206.
284. Oda, O.; Elvezio, C.; Sukan, M.; Feiner, S.; Tversky, B. Virtual replicas for remote assistance in virtual and augmented reality. In Proceedings of the 28th Annual ACM Symposium on User Interface Software & Technology, Charlotte, NC, USA, 11–15 November 2015; pp. 405–415.
285. Piumsomboon, T.; Lee, G.A.; Hart, J.D.; Ens, B.; Lindeman, R.W.; Thomas, B.H.; Billinghurst, M. Mini-me: An adaptive avatar for mixed reality remote collaboration. In Proceedings of the 2018 CHI Conference on Human Factors in Computing Systems, Montreal, QC, Canada, 21–26 April 2018; pp. 1–13.
286. Piumsomboon, T.; Lee, Y.; Lee, G.; Billinghurst, M. CoVAR: A collaborative virtual and augmented reality system for remote collaboration. In Proceedings of the SIGGRAPH Asia 2017 Emerging Technologies, Bangkok, Thailand, 27–30 November 2017; pp. 1–2.
287. Teo, T.; Lee, G.A.; Billinghurst, M.; Adcock, M. Hand gestures and visual annotation in live 360 panorama-based mixed reality remote collaboration. In Proceedings of the 30th Australian Conference on Computer-Human Interaction, Melbourne, Australia, 4–7 December 2018; pp. 406–410.
288. Thanyadit, S.; Punpongsanon, P.; Pong, T.C. ObserVAR: Visualization system for observing virtual reality users using augmented reality. In Proceedings of the 2019 IEEE International Symposium on Mixed and Augmented Reality (ISMAR), Beijing, China, 10–18 October 2019; pp. 258–268.
289. Sodhi, R.S.; Jones, B.R.; Forsyth, D.; Bailey, B.P.; Maciocci, G. BeThere: 3D mobile collaboration with spatial input. In Proceedings of the SIGCHI Conference on Human Factors in Computing Systems, Paris, France, 27 April–2 May 2013; pp. 179–188.
290. Ong, S.; Shen, Y. A mixed reality environment for collaborative product design and development. *CIRP Ann.* **2009**, *58*, 139–142. [CrossRef]
291. Irlitti, A.; Smith, R.T.; Von Itzstein, S.; Billinghurst, M.; Thomas, B.H. Challenges for asynchronous collaboration in augmented reality. In Proceedings of the 2016 IEEE International Symposium on Mixed and Augmented Reality (ISMAR-Adjunct), Merida, Mexico, 19–23 September 2016; pp. 31–35.
292. Azuma, R.; Baillot, Y.; Behringer, R.; Feiner, S.; Julier, S.; MacIntyre, B. Recent advances in augmented reality. *IEEE Comput. Graph. Appl.* **2001**, *21*, 34–47. [CrossRef]
293. Baecker, R.M. *Readings in Groupware and Computer-Supported Cooperative Work: Assisting Human-Human Collaboration*; Morgan Kaufmann: Burlington, MA, USA, 1993.
294. Akussah, M.; Dehinbo, J. Developing a Marker-based Handheld Augmented Reality Application for Learning Mathematics. In *EdMedia+ Innovate Learning*; Association for the Advancement of Computing in Education (AACE): Chesapeake, VA, USA, 2018; pp. 856–866.
295. Roberto, R.; Lima, J.P.; Araújo, T.; Teichrieb, V. Evaluation of motion tracking and depth sensing accuracy of the tango tablet. In Proceedings of the 2016 IEEE International Symposium on Mixed and Augmented Reality (ISMAR-Adjunct), Merida, Mexico, 19–23 September 2016; pp. 231–234.

296. Maimone, A.; Fuchs, H. Computational augmented reality eyeglasses. In Proceedings of the 2013 IEEE International Symposium on Mixed and Augmented Reality (ISMAR), Adelaide, Australia, 1–4 October 2013; pp. 29–38.
297. Mair, E.; Hager, G.D.; Burschka, D.; Suppa, M.; Hirzinger, G. Adaptive and generic corner detection based on the accelerated segment test. In Proceedings of the European Conference on Computer Vision, Heraklion, Crete, Greece, 5–11 September 2010; Springer: Berlin/Heidelberg, Germany, 2010; pp. 183–196.
298. Mandeville, J. A shared virtual environment for architectural design review. In Proceedings of the CVE'96 Workshop Proceedings, Nottingham, UK, 19–20 September 1996.
299. Fernández-Caramés, T.M.; Fraga-Lamas, P. Towards the Internet of smart clothing: A review on IoT wearables and garments for creating intelligent connected e-textiles. *Electronics* **2018**, *7*, 405. [CrossRef]
300. Martínez, H.; Skournetou, D.; Hyppölä, J.; Laukkanen, S.; Heikkilä, A. Drivers and bottlenecks in the adoption of augmented reality applications. *J. Multimed. Theory Appl.* **2014**, *2*. [CrossRef]
301. Chessa, M.; Maiello, G.; Klein, L.K.; Paulun, V.C.; Solari, F. Grasping objects in immersive Virtual Reality. In Proceedings of the 2019 IEEE Conference on Virtual Reality and 3D User Interfaces (VR), Osaka, Japan, 23–27 March 2019; pp. 1749–1754. [CrossRef]
302. Han, D.T.; Suhail, M.; Ragan, E.D. Evaluating Remapped Physical Reach for Hand Interactions with Passive Haptics in Virtual Reality. *IEEE Trans. Vis. Comput. Graph.* **2018**, *24*, 1467–1476. [CrossRef]
303. Fotouhi, J. Augmented Reality and Artificial Intelligence in Image-Guided and Robot-Assisted Interventions. Ph.D. Thesis, The Johns Hopkins University, Baltimore, MD, USA, 2020.
304. Wang, Z.; Bai, X.; Zhang, S.; Billinghurst, M.; He, W.; Wang, Y.; Han, D.; Chen, G.; Li, J. The role of user-centered AR instruction in improving novice spatial cognition in a high-precision procedural task. *Adv. Eng. Inform.* **2021**, *47*, 101250. [CrossRef]
305. Newman, J.; Wagner, M.; Bauer, M.; MacWilliams, A.; Pintaric, T.; Beyer, D.; Pustka, D.; Strasser, F.; Schmalstieg, D.; Klinker, G. Ubiquitous tracking for augmented reality. In Proceedings of the Third IEEE and ACM International Symposium on Mixed and Augmented Reality, Washington, DC, USA, 2–5 November 2004; pp. 192–201.
306. Newman, J.; Schall, G.; Barakonyi, I.; Schürzinger, A.; Schmalstieg, D. Wide-Area Tracking Tools for Augmented Reality. 2006. Available online: http://www.barakonyi.net/papers/ubisense_demo_pervasive06.pdf (accessed on 20 October 2022).
307. Nilsen, T.; Looser, J. Tankwar-Tabletop war gaming in augmented reality. In Proceedings of the 2nd International Workshop on Pervasive Gaming Applications, Munich, Germany, 8–13 May 2005; Volume 5.
308. Nilsson, S.; Johansson, B. Acceptance of augmented reality instructions in a real work setting. In Proceedings of the CHI'08 Extended Abstracts on Human Factors in Computing Systems, Florence, Italy, 5–10 April 2008; pp. 2025–2032.
309. O'Conaill, B. Characterizing, predicting and measuring video-mediated communication: A conversational approach. In *Video-Mediated Communication*; L. Erlbaum Associates: Hillsdale, NJ, USA, 1997.
310. Song, E.; Suaib, N.M.; Sihes, A.J.; Alwee, R.; Yunos, Z.M. Design and development of learning mathematics game for primary school using handheld augmented reality. *Iop Conf. Ser. Mater. Sci. Eng.* **2020**, *979*, 012014. [CrossRef]
311. Oh, Y.; Woo, W. A unified application service model for ubihome by exploiting intelligent context-awareness. In *International Symposium on Ubiquitious Computing Systems*; Springer: Berlin/Heidelberg, Germany, 2004; pp. 192–202.
312. Oh, Y.; Shin, C.; Jung, W.; Woo, W. The ubiTV application for a Family in ubiHome. In Proceedings of the 2nd Ubiquitous Home Workshop, 2005; pp. 23–32. Available online: https://www.researchgate.net/profile/Woontack-Woo/publication/228358612_The_ubiTV_application_for_a_Family_in_ubiHome/links/0fcfd50b7fffbc955a000000/The-ubiTV-application-for-a-Family-in-ubiHome.pdf (accessed on 20 October 2022).
313. Ohshima, T.; Satoh, K.; Yamamoto, H.; Tamura, H. Ar2 hockey: A case study of collaborative augmented reality. In Proceedings of the VRAIS'98: Proceedings of the Virtual Reality Annual International Symposium, Atlanta, GA, USA, 14–18 March 1998; IEEE Computer Society: Washington, DC, USA, 1998.
314. Olsson, T.; Lagerstam, E.; Kärkkäinen, T.; Väänänen-Vainio-Mattila, K. Expected user experience of mobile augmented reality services: A user study in the context of shopping centres. *Pers. Ubiquitous Comput.* **2013**, *17*, 287–304. [CrossRef]
315. Ozuysal, M.; Calonder, M.; Lepetit, V.; Fua, P. Fast keypoint recognition using random ferns. *IEEE Trans. Pattern Anal. Mach. Intell.* **2009**, *32*, 448–461. [CrossRef]
316. Pandey, J.; Liao, Y.T.; Lingley, A.; Mirjalili, R.; Parviz, B.; Otis, B.P. A fully integrated RF-powered contact lens with a single element display. *IEEE Trans. Biomed. Circuits Syst.* **2010**, *4*, 454–461. [CrossRef] [PubMed]
317. Botha-Ravyse, C.; Lähtevänoja, A.; Luimula, M. Collaborative AR application design for early childhood education. In Proceedings of the EdMedia+ Innovate Learning. Association for the Advancement of Computing in Education (AACE), Amsterdam, The Netherlands, 24–28 June 2019; pp. 18–27.
318. Parviz, B.A. For your eye only. *IEEE Spectr.* **2009**, *46*, 36–41. [CrossRef]
319. Jana, S.; Molnar, D.; Moshchuk, A.; Dunn, A.; Livshits, B.; Wang, H.J.; Ofek, E. Enabling Fine-Grained Permissions for Augmented Reality Applications with Recognizers. In Proceedings of the 22nd USENIX Security Symposium (USENIX Security 13, Washington, DC, USA, 14–16 August 2013; pp. 415–430.
320. Ruth, K.; Kohno, T.; Roesner, F. Secure Multi-User Content Sharing for Augmented Reality Applications. In Proceedings of the 28th USENIX Security Symposium (USENIX Security 19), Santa Clara, CA, USA, 14–16 August 2019; pp. 141–158.

321. Pierdicca, R.; Prist, M.; Monteriù, A.; Frontoni, E.; Ciarapica, F.; Bevilacqua, M.; Mazzuto, G. Augmented reality smart glasses in the workplace: Safety and security in the fourth industrial revolution era. In Proceedings of the International Conference on Augmented Reality, Virtual Reality and Computer Graphics, Lecce, Italy, 7–10 September 2020; Springer: Berlin/Heidelberg, Germany, 2020; pp. 231–247.
322. Ahn, S.; Gorlatova, M.; Naghizadeh, P.; Chiang, M.; Mittal, P. Adaptive fog-based output security for augmented reality. In Proceedings of the 2018 Morning Workshop on Virtual Reality and Augmented Reality Network, Budapest, Hungary, 24 August 2018; pp. 1–6.
323. Chen, S.; Li, Z.; Dangelo, F.; Gao, C.; Fu, X. A case study of security and privacy threats from augmented reality (ar). In Proceedings of the 2018 International Conference on Computing, Networking and Communications (ICNC), Maui, HI, USA, 5–8 March 2018; pp. 442–446.
324. Langfinger, M.; Schneider, M.; Stricker, D.; Schotten, H.D. Addressing security challenges in industrial augmented reality systems. In Proceedings of the 2017 IEEE 15th International Conference on Industrial Informatics (INDIN), Emden, Germany, 24–26 July 2017; pp. 299–304.
325. Roesner, F.; Kohno, T.; Molnar, D. Security and privacy for augmented reality systems. *Commun. ACM* **2014**, *57*, 88–96. [CrossRef]
326. Wazir, W.; Khattak, H.A.; Almogren, A.; Khan, M.A.; Din, I.U. Doodle-based authentication technique using augmented reality. *IEEE Access* **2020**, *8*, 4022–4034. [CrossRef]
327. Lebeck, K.; Ruth, K.; Kohno, T.; Roesner, F. Securing augmented reality output. In Proceedings of the 2017 IEEE Symposium on Security and Privacy (SP), San Jose, CA, USA, 25 May 2017; pp. 320–337.
328. Zhang, X.; Slavin, R.; Wang, X.; Niu, J. Privacy assurance for android augmented reality apps. In Proceedings of the 2019 IEEE 24th Pacific Rim International Symposium on Dependable Computing (PRDC), Kyoto, Japan, 1–3 December 2019; pp. 114–1141.
329. McPherson, R.; Jana, S.; Shmatikov, V. No escape from reality: Security and privacy of augmented reality browsers. In Proceedings of the 24th International Conference on World Wide Web, Florence, Italy, 18–22 May 2015; pp. 743–753.
330. Roesner, F.; Kohno, T. Security and Privacy for Augmented Reality: Our 10-Year Retrospective. In Proceedings of the VR4Sec: 1st International Workshop on Security for XR and XR for Security, Online, 6 August 2021.
331. Lebeck, K.; Ruth, K.; Kohno, T.; Roesner, F. Towards security and privacy for multi-user augmented reality: Foundations with end users. In Proceedings of the 2018 IEEE Symposium on Security and Privacy (SP), San Francisco, CA, USA, 20–24 May 2018; pp. 392–408.
332. Dissanayake, V.D. *A Review of Cyber Security Risks in an Augmented Reality World*; University of Sri Lanka, Institute of Information Technology: Malabe, Sri Lanka, 2019.
333. Lebeck, K. Security and Privacy for Emerging Augmented Reality Technologies. Ph.D. Thesis, University of Washington, Seattle, WA, USA, 2019.
334. Marques, B.; Silva, S.; Alves, J.; Rocha, A.; Dias, P.; Santos, B.S. Remote collaboration in maintenance contexts using augmented reality: Insights from a participatory process. *Int. J. Interact. Des. Manuf.* **2022**, *16*, 419–438. [CrossRef]
335. Kang, J.Y.M.; Kim, J.E.; Lee, J.Y.; Lin, S.H. How mobile augmented reality digitally transforms the retail sector: examining trust in augmented reality apps and online/offline store patronage intention. *J. Fash. Mark. Manag. Int. J.* **2022**. [CrossRef]
336. Alimamy, S.; Gnoth, J. I want it my way! The effect of perceptions of personalization through augmented reality and online shopping on customer intentions to co-create value. *Comput. Hum. Behav.* **2022**, *128*, 107105. [CrossRef]
337. Ghafoori, M.; Shadnoosh, N.; Karamati, M.A. The effect of co-creation in the face of augmented reality on perceived risk, perceived trust. *J. Invest. Knowl.* **2022**, *11*, 551–575.
338. Butt, G.Q.; Sayed, T.A.; Riaz, R.; Rizvi, S.S.; Paul, A. Secure Healthcare Record Sharing Mechanism with Blockchain. *Appl. Sci.* **2022**, *12*, 2307. [CrossRef]
339. Djenouri, Y.; Belhadi, A.; Srivastava, G.; Lin, J.C.W. Secure collaborative augmented reality framework for biomedical informatics. *IEEE J. Biomed. Health Inform.* **2021**, *26*, 2417–2424. [CrossRef] [PubMed]
340. Lukosch, S.; Lukosch, H.; Datcu, D.; Cidota, M. On the spot information in augmented reality for teams in the security domain. In Proceedings of the 33rd Annual ACM Conference Extended Abstracts on Human Factors in Computing Systems, Seoul, Republic of Korea, 18–23 April 2015; pp. 983–988.
341. Althewaynee, H.B.; Hamood, M.M.; Hussein, H.A. A systematic review of using augmented reality in tourism between 2017 and 2021. *Res. J. Anal. Invent.* **2022**, *3*, 18–45.
342. Ali, T.; Alam, M.; Nauman, M.; Ali, T.; Ali, M.; Anwar, S. A scalable and privacy preserving remote attestation mechanism. *Inf.-Int. Interdiscip. J.* **2011**, *14*, 1193–1203.
343. Syed, T.A.; Jan, S.; Musa, S.; Ali, J. Providing efficient, scalable and privacy preserved verification mechanism in remote attestation. In Proceedings of the 2016 International Conference on Information and Communication Technology (ICICTM), Bangkok, Thailand, 16–18 December 2016; pp. 236–245.
344. Siddiqui, M.S.; Syed, T.A.; Nadeem, A.; Nawaz, W.; Alkhodre, A. Virtual Tourism and Digital Heritage: An Analysis of VR/AR Technologies and Applications. *Int. J. Adv. Comput. Sci. Appl.* **2022**, *13*, 303–315. [CrossRef]

345. Tola, E.; Lepetit, V.; Fua, P. Daisy: An efficient dense descriptor applied to wide-baseline stereo. *IEEE Trans. Pattern Anal. Mach. Intell.* **2009**, *32*, 815–830. [CrossRef]
346. Träskbäack, M.; Haller, M. Mixed reality training application for an oil refinery: User requirements. In Proceedings of the 2004 ACM SIGGRAPH International Conference on Virtual Reality Continuum and Its Applications in Industry, Singapore, 16–18 June 2004; pp. 324–327.

virtual worlds

MDPI

Article

Enhancing Self-Learning in Higher Education with Virtual and Augmented Reality Role Games: Students' Perceptions

Luis Valladares Ríos [1], Ricardo Acosta-Diaz [2] and Pedro C. Santana-Mancilla [2,*]

[1] Higher Institute of Normal Education of the State of Colima (ISENCO), Colima 28040, Mexico; luis.valladares@isencolima.edu.mx
[2] School of Telematics, Universidad de Colima, Colima 28040, Mexico; acosta@ucol.mx
* Correspondence: psantana@ucol.mx

Abstract: This study investigates how virtual and augmented reality role games impact self-learning in higher education settings. A qualitative research–action approach that involved creating augmented reality micro-stories to encourage creativity and critical thinking was used. Through role-playing, students collaborated and gained a deeper understanding of the course, improving their self-learning abilities. The findings indicate that incorporating virtual and augmented reality into higher education positively affects self-learning, promoting active student engagement and meaningful learning experiences. Additionally, students perceive these immersive educational methods as bridging the gap between virtual and in-person learning environments, ultimately leading to enhanced educational results.

Keywords: virtual reality; augmented reality; role games; higher education; self-learning

Citation: Valladares Ríos, L.; Acosta-Diaz, R.; Santana-Mancilla, P.C. Enhancing Self-Learning in Higher Education with Virtual and Augmented Reality Role Games: Students' Perceptions. *Virtual Worlds* **2023**, *2*, 343–358. https://doi.org/10.3390/virtualworlds2040020

Academic Editors: Radu Comes, Dorin-Mircea Popovici, Calin Gheorghe Dan Neamtu and Jing-Jing Fang

Received: 31 July 2023
Revised: 22 October 2023
Accepted: 26 October 2023
Published: 30 October 2023

1. Introduction

Learning, by nature, is a collaborative process in which students work together and share resources to learn [1]. The teacher guides students in experimentation and exploration; individual learning is derived from group activities. The teacher must design learning problems to be solved in simulated learning environments and promote social participation and sustainable development. They should also consider interaction with the community and social projects and encourage creative and scientific thinking. Using technology and digital platforms in learning should create confidence in students and develop their digital skills. According to [2], virtuality in education responds satisfactorily to the needs of current social, cultural, and economic changes in Latin American digital times. These cultural aspects of student generations interacting with virtuality with their digital devices help create and build an equitable and inclusive society by developing active methodologies that allow learning and trusting of others in an interrelated and complex system. Digital models, which use modern techniques such as virtual reality (VR) and augmented reality (AR), should promote problem-solving that contributes to social well-being and the development of student expertise. Students should be able to interact with natural or very similar environments and apply their knowledge and skills to relevant situations [3].

To generate curiosity and prepare professionals for the future, the emerging education of a resilient, collaborative type that empowers everyone is role-playing, as noted by [4]. It promotes gamification, volunteering, self-motivation, myth, and fantasy; integrates knowledge in a globalizing way; considers creativity and construction of meanings, self-organization of knowledge, and critical thinking; grants the importance of small information, interaction among peers, dialogue, collaboration, teamwork, empathy, tolerance, decision-making and responsibility, personal self-affirmation, motivation to learn, security, and self-esteem; it responds to affective needs; fosters freedom of movement and expression; is therapeutic and liberating of tension, with anticipatory experiences; and is multicultural.

Self-Learning

As part of the learning process, we come across self-learning, which consists of students being able to independently identify, explore, develop, elaborate, observe, apply, analyze, and conclude educational activities. By working in teams in real-time virtual environments, students can interact with technology and their peers in a way that allows them to develop cognitive skills and a connective and virtual vision for learning in collaboration. Students can also be producers, creators, and consumers of their content when learning with role-playing games using AR and VR technologies. By facing situations of analysis and problem-solving in real-world or simulated environments, students can develop skills such as creativity, leadership, and self-management. Students can also develop a critical attitude by evaluating and analyzing information and applying their knowledge and skills to relevant situations [2].

Furthermore, self-learning can foster the development of identity and social responsibility by involving students in projects that benefit the community. In higher education, self-learning can have several problems and benefits [5–7].

Some potential problems of self-learning are

- Lack of motivation: Students may need help motivating themselves to learn independently, especially if they need a clear learning structure or incentives to learn.
- Lack of supervision: Students learning independently may need access to a teacher or tutor who can provide feedback or guidance during the learning process.
- Lack of social interaction: Collaborative learning may only be effective if students can interact with their classmates and discuss and debate ideas.

However, there are also several potential benefits of self-learning in higher education:

- Autonomy and responsibility: Self-learning can foster autonomy and responsibility in students by allowing them to take control of their learning process.
- Flexibility: Self-learning can be more flexible than traditional learning, as students can work at their own pace and in the place of their choice.
- Development of lifelong learning skills: Self-learning can help students develop lifelong learning skills, which can be helpful in their professional and personal lives.
- Increased participation and engagement: Students who participate in self-learning may show increased participation and engagement in their learning process and with learning materials.

The goal of this research is to explore the impact of VR and AR role-playing games on self-learning in higher education. The research question guiding our inquiry is: How do virtual and augmented reality role-playing games influence the self-learning processes of students in higher education? We aim to explore how VR and AR role-playing games can enhance self-directed learning in higher education.

2. Virtual Reality and Augmented Reality in Education

VR and AR have significantly evolved over the years, becoming pivotal technologies in higher education that offer immersive learning experiences and enhance the understanding of abstract concepts [8,9]. The main difference between VR and AR is their level of immersion and interaction. VR completely replaces the real world with a digital environment, providing a fully immersive experience. On the other hand, AR superimposes digital content onto the real world using devices like smartphones or AR glasses, allowing users to interact with both the real and digital worlds simultaneously.

The fundamental theories underpinning the use of VR and AR in education include constructivism, situated learning, and experiential learning, emphasizing the importance of interactive and hands-on learning experiences. These pedagogical theories align with the affordances of VR and AR, providing rich, interactive, and immersive learning environments that foster more profound understanding and engagement among students.

Azuma and Milgram's seminal works fundamentally understand AR and VR. In particular, Azuma's survey on AR laid the groundwork for comprehending how digital information could be overlaid in the real world, resulting in enhanced interactive experiences [10]. Milgram et al.'s classification of displays on the reality–virtuality continuum provides a framework for understanding the different immersive experiences offered by AR and VR [11].

A comprehensive overview of AR and Gamification in Education was provided in a recent systematic review conducted by Lampropoulos et al. [12]. The review showcased a range of applications and empirical studies exploring these technologies' pedagogical benefits. This paper provides valuable insights into how AR and VR can be gamified to enhance learning engagement and outcomes.

Krug et al. [13] proposed a set of evaluation criteria that provide a structured approach for designing and analyzing AR applications in educational contexts. These criteria have been used in recent studies to compare and evaluate the effectiveness of AR applications in education. By doing so, they enabled a better understanding of AR and VR's pedagogical benefits and challenges.

In higher education, VR and AR have been used in a variety of ways:

- Simulation of environments: VR and AR can simulate real-world or hypothetical environments, such as laboratories, hospitals, or extraterrestrial planets. Students can interact with these environments, practice skills, and make decisions in controlled contexts.
- Role-playing games: VR and AR can allow students to put themselves in the place of characters or professionals in different contexts and make decisions that affect the game's outcome.
- Virtual tours: VR and AR can provide students with virtual tours of places that would otherwise be inaccessible or costly to visit in person, such as museums or historical sites.
- Presentations: VR and AR can be used to make presentations more interactive and engaging for students, for example, by adding augmented visual elements to a PowerPoint slide.

In addition, both AR and VR have been used in education to improve self-directed learning. The literature presents several works on this topic.

The study reported in [14] evaluated the use of AR in self-directed learning in special education. The results indicated that students were more excited and enthusiastic about classes during the experiment.

VR and AR can be effective for learning abstract or difficult-to-understand concepts. For example, a study found that students who used VR to learn about the lifecycle of a pipe wrench had a greater understanding of the concept and a higher retention of the information in the long-term [9].

AR has also been helpful in secondary education. For example, in [8], a study was reported in which history was taught to students, and the results showed that the students perceived high usability for this kind of application.

In higher education, AR role-playing games allow students to have the opportunity to assume the roles of characters or professionals in diverse scenarios and take actions that impact the game's final result. Some examples of AR role-playing games used in higher education are:

- Escape rooms: Students must solve problems and decode clues to successfully "escape" the room before the time limit expires [15].
- AMELIO: To complete a mission in a space colony emergency, students must make team decisions using mixed reality games [16].
- Chariot Augmented Reality Medical (CHARM) simulator: In an AR environment, students must use their clinical skills and adhere to proper medical protocols to succeed in a cardiovascular life support (ACLS) simulation scenario [17].

Regarding the students' perceptions, opinions, and attitudes, the literature suggests that students generally favor VR and AR in education. Mikropoulos [18] discovered that education students favor using VR in the educational process. Antonietti [19] investigated students' perceptions of VR use in education and found no differences based on gender or prior VR experience. Matome [20] examined student perceptions of VR in higher education and found several benefits associated with its introduction. However, the diverse population and socioeconomic differences among students may affect these advantages' equitable distribution and utilization. Serin [21] surveyed teachers' perspectives on VR in education. The study revealed that VR was perceived as an exciting tool that enhances students' engagement, facilitates learning, and requires concentration.

According to Sural [22], prospective educators expressed enthusiasm for integrating AR into their learning and believed it would benefit other learning materials. Bower [23,24] discussed how AR can improve education by providing students with information at the exact time and place of need, reducing cognitive overload, and enabling various learning methods. Arguing for the merit of having students design AR experiences to develop higher-order thinking capabilities, Rizov [25] discovered that using AR as a teaching tool in higher education significantly improved student engagement, comprehension, and retention while enhancing educators' teaching experience.

This research highlights the importance of role-playing in higher education, utilizing the capabilities of AR and VR. In the previous section, we discussed how role-playing, AR, and VR can affect the learning experience. The following section outlines the target population, details the implementation of the intervention, and describes the data collection and analysis procedures.

3. Methods

3.1. Research Approach

This study follows a qualitative research–action approach, focusing on describing the didactic impact of AR and VR learning objects during role-playing activities. The research–action methodology [26] consists of four interconnected phases: planning, action, observation, and reflection.

The research–action approach involves thinking about the intervened practice, which contributes to the competence of the research participants, as mentioned by [27]. The study encourages reflective examination of the educational practices of the teacher when using STEM methodologies with critical use of technology to promote inclusion in the classroom.

3.2. Target Population

The present research was conducted with the school subject of "Herramientas básicas de estudios de casos (Basic tools for case studies)" in the HE program "Licenciatura en inclusión educativa (Bachelor in Educational Inclusion)" at the Higher Institute of Normal Education of the State of Colima (ISENCO), campus Cuauhtémoc, Colima, Mexico. This study was carried out during the 4th semester. Due to the non-random nature of this qualitative study, a total of 11 students, who were prospective teachers aged between 18 and 22 years old were selected. Due to the COVID-19 pandemic, we had to adapt the original course plan for hybrid teaching. It involved the virtual delivery of course materials through the G-suite platform and in-person small groups for hands-on activities. Data were gathered with the use of three primary tools: an argumentative journal, a photographic analysis, and a questionnaire.

The decision to select this target population was based on several factors. Firstly, the subject topic is crucial in educational inclusion, as it equips future teachers with essential skills and knowledge to support diverse learners effectively. Secondly, the 4th semester was appropriate for this research, as the students had already acquired some foundational knowledge in the field, making them capable of engaging with the content of the course meaningfully. Additionally, the first author was a professor of the subject. The transition to virtual learning during the COVID-19 pandemic presented a unique opportunity to explore the challenges and opportunities associated with technology-mediated classes in the context of educational inclusion.

By examining the experiences and outcomes of this target population, this study aims to contribute valuable insights to the AR and VR role games field in higher education scenarios.

3.3. *Data Collection*

In order to obtain thorough information for this research, various data collection techniques were used, such as analyzing photographs and a questionnaire.

3.3.1. Photographic Analysis

Photography is a valuable tool for researching social reality, as stated in [28]. In this study, we used photographic analysis to evaluate the educational impact of role-playing activities that utilized AR and VR among students. We captured images at the intervention's beginning, during, and end to document the didactic events and student engagement visually. By analyzing the photos alongside questionnaire responses gathered at the end of each session, we gained valuable insights into the AR environments, digital skill applications, and impact on self-directed learning. This immersive and holistic experience bridges the virtual and in-person realms, examining its effect on students' emotions, interactions, and learning outcomes.

3.3.2. Questionnaire

A questionnaire is a form that contains a series of questions applied to study subjects to gather information [29]. After each session, this study administered a questionnaire to collect first-hand ordinary data from the participating students. The questionnaire (see Appendix A) included open-ended questions related to the a priori research categories. To ensure its validity, an expert reviewed and validated the questionnaire in the field of technologies to eliminate any ambiguities in question phrasing, avoid vague terms, prevent negative question formulations, and use precise and straightforward language for the participants [30].

3.4. *Data Analysis*

The data collected with the abovementioned tools underwent a systematic analysis process to derive meaningful insights and findings. The analysis process consisted of the following key steps:

3.4.1. Photographic Analysis

Images captured at the intervention's beginning and end and throughout were systematically examined for photographic analysis. These images documented the didactic events, student engagement, and interactions in AR environments. A qualitative content analysis approach was used to identify the images' patterns, themes, and significant observations.

3.4.2. Questionnaire Data Analysis

Data collected in the questionnaire responses were analyzed using qualitative content analysis techniques. Open-ended questions allowed for a rich exploration of participants' experiences and perceptions. Responses were categorized to identify common themes, insights, and emerging patterns related to the research categories.

The analysis aimed to uncover connections between the data collected using different methods, providing a comprehensive understanding of the didactic impact of AR and VR learning objects during role-playing activities.

By using this research methodology, this study aims to clarify the didactic impact of AR and VR learning objects during role-playing activities among prospective teachers, providing valuable insights into the integration of technology and STEM methodologies in higher education settings for promoting inclusive teaching practices.

4. Study Design

For this experiment, we used the STEM approach as our instructional framework. It involved several phases, namely:

- Understand;
- Imagine;
- Design;
- Construct;
- Test;
- Improve.

We followed these phases to conduct role-playing activities using AR and VR learning objects.

In the Understand phase, students were introduced to role-playing activities that allowed them to experience the role of researchers. In the Imagine phase, students were assigned specific roles and functions to immerse themselves in the experience fully. During the Design phase, students developed a strategy to implement or develop a project based on their emotions and the knowledge gained from the activity. As a prototype to demonstrate their level of achievement, they created a micro-story in AR, as shown in Figure 1.

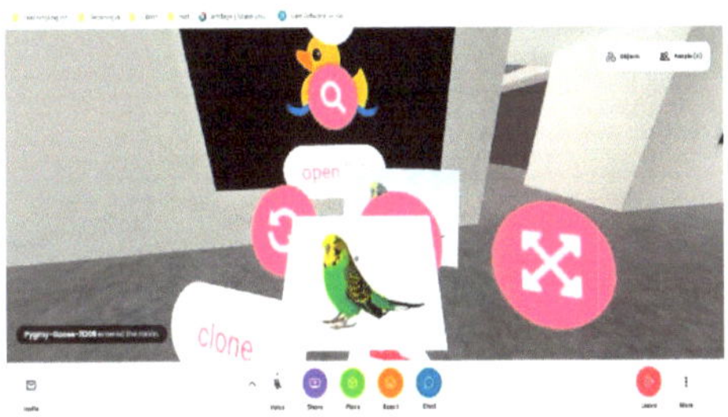

Figure 1. Micro-story in AR.

In the Construct and Test phases, students used 2D and 3D figures to develop the AR micro-story prototype. The design phase visually represented the case studies with drawings that were later animated in AR using the Paint 3D program (see Figure 2).

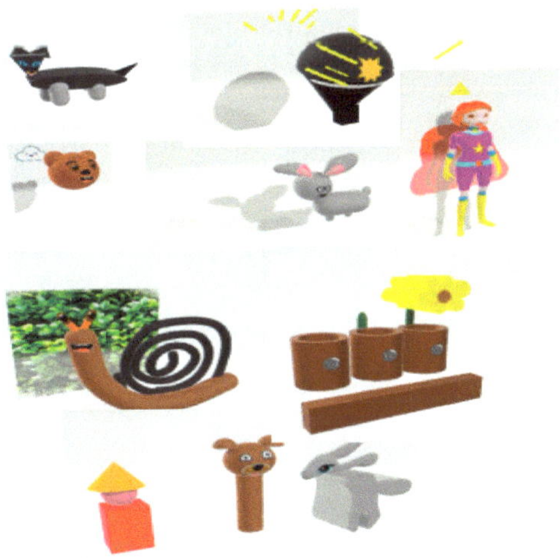

Figure 2. Three-dimensional models created by the students.

As part of an experiment, the students used Oculus Quest 2 to explore AR level 3 and learn about digital design, as seen in Figure 3. By immersing themselves in a virtual story and creating sensory virtual learning objects, they could engage with the content more meaningfully.

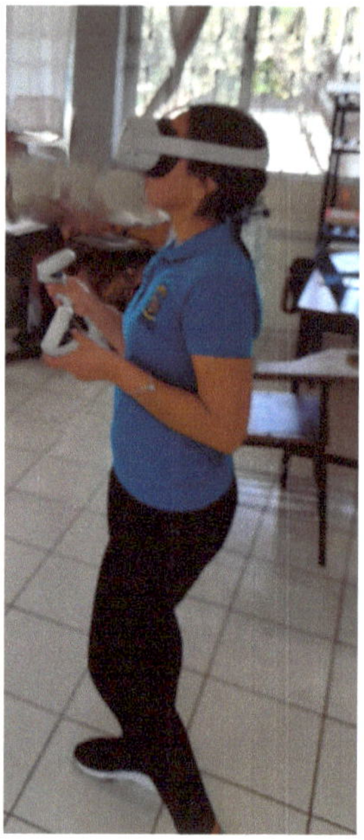

Figure 3. Use of AR level 3 with the Oculus Quest 2 visor.

Finally, to provide a more immersive and interactive experience, the students were introduced to the metaverse of VR using the Mozilla Hubs platform [31]. In this study phase, they were assigned a thrilling role-playing game of "Following Clues", where they had to embark on a quest to find a living being that flies, possesses wings, features green and yellow plumage, and has a beak (see Figure 4). As they followed the clues, the students had to engage in collaborative interactions and navigate through the VR space. This experiment phase aimed to assess the students' adaptability and engagement within an entirely virtual context, promoting teamwork and problem-solving skills in a dynamic and engaging ICT setting.

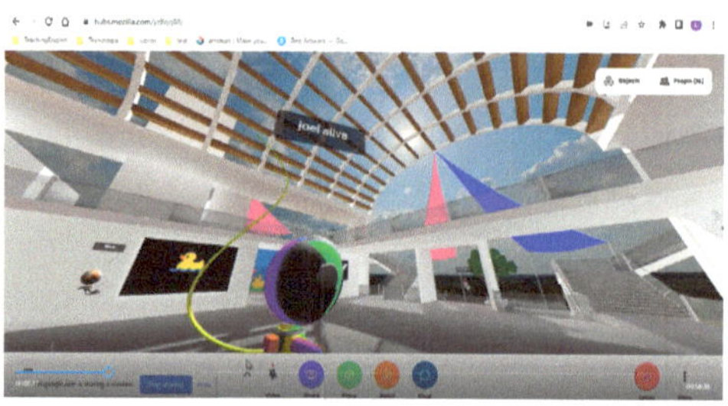

Figure 4. Use of VR with the cardboard visor.

Incorporating the metaverse experience in the experimental study, the investigation sought to delve further into the potential of VR to facilitate more profound learning experiences and foster a more comprehensive understanding of role-playing activities. The Mozilla Hubs platform provided a unique opportunity for the students to interact with the environment in a novel and captivating way, expanding their perspectives on the educational possibilities of immersive technologies. The data collected during this phase complemented the findings from the AR role-playing activities, providing a more holistic understanding of the impact of these technologies on self-learning and skill development in higher education scenarios.

5. Results

5.1. Photographic Analysis

This study's analysis of activities conducted during role-playing sessions involving the use of AR and VR learning objects was undertaken. This analysis primarily focuses on the visual component and participant interactions, offering a detailed view of the didactic influence of technology on the educational process.

5.1.1. Rally Activity and QR Code Usage

During the first session, students formed teams, each representing a group of social researchers (see Figure 5). Their task was to search for clues related to their assigned role-play scenario, which involved exploring different locations and using their mobile devices to scan QR codes. This initial approach centered on levels 1 and 2 of AR, incorporating transmedia storytelling to guide knowledge-seeking.

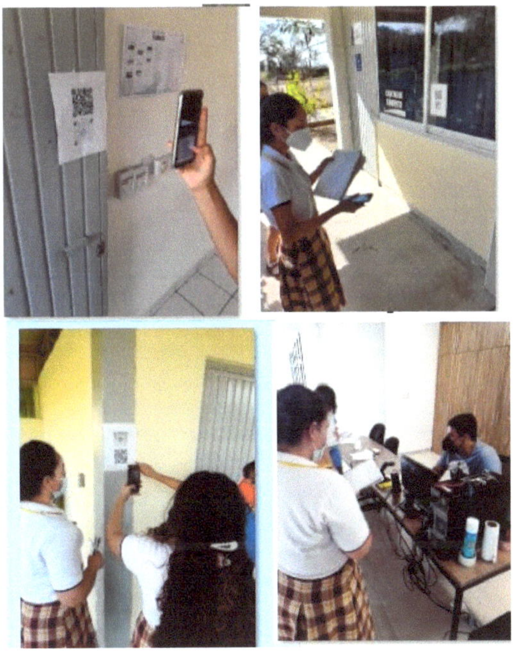

Figure 5. Students during the rally activity.

After analyzing this activity, it was found that the students quickly adapted to the role-play scenario. They organized themselves into teams based on their assigned roles and efficiently used their mobile devices to scan QR codes and access clues. This initial interaction promoted teamwork and critical thinking skills, laying a solid foundation for future activities.

5.1.2. Creation of Micro-Stories and Transmedia Narrative

Analysis of the development process (see Figure 6) at level 1 included the creation of micro-stories in AR. Students formulated research questions about their assigned case study during the investigator role-play. These questions were used to gather information about observed barriers to learning and participation during their professional practice.

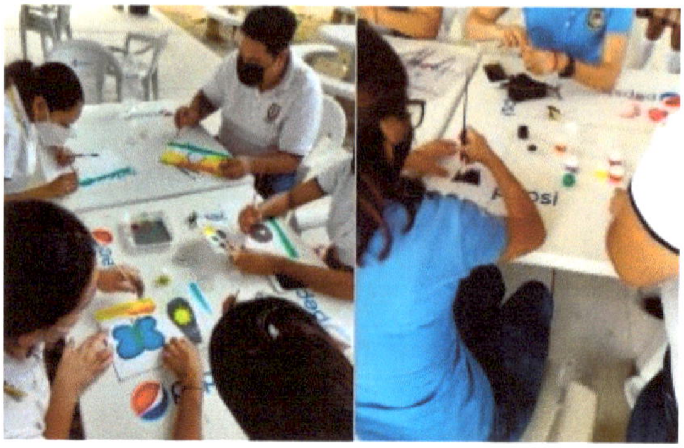

Figure 6. Students creating transmedia materials.

This activity promoted collaboration among students who worked in teams to design drawings related to the selected case studies. Each student recorded observations and interpretations of the drawings, enriching their understanding of the topic. The resulting micro-stories were presented via QR codes, allowing students to access content related to the micro-story, thus enhancing the learning experience.

5.2. Questionnaire Results

By analyzing the responses to the questionnaire, we gained valuable insights into how role-playing activities using AR and VR affect students' learning experiences. According to the research, incorporating AR and VR technology into role-playing situations benefited students' interactions and communication with their classmates. Through the immersive and collaborative nature of the activities, students engaged in effective teamwork, fostering communication and collaboration skills. One student noted, "Yes, there was more communication with peers". Another student shared, "Yes, it allowed us to use our imagination". The combination of the STEM instructional framework and creative thinking encouraged the students to envision and create imaginative AR stories, showcasing their abilities to apply acquired knowledge and skills dynamically and innovatively.

In addition, the interactive nature of the role-playing exercises helped the students fully embody the role of social researchers. It led to an improvement in their ability to present their case studies engagingly and playfully. By using an experiential approach, the students were able to gain a better understanding of the case studies they were studying. This approach also helped the students empathize with the subjects they observed, as a student expressed, "The interaction with classmates, more knowledge, and experience in how to conduct a case study". The transmedia narrative technique in digitalizing the micro-stories provided a unique opportunity for the students to explore and present their findings creatively, fostering a sense of ownership and pride in their work.

While the advantages of AR role-playing activities were evident, this study also uncovered some challenges faced by the students. Due to technical difficulties, some users encountered obstacles while attempting to digitize 2D drawings into 3D using the Paint 3D application. However, the activity allowed the students to develop problem-solving skills as they explored solutions to overcome these obstacles. As one student reflected, "I am not good at creating stories, so it was challenging to come up with ideas or imagine, but when I started drawing the story, it became easy for me". Another student shared, "I think the difficulties I encountered were in writing the story since it is difficult for me to create stories". By overcoming challenges, the students were able to improve their digital skills while also developing perseverance and adaptability.

The creation of AR stories during role-playing activities proved beneficial in fostering reading comprehension. By crafting their stories and reading them aloud to their peers, the students engaged in an interactive and dynamic process that deepened their understanding of the subject matter. This approach allowed them to effectively express complex concepts and emotions, promoting critical thinking and analytical skills. One student explained, "By reading the story, imitating or using different voices, fully engaging in the story, and teaching with creativity the drawing that was created".

The research rally using QR codes was met with enthusiasm by the students, who found it innovative, interactive, and enjoyable. This activity encouraged exploration and independent learning as they searched for clues and answers using QR code reader applications. The combination of technology and gamification made the students' learning experience exciting and engaging. As one student enthusiastically shared, "It was fun because we were moving around, thinking about the answer to the clues".

5.3. Sentiment Analysis

AR in role-playing games has proven to be an immersive tool in higher education, promoting student interaction and collaboration. Two specific questions from the questionnaire were analyzed to comprehend the emotional impact of these activities. The first question, Question 8, asked about the emotions experienced while writing stories in AR. The second question, Question 10, explored the emotions felt during role-playing while developing micro-stories in AR.

Figure 7 shows the frequency of positive and negative emotions mentioned in response to both questions. In Question 8, 13 mentions of positive emotions and four mentions of negative emotions were observed, suggesting a generally positive reception of the AR story-writing task. Similarly, in Question 10, 11 mentions of positive and six mentions of negative emotions were recorded, indicating a diverse emotional experience during micro-story development in the role-playing game.

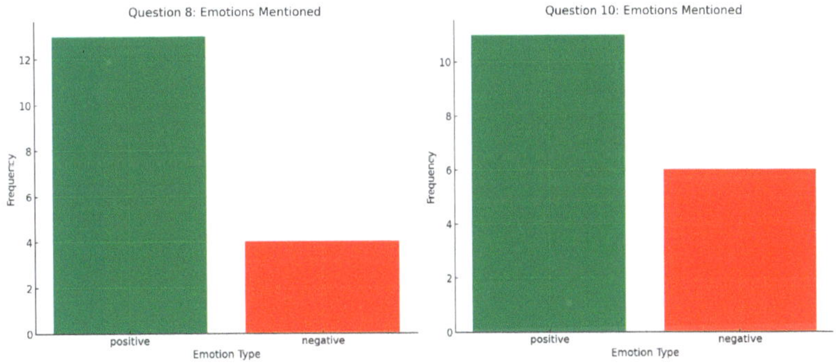

Figure 7. Sentiment analysis of emotions.

Figure 8 presents a word cloud that visually encapsulates the spectrum of emotions articulated by students in response to Questions 8 and 10, spotlighting the emotional undertones experienced during AR storytelling and role-playing activities. Dominating the visual are the words "Joy" and "Emotion", presented in larger fonts, underscoring their frequent mention, and thereby hinting at a generally positive emotional experience among participants. The presence of emotions like "Confusion", "Desperation", and "Nervousness" interwoven with the predominantly positive emotions suggests a complexity in the students' emotional journey, where moments of enjoyment and engagement coexist with instances of challenge and uncertainty.

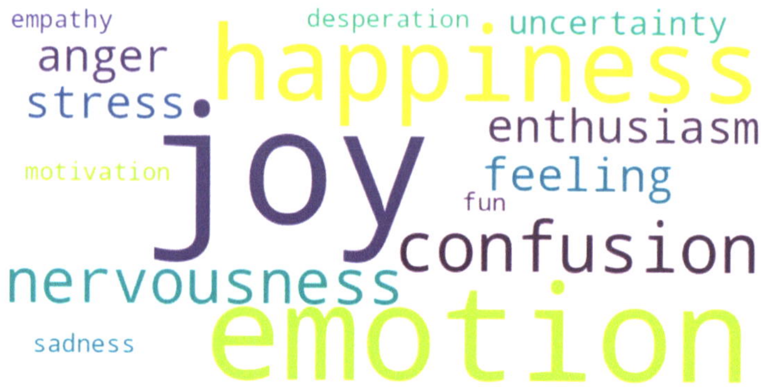

Figure 8. Word cloud of emotions.

Although the prevalence of positive emotions suggests a generally beneficial and pleasant experience for students, the mentions of negative emotions indicate that challenges and difficulties were also presented that emotionally impacted participants. Specifically, these negative emotions may be linked to obstacles and challenges encountered while developing stories in AR, such as technical problems or creative difficulties.

In order to identify a connection with negative emotions, an analysis was conducted to correlate the responses from Question 3, "What difficulties did you experience while developing the AR story during role-playing activities?", as patterns may emerge between the encountered difficulties and the negative emotions from Questions 8 and 10. These relationships could provide insights into how challenges faced during the development of AR stories may have influenced student emotions.

5.3.1. Technical Difficulties

Students expressed challenges with understanding and utilizing AR tools effectively, which could be correlated with feelings of enjoyment, as seen in Table 1.

Table 1. Technical difficulties in relation to emotions.

Difficulties	Emotions Writing Stories	Emotions Developing Micro-Stories
I needed clarification on how the tools worked, possibly with a slightly more detailed explanation to do a better job	Joy	Joy and fun
Lack of experience	Nerves and excitement	Enthusiasm

Participants encountering technical difficulties, particularly in comprehending and using AR tools, exhibited a variety of emotions in the subsequent activities. Despite technological struggles, they expressed predominantly positive emotions like "joy" and "excitement" in Question 8, indicating a positive reception toward writing AR stories. The responses for Question 10 were mostly positive, with words like "fun" and "enthusiasm", indicating that participants enjoyed creating AR micro-stories within role-playing games despite facing technical difficulties.

This suggests that even though technical challenges were encountered, they did not significantly impact the overall emotional experience. This finding could be due to the engaging nature of the AR activities.

5.3.2. Story Creation

Struggles in imagination and structuring the narrative were highlighted as difficulties in developing stories, which can lead to mixed emotions, as shown in Table 2. The stress and confusion of the creative process can overshadow the joy of creation.

Table 2. Story creation in relation to emotions.

Difficulties	Emotions Writing Stories	Emotions Developing Micro-Stories
Developing the story	Joy	Joy and happiness
I am not good at creating stories, so I found it very difficult to think about what to put or imagine, but it became easy for me when I drew the story	Happiness, confusion, and excitement	Desperation, joy, and motivation
I did not know how to shape both the story and the drawing	Nerves	Stress
I had difficulties writing the story since I found it difficult to create stories	Joy and emotion	Emotion, confusion, and stress

Participants who encountered challenges in creating and developing stories conveyed a spectrum of emotions. In Question 8, despite the inherent challenges in developing stories, emotions were notably positive, with expressions like "Joy" and "Happiness" surfacing, suggesting that crafting stories in AR was pleasurable. In contrast, responses to Question 10, such as "Desperation", "stress", and "confusion", indicated a blend of emotions. During the creative process, one can experience both joy and desperation. The latter can arise due to struggles with the creative writing process. This highlights that the challenges of creating a story can elicit a complex emotional response. It intertwines the joy of creation with the potential stress or anxiety that may arise from these challenges.

5.3.3. Creative Expression

Participants pointed out challenges in expressing ideas and choosing characters, potentially linked to feelings of insecurity, confusion, and joy, reflecting a bittersweet experience where creative expression was enjoyable and slightly daunting, as seen in Table 3.

Table 3. Creative expression in relation to emotions.

Difficulties	Emotions Writing Stories	Emotions Developing Micro-Stories
Not knowing exactly how to express myself correctly	Joy and emotion	Happiness, confusion, emotion, and anger
How to create or choose the characters	Emotion and happiness	Joy and uncertainty

Participants who expressed difficulties with creative expression and character creation revealed a range of emotions in their responses. In Question 8, responses such as "Joy and emotion" suggest a wholesome emotional experience. Meanwhile, in Question 10, expressions like "Happiness, confusion, emotion, and anger" unveil a multifaceted emotional response to developing micro-stories, where the happiness derived from creative expression is juxtaposed with confusion and anger, possibly related to struggles with embodying creativity in the AR platform. While creative expression in AR is enriching and enjoyable, it also introduces emotional complexity, where positive emotions coexist with potential emotional struggles tied to the creative process.

This analysis illustrates the importance of considering students' emotional experiences in innovative and technologically advanced learning activities. Although these activities can offer enriching and exciting opportunities for interactive learning and collaboration, they can also present challenges that require adequate support and guidance to ensure positive and effective learning experiences for all students.

Future research could explore the circumstances and factors contributing to negative emotions to develop strategies and supports that minimize these challenges and enhance positive experiences and learning outcomes.

6. Discussion

Using role-playing activities in AR and VR environments was effective in helping students express and reflect on their learning experiences. Students could immerse themselves in various scenarios through these activities, engaging in dynamic interactions with their peers and the digital content. This immersive experience helped bridge the gap between virtual and in-person learning environments, as students felt actively involved in the learning process despite being in a digital setting. Integrating asynchronous and synchronous activities further enriched their skills in using inclusive technology for educational purposes, contributing to their overall digital literacy.

VR and AR have gained increasing interest in higher education, especially in role-playing games that promote self-learning. Oyelere et al.'s systematic review [32] highlights the emergence of Educational VR Games (EVRGs) as a catalyst for transformative educational experiences at different levels, including higher education. Our study supports this trend, demonstrating how role-playing in VR and AR environments enhances self-learning, critical thinking, and creative application among higher education students, in line with current literature.

By incorporating STEM teaching practices, the experiment encouraged critical thinking and problem-solving skills among the students. The creation of AR micro-stories necessitated creative thinking and the application of knowledge to craft engaging narratives. This experiential learning approach allowed students to develop a deeper understanding of the lessons as they become active creators of knowledge rather than passive recipients. Moreover, the use of AR and VR technology provided a unique opportunity for students to explore their creativity and present their findings visually compellingly. Upon further comparison with other studies, it was revealed that although traditional teaching methods have their benefits, the immersive digital experiences offered by VR and AR tend to provide a more engaging learning environment. They allow for a deeper level of engagement with complex materials beyond what can be achieved with conventional lectures and textbooks, providing opportunities for personalized learning experiences [33].

This exploration unveiled a blend of emotions experienced by students, with a generally positive inclination toward AR activities, but not without the presence of negative emotions arising from various difficulties. While the innovative approach of integrating AR in role-playing was found to be engaging and imaginative, it is crucial to acknowledge the emotional and technical challenges encountered by the students. Identifying and developing strategies to minimize these hurdles could enhance the learning experience, ensuring it is innovative, emotionally supportive, and educationally productive.

This complex emotional landscape sheds light on the intricate relationship between technology, creativity, and emotional response in educational activities. It also highlights areas for further exploration and support in future implementations of AR in learning environments.

The positive response from students toward the AR and VR role-playing activities underscores the potential of these immersive educational experiences to enhance self-learning in higher education contexts. This sentiment is supported by the existing literature on the pedagogical advantages of VR and AR [34,35].

Future research and implementations may further focus on providing additional support in areas identified as challenging, such as technical guidance, creative writing workshops, and emotional support, to nurture positive learning experiences in technologically advanced educational activities.

The teacher's role in crafting a comprehensive virtual classroom plan must be considered. The experiment's success relied heavily on the teacher's ability to design and implement various activities and strategies aligned with the learning objectives. With the teacher's guidance and facilitation during role-playing exercises, students could better understand the lessons and connect them to real-world scenarios based on their experiences.

7. Limitations

Although our study provided valuable insights into using AR and VR role-playing activities in higher education, it is essential to acknowledge its limitations. Firstly, this study was conducted in a specific higher education setting, focusing on a particular subject and semester. Thus, the context of our study may limit the generalizability of our findings to other academic institutions or disciplines. Secondly, this study relied on a relatively small sample size, with only 11 students participating. A more extensive and diverse sample could offer a broader perspective on the impact of AR and VR in higher education.

This study evaluated the immediate impact of AR and VR role-playing activities but did not assess long-term effects and sustained learning outcomes. Future studies could investigate the durability of the skills and knowledge acquired through these immersive experiences. Additionally, this study could have provided a more in-depth analysis of students' technical challenges while using AR and VR technology. Developing effective strategies to address these challenges could improve the overall learning experience.

Our research methodology uses an action research approach, but we do not include a control group. There are both advantages and disadvantages to this methodological choice. On the one hand, it allows us to explore the phenomenon under study in a way that enhances our understanding of the processes and dynamics involved. It is important to acknowledge that our findings may need to be generalizable due to the absence of a control group, which limits our ability to establish definitive causal relationships. However, despite this limitation, the action research approach has enriched our research by providing a valuable qualitative perspective that complements our analysis of using AR and VR role-playing activities in higher education.

Although there are some limitations, our research has provided valuable insights into how AR and VR can be utilized in higher education. Further studies can expand on our findings and explore the transformative effects of immersive technologies on self-directed learning and skill development.

8. Conclusions

This project evaluated the impact of AR and VR learning objects on developing both generic competencies related to ICT and professional competencies in inclusive teaching strategies. The evaluation criteria focused on the quality of the learning objects, the effectiveness of collaborative work among students, and the final prototype of the micro-story in AR. The findings showed that the integration of AR and VR technology positively impacted the students' competency development.

In conclusion, combining AR and VR technology with role-playing activities in higher education offers a promising pathway for enhancing self-learning and promoting active student engagement. The immersive and interactive nature of these activities fosters creativity, critical thinking, and collaboration, empowering students to become active participants in their educational journey. As educational institutions continue to embrace innovative technologies, integrating AR and VR in higher education holds immense potential for transforming how students learn and prepare for a technology-driven world.

Author Contributions: Methodology, L.V.R. and R.A.-D.; formal analysis, P.C.S.-M. and R.A.-D.; data curation, L.V.R., R.A.-D. and P.C.S.-M.; writing—original draft preparation, P.C.S.-M. and L.V.R.; writing—review and editing, R.A.-D. All authors have read and agreed to the published version of the manuscript.

Funding: This research received no external funding.

Institutional Review Board Statement: This study was approved by the Higher Institute of Normal Education of the State of Colima (ISENCO), campus Cuauhtémoc, Colima, Mexico.

Informed Consent Statement: Informed consent was obtained from all subjects involved in this study.

Data Availability Statement: The data presented in this study are available upon request from the first author.

Acknowledgments: We thank the program authorities of "Licenciatura en inclusión educativa" at the Higher Institute of Normal Education of the State of Colima (ISENCO), campus Cuauhtémoc, Colima, Mexico. Their support and cooperation were invaluable throughout the research process. We also sincerely thank the students of the "Herramientas básicas de estudios de casos" course for actively participating in this study. Their involvement made this study possible.

Conflicts of Interest: The authors declare no conflict of interest.

Appendix A

This appendix contains the questionnaire used to collect insights from the participants in our study on the impact of augmented and virtual reality role-playing activities. The questionnaire assesses various aspects of creating augmented reality stories during the role-playing sessions, including inquiries about the emotions experienced by the participants. The original questions are in Spanish to ensure a comprehensive understanding for the participating students, who are native Spanish speakers.

1. Did the elaboration of stories in augmented reality during the role-playing games favor the interaction between your classmates?
2. Based on your perception, what did the dynamics during the role-playing activities foster?
3. What difficulties did you experience while developing the augmented reality story during role-playing activities?
4. What advantages did the creation of augmented reality stories during role-playing activities offer?
5. In your opinion, how does the creation of augmented reality stories contribute to fostering reading comprehension?
6. What are your thoughts on the research rally using QR codes?
7. What is your opinion about the digital skills used in developing augmented reality micro-stories during role-playing activities?
8. What emotions did you experience while writing stories in augmented reality during role-playing games?
9. What socioemotional skills were developed while creating micro-stories in augmented reality during role-playing?
10. What emotions did you feel while developing micro-stories in augmented reality during the role-playing game?

References

1. Rodriguez Villamil, H. Del Constructivismo al Construccionismo: Implicaciones Educativas. *Rev. Educ. Desarro. Soc.* **2008**, *2*, 71–89.
2. Fainholc, B. Presente y Futuro Latinoamericano de La Enseñanza y El Aprendizaje En Entornos Virtuales Referidos a Educación Universitaria. *RED Rev. Educ. Distancia* **2016**, *48*, 1–22. [CrossRef]
3. Zambrano-Ramírez, J. Aprendizaje Complejo En La Educación Superior Ecuatoriana. *Rev. Cienc. UNEMI* **2016**, *9*, 158–167. [CrossRef]
4. Grande de Prado, M.; Abella Garcia, V. Los Juegos de Rol En El Aula. *Teoría Educ. Educ. Cult. Soc. Inf.* **2010**, *11*. [CrossRef]
5. Tomlinson, H. (Ed.) *Educational Leadership*; RoutledgeFalmer: London, UK, 2004; ISBN 978-0-415-27651-1.
6. Lee, S.Y.; Kim, Y. The Effects of Self-Efficacy and Self-Directed Learning Readiness to Self-Leadership of Nursing Student. *J. Digit. Converg.* **2016**, *14*, 309–318. [CrossRef]
7. Knowles, M.S. *Self-Directed Learning: A Guide for Learners and Teachers*; Association Press: Chicago, IL, USA, 1975; ISBN 978-0-695-81116-7.
8. Santana-Mancilla, P.C.; Garcia-Ruiz, M.A.; Acosta-Diaz, R.; Juarez, C.U. Service Oriented Architecture to Support Mexican Secondary Education through Mobile Augmented Reality. *Procedia Comput. Sci.* **2012**, *10*, 721–727. [CrossRef]
9. Yee, N.; Bailenson, J. The Proteus Effect: The Effect of Transformed Self-Representation on Behavior. *Hum. Commun. Res.* **2007**, *33*, 271–290. [CrossRef]
10. Azuma, R.T. Survey of Augmented Reality. *Presence Teleoperators Virtual Environ.* **1997**, *6*, 355–385. [CrossRef]
11. Milgram, P.; Takemura, H.; Utsumi, A.; Kishino, F. Augmented Reality: A Class of Displays on the Reality-Virtuality Continuum. In Proceedings of the SPIE—The International Society for Optical Engineering, Boston, MA, USA, 21 December 1995; Das, H., Ed.; pp. 282–292.

12. Lampropoulos, G.; Keramopoulos, E.; Diamantaras, K.; Evangelidis, G. Augmented Reality and Gamification in Education: A Systematic Literature Review of Research, Applications, and Empirical Studies. *Appl. Sci.* **2022**, *12*, 6809. [CrossRef]
13. Krug, M.; Czok, V.; Huwer, J.; Weitzel, H.; Müller, W. Challenges for the Design of Augmented Reality Applications for Science Teacher Education. In Proceedings of the 15th International Technology, Education and Development Conference, Online Conference, 8–9 March 2021; pp. 2484–2491.
14. Cakir, R.; Korkmaz, O. The Effectiveness of Augmented Reality Environments on Individuals with Special Education Needs. *Educ. Inf. Technol.* **2019**, *24*, 1631–1659. [CrossRef]
15. Karageorgiou, Z.; Mavrimmati, E.; Fotaris, P. Escape Room Design as a Game-Based Learning Process for STEAM Education. In Proceedings of the 12th European Conference on Game Based Learning, Sophia Antipolis, France, 3 October 2019; p. 46.
16. Warmelink, H.; Mayer, I.; Weber, J.; Heijligers, B.; Haggis, M.; Peters, E.; Louwerse, M. AMELIO: Evaluating the Team-Building Potential of a Mixed Reality Escape Room Game. In Proceedings of the Extended Abstracts Publication of the Annual Symposium on Computer-Human Interaction in Play, Amsterdam, The Netherlands, 15 October 2017; ACM: Amsterdam, The Netherlands; pp. 111–123.
17. Hess, O.; Qian, J.; Bruce, J.; Wang, E.; Rodriguez, S.; Haber, N.; Caruso, T.J. Communication Skills Training Using Remote Augmented Reality Medical Simulation: A Feasibility and Acceptability Qualitative Study. *Med. Sci. Educ.* **2022**, *32*, 1005–1014. [CrossRef] [PubMed]
18. Mikropoulos, T.A.; Chalkidis, A.; Katsikis, A.; Emvalotis, A. Students' Attitudes Towards Educational Virtual Environments. *Educ. Inf. Technol.* **1998**, *3*, 137–148. [CrossRef]
19. Antonietti, A.; Rasi, C.; Imperio, E.; Sacco, M. The Representation of Virtual Reality in Education. *Educ. Inf. Technol.* **2000**, *5*, 317–327. [CrossRef]
20. Matome, T.J.; Jantjies, M.E. Student Perceptions of Virtual Reality in Higher Education. In Proceedings of the 16th International Conference on Cognition and Exploratory Learning in Digital Age (CELDA 2019), Cagliari, Italy, 7–9 November 2019; IADIS Press: Porto, Portugal; pp. 92–100.
21. Serin, H. Virtual Reality in Education from the Perspective of Teachers. *Amazonia Investig.* **2020**, *9*, 291–303. [CrossRef]
22. Sural, I. Augmented Reality Experience: Initial Perceptions of Higher Education Students. *Int. J. Instruction.* **2018**, *11*, 565–576. [CrossRef]
23. Bower, M.; Howe, C.; McCredie, N.; Robinson, A.; Grover, D. Augmented Reality in Education—Cases, Places, and Potentials. In Proceedings of the 2013 IEEE 63rd Annual Conference International Council for Education Media (ICEM), Singapore, 1–4 October 2013; IEEE: Singapore, 2013; pp. 1–11.
24. Bower, M.; Howe, C.; McCredie, N.; Robinson, A.; Grover, D. Augmented Reality in Education—Cases, Places and Potentials. *Educ. Media Int.* **2014**, *51*, 1–15. [CrossRef]
25. Rizov, T.; Rizova, E. Augmented Reality as a Teaching Tool in Higher Education. *Int. J. Cogn. Res. Sci. Eng. Educ.* **2015**, *3*, 7–15. [CrossRef]
26. Latorre-Beltrán, A. *La Investigación-Acción: Coniocer y Cambiar la Práctica Educativa*, 1st ed.; Graó: Barcelona, Spain, 2010; ISBN 978-84-7827-292-1.
27. Fernández Batanero, J.M. Capacidades y Competencias Docentes Para La Inclusión Del Alumnado En La Educación Superior. *Rev. Educ. Super.* **2012**, *61*, 9–24.
28. Bonetto, M.J. El Uso de La Fotografía En La Investigación Social. *Rev. Latinoam. Metodol. Investig. Soc.* **2016**, *6*, 71–83.
29. Marshall, G. The Purpose, Design and Administration of a Questionnaire for Data Collection. *Radiography* **2005**, *11*, 131–136. [CrossRef]
30. Santana-Mancilla, P.C.; Rodriguez-Ortiz, M.A.; Garcia-Ruiz, M.A.; Gaytan-Lugo, L.S.; Fajardo-Flores, S.B.; Contreras-Castillo, J. Teaching HCI Skills in Higher Education through Game Design: A Study of Students' Perceptions. *Informatics* **2019**, *6*, 22. [CrossRef]
31. Brown, R.; Habibi-Luevano, S.; Robern, G.; Wood, K.; Perera, S.; Uribe-Quevedo, A.; Brown, C.; Rizk, K.; Genco, F.; McKellar, J.; et al. Employing Mozilla Hubs as an Alternative Tool for Student Outreach: A Design Challenge Use Case. In *New Realities, Mobile Systems and Applications*; Auer, M.E., Tsiatsos, T., Eds.; Lecture Notes in Networks and Systems; Springer International Publishing: Cham, Switzerland, 2022; Volume 411, pp. 213–222. ISBN 978-3-030-96295-1.
32. Oyelere, S.S.; Bouali, N.; Kaliisa, R.; Obaido, G.; Yunusa, A.A.; Jimoh, E.R. Exploring the Trends of Educational Virtual Reality Games: A Systematic Review of Empirical Studies. *Smart Learn. Environ.* **2020**, *7*, 31. [CrossRef]
33. Al-Ansi, A.M.; Jaboob, M.; Garad, A.; Al-Ansi, A. Analyzing Augmented Reality (AR) and Virtual Reality (VR) Recent Development in Education. *Soc. Sci. Humanit. Open* **2023**, *8*, 100532. [CrossRef]
34. Bermejo, B.; Juiz, C.; Cortes, D.; Oskam, J.; Moilanen, T.; Loijas, J.; Govender, P.; Hussey, J.; Schmidt, A.L.; Burbach, R.; et al. AR/VR Teaching-Learning Experiences in Higher Education Institutions (HEI): A Systematic Literature Review. *Informatics* **2023**, *10*, 45. [CrossRef]
35. Dick, E. *The Promise of Immersive Learning: Augmented and Virtual Reality's Potential in Education*; Information Technology & Innovation Fundation: Washington, DC, USA, 2021.

sensors

Article

Estrus Detection and Dairy Cow Identification with Cascade Deep Learning for Augmented Reality-Ready Livestock Farming

İbrahim Arıkan [1], Tolga Ayav [1], Ahmet Çağdaş Seçkin [2] and Fatih Soygazi [2,*]

[1] Computer Engineering Department, İzmir Institute of Technology, Izmir 35430, Türkiye; ibrahimarikan064@gmail.com (İ.A.); tolgaayav@iyte.edu.tr (T.A.)
[2] Computer Engineering Department, Aydın Adnan Menderes University, Aydın 09100, Türkiye; acseckin@adu.edu.tr
* Correspondence: fatih.soygazi@adu.edu.tr

Abstract: Accurate prediction of the estrus period is crucial for optimizing insemination efficiency and reducing costs in animal husbandry, a vital sector for global food production. Precise estrus period determination is essential to avoid economic losses, such as milk production reductions, delayed calf births, and disqualification from government support. The proposed method integrates estrus period detection with cow identification using augmented reality (AR). It initiates deep learning-based mounting detection, followed by identifying the mounting region of interest (ROI) using YOLOv5. The ROI is then cropped with padding, and cow ID detection is executed using YOLOv5 on the cropped ROI. The system subsequently records the identified cow IDs. The proposed system accurately detects mounting behavior with 99% accuracy, identifies the ROI where mounting occurs with 98% accuracy, and detects the mounting couple with 94% accuracy. The high success of all operations with the proposed system demonstrates its potential contribution to AR and artificial intelligence applications in livestock farming.

Keywords: artificial intelligence; augmented reality; dairy cow identification; deep learning; estrus detection; image processing; livestock; precision livestock farming; transfer learning

Citation: Arıkan, İ.; Ayav, T.; Seçkin, A.Ç.; Soygazi, F. Estrus Detection and Dairy Cow Identification with Cascade Deep Learning for Augmented Reality-Ready Livestock Farming. *Sensors* **2023**, *23*, 9795. https://doi.org/10.3390/s23249795

Academic Editors: Radu Comes, Dorin-Mircea Popovici, Calin Gheorghe Dan Neamtu and Jing-Jing Fang

Received: 13 October 2023
Revised: 9 December 2023
Accepted: 11 December 2023
Published: 13 December 2023

1. Introduction

In today's context, agricultural and livestock sectors make significant changes in order to increase labor productivity and become more efficient [1–3]. Augmented reality (AR) technology is gaining increasing importance for the success of precision agriculture. Emerging technologies, such as data-driven farming and autonomous agricultural robots, provide substantial advantages in terms of data visualization, animal monitoring, and access to information, suggesting that this technology may find broader applications in agriculture and food supply chain domains in the future [4]. For instance, Caria and others have emphasized the significance of AR technology in the context of precision livestock farming, highlighting its crucial role in enabling the real-time monitoring of animals during farm operations [5]. Augmented reality can enhance farm management by providing farmers with real-time access to details, such as milking, feeding, and breeding of animals, thereby improving efficiency and accuracy in farm operations. Particularly, AR-based smart glasses can display information, like animal identification numbers, health status, genetic characteristics, and production data, making the process of animal selection and management more efficient and precise, thus offering substantial advantages to farmers [6]. AR technologies can also assist farmers in navigation and guidance, especially in large-scale farms. They can be utilized to determine the locations of animals and facilities using GPS and sensors. For example, AR-based smart glasses can provide directions to specific animals or groups of animals, as well as suggest the most optimal routes to reach them, which can reduce the time and effort required for animal tracking and grouping [7]. Another example of the use of AR in the field of livestock is its application in improving the education and training of veterinary students and professionals. AR can provide interactive learning experiences by simulating animal anatomy, physiology, diseases, and treatments [8,9].

Industry 4.0 and precision livestock farming (PLF) have enabled a modern technological approach to animal farming and production, encompassing ethical, economic, and logistical aspects [10]. The advent of Industry 4.0 and the Internet of Things (IoT) have enabled the continued advancement and development of PLF. Everyday farming practices coupled with continuous and real-time monitoring of animal parameters can have significant impacts on welfare and health assessment. The term Agriculture 4.0 emerged from the term Industry 4.0. However, the benefits that Industry 4.0 bring to industrial use cases may not be fully transferable to livestock farming [11]. The presence of individual living animals and the strong environmental impact of livestock farming affect the role of digital individualization and demand orientation. The introduction and adoption of Industry 4.0 concepts and technologies may contribute significantly to transforming agriculture into something that may be called Agriculture 4.0.

AR is still an emerging technology in the field of agriculture [4]. It can potentially help farmers with training by providing an interactive and safe form of training. However, its usage in agriculture is unexplored. AR technologies are employed in agriculture and livestock to enhance data visualization, integrate with Industry 4.0 technologies, support disease detection, facilitate real-time monitoring, and enable individual animal management, as well as improve efficient access to information and animal tracking. These applications aim to enhance overall efficiency, productivity, and sustainability in the agricultural sector. Factors such as monitoring, identification, and estrus detection in animals hold significant importance in dairy cow farming, both in open and closed environments. These processes facilitate the close monitoring of animal health, early disease detection, and timely treatment when needed. Furthermore, animal identification allows for accurate record keeping and data tracking, thereby enhancing efficiency. Estrus detection, when accurately timed, improves reproductive efficiency and enables more effective management of genetic resources. Therefore, animal monitoring and management play a critical role in both animal welfare and production efficiency in dairy cow farming. Traditionally, identification methods such as ear tags, smart collars, and Radio-Frequency Identification (RFID) are commonly used in livestock farming [12]. These systems are suitable for indoor facilities and are typically associated with static infrastructure, such as milking, feeding, or watering units. However, innovative identification methods, such as image-based pattern/spot [13–15], nose prints [16,17], or head/face recognition systems [18], have emerged as alternatives to traditional systems. These new systems can provide more precise, cost-effective, and efficient monitoring and management of cows, and they are also suitable for deployment in mobile setups.

The estrus period in cows refers to the time when a mature cow is most fertile and ready for conception. This period is usually marked by specific movements and behaviors. Cows typically have an estrus cycle that lasts around 21 days, and if they do not become pregnant, they will enter another estrus period approximately 21 days later [19,20]. The estrus period of cows can vary depending on factors such as age, seasonal conditions, diet, etc. Monitoring estrus in cows is important to ensure that pregnancy occurs within a short period of time after giving birth. In Reith and Hoy's classification of estrus signs, both primary and secondary signs of estrus are explained [21]. Primary signs include "standing to be mounted", which is the most prominent behavior, indicating that cows are ready for mating during the estrus period. However, a decrease in the frequency of this behavior has been noted, especially in cows with high milk production. The duration of this behavior may be shorter in high-yielding cows. Secondary signs include mounting behavior, increased activity, changes in rumination time, agonistic interactions, and social interactions. Mounting behavior is a secondary sign that begins before the primary sign of estrus and continues afterward. The frequency of cows mounting each other or attempting to mount during the mating period can be considered a more reliable indicator for estrus detection. These signs are important for accurately detecting the estrus period and determining the optimal time for artificial insemination. Additionally, the text emphasizes the impact of environmental factors such as housing conditions, floor features, and climate on these signs. Observing the estrus period of a cow is important for optimal timing of insemination to increase productivity [19,22]. The estrus cycle seen in cows is shown in Figure 1. Artificial insemination can be performed between the 12th and 24th h of estrus, but the highest conception rate is achieved between the 12th and 18th h.

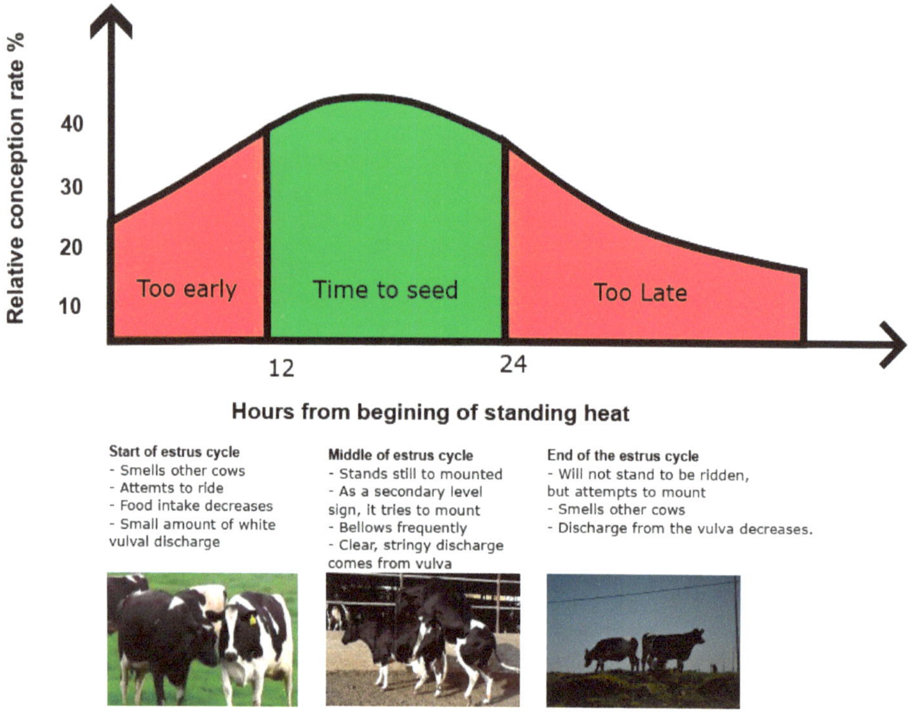

Figure 1. Estrus cycle diagram.

The detection of estrus using traditional methods involves employees on the farm monitoring the mounting behavior of the cows. Missing the estrus period due to any disruptions can result in economic losses for the business. These economic losses can lead to a reduced milk yield, delayed insemination by 21 days, and a one-month delay in calf birth [23–26]. For example, in a farm with 10 cows, if estrus is missed once for each cow, it causes one calf loss in a year in the number of calves that will be born on the farm.

Machine learning and deep learning techniques are among the latest technologies used to automate estrus detection. These techniques detect the estrus period based on the activities, behaviors, and/or physiological characteristics of the cows relying on their video images. This enables increased productivity in farming by preventing the need for employees to spend time on estrus detection and minimizing the risk of inaccurate detections [22].

The mounting behavior of the cow in estrus is shown in Figure 1. Memmedova and Keskin aimed to detect cows' estrus by utilizing the movement characteristics of cows during the estrus period [23]. They aimed to detect estrus using a fuzzy logic model that includes features like the level of activity of a cow and the time elapsed since giving birth. The movement characteristics of the cows were measured by attaching step counters to their front legs. Memmedova and Keskin were able to detect the cows' estrus state at a rate of 98% using the method they used [23].

Yıldız and Özgüven conducted a study that aimed to detect cows' estrus by examining not only the movements displayed by cows during the estrus periods but also the effects of the season [27]. They collected movement data and seasonal information from 186 cows that exhibited estrus, of which 78 were dairy cows. They trained single-layer artificial neural network models on this data and obtained an estrus period detection accuracy of 97% [27]. Arago et al. developed a system that aims to detect cows' estrus by tracking the mounting behavior displayed by cows during the estrus period [28]. In their study, they trained two artificial neural network models using the Tensor Flow Object Detection Application Programming Interface (API) with the goal of detecting the estrus event within 100 m. They carried out the detection process with the trained models by analyzing images taken from cameras installed at specific angles. The system they developed has an accuracy rate of 94%. In addition to these academic studies, there are also products that detect estrus in cows. Actimoo is a commercial estrus tracking system [29]. This product detects estrus based on physical data collected by an activity meter attached to the neck of the cows, and its accuracy rate is defined as 80%. Another product used for estrus tracking is the estrus band. Estrotect bands are attached to the backs of cows, and they change color during the estrus period when another cow mounts the band-wearing cows, indicating estrus [30].

Various methods exist for detecting the estrus period in cows used in production. These methods typically involve attaching a pedometer-like collar or wearable bracelet device [23,27,29,31–33] to the cow or applying painting patches called estrus patches [30] to the tail region of the cows. The main disadvantage of commercial wearable devices used in animal husbandry, namely wristbands, collars, or paint patches, compared to computer vision-based systems, is the necessity of allocating a device to each animal and, therefore, pricing per animal. In addition, painting patches, such as Estrotect [30], are disposable, although they are cheap and practical. Actimoo [29] and SCR [33], which are commercial systems, have a limited usage time (as long as battery life) and require infrastructure because they communicate wirelessly with the intermediary device; that is, they are environment dependent.

Systems supported by deep learning, which could be considered more recent, are still in the research stage, and a commercially matured system has not been encountered. Existing visual systems serve a single purpose, such as estrus detection. This paper proposes the development of a system that sequentially performs both estrus detection and cow identification processes for use in augmented reality applications in dairy cows. The system we propose is not individual based but refers to a volume such as a room, cow pen, or open area, and its mobility is higher, especially for use in devices such as smartphones or drones. The method proposed in this study aims to contribute to the following aspects:

- Introduce a deep learning-based method to visually identify animals on a livestock farm;
- Introduce a deep learning-based method for detecting standing mounted and mounting behaviors, the primary and secondary signs of estrus behavior. This brings new technology to the dynamic structure of modern animal husbandry;
- Present a high-accuracy system by integrating estrus detection and cow identification processes through the proposed method.

2. Materials and Methods

The core idea of the method is shown in Figure 2. The general structure of the method involves the sequential utilization of two deep learning-based detectors for estrus and cow identification, as illustrated in Figure 2. In the general method, the mounting detection process is initially performed using a CNN or VGG, followed by determining the region of interest (ROI) where the mounting action occurs using YOLO. After identifying the ROI, it is cropped with a padding of 20 pixels around it. Cow ID detection is then carried out on this cropped ROI using YOLO. Subsequently, the cow IDs are registered in the system. The details of these procedures are presented in the subsequent subsections.

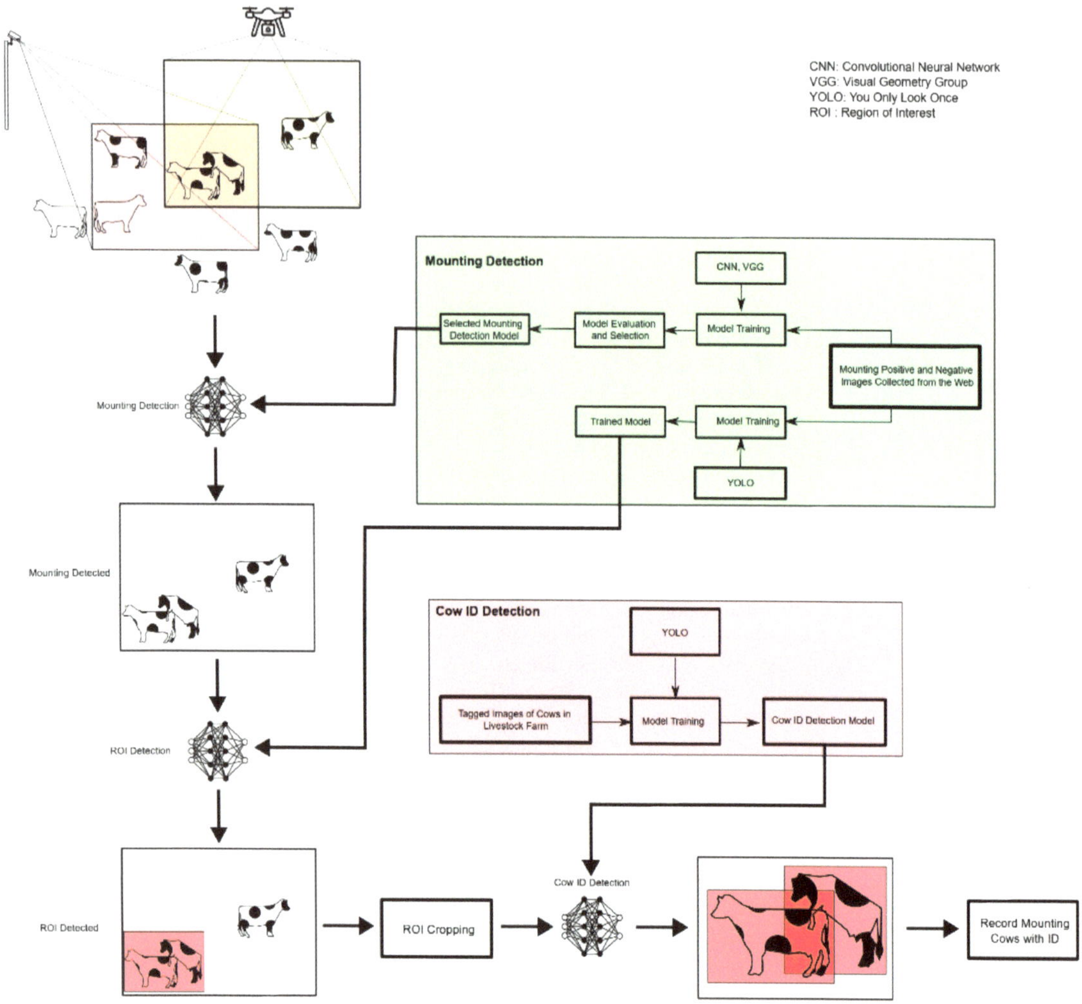

Figure 2. General method.

The estrus detector operates by transferring a model trained on images containing positive and negative cases of estrus periods, collected from the internet to real videos. This method was chosen due to the labor-intensive and time-consuming nature of monitoring and photographing the estrus period. For cow identification, a dataset of images was gathered from various angles of cows present in the livestock facility and manually labeled. The obtained dataset was utilized for this purpose. The two models obtained were tested on images captured from drones, smartphones, and pan-tilt cameras. Initially, estrus detection is performed, followed by the identification of cows during the estrus period, enabling labeling within the facility.

2.1. Dataset and Transfer Learning for Mounting Detection

After the first calving, a dairy cow can be counted in the productive stage [34]. The lifecycle in this stage is a sequence of lactation (up to 305 days), dry period (about 60 days), and calving (about 280 days) [34–36]. Even if samples are collected in an area with many animals due to the fact that obtaining comprehensive data from different animals would take a year and necessitate continuous observation by an individual who tags these moments through video, it has been decided that the process of data collection is both laborious and time consuming. To alleviate the burden on human resources, expedite the process, and expand the dataset, we opted to source images featuring both mounting and non-mounting behavior from the internet. Our research is centered around a dataset comprising cows of diverse breeds, specifically Simmental, Holstein, Jersey, and Brown Swiss (Montofon). This dataset encompasses images of cows engaged in mounting behavior and those not involved in such activities, all captured from various angles. The dataset was curated by collating images from online sources, specifically from search engines where cow images are publicly shared. Importantly, each image underwent a manual labeling process to categorize them appropriately.

The dataset was enriched with data augmentation techniques to prevent the models from overfitting. During the data augmentation phase, techniques such as rotating images by a specific angle and zooming in and out were benefited [37]. The total size of the dataset is 1638. The test data size is 492 (30%), and the training size is 1146 (70%). The distribution is not stratified. The two-class dataset consists of a total of 1638 images, comprising 937 images of cows in estrus and 701 images of cows not in estrus. Figures 3 and 4 display some examples belonging to the positive and negative classes within the dataset. The images in the dataset were preprocessed and normalized prior to training. During the preprocessing stage, images with different pixel dimensions were resized to (224,224) pixel dimensions.

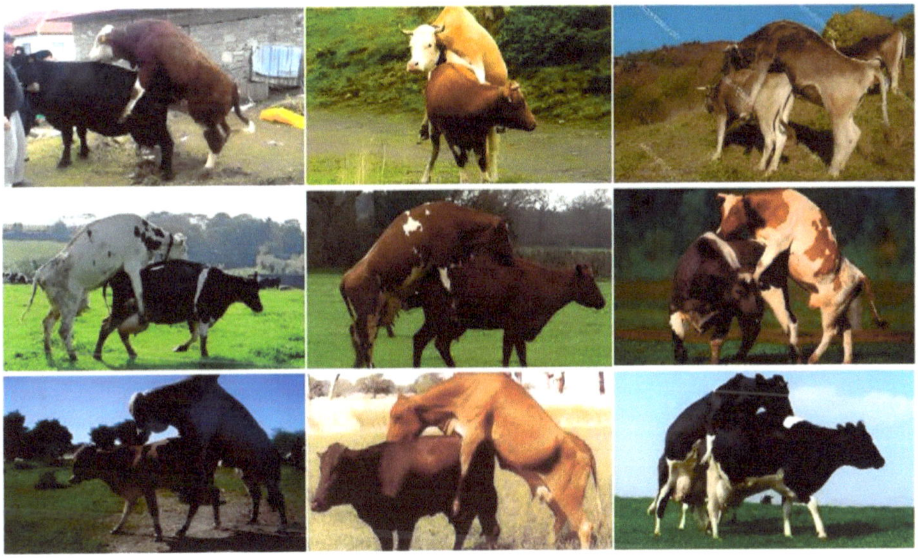

Figure 3. Dataset positive class image collage.

2.2. Dataset and Cow Identification

The dataset was collected from a farm in the Aydın region, and this cow recognition project was enhanced through the use of drone technology. All 300 dairy cows in the full-capacity section of the farm were captured in high-quality images, which were then analyzed using artificial intelligence techniques. The inclusion of cows from different breeds, such as Holstein and Simmental, highlights the ability of artificial intelligence and deep learning to accurately recognize various breeds and characteristics.

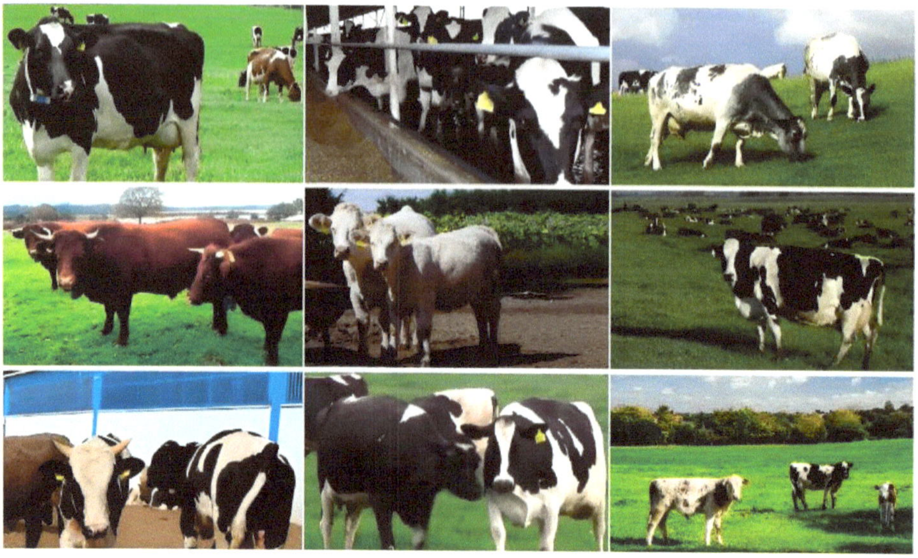

Figure 4. Dataset negative class image collage.

2.3. *Deep Learning Architectures*

2.3.1. Convolutional Neural Network (CNN)

A CNN was used only for mounting detection purposes; therefore, only the estrus dataset consisting of images of mounting or non-mounting situations was used, and the images were collected from the internet. Artificial neural networks are models that are based on the functioning of the human brain. The goal of this structure is to perform the learning process, interpret the acquired knowledge, and make decisions autonomously. Convolutional neural networks (CNNs) are a type of artificial neural network that are used primarily for image recognition and computer vision tasks, although they can also be used for other types of data processing, such as natural language processing. CNNs have revolutionized the field of computer vision and continue to be an active area of research and development [38,39]. Computers must recognize and convert incoming images into a computationally manageable matrix format. The first layer in a CNN is a convolutional layer, which applies a set of filters to the input image to extract features, such as edges and corners. The output of the convolutional layer is then passed through an activation function to introduce non-linearity into the model. The output of the activation function is then passed through a pooling layer, which reduces the dimensionality of the feature maps while retaining the most important information. The final output of the network is typically a fully connected layer that performs classification. It learns the impact of these differences on the label during the training phase and then uses this knowledge to make predictions for new images. In this study, a 9-layer convolutional neural network was used, as seen in Figure 5, and the network was trained for 20 epochs with binary classification.

2.3.2. VGG-19

VGG-19 was used only for mounting detection purposes; therefore, only the estrus dataset consisting of images of mounting or non-mounting situations was used, and the images were collected from the internet. The VGG-19 is a CNN architecture that was introduced by the Visual Geometry Group (VGG) at the University of Oxford [40]. It is a deep CNN with 19 layers that was designed primarily for image classification tasks. The VGG-19 architecture consists of a series of convolutional layers with 3×3 filters, followed by max pooling layers and rectified linear unit activation functions. The convolutional layers are organized into five blocks, with each block containing multiple convolutional layers and a max pooling layer. The final layers of the VGG-19 architecture consist of fully connected layers that perform the classification task. The output of the last fully connected layer is fed into a SoftMax activation function to produce the class probabilities [40,41]. In this study, as seen in Figure 6, we removed the fully connected layer of the pretrained VGG-19 model and added a new connection layer based on the number of classes in the dataset.

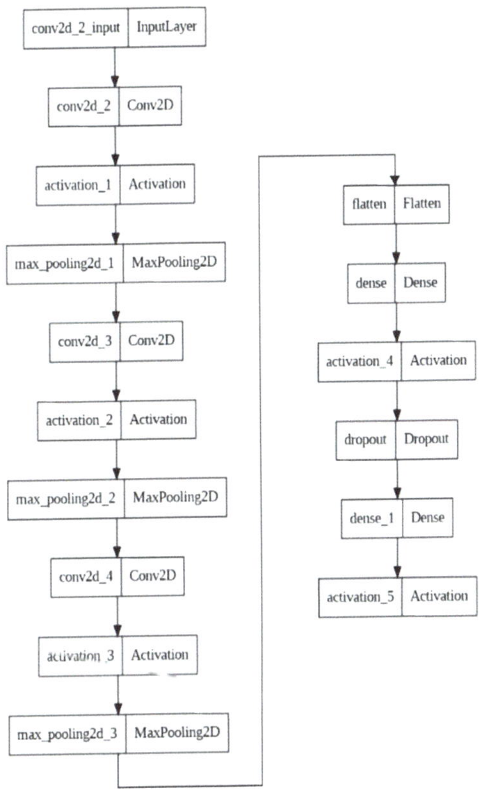

Figure 5. Proposed CNN architecture.

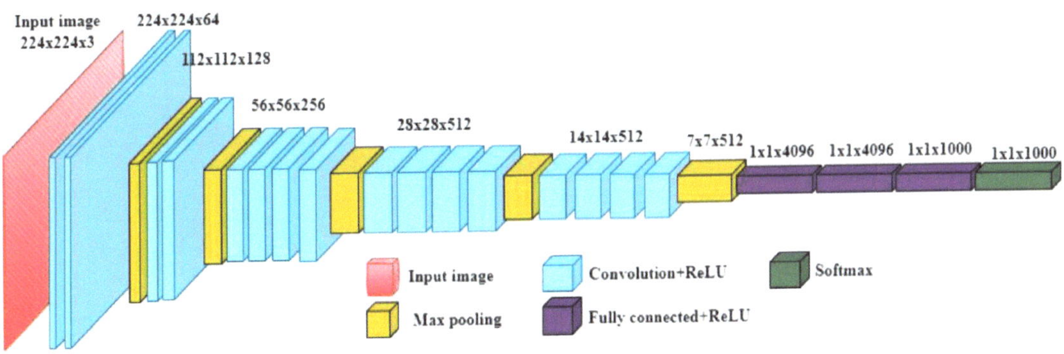

Figure 6. VGG model's architecture.

2.3.3. YOLO

The YOLOv5 method was used for both mounting regions of interest detection and cow identification. For this reason, two models were created separately for each dataset. YOLOv5 is a convolutional neural network (CNN) architecture that was introduced in 2020 as an evolution of the popular YOLO (You Only Look Once) object detection model [42]. YOLOv5 is designed primarily for real-time object detection and recognition tasks, including the detection of people, vehicles, and animals. Its acronym stands for "You Only Look Once", referring to its ability to quickly and efficiently make object detection predictions in a single step. YOLO divides the input image into an N × N grid, and each grid cell determines the presence of an object within its area, considering the object's center. The grid cell that determines the center of the object will also find the class, height, and width of the object and draw a bounding box around it [43]. This simplifies the architecture and improves speed and accuracy. In our study, the dataset was labeled as positive or negative, and the YOLOV5 model, which is the 5th version of YOLO, was trained on this dataset for 150 epochs.

2.4. Deep Learning Performance Evaluation and Model Selection

The hyperparameters of the algorithms used in the study, the optimizer used, the preferred primary performance metric, train test dataset ratios, and loss value are shared in Table 1. Models are focused on a binary classification problem. Models are compiled with the "binary_crossentropy" loss function and "rmsprop" optimizer presented in Table 1. The "accuracy" metric is used to evaluate the model's performance in terms of accuracy. To measure classification performance, accuracy, F1 score, precision, and recall performance metrics, as presented in Table 2, are used. The dataset was split into 70% training data and 30% test data. In our study, we opted not to use k-fold validation for several reasons. Firstly, k-fold validation may present challenges during deployment, as determining which fold to use in real-world scenarios lacks a clear criterion. Additionally, our models demonstrated high performance without the need for extensive hyperparameter tuning, making the application of k-fold validation less crucial in our context. Moreover, the computational cost associated with k-fold cross-validation, which requires training a separate model for each fold, was deemed excessive given the satisfactory performance of our models. In summary, our decision aligns with practical considerations related to deployment, a lack of hyperparameter tuning needs, and the desire to maintain computational efficiency in the field of computer engineering.

Table 1. The model's hyperparameters.

Model	Loss Function	Optimizer	Performance Metric	Train Data (%)	Validation Data (%)	Epoch	Mini-Batch Size	Learning Rate
CNN	Binary crossentropy	Rmsprop	Accuracy	70	30	20	32	0.001
VGG-19	Binary crossentropy	Rmsprop	Accuracy	70	30	20	32	0.001
YOLO	Binary crossentropy	Rmsprop	Accuracy	70	30	150	16	0.001

Table 2. Classification performance metrics.

Metric	Equation
Accuracy	$A = \frac{Number\ of\ True\ Positives + Number\ of\ True\ Negatives}{Number\ of\ Samples}$
Precision	$P = \frac{Number\ of\ True\ Positives}{Number\ of\ True\ Positives + Number\ of\ False\ Positives}$
Recall	$R = \frac{Number\ of\ True\ Positives}{Number\ of\ True\ Positives + Number\ of\ False\ Negatives}$
F1 Score	$F1 = \frac{2 \times P \times R}{P + R}$

3. Results and Discussion

The dataset containing images of cows' mounting movements during the estrus period was used to successfully detect estrus in cows. Three different deep learning models, namely the convolutional neural network, YOLO, and VGG-19, were trained on the dataset.

3.1. Estrus Detection

Performance metric results obtained by the methods used for estrus detection are presented in Table 3. Accordingly, the highest accuracy value was obtained with VGG-19 and is 99%. The findings obtained with each method are discussed in the subsections.

Table 3. Performance metric results of the models.

Model	Accuracy (%)	Precision (%)	Recall (%)	F1 Score (%)
CNN	98	97	98	97
VGG-19	99	99	98	99
YOLO	98	98	98	97

3.1.1. Mounting Detection with CNN

The CNN model, which is a classical approach to image recognition problems, has been developed for this study. The developed CNN model consists of nine layers, and the dataset has been divided into 70% for training and 30% for testing. The CNN training process consists of 20 epochs, with a duration of 25.2 min. While training the CNN model, the GPU services of Google Colab, specifically the T4 GPU, were utilized. In this process, using 32 GB of RAM proved to be sufficient. After training on the training dataset for 20 epochs, Figure 7 shows that the model achieved an accuracy rate of 98%, as represented in Table 3. The model's loss value is calculated to be 0.1. Interpreting the CNN results requires an understanding of the metrics used to measure the model's performance, consideration of the dataset and training parameters used, and careful analysis of the results. Figure 8 presents a confusion matrix, indicating that the CNN model correctly identified 203 out of 207 estrus cases in the test dataset. In the negative cases where the cows did not show estrus, it accurately detected 279 out of 285 cases. Figure 9 includes an example of prediction results from the trained model. It is observed that the second case is the false predictions, and this error seems to stem from the model perceiving the size difference between cows and calves as a feature. In Figure 9, it is observed that errors occur in images predicted as false not mounting when the feet are aligned, in contact, or very close. In images predicted as false mounting, incorrect results are noticeable in crowded situations. However, despite all these errors, only 10 out of a total of 492 test images have been predicted as false.

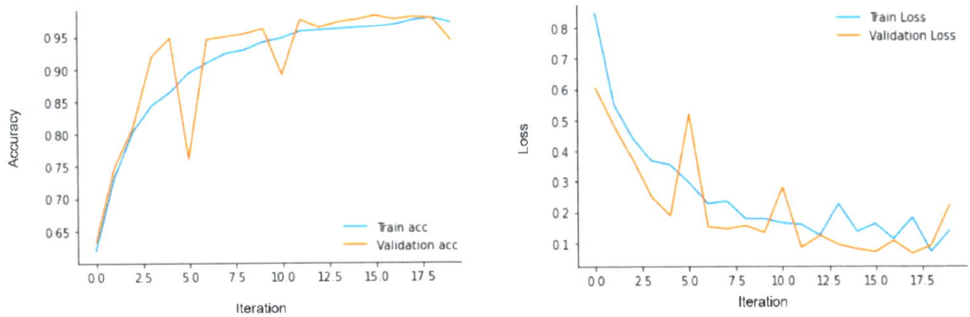

(**a**) (**b**)

Figure 7. CNN training and test: (**a**) accuracy and (**b**) loss.

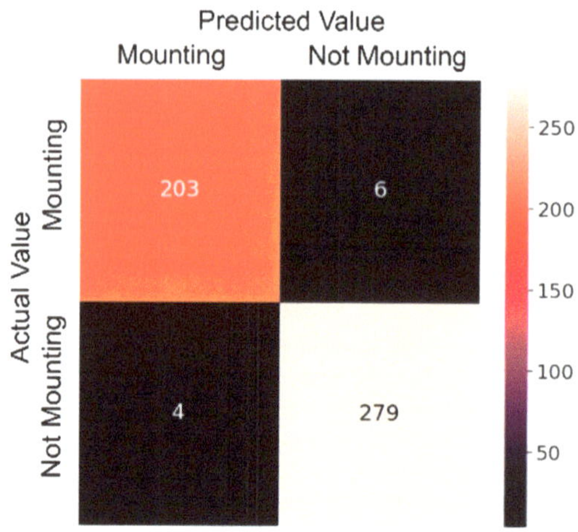

Figure 8. The CNN model's confusion matrix of the test dataset.

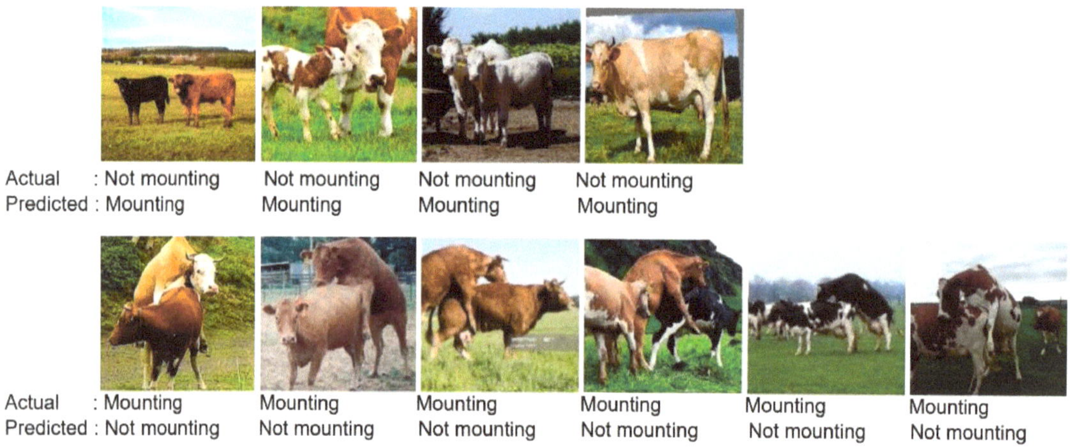

Figure 9. CNN false predictions of the test dataset.

3.1.2. Mounting Detection with VGG-19

The VGG-19 model, which is a transfer learning model, has been trained on the dataset. The dataset has been divided into 70% for training and 30% for testing. Considering the two classes in the dataset, the fully connected layer has been adjusted accordingly, and the model has been trained on the training dataset for 20 epochs with a duration of 28.3 min. While training the VGG-19 model, the GPU services of Google Colab, specifically the T4 GPU, were utilized. In this process, using 32 GB of RAM proved to be sufficient. The interpretation of the VGG model results may vary depending on the task and performance criteria for which the model is used. The VGG model is commonly used for image classification tasks, and accuracy is the most common performance measure for this task. Therefore, the VGG model results are typically presented in the form of a table or graph with high accuracy, indicating that the model is successful in the classification task with high accuracy. The trained model achieved an accuracy rate of 99%, making it the most successful model in our study. Furthermore, the developed model correctly identified 280 out of 283 negative states. Figure 10 shows that the developed model's loss value approaches zero. Figure 11 displays a confusion matrix, which demonstrates that the developed VGG-19 model successfully predicted 209 out of 209 estrus states in the test dataset. Figure 12 includes an example of prediction results from the trained model. The origin of all false predictions made by the VGG-19 model is attributed to the data augmentation techniques applied to prevent overfitting. Due to operations, such as rotation, zooming, and others applied within the dataset, pixel losses occurred, leading to erroneous classifications by our transfer learning model. Similar to the CNN model, in images predicted as false negatives in Figure 12, errors are observed in aligning the feet in close or touching images. However, in the VGG model, there are no images predicted as false mounting, and only three out of 492 test images are falsely predicted.

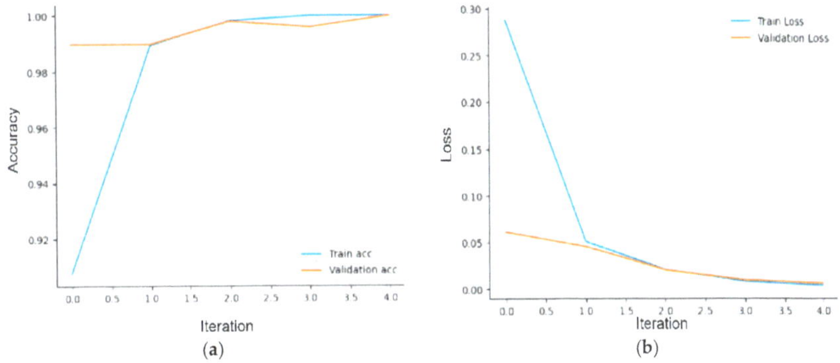

Figure 10. VGG-19 training and test: (**a**) accuracy and (**b**) loss.

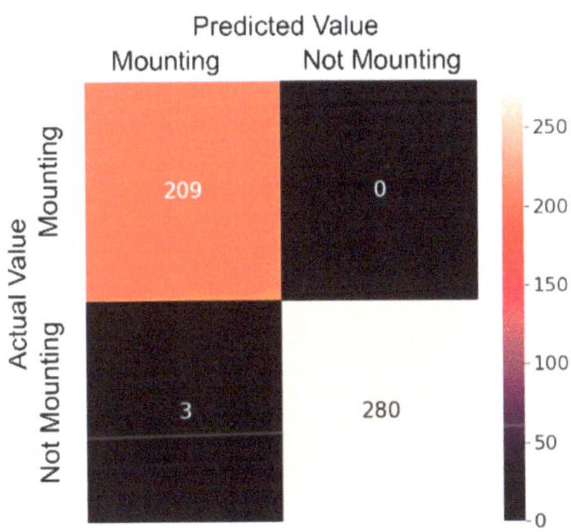

Figure 11. VGG-19 model's confusion matrix of the test dataset.

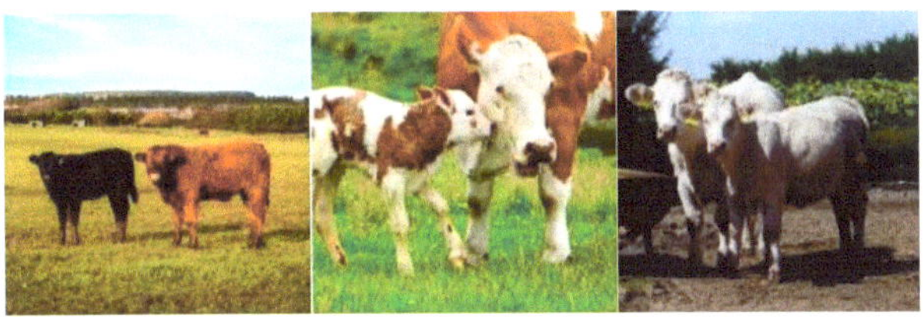

Figure 12. VGG-19 model false predictions of the test dataset.

3.1.3. Mounting Region of Interest Detection with YOLOv5

The YOLOv5 deep learning model was used to detect estrus states by labeling the 937 images in the dataset that show estrus. YOLOv5 can be evaluated using a variety of performance metrics, and these include mean average precision (mAP), accuracy, precision, and recall. mAP is a widely used metric to examine the results of object recognition models. The higher the map of an object recognition model, the more accurate and reliable the model is. Accuracy measures the evaluation of samples, showing that the modeling is correct. Based on Figure 13, the trained YOLOv5 model achieved a 98% accuracy rate in detecting estrus conditions. The "metrics/mAP 0.5" value in this figure shows the accuracy rate of our model. The "loss" values in the figure indicate how many errors the model made during its training. Our model continued its training until we minimized our loss values. The YOLOv5 training process is 150 epochs, and the duration is 32.4 min. While training the YOLO model, the GPU services of Google Colab, specifically the T4 GPU, were utilized. In this process, using 32 GB of RAM proved to be sufficient. Figure 14 includes an example of prediction results from the trained model.

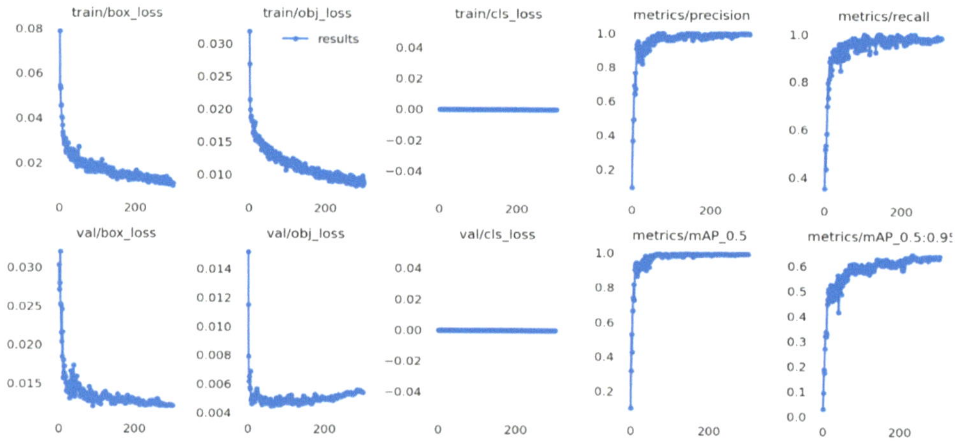

Figure 13. YOLOv5 accuracy.

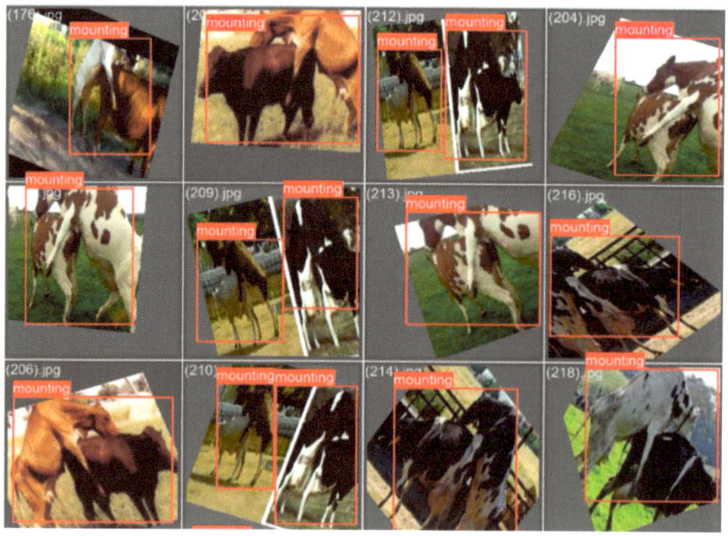

Figure 14. YOLO model prediction examples.

3.2. Cow Identification

All 300 dairy cows in the full-capacity section of a farm in the Aydın region were captured with high-quality images. Sample images obtained for YOLOv5 used are presented in Figure 15, and evaluation results are presented in Figure 16. The YOLOv5 training process is 150 epochs, and the duration is 15.2 min. The cow identification accuracy of the system is about 95%.

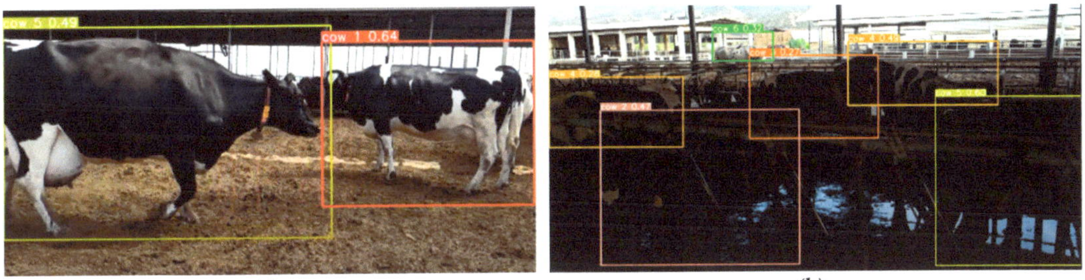

(a) (b)

Figure 15. YOLO cow identification: (**a**) cow identification from a pan-tilt camera; (**b**) cow identification from a drone camera.

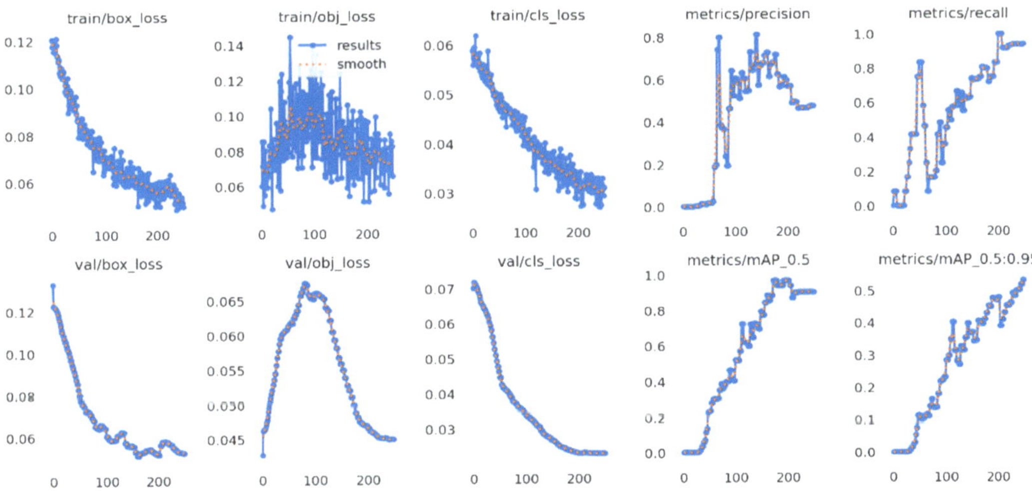

Figure 16. YOLO cow identification evaluation.

3.3. Cascaded System Results

The process of cow identification is illustrated in Figure 17, where cropping is performed around the relevant bounding box after mounting detection, with a 20-pixel padding. Primary and secondary behavioral signs for estrus, such as waiting periods for standing to be mounted and mounting, are depicted in Figure 17a. Subsequently, the identified identifiers for both cows are presented in Figure 17b. Following this detection and animal marking process, relevant information can be sent, and the artificial insemination process can be initiated. Mounting couple detection accuracy is 94%.

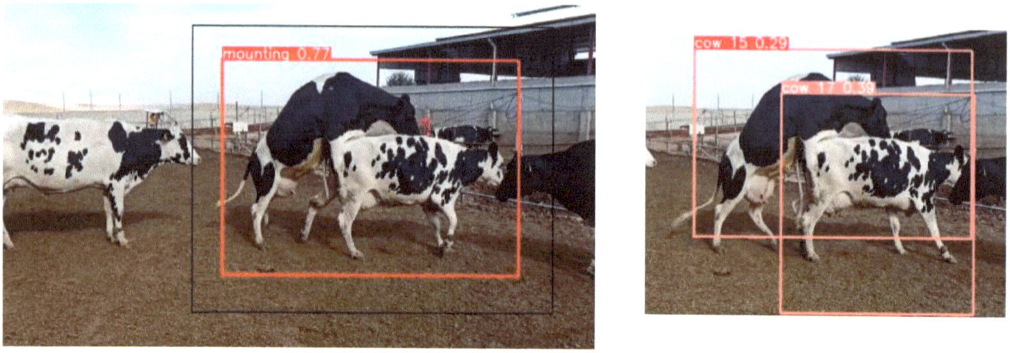

(a) (b)

Figure 17. Cascaded system results: (**a**) mounting detection and (**b**) cow identification after from mounting detection crop.

3.4. Comparison with Similar Studies

Table 4 illustrates the differences between our approach and other common methods. Commercial systems in the literature are designed as wearable smart collars and paint patches, as presented in Table 4. Determining the onset of estrus, which is considered the most suitable time for the beginning of cows' reproductive cycles, and artificial insemination, supports livestock farming that meets a large portion of the increasing country's population's food needs. On the other hand, it will also save the farm owner from the delays and economic losses that occur during these reproductive cycles. If the farm owner misses or incorrectly detects the estrus period, they may face problems such as a loss in milk production, a calf born with a delay of at least a month, and the inability to take advantage of government support. The purpose of our study is to detect the estrus periods and thereby help farm owners avoid economic losses and delays. Traditional methods used to detect estrus in cows include observing physical movements. Among these studies, Memedova and Keskin achieved 98% accuracy in detecting estrus by tracking the physical movements of cows with a fuzzy logic model that they developed [23]. In another study, which was prepared as a doctoral thesis by Yildiz, an artificial neural network model was developed that used not only physical movements but also seasonal data, achieving 97% accuracy [27]. Arago et al. aimed to detect cows in estrus that display mounting behavior, using models trained on images of cows [28]. Although the collected dataset has not been shared, a system that works with a 94% accuracy rate was developed with the help of the trained model. Our study and the results of other studies conducted in the literature are shown in Table 5.

Behaviors such as standing to be mounted and mounting are all just symptoms of the estrus period, and as shown in Figure 1. If these symptoms are detected, only the success rate of artificial insemination increases [21]. While livestock wearables equipped with IMU, painting patches, and visual computing systems successfully identify mounting and/or standing-to-be-mounted behaviors, they are commonly referred to as estrus detection systems [28–33]. The proposed method is a visual system and is used to detect mounting and/or standing-to-be-mounted behaviors. In this way, it is possible to increase the success rate of artificial insemination by identifying only animals that are likely to be in estrus. It is important to mention that false estrus warnings, resulting from social mounting interactions in dairy cows, can also be detected by the system. This limitation has implications for the broader impact of smart estrus detection studies presented in Table 4 as well. In addition, the interactions creating false alerts are short in duration [21,44]. Therefore, it is possible to reduce false alerts by separating longer-term standing-to-be-mounted situations and creating a rule-based system for when the visual system is triggered. If it is desired to determine the exact status of the cows rather than predicting, more comprehensive studies are required that include not only visual or biomechanical data but also physiological data and veterinary examination reports.

Table 4. Comparison of the systems to detect the estrus period and cow identification.

Reference	Sensor	Estrus Detection	Cow Identification	Cost	Lifetime
Actimoo [29]	IMU	Pattern recognition from IMU signals obtained from cow collars	Smart collar matching with the ID of the dairy cow	~EUR 120 per cow	5 years battery life
SCR Heatime [33]	IMU	Pattern recognition from IMU signals obtained from cow collars	Smart collar matching with the ID of the dairy cow	~EUR 200 per cow	7 years battery life
Estrotect [30]	Paint	Patch that changes color when the cow mounts	Accomplished by seeing the painted cow by the farmer	EUR 2.5 per usage	Disposable
[28]	PTZ Camera	Faster R-CNN and SSD cow localization and tracking	NA	NA	No battery
[45]	Camera	Detection of cow images with deep learning (YOLOv5)	NA	NA	No battery
[46]	Multiple cameras	Detection of ewe images with deep learning (YOLOv3)	NA	NA	No battery
[47]	RFID	NA	Yes	Under EUR 1 per cow	No battery
[48]	IMU and RFID	NA	Yes	Under EUR 20 per cow	Rechargeable Li-Po (728 days)
Proposed method	Camera	Detection of cow images with deep learning	Classification of images with deep learning	NA	No battery

Table 5. Comparison of machine learning-based methods in estrus detection and cow identification.

Reference	Sensor	Software	Estrus Detection Accuracy (%)	Cow Identification Accuracy (%)
[23]	IMU	Fuzzy logic model	98	NA
[27]	IMU	Deep learning	97	NA
[29]	IMU	NA	80	NA
[28]	Camera	Deep learning	94	NA
[45]	Camera	Detection of cow images with Deep learning (YOLOv5)	94.3	NA
[49]	Camera	Computer vision	90.9	NA
[50]	Camera	YOLOv3	82.1	NA
[51]	Camera and ear tag	CNN	NA	84
[52]	Camera	YOLO and faster R-CNN	NA	84.4
Proposed CNN model	Camera	Deep learning	98	NA
Proposed VGG-19 model	Camera	Deep learning	99	NA
Proposed YOLO model	Camera	Deep learning	98	95

4. Conclusions and Future Works

This manuscript introduces an innovative approach utilizing machine learning for the identification of individual cows and the detection of estrus behaviors. While previous studies have successfully detected estrus behaviors through machine vision, identifying individual cows in estrus within a herd has proven challenging. This pursuit is deemed valuable, and the development of an algorithm capable of providing such information holds significant importance. In livestock production, various methods exist for detecting the estrus period, such as attaching pedometer-like devices or applying estrus patches. However, these commercial wearable devices pose limitations, including the need for one device per animal, pricing concerns, environmental dependency, and restricted lifespans. This study proposes a deep learning-based system for both estrus detection and cow identification, addressing the shortcomings of existing methods and aiming to contribute to automated livestock management.

The proposed approach seamlessly integrates estrus period detection and cow identification using AR. The process commences with deep learning-based mounting detection, followed by the identification of the mounting ROI through YOLOv5. Subsequently, the ROI is cropped with padding, and cow ID detection is performed using YOLOv5 on the cropped ROI. The system then records the identified cow IDs. Demonstrating exceptional accuracy, the proposed system achieves 99% precision in detecting mounting behavior, 98% accuracy in ROI identification for mounting, and 94% accuracy in detecting the mounting couple. The overall success of these operations underscores the potential of the proposed system in contributing to AR and AI applications within the realm of livestock farming. This research holds significance for automating livestock management through advanced augmented reality systems, showcasing efficiency in estrus period detection and cow identification by integrating CNN and VGG-16 detectors sequentially. This approach addresses the limitations of labor-intensive and time-consuming traditional monitoring methods.

Recognizing the critical importance of accurately determining the reproductive cycles of cows for sustainable livestock farming, this study emphasizes the economic benefits and increased production efficiency that result from informed decision making. By combining augmented reality and deep learning models, the research represents a scientific advancement, offering a non-intrusive alternative to traditional wearable systems. The proposed system also presents cost-effective and durable solutions for veterinary training in large businesses, with potential applications in pasture farming, drone adaptation, and even aspects of robotic shepherding. This study anticipates a positive impact on livestock management by providing a state-of-the-art solution that facilitates automation and enhances productivity in the livestock sector.

In conclusion, this research proposes a cutting-edge solution to enhance livestock management, offering a method that can detect estrus periods in an efficient way. The image-based approach for estrus period detection contributes to the literature and is poised to drive automation and productivity improvements in the livestock sector.

Author Contributions: Conceptualization, İ.A., T.A., A.Ç.S. and F.S.; methodology, İ.A., T.A., A.Ç.S. and F.S.; software, İ.A., T.A., A.Ç.S. and F.S.; validation, İ.A., T.A., A.Ç.S. and F.S.; resources, İ.A., T.A., A.Ç.S. and F.S.; writing—original draft preparation, İ.A., T.A., A.Ç.S. and F.S.; writing—review and editing, İ.A., T.A., A.Ç.S. and F.S.; visualization, İ.A., T.A., A.Ç.S. and F.S. All authors have read and agreed to the published version of the manuscript.

Funding: This research received no external funding.

Institutional Review Board Statement: Not applicable.

Informed Consent Statement: Not applicable.

Data Availability Statement: Please contact the corresponding author for the findings, model, and dataset obtained in the study.

Acknowledgments: This study was prepared as part of the Master Thesis at Izmir Institute of Technology, Graduate Education Institute. The author of the thesis is İ.A., the advisor is T.A., and the co-advisor is F.S.

Conflicts of Interest: The authors declare no conflict of interest.

References

1. Araújo, S.O.; Peres, R.S.; Barata, J.; Lidon, F.; Ramalho, J.C. Characterising the Agriculture 4.0 Landscape—Emerging Trends, Challenges and Opportunities. *Agronomy* **2021**, *11*, 667. [CrossRef]
2. Symeonaki, E.; Arvanitis, K.G.; Loukatos, D.; Piromalis, D. Enabling IoT Wireless Technologies in Sustainable Livestock Farming Toward Agriculture 4.0. In *IoT-Based Intelligent Modelling for Environmental and Ecological Engineering: IoT Next Generation EcoAgro Systems*; Krause, P., Xhafa, F., Eds.; Lecture Notes on Data Engineering and Communications Technologies; Springer International Publishing: Cham, Switzerland, 2021; pp. 213–232, ISBN 978-3-030-71172-6.
3. Liu, Y.; Ma, X.; Shu, L.; Hancke, G.P.; Abu-Mahfouz, A.M. From Industry 4.0 to Agriculture 4.0: Current Status, Enabling Technologies, and Research Challenges. *IEEE Trans. Ind. Inform.* **2021**, *17*, 4322–4334. [CrossRef]
4. Hurst, W.; Mendoza, F.R.; Tekinerdogan, B. Augmented Reality in Precision Farming: Concepts and Applications. *Smart Cities* **2021**, *4*, 1454–1468. [CrossRef]
5. Caria, M.; Todde, G.; Sara, G.; Piras, M.; Pazzona, A. Performance and Usability of Smartglasses for Augmented Reality in Precision Livestock Farming Operations. *Appl. Sci.* **2020**, *10*, 2318. [CrossRef]
6. Caria, M.; Sara, G.; Todde, G.; Polese, M.; Pazzona, A. Exploring Smart Glasses for Augmented Reality: A Valuable and Integrative Tool in Precision Livestock Farming. *Animals* **2019**, *9*, 903. [CrossRef]
7. Zhao, Z.; Yang, W.; Chinthammit, W.; Rawnsley, R.; Neumeyer, P.; Cahoon, S. A New Approach to Utilize Augmented Reality on Precision Livestock Farming. In Proceedings of the ICAT-EGVE, Adelaide, Australia, 22–24 November 2017; pp. 185–188.
8. Lee, S.; Lee, J.; Lee, A.; Park, N.; Lee, S.; Song, S.; Seo, A.; Lee, H.; Kim, J.-I.; Eom, K. Augmented Reality Intravenous Injection Simulator Based 3D Medical Imaging for Veterinary Medicine. *Vet. J.* **2013**, *196*, 197–202. [CrossRef] [PubMed]
9. Little, W.B.; Dezdrobitu, C.; Conan, A.; Artemiou, E. Is Augmented Reality the New Way for Teaching and Learning Veterinary Cardiac Anatomy? *Med. Sci. Educ.* **2021**, *31*, 723–732. [CrossRef]
10. Morrone, S.; Dimauro, C.; Gambella, F.; Cappai, M.G. Industry 4.0 and Precision Livestock Farming (PLF): An up to Date Overview across Animal Productions. *Sensors* **2022**, *22*, 4319. [CrossRef]
11. Kraft, M.; Bernhardt, H.; Brunsch, R.; Büscher, W.; Colangelo, E.; Graf, H.; Marquering, J.; Tapken, H.; Toppel, K.; Westerkamp, C.; et al. Can Livestock Farming Benefit from Industry 4.0 Technology? Evidence from Recent Study. *Appl. Sci.* **2022**, *12*, 12844. [CrossRef]
12. Pandey, S.; Kalwa, U.; Kong, T.; Guo, B.; Gauger, P.C.; Peters, D.J.; Yoon, K.-J. Behavioral Monitoring Tool for Pig Farmers: Ear Tag Sensors, Machine Intelligence, and Technology Adoption Roadmap. *Animals* **2021**, *11*, 2665. [CrossRef]
13. Zhao, K.; Jin, X.; Ji, J.; Wang, J.; Ma, H.; Zhu, X. Individual Identification of Holstein Dairy Cows Based on Detecting and Matching Feature Points in Body Images. *Biosyst. Eng.* **2019**, *181*, 128–139. [CrossRef]
14. Zin, T.T.; Phyo, C.N.; Tin, P.; Hama, H.; Kobayashi, I. Image Technology Based Cow Identification System Using Deep Learning. In Proceedings of the International Multiconference of Engineers and Computer Scientists, Hong Kong, 14–16 March 2018; Volume 1, pp. 236–247.
15. Xiao, J.; Liu, G.; Wang, K.; Si, Y. Cow Identification in Free-Stall Barns Based on an Improved Mask R-CNN and an SVM. *Comput. Electron. Agric.* **2022**, *194*, 106738. [CrossRef]
16. Kumar, S.; Singh, S.K.; Singh, A.K. Muzzle Point Pattern Based Techniques for Individual Cattle Identification. *IET Image Process.* **2017**, *11*, 805–814. [CrossRef]
17. Bello, R.W.; Olubummo, D.A.; Seiyaboh, Z.; Enuma, O.C.; Talib, A.Z.; Mohamed, A.S.A. Cattle Identification: The History of Nose Prints Approach in Brief. *IOP Conf. Ser. Earth Environ. Sci.* **2020**, *594*, 012026. [CrossRef]
18. Yang, L.; Xu, X.; Zhao, J.; Song, H. Fusion of RetinaFace and Improved FaceNet for Individual Cow Identification in Natural Scenes. *Inf. Process. Agric.* **2023**. [CrossRef]
19. Roelofs, J.; López-Gatius, F.; Hunter, R.H.F.; van Eerdenburg, F.J.C.M.; Hanzen, C. When Is a Cow in Estrus? Clinical and Practical Aspects. *Theriogenology* **2010**, *74*, 327–344. [CrossRef] [PubMed]
20. Remnant, J.G.; Green, M.J.; Huxley, J.N.; Hudson, C.D. Associations between Dairy Cow Inter-Service Interval and Probability of Conception. *Theriogenology* **2018**, *114*, 324–329. [CrossRef] [PubMed]
21. Reith, S.; Hoy, S. Review: Behavioral Signs of Estrus and the Potential of Fully Automated Systems for Detection of Estrus in Dairy Cattle. *Animal* **2018**, *12*, 398–407. [CrossRef]
22. Fricke, P.M.; Carvalho, P.D.; Giordano, J.O.; Valenza, A.; Lopes, G.; Amundson, M.C. Expression and Detection of Estrus in Dairy Cows: The Role of New Technologies. *Animal* **2014**, *8*, 134–143. [CrossRef]
23. Memmedova, N.; Keskin, İ. Oestrus Detection by Fuzzy Logic Model Using Trait Activity in Cows. *Kafkas Üniversitesi Vet. Fakültesi Derg.* **2011**, *17*, 1003–1008. [CrossRef]
24. Bayril, T.; Yilmaz, O.; Çak, B. Effect of Timing of Artificial Insemination Relative to Spontaneous Estrus on Reproductive Performance and Calf Gender Ratio in Repeat Breeder Holstein Cows. *JAPS J. Anim. Plant Sci.* **2016**, *26*, 34123459.
25. Kaya, A.; Güneş, E.; Memili, E. Application of Reproductive Biotechnologies for Sustainableproduction of Livestock in Turkey. *Turk. J. Vet. Anim. Sci.* **2018**, *42*, 143–151.
26. Koçyiğit, R.; Yanar, M.; Diler, A.; Aydın, R.; ÖZDEMİR, V.F.; Yılmaz, A. Cattle and Calf Raising Practices in The Eastern Anatolia Region: An Example of Central County of Ağrı Province. *Int. J. Agric. Nat. Sci.* **2021**, *14*, 152–163.
27. Yıldız, A.K.; Özgüven, M.M. Determination of Estrus in Cattle with Artificial Neural Networks Using Mobility and Environmental Data. *J. Agric. Fac. Gaziosmanpaşa Univ. (JAFAG)* **2022**, *39*, 40–45. [CrossRef]

28. Arago, N.M.; Alvarez, C.I.; Mabale, A.G.; Legista, C.G.; Repiso, N.E.; Robles, R.R.A.; Amado, T.M.; Romeo, L.J., Jr.; Thio-ac, A.C.; Velasco, J.S. Automated Estrus Detection for Dairy Cattle through Neural Networks and Bounding Box Corner Analysis. *Int. J. Adv. Comput. Sci. Appl.* **2020**, *11*, 935. [CrossRef]
29. ActimooTM Actimoo Estrus Detection System. Available online: https://www.actimoo.com (accessed on 1 October 2023).
30. EstrotectTM | Breed with Confidence. Available online: https://estrotect.com/ (accessed on 3 September 2023).
31. Benaissa, S.; Tuyttens, F.A.M.; Plets, D.; Trogh, J.; Martens, L.; Vandaele, L.; Joseph, W.; Sonck, B. Calving and Estrus Detection in Dairy Cattle Using a Combination of Indoor Localization and Accelerometer Sensors. *Comput. Electron. Agric.* **2020**, *168*, 105153. [CrossRef]
32. Wang, J.; Bell, M.; Liu, X.; Liu, G. Machine-Learning Techniques Can Enhance Dairy Cow Estrus Detection Using Location and Acceleration Data. *Animals* **2020**, *10*, 1160. [CrossRef] [PubMed]
33. SCR Heatime | Micro Technologies. Available online: https://www.microtechnologies.com/dairy/heatime (accessed on 3 September 2023).
34. Dallago, G.M.; Wade, K.M.; Cue, R.I.; McClure, J.T.; Lacroix, R.; Pellerin, D.; Vasseur, E. Keeping Dairy Cows for Longer: A Critical Literature Review on Dairy Cow Longevity in High Milk-Producing Countries. *Animals* **2021**, *11*, 808. [CrossRef]
35. Sehested, J.; Gaillard, C.; Lehmann, J.O.; Maciel, G.M.; Vestergaard, M.; Weisbjerg, M.R.; Mogensen, L.; Larsen, L.B.; Poulsen, N.A.; Kristensen, T. Review: Extended Lactation in Dairy Cattle. *Animal* **2019**, *13*, s65–s74. [CrossRef]
36. Webster, J. *Understanding the Dairy Cow*; John Wiley & Sons: Hoboken, NJ, USA, 2020; ISBN 978-1-119-55022-8.
37. Shorten, C.; Khoshgoftaar, T.M. A Survey on Image Data Augmentation for Deep Learning. *J Big Data* **2019**, *6*, 60. [CrossRef]
38. LeCun, Y.; Bengio, Y. Convolutional Networks for Images, Speech, and Time Series. *Handb. Brain Theory Neural Netw.* **1995**, *3361*, 1995.
39. Li, Z.; Liu, F.; Yang, W.; Peng, S.; Zhou, J. A Survey of Convolutional Neural Networks: Analysis, Applications, and Prospects. *IEEE Trans. Neural Netw. Learn. Syst.* **2021**, *33*, 6999–7019. [CrossRef]
40. Simonyan, K.; Zisserman, A. Very Deep Convolutional Networks for Large-Scale Image Recognition. *arXiv* **2015**, arXiv:1409.1556.
41. Nguyen, T.-H.; Nguyen, T.-N.; Ngo, B.-V. A VGG-19 Model with Transfer Learning and Image Segmentation for Classification of Tomato Leaf Disease. *AgriEngineering* **2022**, *4*, 871–887. [CrossRef]
42. Redmon, J.; Divvala, S.; Girshick, R.; Farhadi, A. You Only Look Once: Unified, Real-Time Object Detection. *arXiv* **2016**, arXiv:1506.02640.
43. Jiang, P.; Ergu, D.; Liu, F.; Cai, Y.; Ma, B. A Review of Yolo Algorithm Developments. *Procedia Comput. Sci.* **2022**, *199*, 1066–1073. [CrossRef]
44. Gaude, I.; Kempf, A.; Strüve, K.D.; Hoedemaker, M. Estrus Signs in Holstein Friesian Dairy Cows and Their Reliability for Ovulation Detection in the Context of Visual Estrus Detection. *Livest. Sci.* **2021**, *245*, 104449. [CrossRef]
45. Wang, R.; Gao, Z.; Li, Q.; Zhao, C.; Gao, R.; Zhang, H.; Li, S.; Feng, L. Detection Method of Cow Estrus Behavior in Natural Scenes Based on Improved YOLOv5. *Agriculture* **2022**, *12*, 1339. [CrossRef]
46. Yu, L.; Pu, Y.; Cen, H.; Li, J.; Liu, S.; Nie, J.; Ge, J.; Lv, L.; Li, Y.; Xu, Y.; et al. A Lightweight Neural Network-Based Method for Detecting Estrus Behavior in Ewes. *Agriculture* **2022**, *12*, 1207. [CrossRef]
47. Samad, A.; Murdeshwar, P.; Hameed, Z. High-Credibility RFID-Based Animal Data Recording System Suitable for Small-Holding Rural Dairy Farmers. *Comput. Electron. Agric.* **2010**, *73*, 213–218. [CrossRef]
48. Achour, B.; Belkadi, M.; Saddaoui, R.; Filali, I.; Aoudjit, R.; Laghrouche, M. High-Accuracy and Energy-Efficient Wearable Device for Dairy Cows' Localization and Activity Detection Using Low-Cost IMU/RFID Sensors. *Microsyst. Technol.* **2022**, *28*, 1241–1251. [CrossRef]
49. Guo, Y.; Zhang, Z.; He, D.; Niu, J.; Tan, Y. Detection of Cow Mounting Behavior Using Region Geometry and Optical Flow Characteristics. *Comput. Electron. Agric.* **2019**, *163*, 104828. [CrossRef]
50. Fuentes, A.; Yoon, S.; Park, J.; Park, D.S. Deep Learning-Based Hierarchical Cattle Behavior Recognition with Spatio-Temporal Information. *Comput. Electron. Agric.* **2020**, *177*, 105627. [CrossRef]
51. Zin, T.T.; Misawa, S.; Pwint, M.Z.; Thant, S.; Seint, P.T.; Sumi, K.; Yoshida, K. Cow Identification System Using Ear Tag Recognition. In Proceedings of the 2020 IEEE 2nd Global Conference on Life Sciences and Technologies (LifeTech), Kyoto, Japan, 10–12 March 2020; pp. 65–66.
52. Nguyen, C.; Wang, D.; Von Richter, K.; Valencia, P.; Alvarenga, F.A.P.; Bishop–Hurley, G. Video-Based Cattle Identification and Action Recognition. In Proceedings of the 2021 Digital Image Computing: Techniques and Applications (DICTA), Gold Coast, Australia, 29 November–1 December 2021; pp. 1–5.

applied sciences

Article

Three-Dimensional Coordinate Calibration Models for Augmented Reality Applications in Indoor Industrial Environments

Jandson S. Nunes [1], Fabio B. C. Almeida [2], Leonardo S. V. Silva [2], Vinicius M. S. O. Santos [2], Alex A. B. Santos [3], Valter de Senna [3] and Ingrid Winkler [3,4,*]

1 PPGMCTI—Graduate Program in Modeling Computing and Industrial Technology, University Center SENAI CIMATEC, Salvador 41650-010, Brazil; jan.nunes@gmail.com
2 Software Development Department, University Center SENAI CIMATEC, Salvador 41650-010, Brazil; falmeida@fieb.org.br (F.B.C.A.); leeosena21@gmail.com (L.S.V.S.); viniciusmsos@gmail.com (V.M.S.O.S.)
3 Computing Modeling Department, University Center SENAI CIMATEC, Salvador 41650-010, Brazil; alex.santos@fieb.org.br (A.A.B.S.); senna@fieb.org.br (V.d.S.)
4 Institute for Science, Innovation and Technology in Industry 4.0/INCITE INDUSTRIA 4.0, Salvador 41650-010, Brazil
* Correspondence: ingrid.winkler@doc.senaicimatec.edu.br

Abstract: The calibration of three-dimensional (3D) coordinates in augmented reality systems is a complex activity. It involves the recognition of environmental characteristics and technology that models the 3D space of the device, determining its position and orientation. Single markers suffer from numerical instability, particularly when they are small within the camera image. In the industrial environment, it is common for augmented reality applications to cover large spaces, making it difficult to maintain attributes such as precision and accuracy. To address this issue, our study proposes a two-step calibration model that leverages multiple markers for accurate localization in a larger indoor environment. We developed the calibration model using Unity3D, Mixed Reality ToolKit, and Vuforia and evaluated it in terms of precision and accuracy in a proof of concept using the MS Hololens device. Our findings reveal that employing two markers significantly reduces angular discrepancies between points in the real and augmented environments. Moreover, our results underscore that registration accuracy improves as the number of calibration points increases. The results show improvements in determining the axes that define the 3D space, with a direct influence on the position of the points observed in the experiment.

Keywords: HoloLens; calibration; industrial; augmented reality; indoor positioning

Citation: Nunes, J.S.; Almeida, F.B.C.; Silva, L.S.V.; Santos, V.M.S.O.; Santos, A.A.B.; de Senna, V.; Winkler, I. Three-Dimensional Coordinate Calibration Models for Augmented Reality Applications in Indoor Industrial Environments. *Appl. Sci.* **2023**, *13*, 12548. https://doi.org/10.3390/app132312548

Academic Editors: João M. F. Rodrigues, Calin Gheorghe Dan Neamtu, Radu Comes, Jing-Jing Fang and Dorin-Mircea Popovici

Received: 14 September 2023
Revised: 31 October 2023
Accepted: 10 November 2023
Published: 21 November 2023

1. Introduction

The interactivity between real and virtual objects geometrically and temporally aligned in the real environment defines augmented reality (AR) [1]. The technological advances observed over the last decade have stimulated the implementation of several AR applications in industry [2–8]. The rigor of the precision and accuracy requirements for placing virtual elements in real environments combined with the progress achieved by devices in terms of these competencies has driven the development of AR solutions.

Localization and tracking approaches in AR systems can be based on sensors, visual elements, or both [9]. Regardless of the approach used, factors such as the occlusion of markers, moving objects, noise, electromagnetism, and low light are often observed in industrial environments. They hinder or limit the ability to accurately determine the location and orientation of a device, adding tracking failures to an AR system [10]. Given these challenges, the ability to align virtual and real components with precision and accuracy can determine the feasibility of AR systems in industrial environments [9]. The common challenges inherent to this process include the reliability and scalability in the tracking of device movement [5,10], calibration [2], and the precise contextualization of overlapping information in the real environment [10].

Some studies [11] use the recognition of fiducial markers as a strategy in augmented reality applications. However, execution environments are usually restricted to small spaces such as tables or workbenches. Therefore, they disregard or minimize the effects of factors that can negatively affect the experience of AR applications in an industrial environment. Although other studies [12] consider these aspects and cite the relevance of keeping the positioning of holograms precise and accurate as a precondition for standardized scientific experiments, they almost always present qualitative and subjective analyses of the precision and accuracy of the experiments.

The literature describes the basic architectural components of AR systems: cameras, tracking systems, and user interfaces [5]. Although there are several ways to integrate these elements, studies highlight the relevance of head-mounted displays (HMDs) because they allow operators to move around and access information hands-free [5,13].

Of the devices currently available in the market, the Microsoft HoloLens mixed reality device stands out in terms of performance, presenting itself as a complete and self-contained AR tool [14], i.e., an HMD with all the AR architectural elements embedded in a single device. These studies reveal the importance of representing holograms in AR applications with accuracy and precision, list the characteristics of industrial environments that hinder success, and, finally, reveal the demand for scientific productions that measure these parameters objectively. Thus, they contribute to the motivation of this study. Although it is possible to find a few studies, such as [15,16], capable of proposing quantitative methods to measure the accuracy and precision of their AR solutions, the coverage area of the applications is limited to small distances (a few meters) and has low sampling.

Considering the lack of studies related to the calibration of AR systems, specifically examining the challenges facing HoloLens observed in industrial environments in terms of applying AR solutions efficiently, the following question arises: how to develop a calibration method that helps AR systems to maintain the accuracy and precision of their solutions in industrial areas? To answer to that question, the objective of this study is to propose two models of 3D coordinate calibration for AR applications in an industrial indoor environment and compare these solutions' performances based on their accuracy and precision in displaying virtual objects in these scenarios.

This study is divided into four sections including this introduction. Section 2 describes the methods and experiments carried out to evaluate the precision and accuracy of the implemented models, Section 3 presents the proposed calibration model and the outcomes, and Section 4 presents the final considerations and suggestions for future research.

2. Materials and Methods

We adopted the design science research (DSR) paradigm. In addition to a knowledge contribution, DSR contributes to the real-world application environment from which the research problem or opportunity is drawn [17].

Our method parallels that described by Gregor and Hevner [17], which includes six steps: (1) identify the problem, (2) define solution objectives, (3) design and development, (4) demonstration, (5) evaluation, and (6) communication.

In steps 1 and 2, we carried out a systematic literature review to understand the problem and define the solution objectives.

In step 3, we designed and developed the calibration models proposed. We employed the Unity3D ecosystem, which is a popular tool for crafting 2D and 3D simulations, offering support for over 20 different execution platforms, including HoloLens. Its primary function is to provide a basic framework for associating visual elements (such as buttons, text, images, and 3D objects) with their respective behaviors, defined using application programming interfaces (APIs) and software development kits (SDKs).

We also used the Mixed Reality Toolkit (MRTK), which is an SDK developed by Microsoft to assist in the creation of virtual and augmented reality applications, equipped with its own set of components and resources for integration within Unity3D. Several key functionalities of the MRTK played a significant role in the development of the test application in this study, including interfaces for the input and output of data with the potential for interaction with real-world surfaces, real-time access to the spatial mapping results provided by the HoloLens, and management of anchors implemented through the WorldAnchorManager class. The MRTK software architecture is extensible, allowing developers to customize component behaviors through the utilization of its interfaces. In this research, this capability was leveraged to programmatically assign anchor behavior to specific instances of virtual objects within the environment.

Another SDK used in the development of the test application is Vuforia [18], designed to recognize specific features in flat images or 3D objects for runtime tracking. This feature enables developers to position and orient virtual objects concerning real-world objects when they are viewed through the device's camera and recognized by Vuforia's computer vision algorithms. Consequently, it becomes possible to establish a correspondence between the observer's perspective regarding the recognized real object and the virtual object projected onto it, creating the illusion that the virtual object is an integral part of the real-world scene. Vuforia provides APIs in various programming languages and includes support for .NET through an extension for Unity3D. .NET is a Microsoft initiative for unifying executable libraries across language-independent environments. This approach allows developers to write code that is not specific to a particular device and instead create solutions for the .NET platform. As a result, Vuforia can execute its functionalities on HoloLens just as it would on other devices. In this study, Vuforia was employed for the recognition of fiducial markers within the test application, facilitating the creation of virtual object instances on these markers.

The data collected during the test was stored in comma separated value (CSV) format, a simple and widely recognized data format in the field of computing, compatible with numerous software applications. The R language was used to generate graphical visualizations of the collected data. R is a language dedicated to data analysis, manipulation, and visualization, originally developed by Ross Ihaka and Robert Gentleman in the Department of Statistics at the University of Auckland, New Zealand, and is currently maintained by volunteers under the General Public License (GPL). The choice of data format and language for analysis was based on the researcher's familiarity and did not impact the study's outcomes.

Then, in step 4, we demonstrated a proof-of-concept of our proposed calibration models. To meet the challenges inherent to industrial environments, the scenario defined for this stage was a logistics warehouse. This warehouse is approximately 10,000 m^3, contains a large variety of equipment and components, and has characteristics such as dynamism in the composition of its internal layout and variability in lighting, noise, and obstacles.

The International Organization for Standardization (ISO) defines, in ISO 5725-1:2023, accuracy as the closeness of agreement between a test result and the actual value and precision as the closeness of agreement between independent test results obtained under stipulated conditions [19].

In step 5, we evaluated our proposed calibration models in terms of validity criteria, since DSR includes gathering evidence that the artifact is useful, meaning that the artifact works and does what it is intended to do [17]. To measure these indicators, two experiments were carried out. The first experiment was to verify and compare, in an industrial environment, the precision of the proposed two-step calibration model with a simple calibration model. The second experiment was to check if, in fact, the proposed model achieved the objective of locating and assisting in the identification of components within an industrial environment.

To evaluate the precision (i.e., the dispersion of the samples) and accuracy (i.e., the exactness) of the simple and two-step calibrations in an industrial scenario, the prototype was programmed to perform each calibration separately so that, after the calibration step, it would be able to measure the virtual coordinates relative to the calibration system origin of markers placed in different locations within the scenario.

To configure the experimental environment, five points were first selected inside the warehouse. The criteria for choosing these points were as follows:

1. Locations that remained the same throughout the experiment. Changes in these locations would require measurements to be re-performed;
2. Locations where it was possible to measure with a laser tape measure from the point chosen as the origin to obtain a rigorous measurement (gold standard);
3. Locations at different distances from the point chosen as the origin;
4. Locations where all markers could be placed at the same height, facilitating data analysis;
5. Locations where the markers could be viewed from the front, with at least one meter of distance, so that the marker could be viewed by the HoloLens camera.

Once the points were selected, one of them was defined as the origin, a fiducial marker was placed at this point, and the exact center of this marker was used as a reference for the position of origin of both the virtual and the real coordinate systems. In addition to these markers, an additional marker was added at the same height (y-coordinate) in the direction of the negative x-axis and 1.594 m away from the marker of origin. In general, the second fiducial marker should be aligned with the first. This last marker is used for two-step calibration. Lastly, with the laser tape measure, the x and z coordinates of the other markers were measured from the origin. Figure 1 shows the arrangement of the points within the scenario, as well as the measured coordinates of each point and the distance vector from the origin for each of the points.

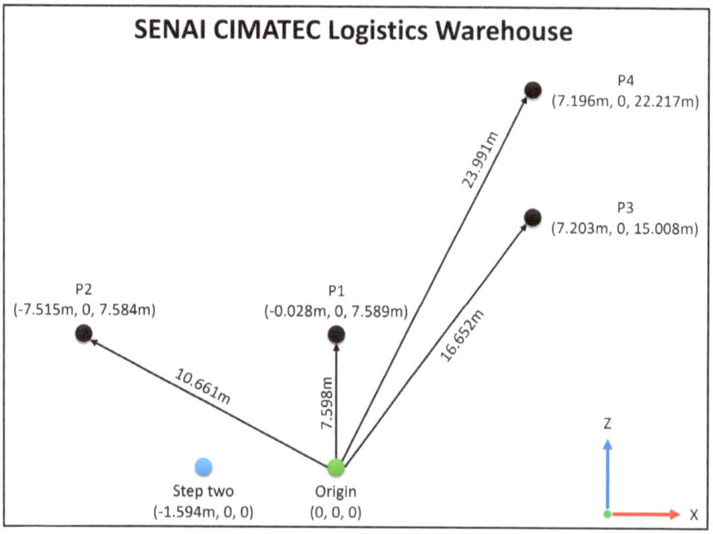

Figure 1. Configuration of the environment for the experiment.

Finally, step 6 of the design science research approach entails communicating our findings in this work.

3. Results

In the sections that follow, we describe our experiment's outcomes.

3.1. Localization and Space Recognition Mechanisms of HoloLens

The HoloLens (1st gen) is an AR device released by Microsoft Corporation in 2016 that has several sensors, lenses, and holographic projectors, as Figure 2 illustrates. This set enables HoloLens to recognize the environment and measure its localization. The system uses depth and environment-understanding cameras to three-dimensionally reconstruct the real environment. Infrared laser projectors, which make up the HoloLens, restrict the use of the device to environments free of sources emitting this light frequency.

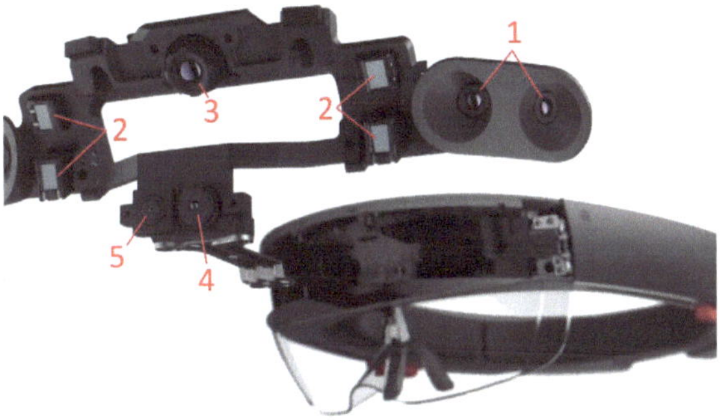

Figure 2. HoloLens sensors. (1) Environment-understanding cameras. (2) Infrared laser projectors. (3) Depth camera. (4) High-definition camera. (5) Light sensor [13].

The process for representing real-world surfaces in the HoloLens is described by a triangular mesh connected to a system of spatial coordinates fixed in the mapped environment. Figure 3 exemplifies the reconstruction as information is captured by the device sensors. The result of this process, continuously updated by the system, causes environmental changes to be reflected in the virtual context, keeping it adapted.

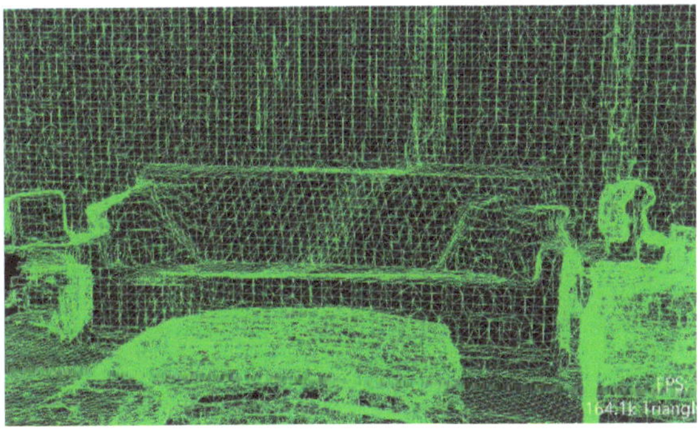

Figure 3. HoloLens sensors. (1) Environment-understanding cameras. (2) Infrared laser projectors. (3) Depth camera. (4) High-definition camera. (5) Light sensor [13].

HoloLens allows associating virtual objects (anchors) with the mesh and reconstructing the real environment to which it is exposed. The function of an anchor is the maintenance of location and orientation metadata relative to the real space. The documentation provided by Microsoft recommends the use of anchors in environments larger than five meters to achieve greater stability in the display of the holograms [14].

3.2. Proposed Calibration Models

HoloLens uses its own method for creating a system of coordinates, mapping, and understanding the environment. When opening an application in HoloLens, it uses its position, i.e., its top, side, and front reference, to create its coordinate system. Thus, if the same application is opened with the device pointing to another direction, for example, the coordinate system will be different. Therefore, when it is necessary for holograms to appear in the same location as the physical environment, a fiducial marker (Figure 4) is used as a calibration point to always generate the same coordinate system.

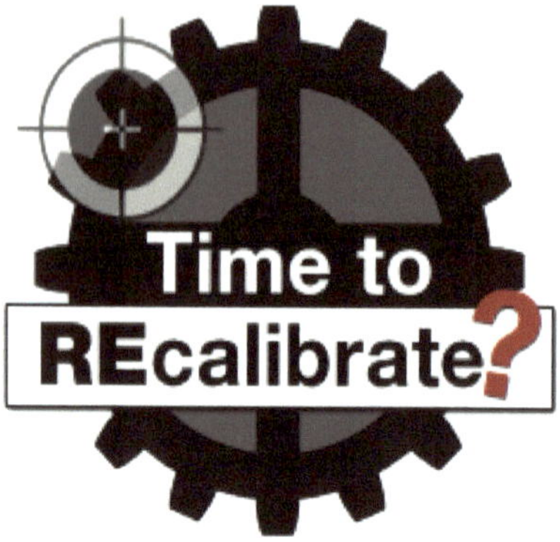

Figure 4. Example of a fiducial marker used in calibration.

When the HoloLens moves through the scenario from a point A to any point B, it uses algorithms for mapping and understanding the world to virtually determine its position in the virtually reconstructed real setting. These algorithms will be called device self-localization. They are proprietary and cannot be modified.

For use of the glasses in spaces larger than five meters, the documentation provided by the HoloLens manufacturer recommends the use of spatial anchors to stabilize the holograms. That is, when instantiating a hologram in space without using a spatial anchor, it is unstable and, consequently, inaccurate. A spatial anchor is a virtual representation of a set of characteristics extracted from the real world over which the system will maintain control over time, and its objective is to provide a more precise position for the hologram [14]. However, to ensure adequate precision, another important manufacturer recommendation is to always position a hologram less than three meters from a spatial anchor.

The use of anchors improves accuracy but does not guarantee high accuracy. There are other variables that influence the results of hologram precision and stability in an industrial scenario. One of these is calibration. As previously mentioned, the calibration strategy proposed in this study is the use of fiducial markers. The quality of the recognition of the markers proportions and orientation is indispensable to ensure the correct alignment between the virtual three-dimensional coordinates with their corresponding real three-dimensional coordinates. However, as accurate as computer vision systems may be, distortions in the dimensions and characteristics used to determine the distance and perspective of the marker add erroneous information in the translation and rotation of points in the virtual environment relative to their equivalent location in the real environment. As a consequence, there is incorrect alignment between the holograms of the virtual environment and their corresponding points in the real environment.

With the objective of mitigating the discrepancy associated with the recognition of the fiducial marker in AR systems developed for HoloLens, in this study a calibration model was developed to address the distortions caused by incorrect recognition of the marker. This model was called two-step calibration and is detailed in the next section.

3.2.1. Simple Calibration

Among the possible ways to translate and rotate the points for the alignment of the virtual coordinates with the real coordinates, a typical method uses calibration, herein called simple calibration. In this calibration, the Vuforia framework is used for marker recognition [19].

Vuforia is used in this context to recognize the fiducial marker through computer vision and then instantiate a hologram that respects the orientation and proportions of this marker. From there, the position and orientation of this hologram are treated as the origin of the virtual coordinate system. Next, previously knowing the coordinates of any fixed point within the physical scenario which will be the origin of the real coordinate system, as well as the orientation and the distance in meters between these two origins, it is possible to determine the orientation and position of the axes of both coordinate systems and thus calibrate the system.

3.2.2. Two-Step Calibration

The identification of the direction of the marker axes through Vuforia has an angular nature. That is, the larger this angle, the greater the divergence between the idealized virtual plane and the virtual plane created by the system. Despite the good quality of computer vision algorithms for marker recognition, distortions are still present, and small divergences in the identification of these angles can generate large inconsistencies as the user wearing the device moves away from the origin. To mitigate this axis angulation problem, we proposed a two-step calibration system. This calibration system consists of adding a second marker with a fixed and known distance and orientation relative to the first marker. This second marker aims to determine angles forming the axes more precisely. In other words, unlike simple calibration, which uses Vuforia to recognize the first marker, instantiate a hologram based on the orientation and proportions of the marker, and use the position and direction of this hologram to create the axes, two-step calibration uses the first marker to determine the position of the hologram and the second marker to rotate the hologram. Only after recognizing the second marker will the axes be generated based on the hologram. It is important that the two markers are facing each other at approximately 1.5 m.

3.3. *The Experiments*

After setting up the environment, the experiment was started. For each type of calibration, five sample collections of spatial coordinates were performed at each point. Each collection consisted of running the application developed for the experiment, performing the calibration procedure, moving toward the point in question, collecting 500 samples of spatial coordinates from the marker, and closing the application. To ensure equality of conditions in the behavior of the application, each time that collection was started at one of the points, the HoloLens mapping information was deleted.

The experiment generated 2500 samples for each point, resulting in 10,000 samples for each type of calibration. To evaluate the accuracy (the mean distance between the virtually measured position and the real measured position) and the precision (the dispersion of the samples) of the simple and two-step calibrations, the following values were measured:

(1) Euclidean distance between the virtual coordinates and the real coordinates;
(2) Magnitude of the error in the evaluation of distances, which in this study is defined as the difference between the absolute value of the measured vector (the actual distance from the origin to the chosen point) and the distance from the origin to the chosen point returned by the HoloLens.

To visualize the angular dispersion of the error, we also mapped the value of the angle formed at the origin between the corresponding vector to the coordinates provided by the HoloLens and the real coordinates of the points (Figure 5). This angle, of course, is determined by the Euclidean distance obtained in (1) and by the absolute values of the real distances and those provided by the HoloLens.

For the Euclidean distance of the samples relative to the real point, magnitude is the difference between the absolute value of the measured vector (the actual distance from the origin to the chosen point) and the distance returned by the HoloLens. Angular distance is the angle formed at the origin between the corresponding vector of the coordinates provided by the HoloLens and the real coordinates of the points.

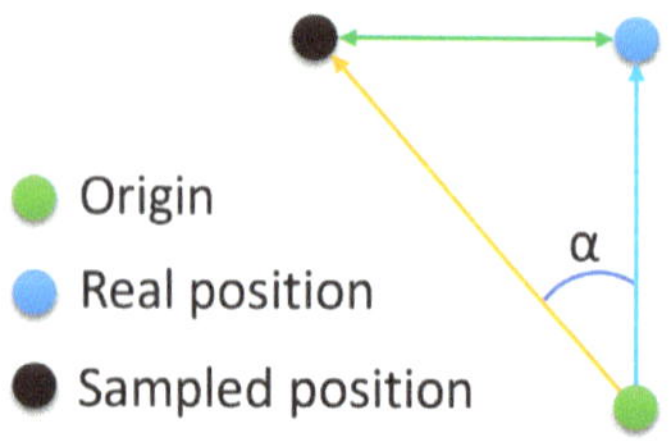

Figure 5. The Euclidean distance between sampled and measured coordinates.

Figure 6 depicts the graph containing the dispersion and the median of the Euclidean distances between the virtual coordinates and the real coordinates obtained from the samples. The graph shows that the two-step calibration was always more precise than the simple calibration at all points. Thus, we conclude that the two-step calibration contributes significantly not only to reducing the Euclidean distance between the virtual and the real coordinates but also to reducing the dispersion of the results.

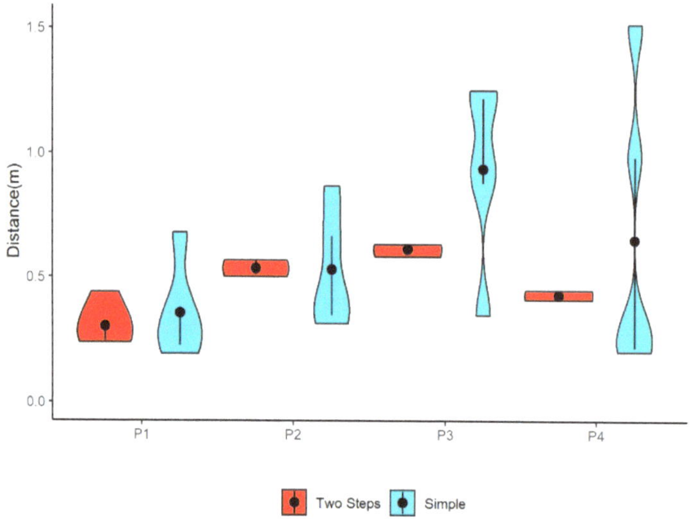

Figure 6. The Euclidean distance between the virtual coordinates and the real coordinates (2500 samples for each point).

Figure 7 shows the dispersion of the difference between the magnitude of the samples and the measured magnitude. Note that at some moments, the two-step calibration had a lower magnitude and/or dispersion; in others, the simple calibration was less dispersed and more precise. This seems to indicate that the error associated with the magnitude is not influenced by the calibration method.

Figure 8 shows how much the two-step calibration contributes positively to reducing the size and dispersion of the angles obtained in the samples.

3.4. Discussion

The absence of indicators for accuracy and precision in related research is evidence of the lack of technical work, highlighted by Bottani and Vignali [2]. Thus, this study contributes to the expansion of technical productions on the adoption of HoloLens in industrial environments, establishing numerical criteria for evaluation and comparison with future solutions. However, it is possible to establish a dialogue between the calibration method proposed in this study and its correlates through the exposure of possible applications and contributions between research fields.

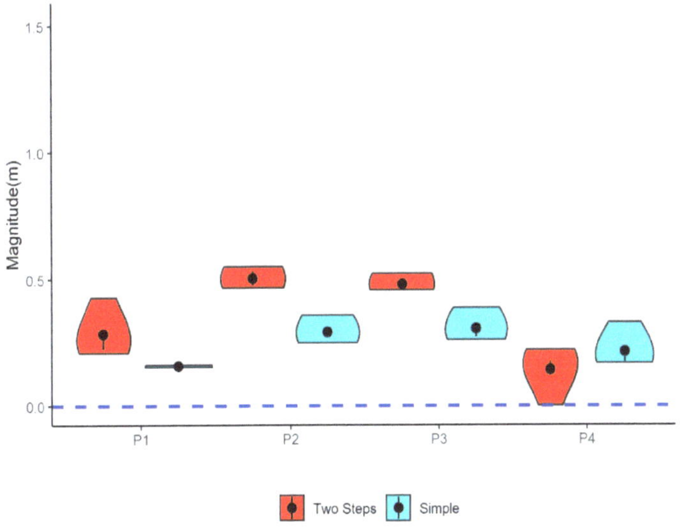

Figure 7. The difference between the sampled and measured magnitude.

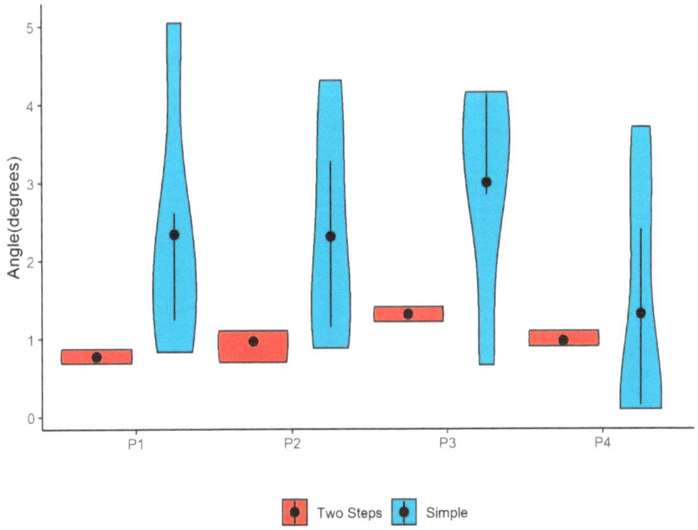

Figure 8. The angular distance between the sampled and measured coordinates.

Bachras, Raptis, and Avouris [20] carried out an empirical study that points to the use of anchors as an instrument to guarantee accuracy and precision in augmented reality applications using HoloLens. Access to the polygon mesh produced by HoloLens during spatial recognition is a necessary condition to generate the executables of these authors' applications. From this mesh, the authors position the virtual objects and assign anchor behavior to them. The use of the two-step calibration method proposed in this study is potentially useful for developing a dynamic system for inserting anchors during run time (i.e., as the polygon mesh is produced by the HoloLens). Given that the application developed by them is a navigation system for some streets in the city of Patras (Greece), the use of two-step calibration would enable the development of generic solutions that can be adapted to various contexts (not just for a specific and previously known environment). Our hypothesis is that applying two-step calibration in the Bachras, Raptis, and Avouris experiment would produce a relatively small average error in the position of the holograms compared to the dimensions of the proposed environment. However, more studies are needed to test this hypothesis.

The assessment of accuracy and precision in the representation of movable virtual objects is an opportunity to extend this research, which is currently limited to measuring these indicators for static virtual objects. The studies by Cýrus et al. [21] indicate that the recognition of fiducial markers is a more suitable alternative for representing mobile virtual objects; however, the analysis of the characteristics that favor the recognition of markers is associated with the field of computer vision and is outside this study scope.

4. Conclusions

Single markers suffer from numerical instability, particularly when they are small within the camera image. To address this, our study introduces a two-step calibration model that leverages multiple markers for accurate localization in a larger indoor environment. We put our model to the test using the MS Hololens AR device, which traditionally relies on SLAM for tracking. Notably, our experiments were conducted in an industrial setting to investigate how markers impact the accuracy of 3D point measurements. We meticulously measured four distinct points in both the physical and augmented reality realms. Our findings reveal that employing two markers significantly reduces angular discrepancies between points in the real and augmented environments. This is made possible by our novel model that deploys two fiducial markers aligned along the x-axis in a virtual space, effectively doubling the measurement data for precise alignment. Moreover, our results underscore that registration accuracy improves as the number of calibration points increases. Thus, our study establishes quantitative forms and parameters to compare the calibration models of AR solutions.

The discussion of the results obtained stimulates the production of studies and quantitative analyses of AR solutions. This study establishes numerical criteria for evaluating the proposed models, enabling direct comparison of results with future experiments and with different devices.

Future generations of HoloLens or other similar AR devices will likely include sensor improvements. However, the calibration and positioning method proposed in this study is based on general concepts and assumptions about AR. Although the experiments were performed on a first-generation HoloLens, the perspective is that future generations of AR devices will also be able to benefit from the results of the two-step calibration process proposed in this study.

One factor that directly influences precision is the angular distance. Here, the two-step calibration proposed in this study has a significant influence. The tests allow us to conclude that the two-step calibration increases the precision compared to the simple calibration, and it also is more suitable for use in industrial scenarios where the localization of objects with high precision is required.

Some hypotheses of contributions of the calibration model proposed in other research [20] help to exemplify the possibilities of practical applications of the two-step calibration model. These hypotheses open new lines of investigation and, consequently, new opportunities for studies.

Some factors may negatively influence HoloLens behavior in specific circumstances, such as the inadequate functioning of the HoloLens in sunlight. These are device limitations reported by Microsoft itself in the equipment documentation. Therefore, this study avoided carrying out the experiment in circumstances that would obviously be frustrated due to the limitations of the equipment (not the proposed calibration model).

Although the research carried out is inspired by the demands of the industrial sector, the calibration method proposed in this study is not limited to this context alone. AR systems with critical precision and accuracy in displaying holograms can benefit from the results achieved in this study.

The two-step calibration model proposed in this study fulfills the general objective of this research and answers the guiding question. Its application in HoloLens presented precision and accuracy values in displaying holograms that were significantly relevant in comparison to the volume of the environment used in the experiment. The two-step calibration model proved to be effective for HoloLens applications in industrial and similar contexts.

Author Contributions: Conceptualization, J.S.N. and F.B.C.A.; methodology, J.S.N. and I.W.; software, J.S.N.; validation, I.W. and V.d.S.; formal analysis, J.S.N. and V.d.S.; investigation, J.S.N., L.S.V.S., V.d.S. and V.M.S.O.S.; resources, A.A.B.S. and I.W.; data curation, J.S.N., F.B.C.A. and V.d.S.; writing—original draft preparation, J.S.N. and I.W.; writing—review and editing, I.W.; supervision, I.W.and V.d.S.; project administration, I.W.; funding acquisition, I.W. All authors have read and agreed to the published version of the manuscript.

Funding: The authors would like to thank the financial support from the National Council for Scientific and Technological Development (CNPq). Ingrid Winkler is a CNPq technological development fellow (Proc. 308783/2020-4).

Institutional Review Board Statement: Not applicable.

Informed Consent Statement: Not applicable.

Data Availability Statement: Data are contained within the article.

Acknowledgments: The authors would like to thank the support from the SENAI CIMATEC University Center.

Conflicts of Interest: The authors declare no conflict of interest.

References

1. Azuma, R.T. A survey of augmented reality. *Teleoperators Virtual Environ.* **1997**, *6*, 355–385. [CrossRef]
2. Bottani, E.; Vignali, G. Augmented Reality Technology in the Manufacturing Industry: A Review of the Last Decade. *IISE Trans.* **2019**, *51*, 284–310. Available online: https://www.tandfonline.com/doi/full/10.1080/24725854.2018.1493244 (accessed on 1 November 2023). [CrossRef]
3. Sanna, A.; Manuri, F.; Lamberti, F.; Paravati, G.; Pezzolla, P. Using handheld devices to support augmented reality-based maintenance and assembly tasks. In Proceedings of the 2015 IEEE International Conference on Consumer Electronics, ICCE 2015, Las Vegas, NV, USA, 9–12 January 2015; pp. 178–179. Available online: www.scopus.com (accessed on 1 November 2023).
4. Funk, M.; Kosch, T.; Schmidt, A. Interactive Worker Assistance: Comparing the Effects of In-Situ Projection, Head-Mounted Displays, Tablet, and Paper Instructions. In Proceedings of the 2016 ACM International Joint Conference on Pervasive and Ubiquitous Computing, ser. UbiComp '16, Heidelberg, Germany, 12–16 September 2016; ACM: New York, NY, USA, 2016; pp. 934–939. Available online: http://doi.acm.org/10.1145/2971648.2971706 (accessed on 1 November 2023).
5. Masood, T.; Egger, J. Augmented Reality in Support of Industry 4.0Implementation Challenges and Success Factors. *Robot. Comput. Integr. Manuf.* **2019**, *58*, 181–195. Available online: https://linkinghub.elsevier.com/retrieve/pii/S0736584518304101 (accessed on 1 November 2023). [CrossRef]
6. Gattullo, M.; Scurati, G.W.; Fiorentino, M.; Uva, A.E.; Ferrise, F.; Bordegoni, M. Towards augmented reality manuals for industry 4.0: A methodology. *Robot. Comput. Integr. Manuf.* **2019**, *56*, 276–286. Available online: http://www.sciencedirect.com/science/article/pii/S0736584518301236 (accessed on 1 November 2023). [CrossRef]
7. Neges, M.; Koch, C.; Konig, M.; Abramovici, M. Combining visual natural markers and imu for improved ar based indoor navigation. *Adv. Eng. Inform.* **2017**, *31*, 18–31. [CrossRef]
8. BIS Research. *Global Augmented Reality and Mixed Reality Market-Analysis and Forecast (2018–2025)*; Tech. Rep.; BIS Research: Noida, India, 2018. Available online: https://bisresearch.com/industry-report/global-augmented-reality-mixed-reality-market-2025.html (accessed on 1 November 2023).
9. Martinetti, A.; Marques, H.C.; Singh, S.; van Dongen, L. Reflections on the Limited Pervasiveness of Augmented Reality in Industrial Sectors. *Appl. Sci.* **2019**, *9*, 3382. Available online: https://www.mdpi.com/2076-3417/9/16/3382 (accessed on 1 November 2023). [CrossRef]

10. Syberfeldt, A.; Holm, M.; Danielsson, O.; Wang, L.; Brewster, R.L. Support Systems on the Industrial Shop-Floors of the Future Operators Perspective on Augmented Reality. In Proceedings of the 6th CIRP Conference on Assembly Technologies and Systems (CATS), Leven, Belgium, 6–8 April 2022; Procedia CIRP: Amsterdam, The Netherlands, 2016; Volume 44, pp. 108–113. Available online: http://www.sciencedirect.com/science/article/pii/S2212827116002341 (accessed on 1 November 2023).
11. Knopp, S.; Klimant, P.; Allmacher, C. Industrial Use Case—AR Guidance using Hololens for Assembly and Disassembly of a Modular Mold, with Live Streaming for Collaborative Support. In Proceedings of the 2019 IEEE International Symposium on Mixed and Augmented Reality Adjunct (ISMAR-Adjunct), Beijing, China, 10–18 October 2019; pp. 134–135. [CrossRef]
12. Keil, J.; Edler, D.; Dickmann, F. Preparing the HoloLens for user Studies: An Augmented Reality Interface for the Spatial Adjustment of Holographic Objects in 3D Indoor Environments. *KN J. Cartogr. Geogr. Inf.* **2019**, *69*, 205–215. [CrossRef]
13. Liu, Y.; Dong, H.; Zhang, L.; El Saddik, A. Technical evaluation of hololens for multimedia: A first look. *IEEE MultiMedia* **2018**, *25*, 8–18. [CrossRef]
14. Spatial Mapping—Mixed Reality. 2018. Available online: https://learn.microsoft.com/en-us/windows/mixed-reality/design/spatial-mapping (accessed on 1 November 2023).
15. Vassallo, R.; Rankin, A.; Chen, E.C.; Peters, T.M. Hologram stability evaluation for Microsoft HoloLens. In *Medical Imaging 2017: Image Perception, Observer Performance, and Technology Assessment*; Proc. SPIE 10136; SPIE: Bellingham, DC, USA, 2017; Volume 1013614. [CrossRef]
16. Radkowski, R.; Kanunganti, S. Augmented Reality System Calibration for Assembly Support with the Microsoft HoloLens. In Proceedings of the ASME 2018 13th International Manufacturing Science and Engineering Conference, College Station, TX, USA, 18–22 June 2018; ASME: New York, NY, USA, 2018; Volume 3, Manufacturing Equipment and Systems. p. V003T02A021. [CrossRef]
17. Gregor, S.; Hevner, A.R. Positioning and presenting design science research for maximum impact. *MIS Q. JSTOR* **2013**, *37*, 337–355. [CrossRef]
18. PTC. Vuforia. 2018. Available online: https://developer.vuforia.com/ (accessed on 1 November 2023).
19. *ISO 5725-1: 2023*; Accuracy (Trueness and Precision) of Measurement Methods and Results-Part 1: General Principles and Definitions. International Organization for Standardization: Geneva, Switzerland, 2023.
20. Bachras, V.; Raptis, G.E.; Avouris, N.M. On the Use of Persistent Spatial Points for Deploying Path Navigation in Augmented Reality: An Evaluation Study. In *Lecture Notes in Computer Science (Including Subseries Lecture Notes in Artificial Intelligence and Lecture Notes in Bioinformatics)*; Springer: Berlin/Heidelberg, Germany, 2019; Volume 11749 LNCS, pp. 309–318. ISBN 9783030293895. ISSN 16113349.
21. Cýrus, J.; Krčmařík, D.; Petrů, M.; Kočí, J. Cooperation of Virtual Reality and Real Objects with HoloLens. In *Advances in Intelligent Systems and Computing*; Springer: Berlin/Heidelberg, Germany, 2020; Volume 944, pp. 94–106. ISBN 9783030177973. ISSN 21945365.

virtual worlds

MDPI

Article

Characterization of Functional Connectivity in Chronic Stroke Subjects after Augmented Reality Training

Gilda A. de Assis [1], Alexandre F. Brandão [2,3], Ana G. D. Correa [4] and Gabriela Castellano [2,3,*]

1 Department of Computing and Systems, Federal University of Ouro Preto, João Monlevade 35931-008, MG, Brazil
2 Institute of Physics Gleb Wataghin, University of Campinas–UNICAMP, Campinas 13083-859, SP, Brazil
3 Brazilian Institute of Neuroscience and Neurotechnology–BRAINN, Campinas 13083-970, SP, Brazil
4 School of Computing and Informatics, Mackenzie Presbyterian University, São Paulo 01302-907, SP, Brazil
* Correspondence: gabriela@unicamp.br

Abstract: Augmented reality (AR) tools have been investigated with promising outcomes in rehabilitation. Recently, some studies have addressed the neuroplasticity effects induced by this type of therapy using functional connectivity obtained from resting-state functional magnetic resonance imaging (rs-fMRI). This work aims to perform an initial assessment of possible changes in brain functional connectivity associated with the use of NeuroR, an AR system for upper limb motor rehabilitation of poststroke participants. An experimental study with a case series is presented. Three chronic stroke participants with left hemiparesis were enrolled in the study. They received eight sessions with NeuroR to provide shoulder rehabilitation exercises. Measurements of range of motion (ROM) were obtained at the beginning and end of each session, and rs-fMRI data were acquired at baseline (pretest) and after the last training session (post-test). Functional connectivity analyses of the rs-fMRI data were performed using a seed placed at the noninjured motor cortex. ROM increased in two patients who presented spastic hemiparesis in the left upper limb, with a change in muscle tone, and stayed the same (at zero angles) in one of the patients, who had the highest degree of impairment, showing flaccid hemiplegia. All participants had higher mean connectivity values in the ipsilesional brain regions associated with motor function at post-test than at pretest. Our findings show the potential of the NeuroR system to promote neuroplasticity related to AR-based therapy for motor rehabilitation in stroke participants.

Keywords: motor imagery; fMRI analysis; augmented reality

Citation: Assis, G.A.d.; Brandão, A.F.; Correa, A.G.D.; Castellano, G. Characterization of Functional Connectivity in Chronic Stroke Subjects after Augmented Reality Training. *Virtual Worlds* **2023**, *2*, 1–15. https://doi.org/10.3390/virtualworlds2010001

Academic Editors: Radu Comes, Dorin-Mircea Popovici, Calin Gheorghe Dan Neamtu and Jing-Jing Fang

Received: 28 November 2022
Revised: 26 December 2022
Accepted: 5 January 2023
Published: 16 January 2023

1. Introduction

Stroke is a serious and common public health problem throughout the world, with high mortality rates [1]. In recent years, advances in the medical treatment of acute stroke have resulted in a decrease in the mortality rate [1–3]. However, many survivors remain with significant commitments [4], with upper limb impairment occurring in up to 77% of cases [5]. This is the major cause of functional dependence and the impossibility of carrying out daily life activities [6]. Therefore, health centers, stroke survivors and their families carry the burden of long-term disability.

The increasing proportion of survivors of stroke is associated with an increase in the number of individuals who persist with sensory motor deficits [3,4]. Despite intensive rehabilitation, more than half of the survivors remain with a disability affecting functional independence [7–9]. Poststroke rehabilitation has been a challenge because it usually requires repetitive and intensive training. Additionally, there is a shortage of health centers and health professionals to deal with this increasing population [10].

Several neurorehabilitation techniques have been used for neuromuscular rehabilitation of these types of patients [11–15]. Technologies such as augmented reality (AR) have been employed as new therapy tools to improve stroke rehabilitation and provide opportunities to promote the repetitive practice of activities as soon as disengagement and boredom threaten the progress in rehabilitation [4]. AR is a technology that combines the real world with virtual objects and can be manipulated by the user and controlled by specialists. AR applications constitute a safe environment for users [16], and they have the potential to be used at home with remote supervision [17].

AR applied to health and wellness fields has been evaluated in recent years and with promising outcomes in some areas, such as rehabilitation [12,16,18]. Moreover, functional magnetic resonance imaging (fMRI) assessment of brain changes resulting from the use of this type of system in rehabilitation has shown that most result in the restoration of activation patterns or relateralization to the ipsilateral hemisphere [19]. fMRI is a noninvasive and safe technique for mapping functional connectivity and brain function. Resting-state fMRI (rs-fMRI) data can be acquired using spontaneous signals obtained while the participant is resting in the scanner [20]. Data from rs-fMRI have been shown to be stable and reproducible across participants [21]. The rs-fMRI experiments are not used to map brain activation/deactivation of the brain regions during a specific task but rather to investigate brain functional connectivity [22].

Usually, functional connectivity is inferred from seed-based analysis or independent component analysis (ICA). Seed-based analysis is performed by correlating the fMRI time signals of chosen regions of interest (ROIs) with the remaining fMRI time series, disregarding other significant neural coactivation patterns [22], while ICA is a data-driven method that does not depend on any chosen ROI [23].

In this work, for AR training, we chose an AR system, NeuroR, that was initially designed to provide a virtual image to stimulate motor imagery [24]. It uses an approach similar to mirror therapy, with a virtual tridimensional arm superimposed on the impaired limb, that is, the user's actual upper limb is substituted in the image by the virtual arm. This AR system seeks to promote neuroplasticity by performing a simple task, where the participant, sitting in front of a projection screen or TV, visualizes him/herself performing exercises of shoulder abduction and flexion with the affected arm, which is replaced by a virtual arm. The virtual arm performs a much larger movement than the real movement the patient is actually capable of executing. Actually, the success of virtual reality and AR games applied to rehabilitation seems to be based on their ability to provide false positive feedback, which is thought to promote appropriate brain reorganization [25,26]. Previous experiments showed that three of four stroke patients physically executed shoulder movement when asked to perform motor imagery from the visual feedback of the animation of the tridimensional virtual arm [24]. Another study, by Brauchle et al., with a multijoint arm exoskeleton reported changes in brain functional connectivity during motor execution and motor imagery of different feedback modalities (visual and proprioceptive) for both healthy participants and stroke survivors [27]. They evaluated the functional connectivity networks from electroencephalography data by defining a seed electrode in the ipsilesional primary motor cortex. In the same way, we hypothesized that changes in brain functional connectivity can occur, as pointed out by [27], since the participants also have visual and proprioceptive feedback while they see themselves on the computer screen and see their virtual arm moving during shoulder exercises for mental practice or motor execution.

The aim of the present work was to explore the use of rs-fMRI data to evaluate possible changes in functional brain connectivity of poststroke participants associated with the use of NeuroR in the context of motor rehabilitation. We also wanted to evaluate the spasticity of the patients and possible changes after therapy in their range of motion (ROM). A pilot study was conducted with an acute stroke participant using rs-fMRI and NeuroR training integrated into the patient's rehabilitation program [28]. Herein, we conducted a case series with three chronic poststroke participants. Functional connectivity analyses were performed to investigate whether functional brain reorganization occurred, triggered by the mental practice of stroke participants using NeuroR. Functional brain connectivity was assessed using the seed-based method. The idea was to investigate whether the integration of the virtual arm image into the AR system stimulates neuroplasticity, making the system a new tool to aid the rehabilitation of poststroke patients.

2. Materials and Methods

Case studies were performed at the Clinics Hospital of the University of Campinas, Brazil. Three male chronic stroke participants with left hemiparesis were enrolled in the study.

2.1. Participants

The inclusion criteria were individuals with a clinical diagnosis of ischemic stroke, with motor sequelae of the upper limb, whose conditions were already clinically stabilized and who had already previously participated in conventional rehabilitation therapy but were not at that moment participating in any such therapy.

The exclusion criteria were individuals diagnosed with stroke who were confused and disoriented, with aphasia of understanding or without motor deficits.

Three chronic stroke participants (mean age 65 +/− 12 years) were screened for eligibility. All participants were informed about the procedures and signed the terms of informed consent approved by the Ethics Committee of the University of Campinas (CAAE 49976315.5.0000.5404), and all study procedures were conducted in accordance with the principles expressed in the Declaration of Helsinki. This study followed the CARE guidelines for case reports. Due to time and funding limitations, it was not possible to recruit more patients for this study.

Participant 1 (P1) is a 49-year-old male who sustained a right-sided ischemic stroke in the middle cerebral right artery four years prior to enrollment in the study, resulting in left hemiparesis. He used a wheelchair propelled by a caregiver. He received botulinum toxin injection to treat spasticity after stroke six months prior to admission in this study. He had earlier exposure to intensive and frequent therapy. The clinical evaluation revealed spastic hemiparesis in the left upper limb, with changes in muscle tone, which impaired the control of the limb in space and movement and facial synkinesis during the exercise without assistance.

Participant 2 (P2) is an 84-year-old male who sustained a right-sided ischemic stroke in the middle cerebral right artery two years prior to participating in the study, resulting in left hemiparesis. He primarily used a wheelchair propelled by a caregiver. He had received prior therapy focusing on functional electrical stimulation. The clinical evaluation showed flaccid hemiplegia affecting the left side and no hint of contraction, with only compensation with the trunk.

Participant 3 (P3) is a 45-year-old male who sustained a right-sided ischemic stroke three years prior to participating in the study, resulting in left hemiparesis. He walked without assistance. He had received intensive and frequent therapy prior to the study. The clinical evaluation revealed spastic hemiparesis in the left upper limb.

None of the patients received any other type of therapy (in addition to NeuroR) during the time span of this study. The last rehabilitation therapy that they had had was at least six months prior to the present study.

2.2. Outcome Measures

Baseline, during- and postintervention measures were performed for all participants. Firstly, spasticity of the shoulder muscles was evaluated using the Modified Ashworth Scale (MAS) at the time of enrollment in the study; more specifically, these were assessed for the impaired upper limb for shoulder adduction, abduction, flexion and extension (Table 1). MAS was evaluated because, in a spasticity condition, the subscapularis muscle remains tonically active, which negatively influences the velocity and ROM of the targets of the intervention (shoulder abduction and flexion). The same physiotherapist assessed all the participants and conducted all AR training sessions.

Table 1. Modified Ashworth Scale (MAS) scores of the enrolled participants at baseline for the impaired shoulder.

Participant	Shoulder Adduction	Shoulder Abduction	Shoulder Flexion	Shoulder Extension
P1	1+	0	2	2
P2	2	0	0	2
P3	1+	1+	1+	1+

Study variables were brain functional connectivity and ROM of shoulder abduction and flexion. Goniometer measurements were obtained at the beginning and end of the sessions. Brain connectivity analysis was performed using rs-fMRI at baseline and after the last training session. Functional connectivity analyses of the rs-fMRI data were performed using a seed placed at the noninjured motor cortex.

2.3. Intervention

The rs-fMRI exams and training sessions were carried out at the Clinics Hospital of the University of Campinas. All three subjects completed one hour of AR training with NeuroR twice a week for four consecutive weeks at the outpatient rehabilitation clinic of this hospital. They also underwent two MRI exams, before the first AR training session and after the last AR training session.

All training sessions were carried out on an individual basis. A licensed physical therapist conducted the training sessions. At the beginning of each session, the physiotherapist showed the participants how to perform the shoulder exercises following the virtual arm. At least two series of ten repetitions of the activities were performed at each training session with 20–40 s of rest after each set. The participants carried out shoulder abduction and flexion exercises with the injured arm, staying seated. At the end of each session, a stretching exercise was performed with the AR arm. Figure 1 shows the visual feedback in front of the participant while the virtual arm is running shoulder abduction.

The training setup comprised the AR software, a camera attached to a tripod, a multimedia projector, a cloth glove and a physical marker. Virtual arm animations were triggered by the physiotherapist using a keyboard. Images mixing the virtual arm and real-time video were projected onto a white wall in front of the participant. The room layout was arranged so as not to have any object cluttering the line of sight, and no extra illumination was needed. A resolution of 640 × 480 was adopted for all video frames, which were generated by the AR system running on a laptop with a refresh rate of 60 Hz.

2.4. Data Acquisition and Analysis

Before the first (pretest) and after the last (post-test) AR training sessions, the participants were scanned in a 3T magnetic resonance scanner (Achieva, Philips, The Netherlands) to acquire resting-state functional images of the brain. First, anatomical images were acquired on the sagittal plane with the following parameters: T1-weighted, voxel size = $1 \times 1 \times 1$ mm^3, image matrix = $240 \times 240 \times 180$, repetition time (TR) = 7.7 ms, echo time (TE) = 3.1 ms and flip angle = 8°. Second, rs-fMRI images were acquired on the axial plane in a 6-min scan with a T2*-weighted echo-planar imaging (EPI) sequence, voxel size = $3 \times 3 \times 3$ mm^3, image matrix = $80 \times 80 \times 40$, gap = 0.6 mm, TR = 2000 ms, TE = 30 ms, ascending acquisition and 180 volumes. During the rs-fMRI exams, the participants were instructed to open their eyes (so as not to fall asleep) and to not think of anything in particular. Figure 2 shows the structural 3D data obtained at baseline for the three participants.

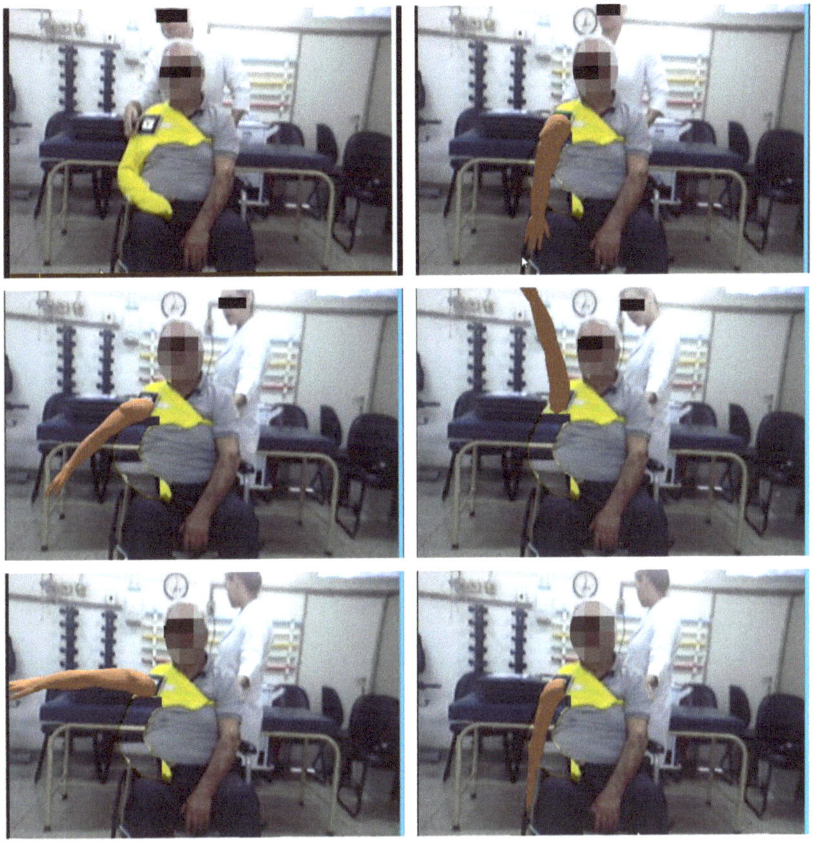

Figure 1. Sequence of frames for shoulder abduction with the NeuroR system. The virtual arm replaces the real, injured arm on the computer screen, which the patient sees as a mirror image. The virtual arm performs a much larger movement than the real movement the patient is actually capable of executing.

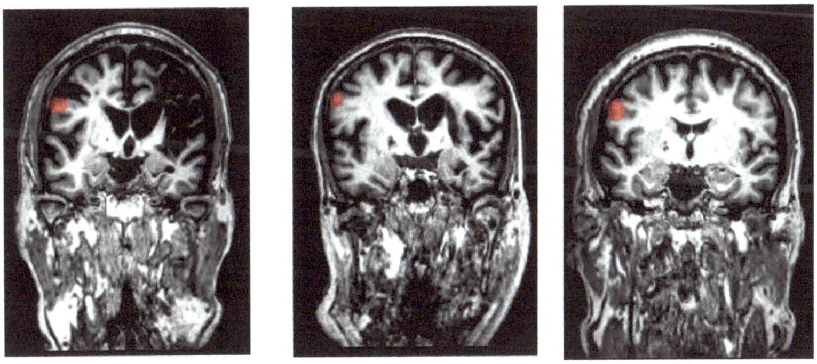

P1 P2 P3

Figure 2. A coronal view of the structural 3D data obtained at the pretest for the three participants. ROIs corresponding to the seed for functional connectivity are shown in red.

Functional connectivity analyses of the rs-fMRI data were performed using a seed placed at the noninjured (left) motor cortex. This is because the injured motor cortex would possibly have little or no signal due to the stroke lesion, particularly before the intervention. Since healthy homotopic motor areas usually have strong connectivity [29], we expected that neuroplasticity in the injured motor cortex after AR rehabilitation would appear as a signal restoration and therefore as an increase in connectivity (with the noninjured motor cortex) in those regions. According to [30], functional connectivity between most motor areas is increased in the motor-planning state, while functional connectivity with the cerebellum and basal ganglia is increased during movement. Therefore, we carried out a statistical analysis between the chosen ROI, motor areas and cerebellum parcellations. Several tools were used to perform rs-fMRI data analysis: MATLAB MathWorks® software, SPM12 software, MRIcron and UF2C [31]. The image data were processed, and statistical analysis was performed according to the UF2C standard pipeline [31], namely, definition of the anterior commissure as the origin of the reference system of the structural T1 and rs-fMRI images; fMRI volume realignment (using the mean image as a reference); image registration (fMRI mean image with structural T1); spatial normalization of all images to a standard space and spatial smoothing of fMRI images; and structural T1 tissue segmentation (gray matter, white matter, and cerebral spinal fluid). Additionally, six head motion parameters (three rotational and three translational) were regressed out of the time series as well as the white matter and cerebral spinal fluid average signals. Finally, the time series were bandpass-filtered (0.008–0.1 Hz).

With all the images in a standard space, the Automated Anatomical Labelling (AAL) atlas [32] was used to segment the images and choose the seed for functional connectivity. This seed was a region of interest (ROI) of $4 \times 4 \times 4$ voxels located in the left precentral area in Brodmann area 4. The ROI was selected in analogous locations for all participants to evaluate functional connectivity related to motor networks. The average time series of all ROI voxels within the participants' gray matter was computed for use as the seed's time series. Pearson's correlation scores were calculated between the seed's time series and the time series of all gray matter voxels of the brain. Subsequently, average correlation values (over the voxels of a given region) were computed for every AAL area. This was performed by converting these values to z scores (Fisher's Z transformation), calculating the mean value and transforming them back to the correlation space. Finally, to evaluate and characterize differences between pretest and post-test data, the average correlation values of the AAL atlas regions related to movement (Table 2) were compared. An intrasubject comparison (for each subject individually) was performed. A paired *t*-test was used with a significance level of 0.05.

Table 2. Motor-related areas of the Automatic Anatomical Labelling (AAL) atlas used to compute functional connectivity values. Odd numbers indicate the left hemisphere (L), while even numbers indicate the right hemisphere (R).

	Label	Abbreviation	Region
Motor areas	1, 2	Precentral_L, R	precentral gyrus
	19, 20	Supp_Motor_Area_L, R	supplementary motor area
Cerebellum	91, 92	Cerebellum_Crus1_L, R	cerebellum crus 1
	93, 94	Cerebellum_Crus2_L, R	cerebellum crus 2
	95, 96	Cerebellum_3_L, R	cerebellum 3
	97, 98	Cerebellum_4_5_L, R	cerebellum 4 and 5
	99, 100	Cerebellum_6_L, R	cerebellum 6
	101, 102	Cerebellum_7b_L, R	cerebellum 7
	103, 104	Cerebellum_8_L, R	cerebellum 8
	105, 106	Cerebellum_9_L, R	cerebellum 9
	107, 108	Cerebellum_10_L, R	cerebellum 10

Additionally, an evaluation of the ROM of the injured shoulder was carried out. Angles of shoulder abduction and flexion were measured before starting and after the end of most AR training sessions to determine the ROM of the injured shoulder, using mechanical goniometers. Goniometer measurements were recorded in a spreadsheet.

3. Results

According to Table 1, P2 had zero MAS scores for shoulder abduction and flexion, which means he had no muscle resistance for the passive execution of these movements [33]. P1 also had a zero score for shoulder abduction but had score 2 for shoulder flexion, indicating "a marked increase in muscle tone throughout most of the ROM, but still being able to move affected part(s) with ease" [33]. Finally, P3 had 1+ MAS score for both shoulder abduction and flexion, meaning he had a "slight increase in muscle tone, manifested as a catch, followed by minimal resistance through the remainder (less than half) of the ROM" [33].

Due to the different degrees of motor impairment of the patients, the only requirements for shoulder exercise during AR were for them to try to raise their arms (in both flexion and abduction movements) as much as they could. All participants underwent all eight NeuroR training sessions. There were no adverse outcomes for any of the patients.

Table 3 summarizes goniometry data for all participants. Data for P2 were equal to zero angles for all sessions since this participant had the most severe degree of hemiplegia. For P3, it is possible to notice that measurements taken after sessions were usually smaller than measures taken before sessions, which is most likely due to participant fatigue.

Table 3. Summary of the goniometry data for range of motion (ROM), measured in degrees. "First" and "Last" represent the first and last training sessions for which these data were acquired, respectively, while "Start" and "End" represent the beginning and end of a given session, respectively. Larger values indicate more flexible movements.

Session	Participant	Abduction		Flexion	
		Start	End	Start	End
First	P1	60	70	40	40
Last		75	70	50	50
First	P2	0	0	0	0
Last		0	0	0	0
First	P3	60	60	70	40
Last		70	70	80	60

Table 4 shows the mean functional connectivity values (considering only positive correlations) over the AAL regions listed in Table 2 at pretest and post-test for all patients. P1 and P2 presented significant differences (t-test, $p < 0.05$) in functional connectivity in motor-related areas between pretest and post-test, but not P3 (Table 4).

Table 4. Mean functional connectivity values (considering only positive correlations) over the AAL motor-related regions (listed in Table 2) and standard deviation, at pretest and post-test.

Subject	Mean Functional Connectivity		*t* Test
	Pretest	Post-Test	*p* Value
P1	0.166 ± 0.085	0.312 ± 0.209	0.004
P2	0.082 ± 0.049	0.141 ± 0.111	0.018
P3	0.037 ± 0.051	0.065 ± 0.125	0.121

Figure 3 shows plots of mean functional connectivity values for each region of Table 2 for each participant at both time points. P1 and P3 showed a clear increase in connectivity for the primary motor cortex (precentral gyrus) and supplementary motor area bilaterally after training with NeuroR, but P2 only had an increase in the supplementary motor area (also in both hemispheres). On the other hand, P1 and P2 had functional connectivity increases at post-test in most cerebellum areas, while P3 had very low connectivity values in the cerebellum before and after training.

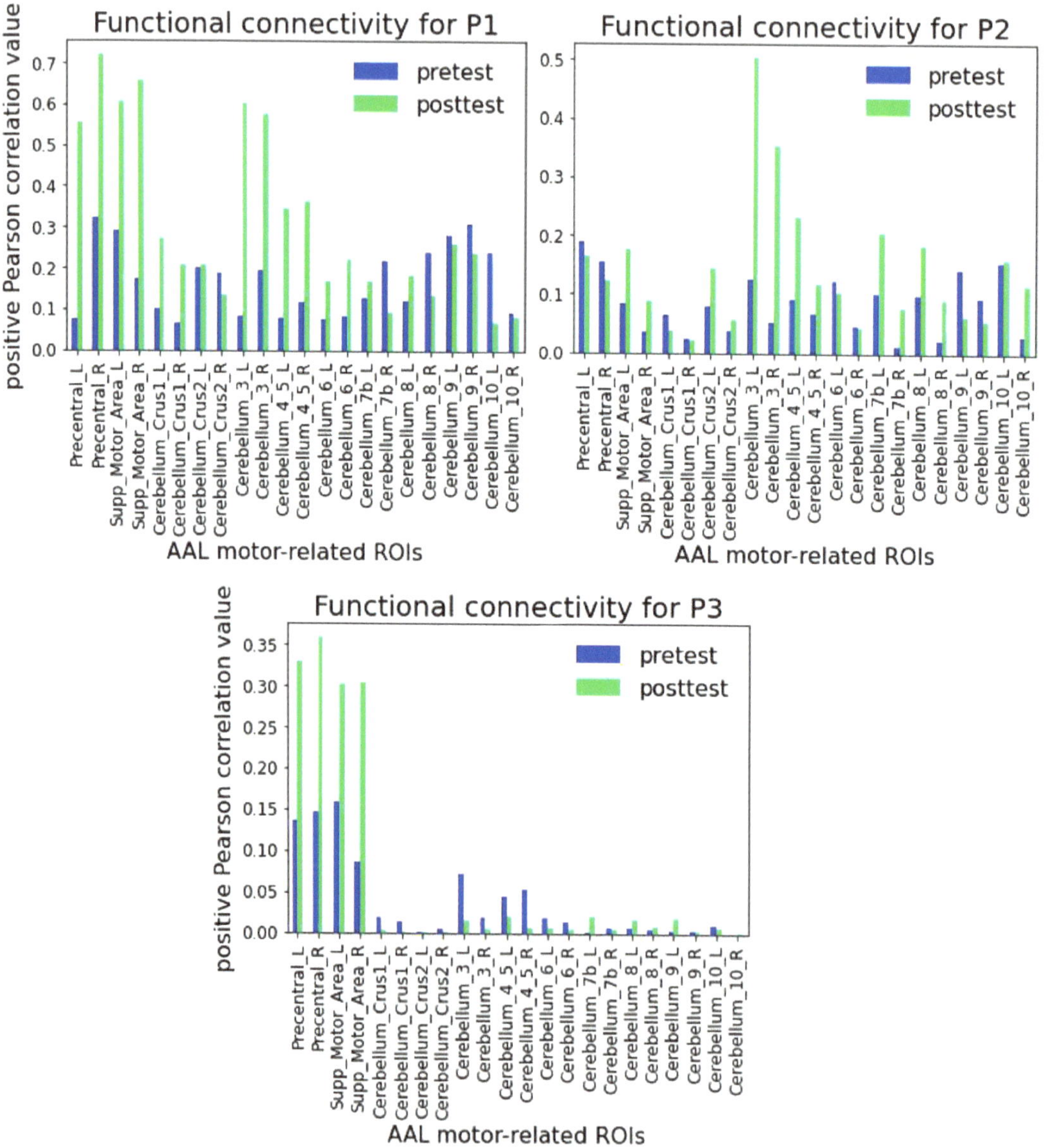

Figure 3. Mean positive correlation of motor-related areas and seed for each participant before (blue) and after (green) training with NeuroR. The AAL areas along the x-axis are listed in Table 2.

Figure 4 shows positive correlation maps for each patient at pretest (left column) and post-test (right column). The increase in correlation values is evident for P1, for whom even the lesioned area presents higher correlation values at post-test. P2 and P3 had subtler lesions, and although the changes at post-test are not as evident, brighter areas can be seen for P2 at the right motor cortex (red arrow), temporal lobes and cerebellum and at both right and left motor cortices for P3.

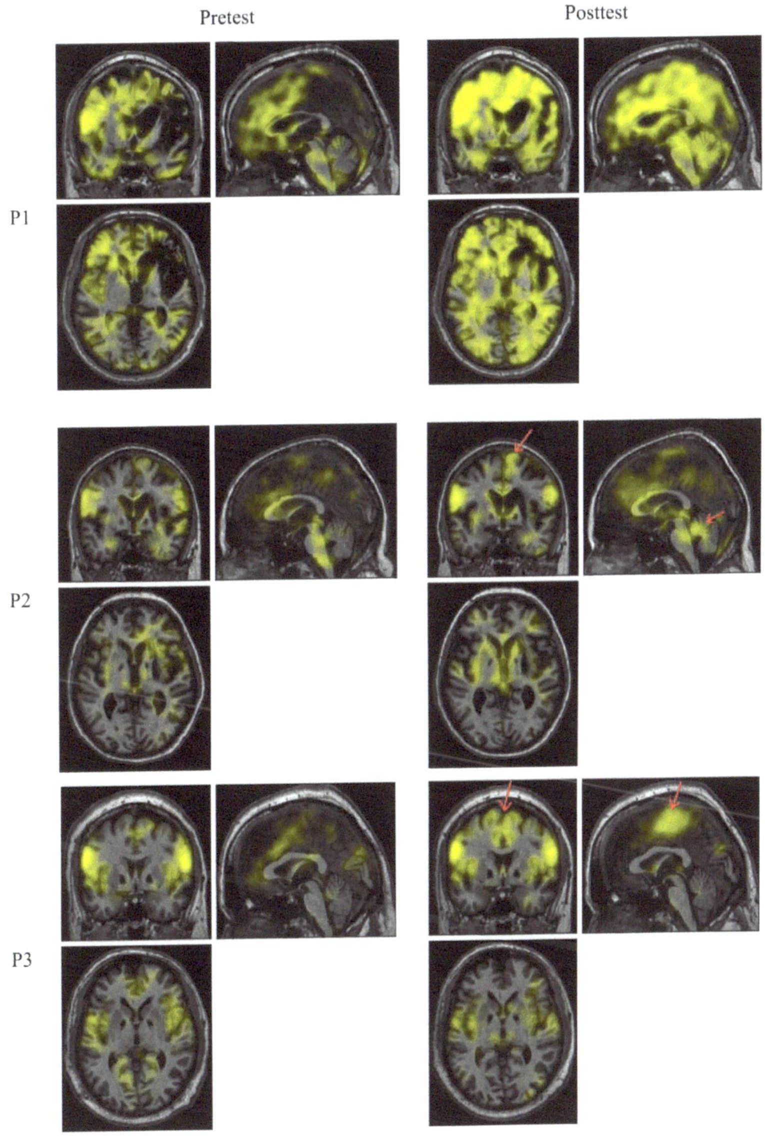

Figure 4. Positive correlation maps with the seed in the left motor area at pretest (left column) and post-test (right column). Each line shows maps for a patient, from top to bottom: P1, P2 and P3. Brighter colors indicate higher correlation values and/or a larger number of correlated voxels. In particular, red arrows for P2 and P3 indicate increases in motor-related areas.

4. Discussion

The aim of this study was to evaluate brain functional connectivity changes in three chronic stroke patients resulting from AR-based upper limb rehabilitation with the NeuroR system and to compare these changes with shoulder ROM changes in those patients. Patients completed up to eight sessions of the NeuroR intervention.

For two individuals (P1 and P2), there was a statistically significant increase in the functional connectivity of motor-related areas (motor cortex plus cerebellar areas; see Table 2) with the seed at the noninjured (left) motor area after the NeuroR training sessions (Table 4). Moreover, four motor areas (left and right primary and supplementary motor areas) had higher correlation values at post-test than at pretest for P1 and P3, while only the supplementary motor areas had higher correlation values for P2 (Figure 3). Particularly, connectivity in the right (injured) motor cortex increased for all patients, although with different amplitudes: P1 and P3 had a substantial increase in connectivity both in the right precentral gyrus (about two-fold) and the right supplementary motor area (about three-fold), while P2 had a moderate increase only in the right supplementary motor area (about two-fold), with a small decrease in the right precentral gyrus (about 20%) (Figure 3). This could possibly indicate the occurrence of neuroplasticity on the injured side, as hypothesized. Regarding the results for P2, since this patient had more movement restrictions (all his goniometry data were zero) than the other patients and flaccid hemiplegia affecting the left side, this could indicate that only his movement planning areas were recruited [34]. The difference for P3 was nonsignificant; however, unlike the others, this participant reported shoulder pain after AR training. Additionally, since this participant had previously received intensive and frequent therapy, he might have been closer to a plateau than the other patients, which could explain the nonsignificant changes observed. Another factor that may explain the outcome is the age of the patients. It has been reported that advanced age is one of the main social factors that can affect stroke recovery [35]. While P1 and P3 were in their forties, P2 was in their eighties, which could help describe their poorer performance.

Other studies have reported similar findings. In the study by Song et al., nine stroke patients with persistent upper extremity motor impairment completed up to fifteen two-hour sessions of rehabilitation therapy using brain–computer interface (BCI) technology, and cortical motor activity was assessed using motor-task fMRI data [36]. They found an increase in corticomotor activity (during finger tapping) associated with worse motor rehabilitation outcomes in the patients. Although rs-fMRI investigates synchronous and spontaneous activity between brain regions occurring in the absence of a task or stimulus, these simultaneous activities have shown close correspondence to brain activation dynamics. Therefore, an rs-fMRI experiment is a potential alternative for mapping motor networks that does not require task performance [36].

In the study by Schuster-Amft and colleagues, two stroke patients with upper limb motor impairments performed nineteen VR training sessions and showed changes in brain activity revealed using fMRI data [37]. Analysis of their fMRI data showed recruitment of secondary motor areas [37]. In our study, three stroke participants with persistent upper extremity motor impairment completed up to eight one-hour sessions of NeuroR training. Rs-fMRI measures showed higher values of functional connectivity in motor areas after AR training for all patients, although for P2, these were only for the supplementary motor areas.

Previous studies using fMRI data have pointed out that increased recruitment of ipsilesional motor areas over the course of treatment is associated with improved outcomes [38,39]. According to [40], brain-based rehabilitation to improve motor function for poststroke patients should promote ipsilesional activity during impaired limb movement for optimal improvement. In our study, P1 and P3 showed higher correlation values/area in the ipsilesional primary and supplementary motor cortices at post-test (Figures 3 and 4).

Brauchle et al. pointed out that the functional connectivity networks between the contralateral motor imagery motor network and the entire brain can be evaluated by defining a seed electrode in the ipsilesional primary motor cortex [27]. Similarly, our outcomes indicated that the functional connectivity of stroke participants can be evaluated by defining a seed of voxels in the noninjured (left) primary motor cortex from rs-fMRI exams.

ROM measures suggested an improvement tendency for two of the participants (P1 and P3), and although the participant with the most severe degree of hemiplegia remained at zero angles (P2), a hint of muscle contraction was observed. Based on this observation, we propose that, in the next study, the muscle strength scale should be used as an evaluation tool rather than goniometry. On the other hand, P3 showed an angle decrease for both shoulder abduction and flexion after sessions compared to before sessions, possibly due to participant fatigue. According to [41], in the presence of an event of fatigue during a rehabilitation session, either the goals are not achieved or the rehabilitation session is abandoned. Therefore, a control scheme to reduce the effects of muscle fatigue must be planned. In our study, we adopted adequate rest between repetition sessions to reduce fatigue during AR training, but it may not have been sufficient for this patient.

Regarding ROM results for P2, it is interesting to note that according to Su and Xu [42], various poststroke interventions seek to promote the plasticity of the remaining neural circuit. Notwithstanding, factors such as a long time since stroke, location and size of the lesion and biological factors such as aging can reduce the neuroplasticity effects. In our study, clinical measures showed that P2 (84 years old), who was much older than P1 (49 years old) and P3 (45 years old), remained without gain in flexion and extension in the injured limb after AR training with NeuroR. Although P2 presented an increase in functional connectivity with motor-related areas from 0.082 (pretest) to 0.141 (post-test) (Table 4), this did not translate into motor improvement for this patient.

Although valuable outcomes were reported in our study, the case series design prevents us from drawing robust conclusions about the impact of augmented reality training exercises on brain connectivity. The design of case series has several limitations and needs further validation from stroke cases with different brain damage features and postonset periods. On the other hand, it is important to draw attention to the difficulties concerning this type of multidisciplinary study, which requires compliance with the subtleties of many different expertise areas, including motor rehabilitation, brain imaging and AR. The main one is that participants are required to come several times to the research facility (be it a clinic, hospital or university) for exams and therapy sessions, but most are impaired and have locomotion problems and thus depend on caregivers to bring them to the sessions. Polese and coworkers [43] reported that individuals with chronic stroke had low rates of recruitment and retention. In our country, research subjects are not paid. A previous study [44] revealed a problem of slow recruitment for Brazilian clinical trials with stroke survivors, in which 150 stroke survivors were screened for eligibility and only 10 agreed to participate. According to these authors, the lack of transport was reported as the main obstacle to participating in and attending the training sessions. We also faced those same recruitment challenges, with the addition of funding and schedule limitations. All this results in a high dropout rate. Another limitation was the fact that the participants were all male. Stroke subjects of both sexes, male and female, were invited to participate in the study. We are aware that the underrepresentation of women in cardiovascular disease research has been a long-standing problem [45]. However, due to schedule constraints, we could not delay the recruitment period to balance the participants' genders in the study.

Yet another problem with our study could be attributed to the fact that the virtual arm in the AR environment does not appear realistic. Nevertheless, in a previous study with the NeuroR system with four participants, three demonstrated perceiving a "matching" of the NeuroR's virtual arm with their actual arm [24]. Only a participant who had suffered an injury in the nucleus of the thalamus and base neglected the relationship between his physical arm and the virtual arm. The authors argued that there is evidence that participants with lesions in the reticular formation or elsewhere in the brain stem may have difficulties in stimulating motor neurons from visual stimuli, affecting their performance in AR-based training [24], but this was not the case for the patients in the present study. Notwithstanding, improvements in the realistic aspect of the virtual arm of the NeuroR system are already underway. Real disembodiment and re-embodiment are important for the participants to feel a sense of attachment to their avatar self, extending their version of selves in the AR world [46,47]. According to [48], in telepresence scenarios, equal-sized avatars are more influential than small-sized avatars. Therefore, a new version of the NeuroR system will detect the skin pixels in a given initial image [49] and will provide an equal-sized virtual arm.

Participants reported that they were mostly sedentary for the last 30 days prior to the study. These reported data agree with the outcomes of the study by Fini and colleagues [50], in which physical activity levels were low at 24 months after rehabilitation discharge for 79 stroke survivors, with no changes over time observed. Further research could investigate the relation between different levels of physical activity and brain connectivity for stroke survivors.

The feasibility of the proposed protocol for AR training was based on the review by Aramaki et al. [51]. The studies reviewed by these authors performed training sessions two or three times a week, with each session lasting from 30 to 60 min, over 2–12 weeks. In our study, AR sessions happened two times a week for four weeks, and the number of repetitions of AR shoulder flexion and abduction was equally sized to be performed in 30 min, including rest periods and AR stretching at the end. ROM and brain connectivity outcomes suggested that the frequency and number of sessions were feasible.

Finally, functional evaluation scales, such as the Fugl-Meyer assessment, should have been included in the study. This was not executed due to time restrictions during the sessions, but the assessment will be included in a future study.

5. Conclusions

In summary, here, we presented three cases of chronic stroke patients who completed up to eight sessions of intervention with the NeuroR system and who were evaluated using functional connectivity obtained from rs-fMRI data and ROM measurements. Each case showed different degrees of change in the ROM of the upper limb and brain connectivity. The analysis of the goniometry measurements showed an increase in the angle in both flexion and abduction of the shoulder for two of the three participants (P1 and P3), comparing the first and last days. P2, the participant with the most severe degree of hemiplegia, remained without a gain in flexion and extension in the injured limb. These outlines of clinical improvement were accompanied by an increase in functional connectivity with the noninjured motor cortex in all participants. Given that these were chronic patients, both ROM and connectivity changes have a chance to be related to the performed NeuroR training. Of course, given that this was a pilot study, these outcomes should be taken with caution. A future study will be carried out with more participants. Since an oversized and distorted virtual arm may be criticized as having a countereffect in neural processing, we will propose a graphics upgrade of the software in future work. Furthermore, functional evaluation scales, such as the Fugl-Meyer assessment, will be included in the study to compare possible changes in the motor function of stroke patients and the functional connectivity findings. Finally, we would like to note that NeuroR is a low-cost solution addressing the global problem of upper limb motor rehabilitation of stroke survivors, which, after more in-depth studies, may eventually be adopted in low-income countries such as ours.

Author Contributions: Conceptualization, G.C. and G.A.d.A.; methodology, G.C., G.A.d.A. and A.F.B.; software, G.A.d.A.; validation, G.C., G.A.d.A., A.F.B. and A.G.D.C.; formal analysis, G.A.d.A., G.C. and A.F.B.; investigation, G.A.d.A. and G.C.; resources, G.A.d.A.; data curation, G.A.d.A. and G.C.; writing—original draft preparation, G.A.d.A.; writing—review and editing, G.C., A.F.B. and A.G.D.C.; visualization, G.A.d.A.; supervision, G.C.; project administration, G.C.; funding acquisition, G.C. All authors have read and agreed to the published version of the manuscript.

Funding: This research was supported by Coordenação de Aperfeiçoamento de Pessoal de Nível Superior-Brazil (CAPES)—Finance Code 001, São Paulo Research Foundation-Brazil (FAPESP)—grant no. 2013/07559-3 and 2015/03695-5, and the Brazilian National Council for Scientific and Technological Development (CNPq)—grant no. 304008/2021-4.

Institutional Review Board Statement: The study was conducted in accordance with the Declaration of Helsinki and approved by the Ethics Committee of the University of Campinas (CAAE 49976315.5.0000.5404).

Informed Consent Statement: Informed consent was obtained from all subjects involved in the study.

Data Availability Statement: fMRI data supporting the findings of this study are available from the corresponding author G.C. upon request.

Acknowledgments: We would like to thank all the participants of the study, physiotherapist Thais de Paulo for her help with the enrolled patients and Corina A. Fernandes for discussions on case series studies.

Conflicts of Interest: The authors declare no conflict of interest.

References

1. Whitehead, S.; Baalbergen, E. Post-Stroke Rehabilitation. *South Afr. Med. J.* **2019**, *109*, 81. [CrossRef]
2. Brewer, L.; Horgan, F.; Hickey, A.; Williams, D. Stroke Rehabilitation: Recent Advances and Future Therapies. *QJM* **2012**, *106*, 11–25. [CrossRef]
3. Jamison, J.; Ayerbe, L.; Di Tanna, G.L.; Sutton, S.; Mant, J.; De Simoni, A. Evaluating Practical Support Stroke Survivors Get With Medicines and Unmet Needs in Primary Care: A Survey. *BMJ Open* **2018**, *8*, e019874. [CrossRef] [PubMed]
4. Tsoupikova, D.; Stoykov, N.S.; Corrigan, M.; Thielbar, K.; Vick, R.; Li, Y.; Triandafilou, K.; Preuss, F.; Kamper, D. Virtual Immersion for Post-Stroke Hand Rehabilitation Therapy. *Ann. Biomed. Eng.* **2015**, *43*, 467–477. [CrossRef] [PubMed]
5. Lawrence, E.S.; Coshall, C.; Dundas, R.; Stewart, J.; Rudd, A.G.; Howard, R.; Wolfe, C.D.A. Estimates of the prevalence of acute stroke impairments and disability in a multiethnic population. *Stroke* **2001**, *32*, 1279–1284. [CrossRef] [PubMed]
6. Duncan Millar, J.; van Wijck, F.; Pollock, A.; Ali, M. Outcome measures in post-stroke arm rehabilitation trials: Do existing measures capture outcomes that are important to stroke survivors, carers, and clinicians? *Clin Rehabil.* **2019**, *33*, 737–749. [CrossRef] [PubMed]
7. Duncan, P.W.; Zorowitz, R.; Bates, B.; Choi, J.Y.; Glasberg, J.J.; Graham, G.D.; Katz, R.C.; Lamberty, K.; Reker, D. Management of Adult Stroke Rehabilitation Care. *Stroke* **2005**, *36*, e100–e143. [CrossRef] [PubMed]
8. Ohannessian, R.; Fortune, N.; Rodrigues, J.M.; Moulin, T.; Derex, L.; Madden, R.; Schott, A.-M. Coding Acute Stroke Care and Telestroke With the International Classification of Health Interventions (ICHI). *Int. J. Med. Inform.* **2017**, *108*, 9–12. [CrossRef] [PubMed]
9. Scheffler, E.; Mash, R. Surviving a Stroke in South Africa: Outcomes of Home-Based Care in a Low-Resource Rural Setting. *Top. Stroke Rehabil.* **2019**, *26*, 423–434. [CrossRef]
10. Cieza, A.; Causey, K.; Kamenov, K.; Hanson, S.W.; Chatterji, S.; Vos, T. Global Estimates of the Need for Rehabilitation Based on the Global Burden of Disease Study 2019: A Systematic Analysis for the Global Burden of Disease Study 2019. *Lancet* **2020**, *396*, 2006–2017. [CrossRef]
11. Belger, J. DC: Clinical Application of Immersive VR in Spatial Cognition: The Assessment of Spatial Memory and Unilateral Spatial Neglect in Neurological Patients. In Proceedings of the 2021 IEEE Conference on Virtual Reality and 3D User Interfaces Abstracts and Workshops (VRW), Lisbon, Portugal, 27 March–1 April 2021. [CrossRef]
12. Escalada-Hernández, P.; Soto Ruiz, N.; San Martín-Rodríguez, L. Design and Evaluation of a Prototype of Augmented Reality Applied to Medical Devices. *Int. J. Med. Inform.* **2019**, *128*, 87–92. [CrossRef] [PubMed]
13. Guerra, Z.F.; Bellose, L.C.; Coelho de Morais Faria, C.D.; Lucchetti, G. The Effects of Mental Practice Based on Motor Imagery for Mobility Recovery After Subacute Stroke: Protocol for a Randomized Controlled Trial. *Complement. Ther. Clin. Pract.* **2018**, *33*, 36–42. [CrossRef] [PubMed]
14. Langan, J.; Subryan, H.; Nwogu, I.; Cavuoto, L. Reported Use of Technology in Stroke Rehabilitation by Physical and Occupational Therapists. *Disabil. Rehabil. Assist. Technol.* **2017**, *13*, 641–647. [CrossRef] [PubMed]
15. Park, S.W.; Kim, J.H.; Yang, Y.-J. Mental Practice for Upper Limb Rehabilitation After Stroke: A Systematic Review and Meta-Analysis. *Int. J. Rehabil. Res.* **2018**, *41*, 197–203. [CrossRef] [PubMed]
16. Peters, T.M. Overview of Mixed and Augmented Reality in Medicine. *Mix. Augment. Real. Med.* **2018**, 1–13. [CrossRef]
17. Adamovich, S.V.; Fluet, G.G.; Tunik, E.; Merians, A.S. Sensorimotor Training in Virtual Reality: A Review. *NeuroRehabilitation* **2009**, *25*, 29–44. [CrossRef]
18. John, B.; Wickramasinghe, N. A Review of Mixed Reality in Health Care. *Healthc. Deliv. Inf. Age* **2019**, 375–382. [CrossRef]

19. Feitosa, J.A.; Fernandes, C.A.; Casseb, R.F.; Castellano, G. Effects of Virtual Reality-Based Motor Rehabilitation: A Systematic Review of FMRI Studies. *J. Neural Eng.* **2022**, *19*, 011002. [CrossRef]
20. Cole, D.M. Advances and Pitfalls in the Analysis and Interpretation of Resting-State FMRI Data. *Front. Syst. Neurosci.* **2010**, *8*. [CrossRef]
21. Griffanti, L.; Rolinski, M.; Szewczyk-Krolikowski, K.; Menke, R.A.; Filippini, N.; Zamboni, G.; Jenkinson, M.; Hu, M.T.; Mackay, C.E. Challenges in the Reproducibility of Clinical Studies With Resting State FMRI: An Example in Early Parkinson. *NeuroImage* **2016**, *124*, 704–713. [CrossRef]
22. De Blasi, B.; Caciagli, L.; Storti, S.F.; Galovic, M.; Koepp, M.; Menegaz, G.; Barnes, A.; Galazzo, I.B. Noise Removal in Resting-State and Task FMRI: Functional Connectivity and Activation Maps. *J. Neural Eng.* **2020**, *17*, 046040. [CrossRef]
23. Fox, M.D. Clinical Applications of Resting State Functional Connectivity. *Front. Syst. Neurosci.* **2010**, *19*. [CrossRef] [PubMed]
24. De Assis, G.A.; Corrêa, A.G.D.; Martins, M.B.R.; Pedrozo, W.G.; Lopes, R.d.D. An Augmented Reality System for Upper-Limb Post-Stroke Motor Rehabilitation: A Feasibility Study. *Disabil. Rehabil. Assist. Technol.* **2014**, *11*, 521–528. [CrossRef]
25. Ballester, B.R.; Nirme, J.; Duarte, E.; Cuxart, A.; Rodriguez, S.; Verschure, P.; Duff, A. The Visual Amplification of Goal-Oriented Movements Counteracts Acquired Non-Use in Hemiparetic Stroke Patients. *J. NeuroEng. Rehabil.* **2015**, *12*, 1–11. [CrossRef]
26. Grealy, M.A.; Cummings, J.; Quinn, K. The Effect of False Positive Feedback on Learning an Inhibitory-Action Task in Older Adults. *Exp. Aging Res.* **2019**, *45*, 346–356. [CrossRef] [PubMed]
27. Brauchle, D.; Vukelić, M.; Bauer, R.; Gharabaghi, A. Brain State-Dependent Robotic Reaching Movement With a Multi-Joint Arm Exoskeleton: Combining Brain-Machine Interfacing and Robotic Rehabilitation. *Front. Hum. Neurosci.* **2015**, *9*. [CrossRef]
28. Assis, G.; Brandao, A.; Correa, A.G.D.; Castellano, G. Evaluation of a Protocol for FMRI Assessment Associated With Augmented Reality Rehabilitation of Stroke Subjects. *J. Interact. Syst.* **2019**, *10*, 1. [CrossRef]
29. Wei, P.; Zhang, Z.; Lv, Z.; Jing, B. Strong Functional Connectivity Among Homotopic Brain Areas Is Vital for Motor Control in Unilateral Limb Movement. *Front. Hum. Neurosci.* **2017**, *11*, 366. [CrossRef]
30. Yeom, H.G.; Kim, J.S.; Chung, C.K. Brain Mechanisms in Motor Control During Reaching Movements: Transition of Functional Connectivity According to Movement States. *Sci. Rep.* **2020**, *10*, 567. [CrossRef]
31. De Campos, B.M.; Coan, A.C.; Lin Yasuda, C.; Casseb, R.F.; Cendes, F. Large-scale Brain Networks Are Distinctly Affected in Right and Left Mesial Temporal Lobe Epilepsy. *Hum. Brain Mapp.* **2016**, *37*, 3137–3152. [CrossRef]
32. Tzourio-Mazoyer, N.; Landeau, B.; Papathanassiou, D.; Crivello, F.; Etard, O.; Delcroix, N.; Mazoyer, B.; Joliot, M. Automated Anatomical Labeling of Activations in SPM Using a Macroscopic Anatomical Parcellation of the MNI MRI Single-Subject Brain. *NeuroImage* **2002**, *15*, 273–289. [CrossRef] [PubMed]
33. Harb, A.; Kishner, S. *Modified Ashworth Scale*; Springer StatPearls Publishing: Berlin/Heidelberg, Germany, 2022.
34. Deecke, L.; Kornhuber, H.H. An Electrical Sign of Participation of the Mesial 'supplementary' Motor Cortex in Human Voluntary Finger Movement. *Brain Res.* **1978**, *159*, 473–476. [CrossRef] [PubMed]
35. Alawieh, A.; Zhao, J.; Feng, W. Factors affecting post-stroke motor recovery: Implications on neurotherapy after brain injury. *Behav. Brain Res.* **2018**, *340*, 94–101. [CrossRef] [PubMed]
36. Song, J.; Young, B.M.; Nigogosyan, Z.; Walton, L.M.; Nair, V.A.; Grogan, S.W.; Tyler, M.E.; Farrar-Edwards, D.; Caldera, K.E.; Sattin, J.A.; et al. Characterizing Relationships of DTI, FMRI, and Motor Recovery in Stroke Rehabilitation Utilizing Brain-Computer Interface Technology. *Front. Neuroeng.* **2014**, *7*. [CrossRef]
37. Schuster-Amft, C.; Henneke, A.; Hartog-Keisker, B.; Holper, L.; Siekierka, E.; Chevrier, E.; Pyk, P.; Kollias, S.; Kiper, D.; Eng, K. Intensive Virtual Reality-Based Training for Upper Limb Motor Function in Chronic Stroke: A Feasibility Study Using a Single Case Experimental Design and FMRI. *Disabil. Rehabil. Assist. Technol.* **2014**, *10*, 385–392. [CrossRef]
38. Dong, Y.; Dobkin, B.H.; Cen, S.Y.; Wu, A.D.; Winstein, C.J. Motor Cortex Activation During Treatment May Predict Therapeutic Gains in Paretic Hand Function After Stroke. *Stroke* **2006**, *37*, 1552–1555. [CrossRef]
39. Ward, N.S. Neural Correlates of Motor Recovery After Stroke: A Longitudinal FMRI Study. *Brain* **2003**, *126*, 2476–2496. [CrossRef]
40. Johnson, N.N.; Carey, J.; Edelman, B.J.; Doud, A.; Grande, A.; Lakshminarayan, K.; He, B. Combined RTMS and Virtual Reality brain–computer Interface Training for Motor Recovery After Stroke. *J. Neural Eng.* **2018**, *15*, 016009. [CrossRef]
41. Xu, W.; Chu, B.; Rogers, E. Iterative Learning Control for Robotic-Assisted Upper Limb Stroke Rehabilitation in the Presence of Muscle Fatigue. *Control. Eng. Pract.* **2014**, *31*, 63–72. [CrossRef]
42. Su, F.; Xu, W. Enhancing Brain Plasticity to Promote Stroke Recovery. *Front. Neurol.* **2020**, *11*. [CrossRef]
43. Polese, J.C.; de Faria-Fortini, I.; Basilio, M.L.; Faria, G.S.E.; Teixeira-Salmela, L.F. Recruitment rate and retention of stroke subjects in cross-sectional studies. *Ciência Saúde Coletiva* **2017**, *22*, 255–260. [CrossRef]
44. Scianni, A.; Teixeira-Salmela, L.F.; Ada, L. Challenges in recruitment, attendance and adherence of acute stroke survivors to a randomized trial in Brazil: A feasibility study. *Braz. J. Phys. Ther.* **2012**, *16*, 40–45. [CrossRef] [PubMed]
45. Carcel, C.; Harris, K.; Peters, S.A.; Sandset, E.C.; Balicki, G.; Bushnell, C.D.; Howard, V.J.; Reeves, M.J.; Anderson, C.S.; Kelly, P.J.; et al. Representation of Women in Stroke Clinical Trials. *Neurology* **2021**, *97*. [CrossRef] [PubMed]
46. Belk, R. Extended Self in a Digital World. *J. Consum. Res.* **2013**, *40*, 477–500. [CrossRef]
47. Ahmed, K.E.-S.; Ambika, A.; Belk, R. Augmented reality magic mirror in the service sector: Experiential consumption and the self. *J. Serv. Manag.* **2023**, *34*, 56–77. [CrossRef]

48. Walker, M.E.; Szafir, D.; Rae, I. The Influence of Size in Augmented Reality Telepresence Avatars. In Proceedings of the 2019 IEEE Conference on Virtual Reality and 3D User Interfaces (VR), Osaka, Japan, 23–27 March 2019; pp. 538–546. [CrossRef]
49. Naji, S.; Jalab, H.; Kareem, S. A survey on skin detection in colored images. *Artif. Intell. Rev.* **2019**, *52*, 1041–1087. [CrossRef]
50. Fini, N.A.; Bernhardt, J.; Churilov, L.; Clark, R.; Holland, A.E. Adherence to physical activity and cardiovascular recommendations during the 2 years after stroke rehabilitation discharge. *Ann. Phys. Rehabil. Med.* **2021**, *64*, 101455. [CrossRef]
51. Aramaki, A.L.; Sampaio, R.F.; Reis, A.C.S.; Cavalcanti, A.; Dutra, F.C.M.S.E. Virtual reality in the rehabilitation of patients with stroke: An integrative review. *Arq. Neuro-Psiquiatr.* **2019**, *77*, 268–278. [CrossRef]

sensors

MDPI

Article

Use of Augmented Reality as a Tool to Support Cargo Handling Operations at the CARGO Air Terminal

Agnieszka A. Tubis *, Anna Jodejko-Pietruczuk and Tomasz Nowakowski

Department of Technical Systems Operation and Maintenance, Faculty of Mechanical Engineering, Wroclaw University of Science and Technology, Wyspianskiego Street 27, 50-370 Wroclaw, Poland; anna.jodejko@pwr.edu.pl (A.J.-P.); tomasz.nowakowski@pwr.edu.pl (T.N.)

* Correspondence: agnieszka.tubis@pwr.edu.pl

Abstract: (1) Background: A current trend observed in the logistics sector is the use of Industry 4.0 tools to improve and enhance the efficiency of cargo handling processes. One of the popular solutions is an augmented reality system that supports operators in everyday tasks. The article aims to present design assumptions for implementing an augmented reality system to support air cargo handling at the warehouse. (2) Methods: Research was carried out based on a five-stage analytical procedure, aiming to analyze the current state and identify the potential for implementing the AR system. The following methods were used to collect data: co-participant observations, process analysis, direct interviews, analysis of internal documentation, and applicable legal regulations. (3) Results: The conducted research allowed for identifying information flows accompanying cargo flows and developing a project to automate selected information flows. The obtained results made it possible to identify operations for which the AR system's implementation will increase their effectiveness and efficiency. (4) Conclusions: The obtained results identified the need to develop a hybrid algorithm for arranging cargo in the warehouse and to build a system supporting self-verification of markings on air cargo.

Keywords: AR technology; air transport; automatization; information flow; logistic processes

Citation: Tubis, A.A.; Jodejko-Pietruczuk, A.; Nowakowski, T. Use of Augmented Reality as a Tool to Support Cargo Handling Operations at the CARGO Air Terminal. *Sensors* **2024**, *24*, 1099. https://doi.org/10.3390/s24041099

Academic Editors: Calin Gheorghe Dan Neamtu, Radu Comes, Jing-Jing Fang and Dorin-Mircea Popovici

Received: 12 December 2023
Revised: 26 January 2024
Accepted: 6 February 2024
Published: 8 February 2024

1. Introduction

A current trend observed in the logistics sector is the use of Industry 4.0 tools to improve and enhance the efficiency of cargo handling processes. This trend, referred to as Logistics 4.0, is now an integral part of the development of the fourth industrial revolution. Logistics 4.0 uses new technologies to support the operation of traditional logistics systems [1]. Implemented cyber–physical solutions allow for improved cargo handling and introduce automation of storage system transportation and decentralized software control [2]. At the same time, the digitization of logistics processes enables companies to monitor material flows in real time and better handle handling units [3,4].

The importance of the Logistics 4.0 concept is growing, as evidenced by the steadily increasing number of publications in this area [5]. An important element of it is the digitization of warehouse-related processes. This is because warehousing is one of the primary logistics processes and is an essential part of the integration of all operations in the supply chain. As Hamdy et al. [6] point out, this process is a crucial part of product flows due to its involvement in achieving optimum and continuous operation of the production and distribution processes. For this reason, the digital solutions of Industry 4.0 are finding numerous applications in warehouse processes, and their implementation makes it possible to create smart warehouses, called Warehouses 4.0. According to the research presented in [7], the following solutions are most commonly used in these facilities: augmented reality (AR), RFID, Internet of Things, visual technology, and automated storage systems. Characteristics of storage facilities based on these solutions include, in particular, interoperability, virtualization, decentralization, real-time aspects, service orientation, modularity, and reconfigurability [8].

The implementation of improvements using Industry 4.0 solutions assumes particular importance in the case of handling cargo moved in transportation systems. In this handling, fast and precise identification of a shipment, real-time monitoring of its flow, coordinated operations performed in a fixed order according to an established procedure, and accurate information delivered to the operator in a readable form are of particular importance. In addition, in the case of air cargo handling, a critical element is the maintenance of safety procedures, short time slots for handling operations, and identification of markings for specific types of shipments that determine the application of specific handling procedures. For this reason, CARGO air cargo handling terminals are reporting a need for dedicated digital solutions to eliminate human error, reduce turnaround times for handling operations, and increase service efficiency.

The article's purpose is to present the design of functionality for an augmented reality system that will support the storage handling of air cargo. The published results are part of the research conducted under the project "A virtual support system for Cargo handling processes at airports, based on augmented reality technologies". The research was conducted in cooperation with a selected airport in Poland, which handles cargo in domestic and international distribution. The results presented in the article allow us to formulate the following main contributions:

- Identification of information flows related to air cargo handling at the CARGO terminal, along with identification of potential for automation.
- Formulation of the research procedure stages for the design of AR tools supporting air cargo handling.
- Presentation of the functionality design of an AR tool to support warehouse operators.
- Identification of challenges associated with the application of AR technology in air cargo handling.

Figure 1 shows the adopted structure of the article.

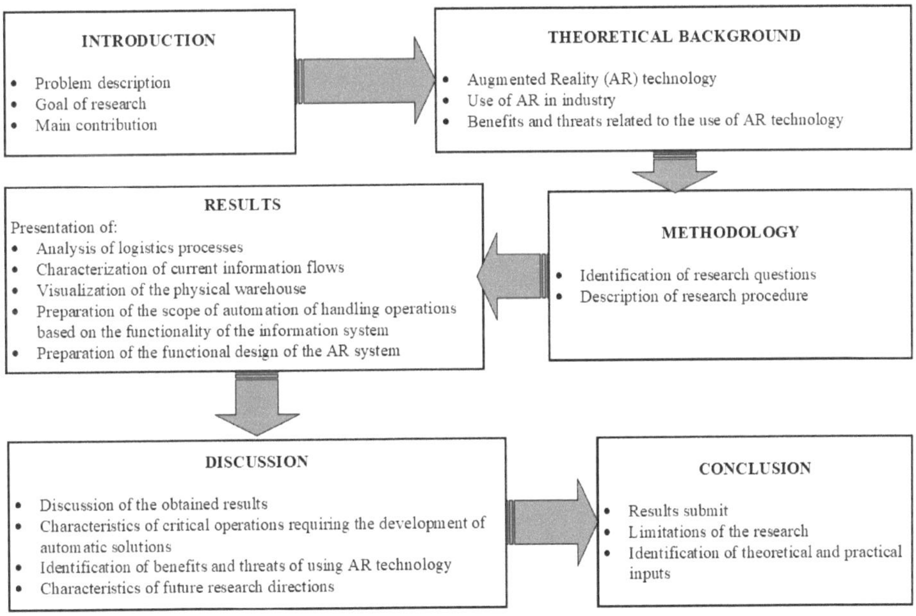

Figure 1. Structure of the article.

2. Theoretical Background

Augmented reality technology is one of the primary tools of Industry 4.0, the application of which is described in the areas of manufacturing [9], maintenance [10], and internal logistics systems [7]. AR technology allows a person to see a computer-generated virtual world that is simultaneously integrated with the real world. Thus, it can be said that AR tools can be used as an interface providing a link between digital information and the physical world [11]. Van Krevelan and Poelman went a step further in their definition, stating that AR "is an emerging technology with which a person can see more than others see, hear more than others hear, and perhaps even touch, smell and taste things that others cannot [12]". Daponte et al. [13], on the other hand, proposed a measurement approach to the definition of AR, defining it as a technology that enriches the user's sensory perception by showing information about the surrounding environment (e.g., physical quantities) that cannot be perceived with the five senses.

AR is a part of mixed reality [12]. That is, it is a form that combines real and virtual environments. Azuma et al. [14] pointed out three primary characteristics of an AR system: (a) it combines real-world and virtual objects, (b) it runs in real time, and (c) it allows interaction between users and virtual objects. The basic structure of an AR system consists of four elements [13]:

- A video camera that transmits an actual image of the environment in which the user is located.
- Tracking Module, which monitors the relative position and orientation of the camera in real time. This module can be based on every type of sensor technology: (1) 9D IMU (3-axis accelerometer, 3-axis gyroscope, and 3-axis magnetometer), (2) ultrasonic sensors, (3) video cameras, (4) GPS modules, and (5) RFID devices.
- Graphic Processing Module processes images captured by the video camera and adds virtual objects to them.
- Display provides users with an integrated image of the physical world combined with virtual objects.

Four visualization technologies are available on the market for AR systems [15]: head-mounted displays (HMDs), handheld devices (HHDs), static screens, and projectors. These systems can be stationary or mobile devices depending on the defined visualization task. The research results presented in [16] indicate that HMDs are the most applicable. Also, Masood et al.'s [15] research indicates that HMDs are the focus of research work and solutions implemented in industry. This is mainly due to the fact that their use does not restrict the operator's movement but instead allows hands-free access and reading of information, which significantly speeds up operations [17]. Nowadays, AR smart glasses (ARSGs) are increasingly being used, showing good potential for industrial applications [18]. ARSGs support the operator's work as they are equipped with numerous functions—from displaying information to tracking, distributing, and storing data about the surrounding environment and the user [19]. It is worth noting, however, that research results show (among others [16]) that most AR deployments occur on various devices. This is because many implementations render in a fixed computer and synchronize the real and virtual objects in a mobile device [16]. It should also be noted that creating an AR system from scratch is difficult and time-consuming. For this reason, several frameworks and platforms are available on the market that allow developers to focus on higher-level applications rather than low-level implementations. An example collection of such platforms is presented in [20].

Research by de Souza Cardoso et al. [16] shows that the primary areas of application of AR technology in industry are manual assembly, robot programming and operations, maintenance, process monitoring, training, process simulation, quality inspection, picking process, operational setup ergonomics, and safety. AR is therefore primarily used in processes for which it is possible to increase productivity by

- Providing flexible, hands-free, and real-time information delivery [21,22];
- Reducing the incidence of human error (e.g., incorrect picking, assembly, or maintenance) [23].

At the same time, the results show that most of the described applications did not consider the specifics of a particular sector but were concerned with supporting general industrial processes. There are, of course, AR solutions dedicated to the specifics of a particular industry. According to Cardoso et al.'s research, these usually apply to architecture, engineering, construction and facilities management (AEC/FM), aeronautics, automotives, electronics/automation, energy, government, logistics, marine, or mechanical aspects [16].

In logistics, the leading application area for AR is the picking process [24]. In this process, AR tools typically support the operator in reaching the right location and indicating the quantity to be picked [21,25,26]. Research indicates that using augmented reality to communicate order completion information improves time efficiency and picking accuracy (among others [27]). Stoltz et al. [28] prove in their research that the three other key warehouse processes also have great potential regarding use of AR. Although publications on the implementation of AR in receiving, storing, and shipping processes are currently very limited, according to Stoltz et al. [28], implementing this technology, in their case, will provide similar effects to those observed in the picking process.

Several publications have appeared in recent years to review the literature focused on using AR technology in logistics. Examples of such publications include [29,30]. These reviews argue that the main benefit of using AR in warehouse operations is primarily to increase visualization and product identification. Rejeb et al., based on their results, identified the main benefits of improving visualization and identification in warehouse processes [30]:

- Increased visual control and monitoring of products and stock-keeping units;
- Efficiency and potential cost savings through minimization of errors during product identification, losses, and damages;
- Increased efficiency and productivity through minimization of search time, mis-picks, fatigue, and errors;
- Efficient inventory management and order-picking processes through better visualization and guidance.

In addition, ref. [29] presented the benefits of using ARSGs in warehouse operations. The results of the analyses have made it possible to identify four areas where smart glasses add value to logistics processes. These include improvements in the following:

- Visualization: (a) the information displayed in the operators' field of view decreases task completion times by eliminating unnecessary head and body movement; (b) documenting all operator actions, continuous monitoring, naturally following the user's attention, providing more information;
- Interaction: (a) building safer and more productive work environments by promoting beneficial uses of technology for people; (b) being able to identify and mitigate risks with ARSGs; (c) improving human–environment interaction and human perception to complete tasks;
- User convenience: (a) efficient, versatile, and comfortable to wear; (b) does not distract workers; (c) enables hands-free access to information;
- Navigation: (a) ability to move quickly along optimized paths; (b) precise location and the ability to track position at all times; (c) easily find physical targets.

Several publications also present challenges and risks associated with implementing AR technology. According to the study in [29], many articles group these risks into three categories: technical, organizational, and ergonomic aspects. A more elaborate classification of challenges and constraints was formulated by de Souza Cardoso et al. [16], according to which there are five categories: users' health and acceptance; tracking methods; projection quality, accuracy, and interaction; hardware; and development complexity. Also noteworthy is the barrier classification presented by Stoltz et al. [28], who distinguish hardware limitations, software challenges, acceptance, and cost.

The literature review confirms that our research and the defined cognitive goal align with the current research trends. In turn, the adopted specification of the developed tool and its adaptation to the needs of air cargo handling processes fill the current research gap related to the need for more publications on adapting AR systems to the specifics of the studied sector.

3. Methods

The research team's task was to visualize the actual system handling cargo flow within the CARGO air terminal and identify logistics operations that can be supported by information technology, including AR technology. During the research, team members worked closely with air terminal employees from all levels of the organization—operators, team leaders, managers, and management. The research approach adopted made it possible to gather information on logistics processes, which were verified at different levels of management. As a result, the mapped processes and developed system recommendations considered the perspective of the operational position and the management of the entire supply chain.

The research procedure included five stages, which are shown in Figure 2. The research procedure was conducted to answer the following questions:

- RQ1: How is the air cargo handling process carried out at the CARGO terminal, what factors regulate its execution, and what information flows accompany the logistics operations performed?
- RQ2: Which information flows can be automated using an appropriate information system?
- RQ3: Which handling operations can be supported by augmented reality solutions, and how will this affect process execution?

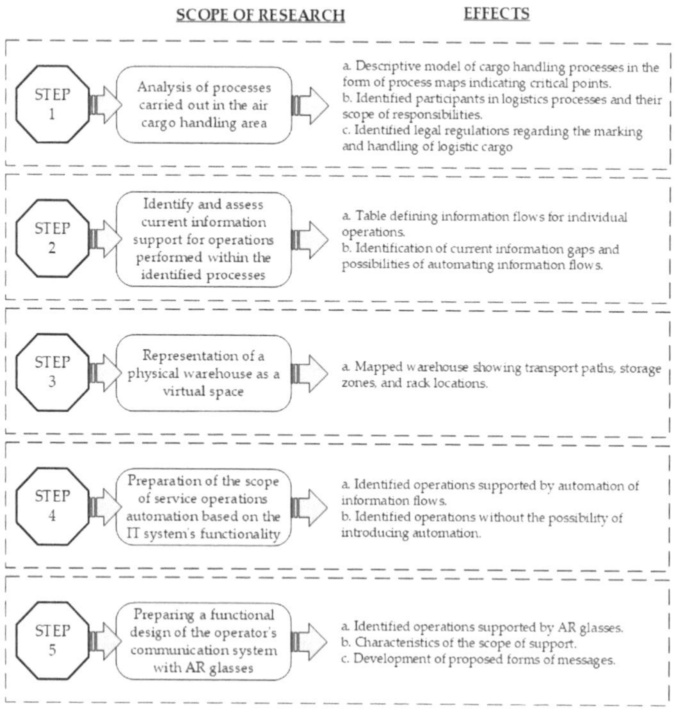

Figure 2. Research procedure.

For each step, the expected sub-results were formulated, the achievement of which was critical to achieving the formulated research objective.

Identification of the current model of the process information system, followed by its analysis from the point of view of the flows and form of transmitted information, were necessary to develop a system of support for the operator by AR technology in the process of cargo handling. Based on the process analysis, the main processes were identified in which the coordination of individual operations should be supported by the information system being developed. Organizational requirements and applicable operating procedures were determined for these processes based on training documentation for warehouse workers. Process maps and organizational requirements were established based on observations accompanying warehouse employees, face-to-face structured interviews conducted among team leaders and managers, and internal documentation of the CARGO terminal and applicable legislation.

Subsequently, the current level of information support for the various operations of the analyzed processes was identified and evaluated. Accompanying observations, direct interviews with employees and analysis of internal documentation were used to identify information flows. The scope of the identification carried out made it possible to create a knowledge base of information flows accompanying logistics operations and included

- Information feeding the implementation of operations;
- The current form of obtaining in-feed information;
- The person carrying out operations at the terminal;
- The type of authorization required to carry out the operation;
- Information generated as a result of the execution of the operation;
- The current form of the generated output information.

All identified feed information should be evaluated as necessary to implement the operation under analysis correctly. Thus, based on the compilation created, it was possible to identify the information gaps present and the potential for automating the process of information flow that accompanies cargo handling operations.

The conducted process analysis was the basis for designing the functionality of the information system, including the operator's communication with AR glasses. However, to ensure the system's required functionality, it is necessary to supplement the process map with a visualized physical object of the warehouse. The task of the information system is to support employees in managing the cargo flow in the warehouse area. Therefore, it is necessary to feed it with knowledge of available warehouse locations, dimensions, and locations in defined service zones. For the AR tool being created, the transport paths operators will use must also be mapped in the system. This necessitates the creation of virtual mapping of the warehouse with the marking of important points that are critical from the point of view of the moving operators and the loads handled.

In the following research stage, operations were specified for each of the processes identified in Stage 1, for which an automated cargo flow support system could be introduced. The scope of automation was determined for the highlighted operations, and the characteristics of the improvement to be introduced were prepared. The scope of automation was determined based on (1) the identified functionality of the WMS system, (2) potential opportunities identified in the analysis of similar market solutions, and (3) the identified demand resulting from the implementation of the AR tool. In addition, face-to-face interviews were conducted with experienced warehouse operators, based on which their information needs in handling operations were identified.

The following research stage focused primarily on developing guidelines for communication between the operator and AR glasses. To this end, critical operations (from the point of view of process continuity) and complicated operations (especially for a new employee) were identified, the implementation of which could be supported by AR technology. The extent of this support was determined based on the operations' characteristics and the demand reported by operators in the face-to-face interviews conducted. On this basis, the proposed functions of the AR system were formulated, along with their characteristics and the proposed form of messages.

4. Results

The project aims to develop a system to support air cargo handling using augmented reality technology. The developed AR system is to correspond to the specifics of the logistics processes carried out at air cargo terminals and the security requirements of air transport. Therefore, the first research stage concerning formulating assumptions for the created information system and AR-supporting cargo handling processes required testing in a real environment. For this purpose, a regional CARGO terminal handling air cargo in domestic and international transport was selected for the study. The terminal offers comprehensive air freight service, including special shipments, cargo security checks, and customs handling. However, it should be noted that the results obtained additionally included consultation with experts from other airports to ensure the conclusions' universality.

4.1. Stage 1—Analysis of Logistics Processes

The study identified two basic cargo handling processes carried out in the CARGO terminal area: (1) the process of handling imported air shipments and (2) the process of handling exported air shipments. Both of these processes were distinguished: eight logistics sub-processes for handling imported shipments (Figure 3) and nine sub-processes for handling exported shipments (Figure 4), which were described at the level of handling operations. Due to the formulated purpose of the article and the level of detail required in further research steps, the presented results do not present detailed process maps at the operational level but only present diagrams showing the order of the distinguished logistics sub-processes implemented within the two distinguished core processes. However, in presenting the results obtained in further research steps, references will appear already at the operational level.

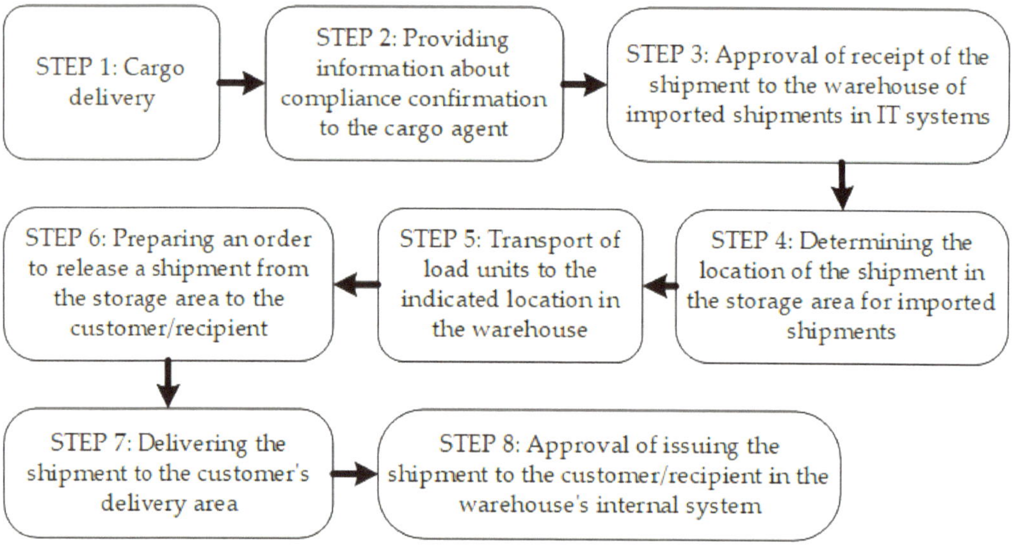

Figure 3. Sub-processes for handling imported shipments.

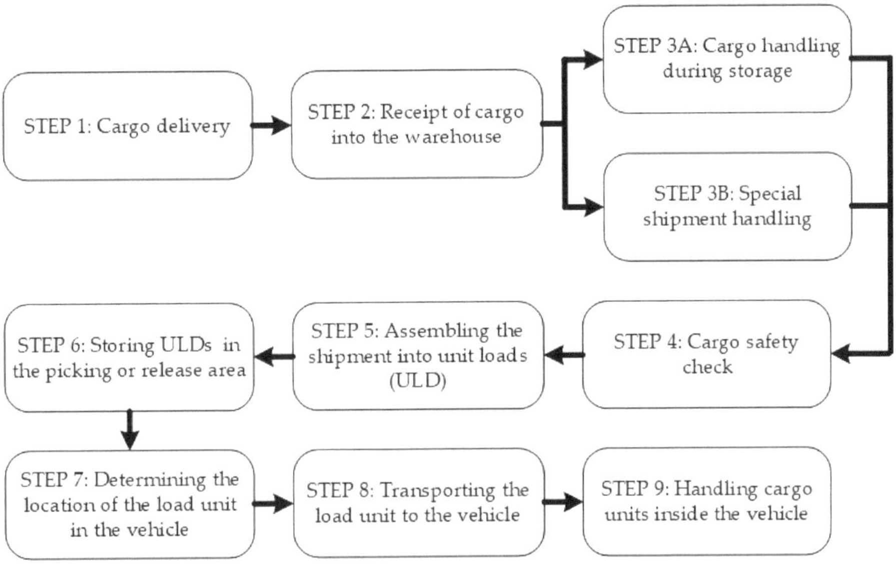

Figure 4. Sub-processes for handling exported shipments.

The analysis also made it possible to distinguish the primary actors involved in handling processes in the warehouse zone and to identify the roles assigned to them that are performed in the processes. These include the following:

- Shipper—a shipping company or direct shipper (e.g., a manufacturing company or an individual) responsible for handling the shipment in terms of booking a seat on the aircraft;
- Cargo agent—a person with the authority to handle shipments: WHA and/or LAR and/or DGR in category six and handling the respective internal transport and with authority to handle goods after security screening;
- Operator—a person with the authorization to handle the given internal transport and the mandatory Basic Cargo authorization and possible additional WHA and/or DGR category seven and/or eight authorizations to handle consignments after security control;
- Security Control employee—a person with DGR authorization in category 12 and to operate the Heimann X-ray viewer;
- Customs and Revenue employee—a person with authorization for customs and revenue handling of imported and exported shipments.

Based on Basic Cargo's training documentation, the documents applicable to air cargo handling were defined. The air waybill (AWB), Cargo Manifest, Cargo Damage Report—CDR, and other documents accompanying air cargo handling were analyzed. At the same time, the general conditions for acceptance of goods and the applicable rules for the classification of cargo according to the IATA guidelines were defined. In accordance with them, air transport distinguishes shipments of, among others, general cargo, AVI—Live Animals, DG—Dangerous goods, HUM—Human Remains, PER—Perishable Cargo, TCR—Temperature Control, DIP—Diplomatic, and VAL—Valuable cargo. These shipments are specially marked with graphic symbols and subject to special packaging procedures, which are inspected in detail before the shipment is released for export. In particular, this applies to hazardous materials, which are marked with additional symbols and letter markings, the identification of which should be assisted by AR technology. Classification of shipment types is important from the point of view of the handling procedures implemented, which will have to be mapped in the augmented reality system.

Guidelines have also been developed for labeling and information that should be placed on cargo packages. These are critical elements for the designed AR system, which these markings must identify to support the operator.

4.2. Stage 2—Characterization of Current Information Flows

All information flows were identified according to the knowledge base structure presented in Section 2. A spreadsheet was used to record the data, which allowed quick analysis and grouping of the collected characteristics. A separate spreadsheet was created for each of the identified sub-processes. Sample characteristics for the selected process are shown in Table 1.

Table 1. Knowledge base about information flows accompanying logistics operations in the CARGO terminal.

PROCESS: DELIVERY OF THE SHIPMENT TO THE WAREHOUSE			
Operation: Verification of shipment data delivered to the warehouse			
Person performing the operation (current form): Cargo agent			
Information supporting the implementation of operations	The current form of obtaining supporting information	Information generated after the operation is completed	The current form of the output information generated
details of the person transporting the shipment/driver	sent e-mail from the sender—no standard form	confirmation of data compliance/determination of inconsistency	verbal message given to the operator along with the order to unload the shipment/telephone contact with the sender of the shipment
registration number of the long-distance transport vehicle	CMR (road transport document) or other consignment note		
shipper			
number of loading units in the shipment			

Analysis of the collected data made it possible to identify current information gaps that may be the source of adverse events. The results also made it possible to assess the efficiency and resilience of the process to the disruptions occurring. The potential for improvement and opportunities for automation of selected operations were identified on this basis.

4.3. Stage 3—Visualization of the Physical Warehouse

Visualization of the warehouse means a digital representation of its volume (length, width, and height) but also the adopted scheme of organizational flows, considering the people involved, the equipment, and the specifics of the cargo handled. The visualization of the studied object is shown in Figure 5.

The visualization of the investigated warehouse includes ten storage zones, which have been designated as blocks in the system, a collection of adjacent storage locations. Each block in the system has its characteristics, including (a) the number/name of the block; (b) the number of rack spaces in the X dimension (rack depth); (c) the number of rack spaces in the Y dimension (block width); and (d) the number of rack spaces in the Z dimension (block height). Designated storage zones refer to

- storage of export goods without SPX (Block M, Block O, and Block P);
- storage of export goods with SPX (Block A and Block T);
- refrigerated goods warehouse (Block G);
- frozen goods warehouse (Block H);
- customs warehouse (Block J);
- storage of radioactive goods and valuable shipments (Block S).

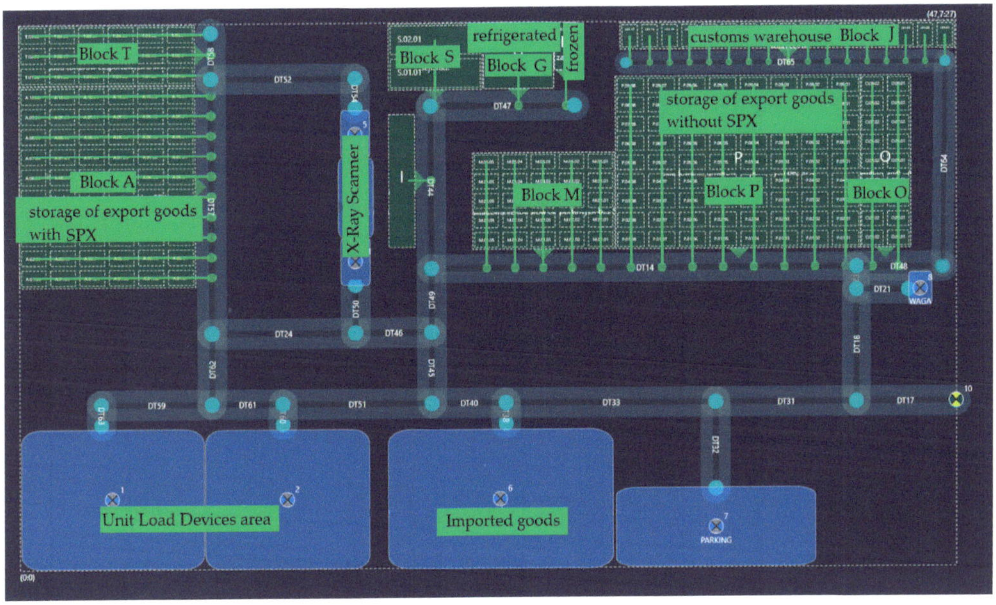

Figure 5. Visualization of the warehouse.

To serve the designed warehouse, 30 transport routes have been defined. Each road has its characteristics in the system, including (a) name/number of the transport road; (b) X and Y coordinates for marking the beginning and end of the road; (c) numbers of blocks and storage areas accessible from the road; and (d) numbers of other transport roads accessible from the road.

In addition, within the warehouse, the zones for construction of air pallets, preparation and unloading of air pallets, security check station, security check end locations, security check start location, import storage, parking, scale, and warehouse gate were designated. Points identified in these zones were noted with X and Y coordinates.

4.4. Stage 4—Preparation of the Scope of Automation of Handling Operations Based on the Functionality of the Information System

Logistics operators use various ERP and WMS systems. Therefore, in determining the potential opportunities for automation, the research team was guided by best practices in various warehouse systems and the specifics of cargo handled in air transportation. At the same time, the potential to automate information flows was validated by the functionality of available IT solutions, the analysis of which was carried out in preparation for the study.

The design of the functionality of the information system supporting cargo flow management was considered separately for export and import shipments. The scope of the automation of handling operations for export shipments concerned the analysis of six logistics processes related to handling such cargo, while five processes were analyzed for import shipments. For each process, operations were identified where automation of information flow was proposed. For each proposal, the expected effects of improving process execution were indicated. Table 2 shows the proposed scope of automation for the process "Receipt of cargo to the warehouse". Analogous studies were prepared for the other processes.

As a result of the analysis, it was also possible to identify currently impossible operations to automate for the warehouse under study. An example of such an operation in the described process of receiving cargo to the warehouse was entering comments and signing the CMR document. However, it should be noted that such results of the analysis do not exclude the possibility of introducing automatic solutions in the future. Their introduction requires one in many cases, procedural changes (often resulting from existing regulations), as well as costly infrastructure changes.

Table 2. Proposed scope of automation for the process "Receipt of cargo to the warehouse".

Operation	Scope of Automation	Justification
Checking whether the vehicle's seal has not been broken	Automatic ticket generation when a seal violation is detected	Ensuring registration of information on verification processes carried out in the system. Possibility to archive information about detected nonconformities and actions taken.
Checking for damage in each load unit	Identification of damaged load units in the process—e.g., an automatically printed sticker with a local shipment number confirming its damage	Ensuring registration of information on verification processes carried out in the system. Possibility to archive information about detected nonconformities and actions taken
Measurement of the maximum length, width, height, and weight of each accepted load unit and verification of shipment parameters.	Automatic ticket generation with detected damages (connection to the sender's key)	Registration of order status. Possibility to archive information about detected inconsistencies. Tracking the history of changes.
Preparation of the admission protocol	Assigning data to the shipment_id in the system and automatic redirection to verification of parameters	The measurement results of the unit after entering the system are the basis for verifying the data contained in the notification. The data are used to indicate the location of the warehouse.
Checking whether the vehicle's seal has not been broken	Automatic ticket generation in case of non-compliance	Registration of order status. Possibility to archive information about detected inconsistencies. Tracking the history of changes.
Checking for damage in each load unit	Automatic generation of the admission report	The cargo agent's acceptance of the entered and verified data in the system results in the automatic generation of an acceptance protocol

4.5. Stage 5—Preparation of the Functionality Design of the AR System

The functionality design of the AR system was developed based on the results of the process analysis, the scope of implementation of automation of handling operations, and the analysis of the functionality of AR tools available on the market. For each operation indicated to be handled using AR technology, the scope of support, the characteristics of the support, and the form of communication between the operator and the glasses were defined. Table 3 presents a summary of all the operations supported by the AR tool.

Table 3. Operations supported by the AR tool.

Operation	Scope of Support	Description	Message Proposal
PROCESS: DELIVERY OF THE SHIPMENT TO THE WAREHOUSE			
Verification of shipment data delivered to the warehouse	Displaying to the operator a message about an order to unload a shipment with the specified CMR or AWB, along with an indication of the place of unloading the goods	Message about an unloading order should appear in an additional panel (e.g., in the form of an upper bar with icons), along with the date and time of receipt, status, and place of unloading. After selecting the order, navigation to the unloading place should be started.	Graphic form to signal a new order (icon notifying about a new order). Navigation (e.g., showing the way with arrows)
PROCESS: RECEPTION OF LOADS INTO THE WAREHOUSE			
Checking whether the vehicle's seal has not been broken	Reporting the need to check the seal	Message about the next step in the service procedure	Text message: "Check the seal". Graphic icon indicating task completion (e.g., thumbs up)
Checking for damage in each load unit	Registration of information about damaged cargo. Possibility to take a photo of the damage.	Message about the next step in the service procedure. Function of taking a photo of the damage using AR glasses and sending it to the system	Text message: "Damaged?" with the option to select "YES/NO". A graphic form of the "take a photo of the damage" message after selecting the YES option
Measurement of the maximum length, width, height, and weight of each accepted load unit and verification of shipment parameters.	Reporting the need to perform a measurement	Message about the next step in the service procedure. Delivering cargo to measuring devices.	A graphic icon indicating the need for measurement. Navigate with arrows. A graphic icon indicating that the task has been completed
Preparation of the admission protocol	Preparation of the admission protocol	Message about the generated protocol with the option to confirm or report an error	Graphic icons: Green for acceptance and red for rejection (in case of rejection, you must indicate the protocol field that requires change)
PROCESS: STORAGE			
Determining the location and transport of the load to the storage area	Indicating the storage area and leading to the indicated location	Message with the designation of the storage area. Delivery to the indicated location.	Text message: "Transport to" + storage box symbol. Navigate with arrows.
Special shipment verification	Verification of graphic markings on the shipment (e.g., checking whether the shipment contains all required markings)	Message about the required graphic markings on the shipment in accordance with its specifications.	Graphic icons: green—complete marking; red—incomplete
PROCESS: SAFETY CONTROL			
Transport of the shipment to the X-ray machine	Identification of a free X-ray machine and delivery to its location	Message informing about the need to perform a security check. Delivery to the indicated location.	Graphic icon of an X-ray machine. Navigate with arrows.
Determining the location and transport of the load to the storage area	Indication of the storage area and delivery to the indicated location	Message with the designation of the storage area. Delivery to the indicated location.	Text message: "Transport to" + storage box symbol. Navigate with arrows.

Table 3. *Cont.*

Operation	Scope of Support	Description	Message Proposal
PROCESS: PICKING			
Printout of the picking list	Display of items from the picking list with status	The system should include a module of picking lists with their implementation status (e.g., to be implemented, in progress, or completed) and priority. For each list, there should be an "Execute" option, which will open the given list	The list is presented in text form. Graphical icon for "Execute"
Collection of empty ULDs and their transport	Indication of the need for ULD	Displaying the number of ULDs needed to be downloaded (continuously updated)	Text message: "Download X ULDs"
Transport of shipments to the picking zone	Indicating the storage area and leading to the indicated location	Message with the designation of the storage area. Delivery to the indicated location.	Text message: "Transport to" + storage box symbol. Navigate with arrows.
Placing the shipment on ULD	Indicating the location of the shipment on the ULD	The place of storage is indicated by the displayed solid outline. Updating the picking list after the shipment has been placed in the indicated place.	Graphic icon indicating task completion (e.g., thumbs up)
ULD protection	Indication of required security measures for ULD	Display a reminder to apply security measures. The system should include requirements regarding the security measures used for particular types of cargo.	List of requirements presented in text form. A graphic icon symbolizing a security check
Storage of completed ULDs	Indication of the storage area and delivery to the selected location	Message with the designation of the storage area. Delivery to the indicated location.	Text message: "Transport to" + storage box symbol. Navigate with arrows.
PROCESS: RELEASE FOR TRANSPORT			
Transporting the ULD to the vehicle	Delivery to vehicle	Message of release for transport. Support for delivery to the vehicle parking location	Graphic icon indicating release for transport. Navigation by arrows.
Placement and securing of ULDs inside the vehicle	Support for correct ULD stowage and verification of correct cargo securing	Message about the ULD stowage location and verification of correct stowage, displaying a message about the need to secure the cargo	Indicating the location of stowage with the help of the outline of the lump. Text message: "Check ULD security". Graphic icon indicating the completion of the task

5. Discussion

The results presented in Section 4 allow us to conclude that the article's aim has been achieved. Based on the analyses and observations, the air cargo handling process at the CARGO terminal was characterized. On this basis, the specifics of the handling operations and the conditions under which they are carried out were identified. This made it possible to identify those parts of the process that generate a need for information support, often in real time, and for which the introduction of an AR system would be justified. Among the most important issues concerning the specifics of air cargo handling processes are the following:

- the lack of fixed storage locations, causing difficulties in the distribution and picking of cargo in a short period;
- the large number of variables determining the location of cargo in the warehouse—(a) the timing of cargo release for transport; (b) the location of cargo from other sources that will be placed in common transport packages; (c) the weight, size, and type of cargo;
- the wide range of markings used for goods transported by air.

Considering the specificities of air cargo handling in the CARGO zone identified in this way, a functionality was proposed for the AR system that would support the execution of selected operations in the five defined phases of warehouse handling.

First of all, it should be emphasized that the results obtained in the research indicate a high demand for the automation of information flows and a high potential for AR technology to support warehouse service personnel. The process analysis and the identified need for real-time information delivery made it possible to identify critical operations whose support in the form of automation of collection, sharing, and processing will significantly affect the effectiveness and efficiency of the implementation of the entire process. Operations related to identifying air cargo were considered critical, particularly aspects related to recognizing markings for special shipments, which require an appropriate handling procedure. Therefore, it is necessary to develop a system to support the verification of the correctness of air cargo markings. This system should have the following functionality:

- detection of markings applied to a given shipment or baggage;
- indication of missing markings;
- identification of irregularities in applied markings (e.g., incorrect orientation, mislabeling, soiling, and damage).

The second critical operation is to identify and guide the operator to the correct location where the cargo should be stored. The distribution of cargo in warehouses handling air cargo is an NP hard problem due to the complexity and multidimensional nature of the processes involved. The process analysis indicated that the optimization of cargo distribution in the storage area cannot be based on traditional methods described in the literature due to the specificity of cargo flows in air cargo handling. Specific handling conditions determine all the logistical processes related to air cargo deployment, storage, picking, and loading. Important factors determining these processes include the following:

- varying handling requirements resulting from, among other things, the physical characteristics of shipments (e.g., maximum pressures), but also specific customer requirements;
- heavily heterogeneous cargoes that make it difficult to group and distribute cargoes in a shared space—including irregularity of shape and the need to ensure isolation of cargoes from other cargo groups;
- organizational impediments—taking into account the priority of the shipment due to the timing of transport and the need to load several shipments on one ULD (e.g., described by one AWB or sent to one intermediate or final destination).

At the same time, the loading stage was considered to be a critical process for handling air shipments. This is because, in the case of air transport, there is the problem of optimizing loading in a limited space, in which a known set of heterogeneous cargo units must be loaded into a known number of (usually) heterogeneous containers (available ULDs) under additional constraints arising from the specifics of air transport and with the most uniform loading of all ULDs. Therefore, considering the identified air-transport-specific requirements, developing a hybrid algorithm to optimize cargo flows in the service area is necessary. Both of the above scopes of required research will be the subject of further analysis by the project team. These studies complement the AR system under development but are critical to optimizing the handling process and will primarily provide the developed solution functionality that reflects the specifics of air cargo handling at the CARGO terminal.

Preliminary tests conducted to assist warehouse operators with smart AR glasses confirm the results of studies reported in the literature (e.g., in [21,25,26,29,30]). Workers with little experience get to the designated location faster and make fewer mistakes when handling cargo. Above all, the operation of verifying a special shipment is shortened, which also has a positive effect on the safety of the operations undertaken. The accompanying observations and interviews with test participants also identified potential risks and limitations to using ARSG. They also align with the limitations described in the literature (e.g., in [15,16,28,29]) and concern technical, organizational, and ergonomic aspects. In particular, emerging fatigue in operators using ARSGs and the operator's limited field of vision with AR glasses are significant risks. The battery life with which ARSGs are equipped also proved to be a significant barrier. On the other hand, the formulated challenge for the tool under development is developing a suitable visualization method to ensure the readability of the messages delivered and enable smooth tracking of the operations performed.

6. Conclusions

The results presented in the article answer the research questions posed in Section 3. The process analysis made it possible to determine the sequence and scope of handling operations and define the specific conditions for air cargo logistics handling. Thanks to the created map of information flows, the currently existing information gaps in the studied processes were determined, and, above all, the scope of the required automation of information flows supporting the work of operators in the warehouse was formulated. At the same time, the potential for applying AR technology as a tool to support air cargo handling in individual logistics procedures was defined.

The limitation of the presented results is the focus of attention on the studied physical system, taking into account the specifics of the selected air terminal. The authors tried to include a broader view in their analysis by verifying the obtained results with experts employed at other air cargo terminals, but the identified information gaps and potential for automation were formulated based on the evaluation of this specific case. Therefore, future research needs to verify the assumptions made for other real-world facilities where logistics processes may be more complex and diverse.

The results presented provide knowledge for the scientific and business community. From a scientific point of view, the article provides knowledge regarding the specifics of handling cargo flows in air cargo warehouse operations and the challenges of considering them in the developed AR solutions to be applied to the described system. For industry representatives, the results regarding the formulated design assumptions and the scope of possible application of AR tools in the ground handling of air cargo may be of interest. Preliminary results were also presented as part of the discussion, confirming a reduction in the time taken by operations and eliminating operator errors. These arguments may encourage industry representatives to implement augmented reality in their logistics systems. Attention was also drawn to the risks and limitations involved. This information may be relevant for managers formulating functional assumptions for the AR tool under development.

Author Contributions: Conceptualization, A.A.T. and A.J.-P.; methodology, A.A.T. and A.J.-P.; validation, A.A.T. and A.J.-P.; formal analysis, A.A.T., T.N. and A.J.-P.; investigation, A.A.T. and A.J.-P.; data curation, A.A.T. and A.J.-P.; writing—original draft preparation, A.A.T., T.N. and A.J.-P.; writing—review and editing, A.A.T. visualization, A.A.T.; project administration, A.J.-P. All authors have read and agreed to the published version of the manuscript.

Funding: This research was funded by the National Centre for Research and Development, grant number POIR.04.01.04-00-0065/20.

Institutional Review Board Statement: Not applicable.

Informed Consent Statement: Not applicable.

Data Availability Statement: Data are contained within the article.

Conflicts of Interest: The authors declare no conflicts of interest.

References

1. Facchini, F.; Oleśków-Szłapka, J.; Ranieri, L.; Urbinati, A. A Maturity Model for Logistics 4.0: An Empirical Analysis and a Roadmap for Future Research. *Sustainability* **2019**, *12*, 86. [CrossRef]
2. Winkelhaus, S.; Grosse, E.H. Logistics 4.0: A Systematic Review towards a New Logistics System. *Int. J. Prod. Res.* **2020**, *58*, 18–43. [CrossRef]
3. Tubis, A.A.; Grzybowska, K. In Search of Industry 4.0 and Logistics 4.0 in Small-Medium Enterprises—A State of the Art Review. *Energies* **2022**, *15*, 8595. [CrossRef]
4. Tubis, A.A.; Grzybowska, K.; Król, B. Supply Chain in the Digital Age: A Scientometric–Thematic Literature Review. *Sustainability* **2023**, *15*, 11391. [CrossRef]
5. Bigliardi, B.; Casella, G.; Bottani, E. Industry 4.0 in the Logistics Field: A Bibliometric Analysis. *IET Collab. Intell. Manuf.* **2021**, *3*, 4–12. [CrossRef]
6. Hamdy, W.; Al-Awamry, A.; Mostafa, N. Warehousing 4.0: A Proposed System of Using Node-Red for Applying Internet of Things in Warehousing. *Sustain. Futures* **2022**, *4*, 100069. [CrossRef]
7. Tubis, A.A.; Rohman, J. Intelligent Warehouse in Industry 4.0—Systematic Literature Review. *Sensors* **2023**, *23*, 4105. [CrossRef] [PubMed]
8. Zoubek, M.; Simon, M. Evaluation of the Level and Readiness of Internal Logistics for Industry 4.0 in Industrial Companies. *Appl. Sci.* **2021**, *11*, 6130. [CrossRef]
9. Zigart, T.; Schlund, S. Evaluation of Augmented Reality Technologies in Manufacturing—A Literature Review. In *Advances in Human Factors and Systems Interaction. AHFE 2020. Advances in Intelligent Systems and Computing*; Nunes, I., Ed.; Springer: Berlin/Heidelberg, Germany, 2020; Volume 1207, pp. 75–82.
10. Palmarini, R.; Erkoyuncu, J.A.; Roy, R.; Torabmostaedi, H. A Systematic Review of Augmented Reality Applications in Maintenance. *Robot Comput. Integr. Manuf.* **2018**, *49*, 215–228. [CrossRef]
11. Song, Y.; Koeck, R.; Luo, S. Review and Analysis of Augmented Reality (AR) Literature for Digital Fabrication in Architecture. *Autom. Constr.* **2021**, *128*, 103762. [CrossRef]
12. Van Krevelen, D.W.F.; Poelman, R. A Survey of Augmented Reality Technologies, Applications and Limitations. *Int. J. Virtual Real.* **2010**, *9*, 1. [CrossRef]
13. Daponte, P.; De Vito, L.; Picariello, F.; Riccio, M. State of the Art and Future Developments of the Augmented Reality for Measurement Applications. *Measurement* **2014**, *57*, 53–70. [CrossRef]
14. Azuma, R.; Baillot, Y.; Behringer, R.; Feiner, S.; Julier, S.; MacIntyre, B. Recent Advances in Augmented Reality. *IEEE Comput. Graph. Appl.* **2001**, *21*, 34–47. [CrossRef]
15. Masood, T.; Egger, J. Augmented Reality in Support of Industry 4.0—Implementation Challenges and Success Factors. *Robot Comput. Integr. Manuf.* **2019**, *58*, 181–195. [CrossRef]
16. de Souza Cardoso, L.F.; Mariano, F.C.M.Q.; Zorzal, E.R. A Survey of Industrial Augmented Reality. *Comput. Ind. Eng.* **2020**, *139*, 106159. [CrossRef]
17. Syberfeldt, A.; Holm, M.; Danielsson, O.; Wang, L.; Brewster, R.L. Support Systems on the Industrial Shop-Floors of the Future—Operators' Perspective on Augmented Reality. *Procedia CIRP* **2016**, *44*, 108–113. [CrossRef]
18. Danielsson, O.; Holm, M.; Syberfeldt, A. Augmented Reality Smart Glasses in Industrial Assembly: Current Status and Future Challenges. *J. Ind. Inf. Integr.* **2020**, *20*, 100175. [CrossRef]
19. Hofmann, B.; Haustein, D.; Landeweerd, L. Smart-Glasses: Exposing and Elucidating the Ethical Issues. *Sci. Eng. Ethics* **2017**, *23*, 701–721. [CrossRef]
20. Devagiri, J.S.; Paheding, S.; Niyaz, Q.; Yang, X.; Smith, S. Augmented Reality and Artificial Intelligence in Industry: Trends, Tools, and Future Challenges. *Expert Syst. Appl.* **2022**, *207*, 118002. [CrossRef]
21. Guo, A.; Raghu, S.; Xie, X.; Ismail, S.; Luo, X.; Simoneau, J.; Gilliland, S.; Baumann, H.; Southern, C.; Starner, T. A Comparison of Order Picking Assisted by Head-up Display (HUD), Cart-Mounted Display (CMD), Light, and Paper Pick List. In Proceedings of the 2014 ACM International Symposium on Wearable Computers, ACM, New York, NY, USA, 13 September 2014; pp. 71–78.
22. Hou, L.; Wang, X. A Study on the Benefits of Augmented Reality in Retaining Working Memory in Assembly Tasks: A Focus on Differences in Gender. *Autom. Constr.* **2013**, *32*, 38–45. [CrossRef]
23. Wang, X.; Ong, S.K.; Nee, A.Y.C. Multi-Modal Augmented-Reality Assembly Guidance Based on Bare-Hand Interface. *Adv. Eng. Inform.* **2016**, *30*, 406–421. [CrossRef]

24. Egger, J.; Masood, T. Augmented Reality in Support of Intelligent Manufacturing—A Systematic Literature Review. *Comput. Ind. Eng.* **2020**, *140*, 106195. [CrossRef]
25. Hanson, R.; Falkenström, W.; Miettinen, M. Augmented Reality as a Means of Conveying Picking Information in Kit Preparation for Mixed-Model Assembly. *Comput. Ind. Eng.* **2017**, *113*, 570–575. [CrossRef]
26. Zywicki, K.; Bun, P. Process of Materials Picking Using Augmented Reality. *IEEE Access* **2021**, *9*, 102966–102974. [CrossRef]
27. Reif, R.; Günthner, W.A.; Schwerdtfeger, B.; Klinker, G. Evaluation of an Augmented Reality Supported Picking System Under Practical Conditions. *Comput. Graph. Forum* **2010**, *29*, 2–12. [CrossRef]
28. Stoltz, M.-H.; Giannikas, V.; McFarlane, D.; Strachan, J.; Um, J.; Srinivasan, R. Augmented Reality in Warehouse Operations: Opportunities and Barriers. *IFAC-PapersOnLine* **2017**, *50*, 12979–12984. [CrossRef]
29. Rejeb, A.; Keogh, J.G.; Leong, G.K.; Treiblmaier, H. Potentials and Challenges of Augmented Reality Smart Glasses in Logistics and Supply Chain Management: A Systematic Literature Review. *Int. J. Prod. Res.* **2021**, *59*, 3747–3776. [CrossRef]
30. Rejeb, A.; Keogh, J.G.; Wamba, S.F.; Treiblmaier, H. The Potentials of Augmented Reality in Supply Chain Management: A State-of-the-Art Review. *Manag. Rev. Q.* **2021**, *71*, 819–856. [CrossRef]

virtual worlds

MDPI

Article

An Augmented Reality Application for Wound Management: Enhancing Nurses' Autonomy, Competence and Connectedness

Carina Albrecht-Gansohr, Lara Timm, Sabrina C. Eimler and Stefan Geisler *

Institute of Positive Computing, Hochschule Ruhr West—University of Applied Sciences, 46236 Bottrop, Germany; carina.gansohr@hs-ruhrwest.de (C.A.-G.); lara.timm@hs-ruhrwest.de (L.T.); sabrina.eimler@hs-ruhrwest.de (S.C.E.)

* Correspondence: stefan.geisler@hs-ruhrwest.de

Abstract: The use of Augmented Reality glasses opens up many possibilities in hospital care, as they facilitate treatments and their documentation. In this paper, we present a prototype for the HoloLens 2 supporting wound care and documentation. It was developed in a participatory process with nurses using the positive computing paradigm, with a focus on the improvement of the working conditions of nursing staff. In a qualitative study with 14 participants, the factors of autonomy, competence and connectedness were examined in particular. It was shown that good individual adaptability and flexibility of the system with respect to the work task and personal preferences lead to a high degree of autonomy. The availability of the right information at the right time strengthens the feeling of competence. On the one hand, the connection to patients is increased by the additional information in the glasses, but on the other hand, it is hindered by the unusual appearance of the device and the lack of eye contact. In summary, the potential of Augmented Reality glasses in care was confirmed, and approaches for a well-being-centered system design were identified but, at the same time, a number of future research questions, including the effects on patients, were also identified.

Keywords: positive computing; augmented reality; wound management; interaction work; HoloLens 2; self-determination theory; autonomy; competence; connectedness

Citation: Albrecht-Gansohr, C.; Timm, L.; Eimler, S.C.; Geisler, S. An Augmented Reality Application for Wound Management: Enhancing Nurses' Autonomy, Competence and Connectedness. *Virtual Worlds* **2024**, 3, 208–229. https://doi.org/10.3390/virtualworlds3020011

Academic Editors: Radu Comes, Dorin-Mircea Popovici, Calin Gheorghe Dan Neamtu and Jing-Jing Fang

Received: 2 February 2024
Revised: 20 March 2024
Accepted: 29 May 2024
Published: 3 June 2024

1. Introduction

Nowadays, employees in the nursing profession are confronted with an immense workload resulting from rising patient numbers [1] and a shortage of skilled professionals [2]. Economic requirements, compliance with standards and bureaucratic regulations are making the nursing processes increasingly complex [3,4]. All these factors have to be reconciled with the need to provide good, humane care that responds to patients' individual needs [5]. Digitalization holds opportunities to improve the situation as an adequate solution that can release resources for individual patient care, and result in a higher quality of work and relief of secondary tasks.

In line with this, new approaches to use technologies, such as extended reality, are now entering the healthcare sector [6–9]. Among them, Augmented Reality (AR) glasses are a promising technology to support nursing processes [7]. Based on the framework for task–technology fit, a model which suggests a strong connection between the requirements of a task and the characteristics of a technology when it comes to adoption and human performance, AR glasses are advantageous to optimize the use of space, as well as for tasks that need to be performed in a timely, hands-free manner, and with continuous attention [10]. In relation to nursing, this gives rise to a wide range of applications, such as to support medication dispensation [11–14] or wound care [9,15]. Information can be retrieved in a timely manner in front of the patient, or while performing a nursing task. Hands-free interaction allows nurses to fulfill hygienic standards while controlling the system. However, using AR might also have negative effects, such as motion sickness or raising privacy concerns [16].

Although both researchers and nursing staff expect many opportunities for the use of AR, many questions remain unanswered: What are the most promising and accepted application scenarios? How does the technology affect the interaction work of nurses and patients? Can it effectively reduce the workload? And, most importantly, as it can be considered an essential requirement, how does it affect well-being (in the sense of supporting important preconditions like autonomy, competence and connectedness) [17,18]?

Following the idea of the positive computing framework [17–19], the presented research uses an exploratory approach to see if and how an AR application can contribute to users' feelings of autonomy, competence and connectedness, and to determine important factors influencing this experience. In doing so, a prototype was developed in a participatory process and tested in a simulated hospital environment with nursing staff.

2. Related Work

2.1. The Positive Computing Framework

As it is important for the acceptance and value-adding of new technology for it to have positive effects on people's well-being, we follow the positive computing framework, which aims to design and develop technology to support psychological well-being and human potential [17]. It extends beyond the common goals of effectiveness and efficiency to also consider the quality-of-life and well-being of the users of a digital system and its impact on society [18]. Based on the Self-Determination Theory (SDT) [20], Peters [19] designed strategies for how technology can be developed to meet individuals' needs for autonomy, competence, and connectedness:

Autonomy is the need to operate in compliance with one's goals and values [19]. Accordingly, Peters claims that technology has to be accessible, embed optional levels of help, and users should be able to choose their own goals and strategies. Individuals should be able to interact independently with the system and decide how to use it in a simple way. Instead of giving strict instructions, it is important to provide guidance and the constant opportunity to correct data. Users should be in control of the communication. The design of the interface should be simplistic, to bring focus and concentration to the essentials. Lastly, users should decide for themselves when and how often to use the system [19].

Competence describes a person's desire to perceive themselves as in control of their environment, and to be able to anticipate it [21]. According to Peters, in order to generate a high degree of competence, it is important to divide larger tasks into sub-tasks. In addition, the system has to be updated constantly and offer the possibility of a simplified presentation of the information. It is beneficial to have informative feedback that guides users through the process [19].

Connectedness refers to the desire to experience interaction with other people. It is characterized by the connectedness and the feeling of caring for others [22]. Peters states that this can be supported by ensuring that the technological interactions with others are seamless. Communication should also continue to happen offline and ensure that both intrinsic and extrinsic motivation is provided. The sense of community should be emphasized, and all involved should be given the opportunity to contribute. Finally, the communication of kindness and positive influence should be emphasized [19].

The basic requirements regarding autonomy, competence and connectedness provide initial guidance on how an AR application could be designed to improve well-being and the quality of work. However, in order to develop a tailored solution for nursing, it is necessary to understand the users and their work environment.

2.2. Specific Requirements Based on Nurses' Needs

Although there has been a change in recent decades, van der Cingel et al. [5] report that the profession of nurses is still being seen as compassionate helpers who perform simple and straightforward tasks to care for patients. Due to the advancing professionalization and versatility of tasks, employees see themselves as an important group that does not simply follow doctors' instructions strictly, but also wants to contribute its own needs and knowledge [5]. An AR application should, therefore, provide the ability to support different skill levels and empower users to make decisions on their own. Economic pressure on the healthcare system, bureaucratic regulations, increasing patient numbers, and less contact time with patients are leading to higher workloads, stress, and emotional exhaustion [4]. With regard to the use of AR glasses, nurses surveyed indicated that they hoped to save time and protect themselves through documentation that might become easier, as information and communication with others could be available in a timely manner, regardless of location [23]. Accordingly, it can be summarized that an AR application has to have a high degree of user friendliness, particularly providing exactly the right information in the respective situation to support nursing and documentation tasks.

There is a growing recognition that interacting with people is an essential part of today's work that requires much closer attention. Interaction work involves establishing a cooperative relationship, dealing with one's own feelings, influencing the feelings of customers, clients and patients, and dealing with the imponderables that are part of working on and with people [24]. For example, many nursing interventions require the patient to be calm and relaxed. This can be impaired by the patient's anxiety, but enabled and encouraged by the nurse's composure and confidence [24].

Accordingly, besides using the AR glasses for documentation or treatment purpose, nurses have to continuously respond to the patient. They have to (1) control their own feelings as they influence the patients emotions, and (2) be able to interpret the patient's emotions and sense the situation, in order to (3) prove to be competent and trustworthy to (4) establish a cooperative relationship.

2.3. Factors That Must Be Considered When Using AR Glasses in Interaction Work

Showing and interpreting emotions is crucial to establishing a trustful connection. Non-verbal communication is used to express emotions, convey attitudes, and demonstrate character traits. Humans are able to decode these subtle signals and interpret them in a culture-specific way [25,26]. Eye contact and glances are particularly effective nonverbal signals for building trust in the Western world [27]. Overall, emotions are perceived and interpreted through several of these channels. If one of the channels is not available (e.g., in the absence of eye contact), it is still possible to assess situations correctly through other signals [28]. Hence, there are multiple opportunities for nurses to express emotions, and multiple ways to decode these emotions for patients. However, many AR glasses cover large parts of the nurse's face, and lenses are often tinted, making eye contact less likely to be made. In previous studies, nurses indicated concerns about the negative impact on the relationship between them and the patient, fearing that AR glasses will be distracting rather than supportive, as eye contact is broken [23]. From the patients' perspective, AR glasses can significantly reduce their estimates of healthcare workers' abilities, and decrease their willingness to opt-in to medical procedures [16]. Many AR glasses can be operated by gesture control. However, it is not obvious to outsiders whether a pointing gesture is used for operation or for communication, for example. The interpretation of non-verbal behavior could therefore be made more difficult by the glasses. Here, it is important to examine the ways in which nurses deal with the various interaction possibilities in order to meet the patient's situation.

According to Böhle and Weihrich [24], it is fundamental in this subjectifying action to sense and feel (e.g., soft skin, acrid odor, or a nervous patient). Thinking and sensing are not performed from a distance, but are directly connected to the service. This leads to an explorative, dialogic-interactive approach, where action and reaction are interwoven [24]. The integration of new technologies in such processes could serve as a facilitator, as digital information could be consulted to better assess the patient's condition and make decisions based on it. However, it also harbors the risk of triggering stress, since operating might be difficult at first and another parallel work thread that demands attention is added. With regard to AR glasses, it is also uncertain how the superimposed digital information influences the perception of the real environment. Is it still possible to sense and feel authentically, as described by Böhle and Weihrich [24], while using AR glasses?

The nurse's external impact on the patient might be influenced by AR glasses. During the interaction, the patient observes the nurse's behavior and makes assumptions about their feelings, traits, and motives. According to the attribution theory, people try to determine why others act in a certain way in order to uncover the feelings and traits behind their actions, distinguishing between internal personality-related attributions or external, situation-related attributions [29].

It is, therefore, questionable as to how caregivers themselves and patients evaluate the care situation mediated with AR glasses. Do they attribute the gain or loss of competence to the AR glasses, or to their own ability?

A lack of common ground might be another issue using AR glasses. By common ground, Clark and Brennan [30] mean the knowledge that is shared by two or more individuals. Three heuristics allow one to infer the shared knowledge: (1) group membership (e.g., belonging to a certain profession), (2) physical co-presence (e.g., objects that everyone can see and know about), and (3) linguistic co-presence (e.g., content of the course of the conversation) [30]. Regarding AR glasses particularly, the second point might be critical, as patients are not able to see the digital content the caregiver is seeing trough the glasses. Also, heuristic three needs to be considered when choosing control opportunities for the AR glasses application, such as voice interfaces that cannot be heard by patients.

2.4. Summary and Research Questions

In summary, by using a participatory, user-oriented approach, this exploratory work studies the design and use of an AR-glasses prototype in a user study, observing the complexities in the interaction work of nurses with patients. It thereby considers factors from the positive computing framework, with the goal of supporting nurses in their autonomous and competent fulfillment of their work, while preserving their connectedness with patients.

Along the previously outlined research, we pose the following research questions:

Research question 1: what strategies for using AR glasses do nurses map out in order to autonomously and competently establish a connection to patients in nursing interaction work?

Research question 2: what ambivalences emerge from empirically identified chances and risks in relation to a successful integration of AR glasses in nursing interaction work?

3. Prototype, Materials, Methods and Procedure

To answer the research questions, a prototype was developed in a participatory process and evaluated in a qualitative study, using behavioral data from a simulation study and semi-structured interviews.

3.1. Prototype

In line with positive computing and participatory design, it is crucial for a successful integration of AR glasses to continuously involve the users of the system in the development process [17,31]. Emergent technologies, such as AR, come with unfamiliar interaction forms. How it works and how the technology is experienced might often be vague and abstract, because users cannot refer to mental models yet. This makes it hard for first-time users to state requirements and to formulate ideas on application areas.

According to the guiding principals of participatory design, it is important for democratic and hierarchy-less teamwork to discuss situations based actions that are understandable, rather than abstract, and to use tools and techniques that help to express needs and visions to be able to participate and achieve a mutual understanding [32]. Hence, tight feedback loops with two co-designing nurses allowed us to pick up the mental model of the caregivers, use plausible (still fictional) patient information, and integrate it meaningfully into a realistic use-case scenario by following the design thinking framework [33,34]. To create an AR application that meets the previously stated requirements and fits in smoothly in a realistic patient scenario, we followed the participatory design approach, using contextual inquiries, interlocking workshops, and co-design techniques to develop a prototype in close coordination with nurses [35].

3.1.1. Use Case and Device Decision

In an early phase of the participatory process, nursing staff were very committed to developing a series of application scenarios in which they expected AR glasses to make their work significantly easier. At the end of the workshop series, the documentation of wounds was chosen as the most interesting use case.

Wound care with simultaneous documentation emerged as an important scenario for the use of AR glasses within surveys conducted with nurses with different levels of expertise and experience [23]. The respondents of [23] mentioned the availability of information regardless of location as the main advantage, as it is important to interact continuously with the patient. It is, therefore, well-suited to test the effects of AR glasses on interaction work. Adherence to hygiene standards is a high priority, which means that non-contact work with the AR glasses could be advantageous. Klinker et al. [36] already investigated wound management by testing an AR-based tablet application, and came to the conclusion that the provided information is beneficial, but handheld-based AR applications are impractical for medical professions, as they can not be used without physical contact. This supports the idea of using AR glasses.

After jointly testing several AR glasses and discussing their system characteristics, the Microsoft HoloLens 2 (HL2) was chosen. In contrast to other devices, the HL2 allows users to interact with digital 3D-holograms via gesture control and, therewith, without a physical control device, whereby the hygienic requirements can be met. Caregivers prefer discreet AR glasses models, as they assume that these are less disconcerting for the patient [23,37]. However, these models have the disadvantage that they usually cannot be operated without physical contact, and they are unsuitable for people who wear glasses. They also usually sit less firmly on the head, and could slip during treatment. The HL2 compensates for these disadvantages, but is heavier, bulkier, and more conspicuous. However, a visor that can be folded up and down allows eye contact with the patient.

The prototype was developed with Unity (according to Microsoft's recommendations version 2021.3 (LTS)) and the mixed reality toolkit MRTK 2.7. All UI elements used originate from this toolkit.

3.1.2. Aim and Scope of Functions

Based on the results of the former section, the prototype is designed to enable nurses to achieve three key objectives while using AR glasses:

- *Competence:* the prototype's structure supports common processes in nursing, and provides information to competently and safely assess, care for, and document the patient's wound.
- *Autonomy:* users are able to set up and use their own digitally augmented workspace autonomously and flexibly according to their individual needs and preferences.
- *Connectedness:* the prototype allows nurses to stay close to the patients and to involve them in the care process.

Different types of features are installed to meet these objectives. The navigation structure and information architecture are based on existing nursing routines and the documentation system currently used by the co-designing nurses. Selected screenshots of the prototype are shown in Figure 1. By picking up on dialog structures, labels, and input options of the existing patient file, we take up the mental model of the nurses and place these building blocks in a new workflow adapted to wound care. In addition to the familiar contents, further information materials on the patient and auxiliary materials for the assessment of wounds are integrated into the concept. For this purpose, the wound care process is sorted into chronologically sequenced tabs (visible in Figure 1a,c). Necessary information is integrated into the main dialogues, and supporting content is incorporated with progressive disclosure mechanisms (Figure 1a,b). This allows the nurse to decide for him/herself whether, when, and where to use the support material.

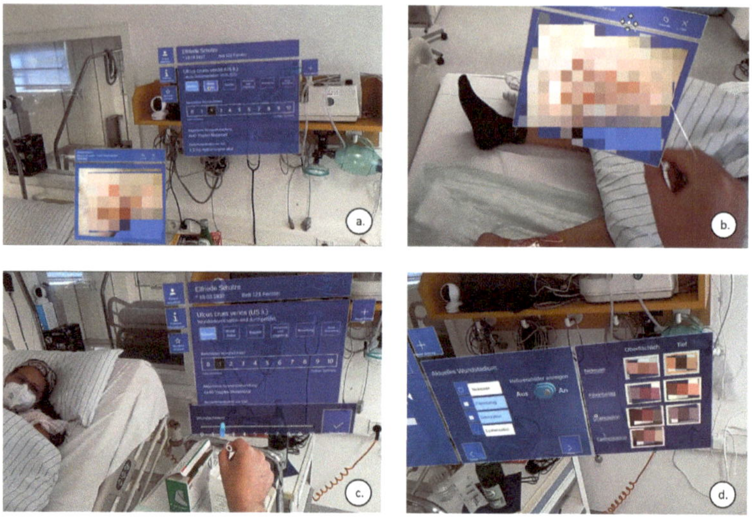

Figure 1. Screenshots from the prototype. The wounds are only pixelated for publication. (**a**) shows the last documented status. The top button bar can be used to call up the individual steps in wound treatment and documentation as described by the nursing staff involved. (**b**) The nurse moves the window to the position where she needs it for her work. (**c**) shows how a new pain score is documented. (**d**) An additional window to document the wound stage is activated. A video of the prototype is available at https://parcura.de/media/parcura_hrw_simulationsstudie_prototyp_promo.mp4 (accessed on 20 May 2024) [38].

Besides retrieving information, it is also possible to create a new documentation entry (Figure 1c). Step-by-step, each documentation entry can be adjusted by selecting pre-defined options. This way, standardized and quick documentation can be made while treating the patient's wound. Additional material, such as reference pictures, can be faded-in to support the wound assessment correctly (Figure 1d). To be able to flexibly adapt the augmented workspace to the spatial conditions, the prototype is divided into two areas that can be separately positioned in the environment. In addition to the patient file, a second window displays a picture of the patient's wound as previously documented, which can be aligned to the actual wound in the real world (Figure 1b). Accordingly, a change in wound status can directly be observed and documented. These features in combination allow the users to receive and document the individually needed information directly within the treatment procedure.

In the implemented prototype, users can choose between far (Figure 1b) and near (Figure 1c) gestures to control the system. This allows them to interact with the system from a distance (e.g., pointing to a window) or from close (e.g., clicking on a button). This way of control is more intuitive, deliberate, and intentional compared to eye-tracking methods. Voice control, as another alternative, was dismissed because of its potential susceptibility. Conversations with the patient might be interpreted as an input by the system, and could lead to unintended actions. By using near and far gestures, the nurses are also able to arrange the windows from a position in the room that allows them to create physical closeness or distance to the patient (Figure 1c). The visor of the HL2 can also be used to maintain eye contact. By providing detailed information about the patient and their current health condition, the user can easily refer to it while being in a dialogue with the patient.

With this first set of functionalities, nurses already have several options to develop their own strategies on how exactly to use the augmented information in a patient situation. The following section presents the study we conducted to simulate realistic nurse–patient interactions, test the prototype in this context, and investigate our research questions.

3.2. Study

The study conducted consisted of two main phases. In the first phase, the participants were given the opportunity to test the AR glasses using the developed prototype in a realistic patient situation. In the second phase of the study, they were asked to reflect on their experiences and impressions of the use in an qualitative interview.

To investigate the use of AR glasses in as realistic a context as possible, a plausible case study was developed with the two co-designing nurses. Therefore, a fictitious patient was created, including all relevant patient data needed for documentation purposes, as well as handover information typically used at shift changes. This information was used as mock data in the prototype. The fictitious patient suffers from a chronic wound on the left lower leg, and was acted out by one of the co-designing nurses. Participants testing the prototype were asked to learn about the patient, care for the wound, and document the procedure.

The patient interaction situation took place in a simulation center. The participants were located in a typically furnished patient room. They were equipped with materials that they could use for the treatment (e.g., painkillers, bandages, and gloves). The researchers were in the control room next door, which allowed a view into the observation room through a mirrored window. Additionally, three cameras were set up in the patient room to observe and record the situation from multiple perspectives. To trace what the participant sees and experiences in the HL2, a live stream was transmitted in the control room, which was recorded as well. Both rooms were connected with an intercom system that allowed the researchers to give instructions to the participants. The subsequent interview took place in a meeting room, and questions were asked face-to-face by a researcher. Screenshots illustrating the main components of the prototype were used as reference materials.

Figure 2 provides an overview of the study's individual steps, methods used, and locations in which it took place. The individual steps will be described in more detail in the following.

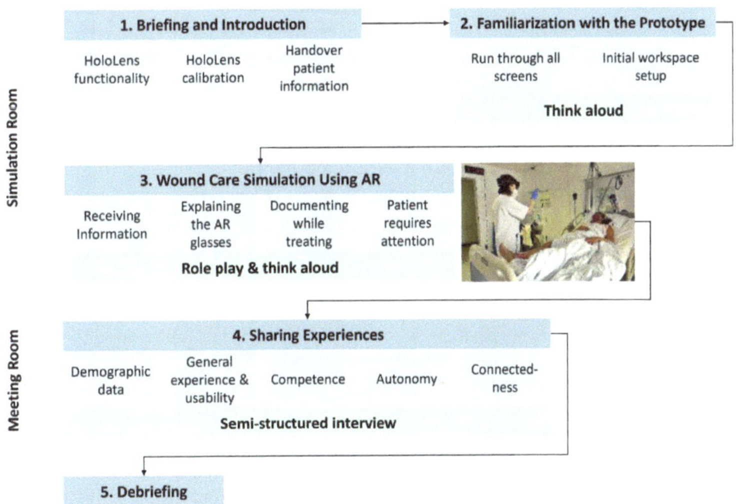

Figure 2. Study setup: overview of the steps of the study and methods used.

3.2.1. Briefing and Introduction

Participants were welcomed and introduced to the study, its procedure, and privacy policy. They were informed that the trial was voluntary, and could be stopped at any time without giving a reason. Emphasis was placed on informing them that the aim was not to test their performance, but rather the usefulness of the prototype. What counts is their subjective opinion. Afterwards, an informed consent form was signed by all participants. They were brought to the simulation room by a researcher, where they were briefly introduced to the HL2 by explaining the main functions and how to use the visor. The main interaction patterns (near and far gesture) were explained, and eye calibration was performed to ensure the best individual experience possible. Afterwards, they were introduced to the patient's case study by using a pre-recorded video on a laptop in which a nurse provides handover information from the previous shift. Finally, they were prompted to start the prototype on the HL2, and the researcher moved to the control room.

3.2.2. Familiarization with the Prototype

In the first phase, the test subjects were able to familiarize themselves with the prototype and its functionalities step-by-step to be prepared for the upcoming patient situation. First, they were encouraged to click on buttons, walk around the three-dimensional holograms, and re-position them. This situation was used to collect direct feedback on the prototype, its screens, and components using the think-aloud technique. Participants were asked to comment on anything coming to their mind while using the prototype to uncover misinterpretations. Furthermore, participants were prompted to express what they like or dislike, and to make suggestions for improvement. To obtain feedback on all screens, users were given the same tasks that subtly navigated them there. The guide was semi-structured, and allowed for flexible responses. The tasks were coordinated in a way that the user could prepare for the patient situation step-by-step and explore the prototype independently beforehand, covering all central components and screens.

After the participants had familiarized themselves with the prototype, they were asked to place the screens in the simulation room. They were free to decide where to place the one with the wound documentation and where the wound image should be displayed while explaining what advantages they expected from which positioning.

3.2.3. Wound Care Simulation Using AR

If participants were ready to receive the patient, they were encouraged to behave as they usually would in a real situation. However, the patient was acted out by one of the co-designing nurses, who followed a behavioral script to create comparable situations. The participants received information about the patient's condition and the perceived wound pain through a simulated handover briefing. Afterwards, the patient was brought into the room and gave the same information about her state of health, so that the participants were able to react accordingly. If the participants did not introduce the AR glasses on their own, the patient addressed them at a specific time, so that all participants were encouraged to explain the use of the AR glasses in their own words. A wound was simulated on the patient's leg with the help of a glued-on photo and makeup. The wound was initially bandaged, and had to be uncovered and treated by the participants. This created a situation in which the hygienic conditions could be addressed. During wound documentation, the patient learns that the wound condition has worsened, subsequently panics and demands the nurse's attention. Due to that, all participants were confronted with an increasingly stressful and distracting situation.

During the interaction with the fictitious patient, participating nurses were asked to treat the wound and provide documentation at the same time (not afterwards) to test the confidence and the ability to work with the hologram in realistic situations. In this situation, the participants could continue to provide comments and suggestions for optimization of the prototype at any time. From the observation room, they received assistance when necessary. In the case of surprising actions or difficulties, the participants were also asked to comment on the situation. The trial ended when the participants reached a pre-defined point in the documentation process, or when the maximum time slot of 60 min was reached.

3.2.4. Sharing Experiences in Semi-Structured Interviews

The subsequent interview was semi-structured and followed a flexible guideline within approximately 30 min. The following topic areas were included: (a) demographic data and current role, (b) usability and overall experience, (c) applicability and integration in interaction work, and (d) perception of the SDT determinants autonomy, competence and connectedness.

Demographics included questions regarding the age and professional experience of each participant, their position in the respective hospital, and whether they had previously been involved in the project or had been using AR glasses before. Subsequently, the subjects were asked to describe their experiences and emotions while using the AR glasses. Participants were asked to relate to specific features and information provided by the prototype, and to share their preferences, criticisms, and suggestions for improvement.

In terms of autonomy, they were particularly asked to describe their regular wound care routine, and to compare it with their experiences during the simulation. If not mentioned by themselves, they were asked how functionalities like the flexible window positioning were perceived with regard to autonomy, and how they used it to create an individual work environment. This served to determine what strategy they chose, and what advantages and disadvantages they perceived as a result.

Concerning competence, the participants' own perceptions were examined, as well as their evaluation of how competent they were considered by the patient during the simulation. On the one hand, technical competence and statements regarding the control and the handling of the glasses were collected. On the other hand, questions were aimed at nursing competence and to what extent the glasses support or hinder nursing care.

With regard to connectedness to the patient, the participants were first instructed to reflect their own feelings during the wound treatment and how they perceived the interaction with the patient. Additionally, we asked them to imagine themselves in the patient's position, in order to recapitulate how they thought the patient might have felt during the treatment. They were questioned if and how the AR glasses had an effect on the interaction work and the perceived connection. This topic area also concluded with a request for suggestions to evaluate advice on how to increase connectedness. In this way, they were encouraged to identify strategies that they would use to improve their connection with the patient.

Finally, they were asked to imagine that AR glasses would be introduced into daily hospital routine in the next one or two months. The subjects were requested to express their feelings towards this situation. We wanted to find out concerns, limitations and necessary improvements.

3.2.5. Debriefing

Following the interviews, the participants were accompanied back to the initial area. They had another opportunity to ask questions and receive further information about the development of the project in future. Afterwards, they were dismissed.

3.3. *Participants*

The participants ($N = 14$) are or have been active in nursing, and were recruited from two different hospitals that previously supported the participative development of the AR application. One of the hospitals is located in a rural area, and the other in the city. Since people from both institutions participated in the design, some of the participants had previous involvement with the project. In addition, they have different levels of knowledge regarding wound management, and different levels of job experience. All participants are trained nurses, although some of them are currently employed as supervisors or division managers. However, they were all familiar with wound treatment. On average, they were

38.93 years old (SD = 10.05), ranging from 22 to 55, and had about 18.25 years (SD = 10.84) of professional experience. Two participants were male, twelve were female.

We reached saturation after 11 participants, meaning that no additional aspects related to the research questions were expressed in the think-alouds and semi-structured interviews by participants 12–14. To this end, we consulted the findings of [39] to confirm that we have a reasonably large sample. Subsequently, we were able to start analyzing the data, which will be described in greater detail in the following section.

3.4. Coding Scheme Development

To evaluate the study, the recorded material of the 14 participants was processed by transcribing the audio recordings of the observations and interviews, and summarizing and synchronizing the video streams. All data were then imported into MAXQDA software (2022, VERBI Software, Berlin, Germany) for further analysis. Qualitative content analysis was performed according to [40]. The coding system resulted from a combination of deductive and inductive procedures. An excerpt of our coding scheme can be viewed in greater detail in Table 1. This form of coding is increasing in preference in current research, as it allows for subjective interpretation of the data and makes it possible to map new and unforeseen findings [41]. Deductive main and subcategories provided a basic structure for the content analysis. Inductive codes were then generated within each thematic block. For example, we used deductive coding to pre-sort the participants' statements (positive, neutral, and negative statements) and assignment to the principals of positive computing (autonomy, competence, and connectedness). Points of discussions, concerns, and suggestions for optimization were coded in an inductive manner based on evolving themes and their similarity to each other. In the further qualitative analysis of the coded segments, multiple responses were clustered. Instead of counting each individual statement made by a person, we only counted whether a person made this statement or not. In addition to the transcript fragments, video excerpts and representative screenshots were collected for further coding: patient–participant interaction, initial window positioning, repositioning of windows, and flipped up visor.

Table 1. Coding scheme.

Inductive Codes	Deductive Codes
Screen 1: Patient selection	Autonomy
Screen 2: Wound selection	Competence
Screen 3: Patient information	Connectedness
Screen 4: View of tabs	Neutral statement
Screen 5: Wound image	Positive statement
Screen 6: Documentation input	Negative statement
Concerns	Motion Sickness
Suggestions	Successful interaction
Expectations	Interaction with problems

4. Results

In order to find answers to both research questions, we first give an overview of the general feedback on the prototype and how differently participants used it to create their work environment. We then go into more detail about how they perceived the situation in terms of autonomy, competence and connectedness with the patient. Afterwards, we discuss the assumed patient perception, and focus on the aspects that lead to different strategies to support interaction with the patient. Finally, we present concerns and suggestions for improvement that participants stated with regard to an integration of AR glasses in nursing interaction work.

4.1. General Feedback and Overall Experience with the Prototype

General feedback on the experience with the HL2 provides both positive and negative statements. In summary, we counted 411 positive statements, 153 neutral statements, and 356 negative statements from all participants, including data from both the simulation and the interview. Negative statements refer to the *wearing comfort* of the HL2, which was perceived as too big and too heavy. It also became warm under the AR glasses, and some subjects began to sweat. A few participants complained about dizziness and the first signs of motion sickness. With regard to *usability*, participants pointed out the poor performance of gesture control in the think-aloud-parts as well as in the interview. The video recordings show a high number of operating problems while using the near and far gestures. Video passages were coded as to whether the gesture successfully triggered the desired interaction, whether it was problematic, or whether it did not trigger the desired interaction at all (failure). Only interactions that were canceled by an interruption (e.g., the patient asked for attention) were ejected from the data set. In 70% (N = 392) of all observed interactions (N = 560), participants used the far gestures. In only 30% of all cases, the near interaction (N = 168) was used. However, the use of near gestures achieved slightly better interaction results compared to the far gestures: 54% of interactions were successful while using the near gestures, whereas it was only 44% of interactions using the far gesture. Accordingly, working with the HL2 was found to be exhausting and frustrating in large parts.

The application and the concept of the prototype, on the other hand, were evaluated positively. The interviewees described the use of the application as exciting, work-saving, self-explanatory, clear, simply structured, and practical, since one has all the information directly at hand. In total, 12 of the 14 subjects indicated that they would fully trust the prototype. Incorrect data are attributable to nurses input errors and not to the glasses (P01, P04). The prototype was conceptually based on the well-known PC-based hospital information system in several aspects (terms, structure of information, etc.). Seven participants said that they recognized the parallels. However, these parallels also raised expectations, some of which are not yet covered by the prototype. During the administration of medication and the wound assessment, some subjects wanted more detailed information.

4.2. Creating the Individual Work Environment by Initial Window Positioning

Based on the video fragments demonstrating the initial window positioning, we were able to derive three recurring patterns (see Figure 3).

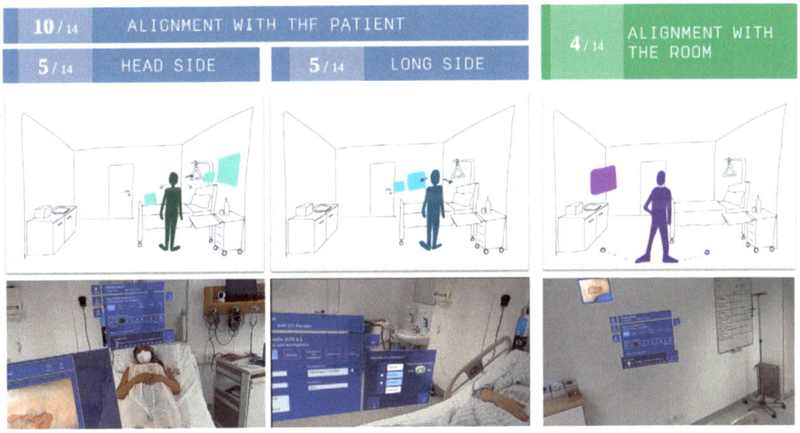

Figure 3. The three found window positioning patterns and their distribution in the sample.

Most participants chose an initial window alignment with the patient (N = 10). In this group, half of the participants opted for an alignment at the head side of the bed (N = 5) or at the long side of the bed ($N = 5$). In the associated think-alouds the participants, those who chose the head side of the bed reasoned that they moved the patient file window to where the information is directly needed. With this positioning, they have the patients' name in view (P02, P11) when speaking to them, but are also able to take another look at the bandage material that they usually prepare on the service desk (P08, P11). This combination was perceived as particularly practical:

> *"I think that's just great because you always have so many patients in your head and you forget so many little things. Which foam dressing and what size was it? I think it's just super practical that you can combine that now [with the room]."* (P11, video transcript, pos.97)

Staying in contact with the patient was important. Participants pointed out that patients remain in the field of view when looking at the patient file (P03, P11), and that that this position is less disturbing (P08) during conversations. P10 points out that the windows must not cover the patient's face.

Participants who chose the long side of the bed for window alignment focused more on the patient's wound. The information is in view during wound treatment, and can be referred to for direct comparison (P04, P14). In addition, the nurse can switch between the patient, the wound, and the information without having to change the body position or turn the head too much (P05). P12 weighs up between a position where a light background allows good legibility for herself, but where she would be standing with her back to the patient, and decides to move the windows to the side of the bed as a compromise in order to be able to make eye contact with the patient by moving her head.

The remaining four participants decided to place (parts of) the application on the opposite wall where the bandage material is stored. One reason is that they will need the information about the bandage material as a check list. However, they verify whether they can still see the information from the bed where they are communicating with the patient. During the dialogue, they are still close to the patient.

In total, half of the participants ($N = 7$) chose to re-position the windows during the patient interaction scene. This behavior could be observed in all three initial groups. However, the participants who initially positioned the windows on the head side of the bed took the wound picture (P02, P03 and P08) and the documentation screens (P02 and P03) to the patient's wound. From this position, we could observe fine tuning. On the one hand, participants pulled screens containing pictures closer to the wound for a better reference. On the other hand, they pulled the screens closer to themselves to use near gestures more comfortably while documenting.

Furthermore, participants recognized that the window positioning influenced the way in which they interacted with the patient. Two contrasting examples provide insights on what was perceived as "too close" or "too distant". During the wound documentation of P12, the hologram hovered very close above the patient. When she used near gestures, she had to reach over the patient and the bed, which she perceived as disturbing (see Figure 4a).

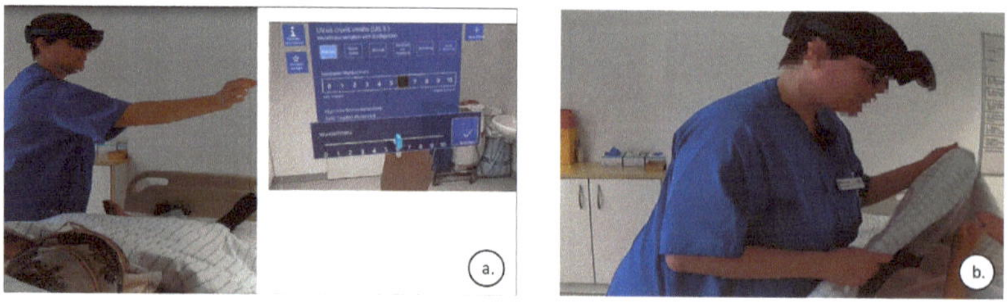

Figure 4. Special work situations at the bedside with the HoloLens 2: (**a**) Participant reaches over the patient to interact with the system by near gestures. (**b**) Participants raises visor to maintain eye contact with the patient.

In the other extreme, P13 was dissatisfied with her initial window position, because she had to write the documentation with her back to the patient. While documenting the wound, she communicated with the patient, but was not able to maintain eye contact. In addition, all participants described the setup of their individual workplace as very positive (*N* = 14).

4.3. Autonomy

Overall, participants felt very autonomous while interacting with the AR glasses. In total, 13 participants stated that they were free in any decisions. During the interviews, it was mentioned that the documentation of wounds must cover certain aspects, so that the hologram does not have a dominating effect.

> *"Being more autonomous means that I can decide freely. It does not tell me what I have to do. I can click my way through as I wish. I am still free to make my own decisions."* (P02, interview, pos. 255)

In addition, when asked to what extent they felt dominated by the glasses, one participant commented that she could always take them off.

The fact that the AR glasses combine various functions and devices enabled the participants to feel more autonomous in their actions. Since the HL2 provides detailed information directly in the situation, the nurses are no longer dependent on their colleagues or the availability of a PC to finish their work. Participant 5 describes this as follows:

> *"Instead of how we are doing it now, having seen the picture before, going into the patient's room and thinking, 'Hm. Did that really look like this?'. Must return to the mobile PC again. This way I had it directly and could continue swiping to see what it looked like."* (P05, interview, pos. 95)

Despite all of the benefits in terms of perceived autonomy, two participants pointed out that the use of the AR glasses must be voluntary. Therefore, documentation via computer would still have to be available. Reference was made to the issues of motion sickness or the constricting feeling when wearing the glasses.

4.4. Competence

The participants commented positively on the AR glasses with regard to their own competence. Twelve participants reported that the glasses enabled them to work more efficiently. For example:

> *"While treating the wound, I would be able to document it immediately and would not have to do it two hours later, as it can happen in clinical practice sometimes."* (P03, interview, pos. 145)

Another important aspect were the reference images. Some participants perceived these as particularly competence-enhancing, since they were confident of evaluating the wound correctly by reviewing the images (*N* = 7). Participant 2 stated:

> *"Personally, I would have been even more uncertain in the evaluation of the wound. Because of the pictures, I was 100 % sure of how to describe them"* (P02, interview, pos. 221)

Additionally, half of the participants recognized the similarity to systems they already knew from their own routine at work. As a result, it promotes their competence, since they do not have to familiarize themselves with a completely new scheme and can start documenting immediately.

Even though the application was rated as very positive and competence-enhancing, six nurses stated that it would limit their interaction work (P04–P06, P09, P13 and P14). More specifically, they indicated that their focus was on the glasses rather than the patient. Additionally, the tinted visor was problematic for two participants. They described that the wound could not be assessed correctly.

In addition, a major negative factor was the limitation of competency in terms of prioritization. In total, seven participants stated that they had focused more on the glasses than on nursing activities (P01, P03, P05–P07, P09–P13). Thus, there is a concern that the interaction with the patients could be neglected.

Another important element was the unavailability of different user profiles ($N = 9$). The subjects stated that wound experts needed different information than certified nurses or nursing students. In addition, they described the wish that the software was designed for ward-specific topics. For example, nurses in the intensive care unit need different information than those in the cardiology unit.

4.5. Connectedness

In the following, we focus more on the feeling of connectedness with the patient. Four participants explicitly stated that they perceived a "distance" between them and the patient (P01, P03, P05, P08). One argument was the reduction of eye contact or loosing sight of the patient (P03, P05, P07, P10, P12, P13). P07 explains:

> *"For patients, it is important to at least be able to see the eyes and to see a little facial expression. That is totally important. Especially when we also wear this FFP2 mask."* (P07, interview, pos. 145)

Another participant referred to the distraction by the holograms that caught their visual attention (P05). Establishing a personal connection to the patients and interacting with them is a key attribute in nursing, as P01 describes:

> *"So in my field, it's very much about having a relationship with patients and being able to cater to patients. Even before competence, before basic care and so on."* (P01, interview, pos. 238)

Accordingly, participants stated that they would establish a relationship with the patients first, before introducing the AR glasses. For example, P13 would feel more comfortable if patients had already been treated by her and knew how she "normally" delivered care (interview, pos. 68–70). P01 believes that once the patients realize that they are nevertheless being well looked after, then it is no longer a problem to use AR glasses (interview, pos. 273). For the subjects, the simulated scene represented an exceptional situation in several respects. As a result, some participants refer to the AR glasses, others to the application, and still others to the overall experience when talking about the impact on feelings of connectedness. The nurses were using the AR glasses for the first time, and had difficulties working with them. Accordingly, three participants pointed out technical difficulties with the HL2 that negatively influenced the patient interaction, as they felt distracted or insecure (P04, P07, and P11). However, all of them assumed that these problems would disappear after a certain period of familiarization and practice.

As the documentation of the wound usually takes place after the treatment, and not simultaneously with it, participants in our study struggled to concentrate on both at the same time. They mentioned that they focused and concentrated on the AR glasses and their content much more and on the patient much less (P01, P03, P05–P07, P09–P13). Here, again, some participants assumed that with a little practice, it will be easier to interact with the patient while documenting.

4.6. Assumed Patient Perception

The participants were concerned about how they would be perceived by the patients when wearing and handling the AR glasses and what effect this might have on the patients:

> *"It takes some getting used to, When you're flailing around in the air. I think that's weird for the patient at first, too, when there's someone standing there waving in the air like crazy."* (P05, interview, pos. 15)

Participants in this study drew a connection between their ability to establish a connection with the patient and the perception of their competence as a nurse. In their assessment, they often refer to their interaction work and that they managed to connect with the patient with or despite the AR glasses. P07, on the one hand, was concerned that the patients might loose trust, as they might equate poor technical skills in using the AR glasses with nursing skills in general.

Participants stated that because of the information inherently provided, they were able to address the patients in a more targeted way and to react more confidently: for example, addressing the patient by the correct name (P02) or referring to more complex details, like the ones that are usually documented on the handover cheat sheet, the patient's file or the medication reference book (P03). It was also assumed that the usage of AR glasses would lead to quality control that would provide reassurance to the patient and enable the nurse to appear more professional:

> *"If someone comes in who wears AR glasses, then you assume that they will be checked, that [. . .] they have guidelines. Control is perhaps the wrong word, but [the nurses] can double check and look at everything again and it all looks professional. That would give me [as a patient] a bit of security."* (P02, interview, Pos. 176)

In total, we found more negative comments (28 segments) related to the assumed patient perception in our sample than positive (5 segments) or neutral (8 segments) comments. Among the negative statements, the most common theme was that patients might feel neglected ($N = 8$). Participants reasoned that they were more preoccupied with the new and unpracticed technique of using the AR glasses, or doing the documentation in parallel with the wound treatment and patient interaction ($N = 6$). The patients' feeling of being neglected was assumed to be caused by losing contact with the patient due to the AR glasses (P10, P12, P13). References were made to the lack of eye contact, and to the fact that patients cannot see what one sees oneself and may not dare to ask about it (P12, P13). One participant wishes "that the patient has the feeling that when I look at him, I am really looking at him and not seeing any pictures." (P04, interview, pos. 171).

Nurses were particularly concerned about patients with dementia and elderly, disoriented, or delirious patients ($N = 7$). Here, they see the use of AR glasses critically, as it could worsen the mental health status of these patients.

However, despite the many critical voices, some participants put their negative statements into perspective. In doing so, they mainly pointed to the still unpracticed situation and the fact that they were using the AR glasses for the first time. If the use of the AR glasses and the procedure of parallel documentation is practiced, the interaction with the patient will be different, and might be easier (P05, P09, P11). Subjects stated in the context that it was important to inform the patients about the AR glasses and how they work (P11, P13).

4.7. Strategies to Support Interaction Work with Patients

Within the role play scene, we were able to observe how the nurses managed to balance interaction work, documentation duties and taking care of the wound. We found different approaches for how participants tried to maintain a connection with the patient.

All participants were informed about the flip-up visor of the HL2 within the introduction, but less than half of the nurses made use of it to establish eye contact. Four participants were using the visor selectively over short amounts of time. In these shorter sequences, they raised the visor, usually at the beginning of the interaction scene, to greet the patient and to introduce themselves, to explain the AR glasses, or in case the patient demanded their attention (see Figure 4b). Two participants raised the visor over an extended period of time, and must have been remembered by the researcher to document the condition of the wound with the AR application. They flipped up the visor while collecting materials and treating the wound.

However, care must be taken when using the visor to ensure that the general hygienic conditions are met. Accordingly, one participant expressed the wish that the HL2 should offer the possibility to flip up the visor without physical contact. One participant found another compromise to deal with the tinted visor. She folded it down only halfway, so that she could squint at the information during the treatment.

Another way to better connect with the patient was to have the patient participate in the procedure. We observed that, similarly to traditional caregiver routines, participants commented in 26 cases on what they saw or did in the AR glasses.

> *"(to the patient:) I would just look at the picture again. I'll put the glasses on now. I think that's a little bit more extraordinary than usual."* (P13, video transcript, pos. 98)

However, only two participants started to introduce the AR glasses and its functioning initially. The other twelve nurses did not explain it until the patient actively asked them about it. All participants involved the patient in different ways. One participant (P02) explained that, during wound treatment without the HL2, some information is not available or incomplete, and thus the patient is frequently asked about it. This creates a continuous dialog in which the patient is involved. Based on this, he/she has concerns that the patient could take on a more passive role, being limited to a subject of documentation, when he/she is using the AR glasses. Another challenge arises from the patient's presence during documentation, as they could notice the entries. Depending on the patient's state of health, this information should be expressed with caution, and nurses were uncertain as to how to react adequately:

> *"I wouldn't say that out loud either: 'this is infected, looks totally bad, etc.'. But I just thought out loud, what should I click here? And then I wasn't sure either, should I continue thinking out loud?"* (P14, interview, pos. 65–68)

5. Discussion

5.1. Factors Influencing Autonomy

The results of our study clearly show that the nurses used different ways to control the prototype autonomously. These observations can be corroborated by the statements of the qualitative interviews. Here, the participants described the operation and set-up of their own work environment as autonomy-promoting. They particularly emphasized the independent positioning of the individual windows, which enabled a high degree of flexibility. Through progressive disclosure mechanisms and the display of additional reference images, the application provided sufficiently graded support material that could be consulted as needed. The sequence of steps could also be customized through the use of tabs, providing the ability to tailor the process to one's own needs and routines. Based on this positive feedback, we conclude that the application and the AR concept, as such, meet the requirements postulated at the beginning regarding autonomy [19]. Nevertheless, suggestions for improvement were also expressed, which can be derived well from window positioning and progressive disclosure. Some reference images were displayed by extending an existing window. At this point, a decoupling of the information in a separate window would have allowed even more flexibility (e.g., in which only these images are aligned to the wound). Based on these findings, we recommend presenting topics that are related in content as modular units. Similar to widgets on a desktop, individual window elements and holograms can be plugged together to form an individual workspace. Compared to the current situation, the subjects stated that this form of documentation allowed for more flexibility.

5.2. Factors Influencing Competence

Regarding the perception of competence, the impressions on the AR experience were diverse. Generally, the caregivers considered themselves competent, although they sometimes had major problems with the operation. However, they attributed this to the AR glasses' maturity level, and not to their own abilities.

On the basis of the constantly retrievable information, the nurses became increasingly informed about the respective medical conditions, and were able to provide more efficient decisions with regard to treatment. Additionally, they assumed that it provides patients with a sense of security, as the nurses are monitored eventually. Thereby, the AR glasses support the professionalization of the nursing care. These findings are in line with the statements made by van der Cingel and Brouwer [5], who said that the self-image of caregivers has changed in recent years. Due to the increased autonomy, the prototype can contribute to enabling nurses to adopt more complex tasks and, thus, to changing the perception of patients and medical doctors towards them.

On the other hand, the subjects criticized the AR glasses' handling with regard to competence. Besides difficulties in usability, they referred to tapping in the air as being ridiculous, thus assuming that the patients would perceive them as less competent. We conclude that, despite the option to use near or far gestures, the way of operation should be improved further to increase the nurses' feeling of competence.

Lastly, participants pointed out the importance of connecting to the patients and making them feel comfortable, as they assumed that was what made a competent nurse.

5.3. *Factors Influencing Connectedness*

By surveying the nurses' perceived connectedness to the patient, it became evident that establishing a connection to patients is considered a core competence in nursing, and that using AR glasses has an influence on this perception. We discovered both promoting and impairing influencing factors.

A feeling of connectedness can be promoted by accessing all of the required information about the patient at any time. It enables nurses to respond to the patient's needs as the situation demands (e.g., referring to pain assessment and providing medication). In addition, the flexible workplace arrangement allows the caregivers to vary the amount of attention they pay to the patient. However, the test subjects pointed to the bulkiness of the HL2. Particularly in combination with a surgical mask, it was seen as a hindrance to connectedness, as nonverbal signals can be shown and interpreted less obviously. This issue is the main criticism of the nurses, as they see the danger of not establishing sufficient eye contact with the patient through the glasses and, as a result, not creating an effective connection. However, the visor could have been a solution to this problem, but was used only by a few participants. The reasons were diverse, ranging from hygienic concerns to forgetting about this functionality at all. How to use this functionality properly should therefore be first re-designed to meet hygienic standards. The participants proposed using the voice function by suggesting raising or lowering the visor by voice commands. Additionally, they wished to use voice commands to bypass the gesture control or to use speech input for documentation. This was assumed easier and faster than the gesture control. An uncertainty was observed on how transparently the documentation should be completed in front of the patient. Loudly expressed documentation content or input commands could make the patient uncomfortable or anxious. This contrasts with statements from [24], which advocate maximizing transparency in order to create a common ground. Concerns were also raised about inadvertently activating voice control when talking to the patient—especially if this input is not perceived consciously.

5.4. *Strategies of the Nurses to Support Interaction Work*

To ensure successful interaction work, the nurses considered it more important to convey a positive feeling to the patients than placing the hologram in the most comfortable position for them. These strategies should be presented and discussed with the nurses to shed more light on the underlying motives and their changing role, as described in [5]. In addition, the interaction concept should be further developed so that it meets both demands.

Similarly to the concept of Klinker et al. [15], our prototype was designed to document and care for the wound simultaneously. However, some nurses did not complete the documentation during wound care initially, but preferred to complete it afterwards as usual. In this case, we prompted them to complete it directly, so that they can gain experience with the HL2. Nurses pointed to this change in procedure and revealed that it incorporates a stress factor. Additionally, if the interaction concept of Böhle and Weihrich [24] is taken into account, it became apparent that not only two, but several, complex tasks need to be performed simultaneously by the nurses: (1) referring to patient's needs, (2) treating the wound, (3) documenting the status, (4) exploring how to individually use the HL2, (5) making the process transparent to the patient to establish common ground and, finally, (6) managing their own emotions to make a calm, competent and trustworthy impression. For further development, it will be crucial to figure out how to best support balancing these tasks. On the one hand, information can be brought much closer to the specific situation, both in time and space. On the other hand, the influence of AR operations that are visible to the outside world, but not comprehensible to outsiders, must be given greater consideration.

5.5. Chances and Risks for Integration

Overall, our study provided a realistic impression of what a nursing situation with AR technology could feel like in the future, which enabled the participants to provide meaningful feedback on the opportunities and risks of integration. In general, the use of AR was seen positively. However, some areas of tension were identified, which revealed fundamental conditions that need to be considered more strongly in the further development of such a system. Besides technical inaccessibility and getting used to the still unfamiliar handling, the integration of the glasses into nursing interaction work with the patients represents a particularly complex challenge. With regard to the on-boarding process, it was stated that both nurses and patients need to be informed about the AR glasses, its functionality, and the context of usage. Nurses emphasized that patient information cannot be their sole responsibility, and that patients need to be kept informed through other channels, such as brochures. In particular, the camera was mentioned in this context, as it could endanger the patient's privacy.

The prototype's concept, content and functionalities were rated as useful, helpful, and facilitating work. Nevertheless, it also became apparent that providing a lot of information and documentation functionalities leads to increasing parallelization of previously linear tasks, with the risk of switching the focus from the patient to the documentation.

Referring to the involvement of patients, our results indicate that the bulky HL2 has to be seen as a disruptive factor in interaction work between nurses and patients. Participants in our study suspected that some patients might feel uncomfortable if they, as caregivers, wore AR glasses. This assumption can be supported by Klinker et al. [16], who investigated, from the patient's perspective, to what extend they would opt-in to a treatment with the HL2. Here, some surveyed participants found that caregivers wearing smart glasses look inhumane, as their eyes can hardly be seen, and found it difficult to build a trusting relationship with this person [16]. However, in the study conducted by Janssen and Prilla [9], in which caregivers tested AR glasses in a comparable nursing scenario, participants expressed less concerns regarding the patient's acceptance towards AR glasses. Interestingly, none of the interviewees expected patients to have severe problems with the nurses wearing AR glasses if they explain this properly to the patient before [9]. In contrast to [16] and our study, [9] used another device, which is far less bulky, has no shades, and reminds one more of a pair of conventional glasses. Additionally, the ongoing technological improvements in hardware could resolve this obstacle in the future. Hence, eye contact is not disturbed, and technical features, such as cameras, are less obvious.

However, with regard to trust, Klinker et al. [16] also reported positive aspects of smart glasses, as some patients mentioned the reduction of errors and higher productivity of the caregivers. This maps well to statements from nurses in our study, who obtained competence from the possibility to check augmented information and to verify their decisions based on it. The information directly provided by AR can also help nurses to respond more quickly to patient's questions. Feeling competent is highly influenced by the ability to establish a trustful relationship with the patient, as was explained in [5,24,42] and also reported by our participants.

6. Limitations and Implications for Future Research

In the further development of AR systems for wound management, the first step should be to ensure that the nurses perceive themselves as competent and autonomous. Good usability must be ensured so that the nurse can use the contents and functions of the application optimally in the nursing situation. Technical difficulties during usage led to frustration when the prototype did not respond to the nurse's input instantly. Since the study only contained a prototype implementation, not all usability problems could be eliminated in advance. We countered this limitation by informing the participants that they would only be working with a prototypical version. In addition, participants' statements were, therefore, evaluated under this restriction. Furthermore, the analysis of the study indicated that some participants had difficulties navigating through the hologram, leading to a number of operating errors. Although we have integrated the option for near and far gestures, a more robust system needs to be implemented in the future to maximize usability and user experience. Therefore, we suggest removing elements like the slider and replacing it with buttons or text input fields. In addition, the menu structure needs to be designed more intuitively, and drop-down buttons should be labeled more explicitly. In the second step, consideration should also be given to how these multimodal forms of interaction, like gestures or voice commands, can be perceived and interpreted by outsiders. This plays a central and complex role, especially in interaction work on and with humans, which has not yet been investigated in sufficient detail. Accordingly, future research should examine the impact of different AR glasses models on the self-perception and perceptions of others by the caregivers who wear them. Special focus should be laid on the impact of eye-contact, as it might have stronger effects on trust than other nonverbal behavior, such as body posture [43]. We observed additional strategies, like involving the patient by explaining what is presented via AR to establish common ground and to inform the patient of what is happening, which can be opposed to eye-contact. As a result, special emphasis should be laid on how a trustful connection between the patient and the caregiver can be realized using AR technology. Nonverbal and verbal communication take place not only among people but, in this case, also between people and technology. The participants highlighted that the information and processes through the HL2 were mapped more clearly than in the system currently used. A direct comparison between traditional documentation and AR-assisted documentation was not made, and could be explored in subsequent studies to prove this impression.

Complicating matters with AR is the lack of common ground, as only the caregiver, not the patient, can see content. Interpersonal misunderstandings, as well as unintentional inputs, can quickly arise in these situations, as our results indicate, and must be adequately addressed by future application concepts. When designing interaction patterns, designers should not only consider intended inputs made by the users, but also inputs that were unintended—either by the user or the patient. We recommend that future research should not only consider the perceptions of nurses, but also those of the patients. Both in our study, as well as in [9,16], the need for introducing and explaining AR glasses to the patient evolves as a key requirement for a successful integration in practice. Thus, we recommend extending the design process beyond the digital product itself and to complementing with service design methods that integrate additional artifacts, instructions and routines. Additionally, Friemer et al. [44] already suggested that nurses need training not only to learn how to operate a new technology, but also how to build an understanding about the context of its usage. A next step should be to investigate the effects of the changed workflow in longer work phases, for example when treating several patients in succession.

Additionally, some participants experienced motion sickness. According to the findings of [16], this is a common accompaniment when using AR glasses. In order to avoid this limitation, we provided the participants with a familiarization period with the glasses at the beginning, and offered them the opportunity to sit down to ensure that no one had to terminate the study. Future research should focus on how AR holograms can be designed to maximize usability and minimize the feeling of dizziness.

7. Conclusions

In conclusion, it can be stated that the approach of the well-being-centered system design with the positive computing framework, an intensive observation of the work task's characteristics, and the involvement of domain experts led to a promising prototype, but also to the identification of further needs for research and development. The perceived autonomy of the nurses could be affirmed based on the option to control the glasses by both near and far gestures, and to be able to set up the workplace independently. Furthermore, it was observed that the presumed patient perception influenced the perceived personal competence. In addition, the hardware was considered too bulky. Future developments are expected to result in smaller devices less disruptive for the connectedness to the patient. We recommend that future research needs to focus on patients' perceptions. Their perspective should also be considered and integrated into the design of applications, in order to ensure that all requirements are covered. In addition, technical and organizational framework conditions for integration into real hospital operations must be investigated. The basic conceptual approaches of this work suggest transferability to other fields of application. This should be investigated in more detail in future work.

Author Contributions: Conceptualization, C.A.-G., L.T., S.C.E. and S.G.; methodology, C.A.-G. and L.T.; software, C.A.-G.; validation, S.C.E. and S.G.; formal analysis, C.A.-G. and L.T.; investigation, C.A.-G. and L.T.; resources, C.A.-G., L.T. and S.G.; data curation, C.A.-G. and L.T.; writing—original draft preparation, C.A.-G. and L.T.; writing—review and editing, S.C.E. and S.G.; visualization, C.A.-G. and L.T.; supervision, S.C.E. and S.G.; project administration, S.C.E. and S.G.; funding acquisition, S.C.E. and S.G. All authors have read and agreed to the published version of the manuscript.

Funding: This work is part of the PARCURA project, funded by the Federal Ministry of Education and Research Germany and the European Social Fund of the EU (grant no. 02L18A164).

Institutional Review Board Statement: Ethical review and approval was not required for the study on human participants in accordance with the local legislation and institutional requirements. The participants provided their written informed consent to participate in this study.

Informed Consent Statement: Informed consent was obtained from all subjects involved in the study.

Data Availability Statement: The data are presented in aggregated format within this manuscript and throughout the results section. Further inquiries can be directed to the corresponding author. The data are not publicly accessible for the protection of the test subjects.

Acknowledgments: We would like to thank partners and participants from the hospitals, especially the co-designers, involved for their valuable contributions.

Conflicts of Interest: The authors declare no conflicts of interest.

References

1. Fendrich, K.; Hoffmann, W. More than just aging societies: The demographic change has an impact on actual numbers of patients. *J. Public Health* **2007**, *15*, 345–351. [CrossRef]
2. Michel, J.P.; Ecarnot, F. The shortage of skilled workers in Europe: Its impact on geriatric medicine. *Eur. Geriatr. Med.* **2020**, *11*, 345–347. [CrossRef] [PubMed]
3. Rössler, W. Stress, burnout, and job dissatisfaction in mental health workers. *Eur. Arch. Psychiatry Clin. Neurosci.* **2012**, *262*, 65–69. [CrossRef] [PubMed]
4. Zander, B.; Dobler, L.; Busse, R. The introduction of DRG funding and hospital nurses' changing perceptions of their practice environment, quality of care and satisfaction: Comparison of cross-sectional surveys over a 10-year period. *Int. J. Nurs. Stud.* **2013**, *50*, 219–229. [CrossRef] [PubMed]
5. van der Cingel, M.; Brouwer, J. What makes a nurse today? A debate on the nursing professional identity and its need for change. *Nurs. Philos.* **2021**, *22*, e12343. [CrossRef] [PubMed]
6. Prilla, M.; Recken, H.; Janßen, M.; Schmidt, A. Die Pflegebrille als Instrument der Digitalisierung in der Pflege: Nutzenpotentiale. In *Assistive Technologien im Sozial- und Gesundheitssektor*; Luthe, E.W., Müller, S.V., Schiering, I., Eds.; Springer Fachmedien: Wiesbaden, Germany, 2022; pp. 735–752. [CrossRef]
7. Wüller, H.; Behrens, J.; Garthaus, M.; Marquard, S.; Remmers, H. A scoping review of augmented reality in nursing. *BMC Nurs.* **2019**, *18*, 19. [CrossRef] [PubMed]

8. Park, S.; Bokijonov, S.; Choi, Y. Review of Microsoft HoloLens applications over the past five years. *Appl. Sci.* **2021**, *11*, 7259. [CrossRef]
9. Janßen, M.; Prilla, M. Investigating the use of Head Mounted Devices for remote cooperation and guidance during the treatment of wounds. *Proc. ACM Hum.-Comput. Interact.* **2022**, *6*, 1–27. [CrossRef]
10. Klinker, K.; Berkemeier, L.; Zobel, B.; Wüller, H.; Huck-Fries, V.; Wiesche, M.; Remmers, H.; Thomas, O.; Krcmar, H. Structure for innovations: A use case taxonomy for smart glasses in service processes. *Multikonferenz Wirtsch. Lünebg. Dtschl.* **2018**, *4*, 1599–1610.
11. Aicher, S.; Klinker, K.; Wiesche, M.; Krcmar, H. Augmented Reality im Gesundheitswesen—Entwurf und Auswertung einer HoloLens-Anwendung zur Verteilung von Medikamenten. In *Systematische Entwicklung von Dienstleistungsinnovationen*; Wiesche, M., Welpe, I.M., Remmers, H., Krcmar, H., Eds.; Research, Springer Gabler: Berlin/Heidelberg, Germany, 2021; pp. 287–306. [CrossRef]
12. Schneidereith, T. Seeing Through Google Glass: Using an Innovative Technology to Improve Medication Safety Behaviors in Undergraduate Nursing Students. *Nurs. Educ. Perspect.* **2015**, *36*, 337–339. [CrossRef]
13. Othman, S.B.; Foinard, A.; Herbommez, P.; Storme, L.; Décaudin, B.; Hammadi, S.; Odou, P. Augmented reality for risks management in injectable drugs preparation in hospital pharmacy. In Proceedings of the GERPAC, Hyères, France, 5–7 October 2016.
14. Chang, W.J.; Chen, L.B.; Hsu, C.H.; Chen, J.H.; Yang, T.C.; Lin, C.P. MedGlasses: A Wearable Smart-Glasses-Based Drug Pill Recognition System Using Deep Learning for Visually Impaired Chronic Patients. *IEEE Access* **2020**, *8*, 17013–17024. [CrossRef]
15. Klinker, K.; Wiesche, M.; Krcmar, H. Digital transformation in health care: Augmented reality for hands-free service innovation. *Inf. Syst. Front.* **2020**, *22*, 1419–1431. [CrossRef]
16. Klinker, K.; Wiesche, M.; Krcmar, H. Smart Glasses in Health Care: A Patient Trust Perspective. In Proceedings of the Hawaii International Conference on System Sciences, Maui, HI, USA, 7–10 January 2020.
17. Calvo, R.A.; Peters, D. *Positive Computing: Technology for Wellbeing and Human Potential*; MIT Press: Cambridge, MA, USA, 2014. [CrossRef]
18. Pawlowski, J.M.; Eimler, S.C.; Jansen, M.; Stoffregen, J.; Geisler, S.; Koch, O.; Müller, G.; Handmann, U. Positive computing: A new trend in business and information systems engineering? *Bus. Inf. Syst. Eng.* **2015**, *57*, 405–408. [CrossRef]
19. Peters, D.; Calvo, R.A.; Ryan, R.M. Designing for motivation, engagement and wellbeing in digital experience. *Front. Psychol.* **2018**, *9*, 797–812. [CrossRef] [PubMed]
20. Ryan, R.; Deci, E. Self-Determination Theory and the Facilitation of Intrinsic Motivation, Social Development, and Well-Being. *Am. Psychol.* **2000**, *55*, 68–78. [CrossRef] [PubMed]
21. Diener, E.; Diener, C. Monitoring psychosocial prosperity for social change. In *Positive Psychology as Social Change*; Springer: Dordrecht, The Netherlands, 2011; pp. 53–71 [CrossRef] [PubMed]
22. Gaggioli, A.; Riva, G.; Peters, D.; Calvo, R.A. Chapter 18—Positive Technology, Computing, and Design: Shaping a Future in Which Technology Promotes Psychological Well-Being. In *Emotions and Affect in Human Factors and Human-Computer Interaction*; Jeon, M., Ed.; Academic Press: San Diego, CA, USA, 2017; pp. 477–502. [CrossRef]
23. Wüller, H.; Behrens, J. Anforderungen an Augmented Reality in der Pflege. In *Systematische Entwicklung von Dienstleistungsinnovationen: Augmented Reality für Pflege und Industrielle Wartung*; Wiesche, M., Welpe, I.M., Remmers, H., Krcmar, H., Eds.; Springer Fachmedien: Wiesbaden, Germany, 2021; pp. 153–169. [CrossRef]
24. Böhle, F.; Weihrich, M. Das Konzept der Interaktionsarbeit. *Z. Arbeitswissenschaft* **2020**, *74*, 9–22. [CrossRef]
25. Ekman, P.; Friesen, W.V. Constants across cultures in the face and emotion. *J. Personal. Soc. Psychol.* **1971**, *17*, 124–129. [CrossRef] [PubMed]
26. Ekman, P.E.; Davidson, R.J. *The Nature of Emotion: Fundamental Questions*; Oxford University Press: Oxford, UK, 1994.
27. Argyle, M. Rules for social relationships in four cultures. *Aust. J. Psychol.* **1986**, *38*, 309–318. [CrossRef]
28. Archer, D.; Akert, R.M. Words and everything else: Verbal and nonverbal cues in social interpretation. *J. Personal. Soc. Psychol.* **1977**, *35*, 443–449. [CrossRef]
29. Heider, F. Social perception and phenomenal causality. *Psychol. Rev.* **1944**, *51*, 358. [CrossRef]
30. Clark, H.H.; Brennan, S.E. Grounding in communication. In *Perspectives on Socially Shared Cognition*; Resnick, L.B., Levine, J.M., Teasley, S.D., Eds.; American Psychological Association: Washington, DC, USA, 1991; pp. 127–149. [CrossRef]
31. Robertson, T.; Simonsen, J. Participatory Design: An introduction. In *Routledge International Handbook of Participatory Design*; Simonsen, J., Robertson, T., Eds.; Routledge: New York, NY, USA, 2012; pp. 1–17. [CrossRef]
32. Greenbaum, J.; Loi, D. Participation, the camel and the elephant of design: An introduction. *CoDesign* **2012**, *8*, 81–85. [CrossRef]
33. Brown, T. Design thinking. *Harv. Bus. Rev.* **2008**, *86*, 84–92. [PubMed]
34. Ball, J. The Double Diamond: A Universally Accepted Depiction of the Design Process. 2019. Available online: https://www.designcouncil.org.uk/our-resources/archive/articles/double-diamond-universally-accepted-depiction-design-process/ (accessed on 30 April 2024).
35. Albrecht-Gansohr, C.; Geisler, S.; Eimler, S.C. Playful Co-Design: Creating an AR-Prototype with Nurses in Interlocking Remote and On-Site Workshops. In Proceedings of the Extended Abstracts of the 2023 CHI Conference on Human Factors in Computing Systems, Hamburg, Germany, 23–28 April 2023; pp. 1–8. [CrossRef]

36. Klinker, K.; Przybilla, L.; Huck-Fries, V.; Wiesche, M.; Krcmar, H. Wundmanagement mittels Tablet-basierter Augmented Reality Anwendungen. In *Systematische Entwicklung von Dienstleistungsinnovationen: Augmented Reality für Pflege und Industrielle Wartung*; Wiesche, M., Welpe, I.M., Remmers, H., Krcmar, H., Eds.; Springer Fachmedien: Wiesbaden, Germany, 2021; pp. 245–262. [CrossRef]
37. Klinker, K.; Przybilla, L.; Wiesche, M.; Krcmar, H. Augmented Reality für das Wundmanagement: Hands-Free Service Innovation mittels Datenbrillen. In *Systematische Entwicklung von Dienstleistungsinnovationen: Augmented Reality für Pflege und Industrielle Wartung*; Wiesche, M., Welpe, I.M., Remmers, H., Krcmar, H., Eds.; Springer Fachmedien: Wiesbaden, Germany, 2021; pp. 263–285. [CrossRef]
38. PARCURA Consortium. Der Erste Prototyp. 2022. Available online: https://www.parcura.de/media/parcura_hrw_simulationsstudie_prototyp_promo.mp4 (accessed on 30 April 2024) .
39. Hennink, M.; Kaiser, B.N. Sample sizes for saturation in qualitative research: A systematic review of empirical tests. *Soc. Sci. Med.* **2022**, *292*, 114523. [CrossRef] [PubMed]
40. Mayring, P.; Fenzl, T. Qualitative Inhaltsanalyse. In *Handbuch Methoden der Empirischen Sozialforschung*; Baur, N., Blasius, J., Eds.; Springer Fachmedien: Wiesbaden, Germany, 2019; pp. 633–648. [CrossRef]
41. Ruin, S. Categories as an Expression of an Identified Observer Perspective? A Constructive Proposal for a more Qualitative Qualitative Content Analysis. *Forum Qual. Sozialforschung/Forum Qual. Soc. Res.* **2019**, *20*, Art. 37. [CrossRef]
42. Crigger, N.; Godfrey, N. From the Inside Out: A New Approach to Teaching Professional Identity Formation and Professional Ethics. *J. Prof. Nurs.* **2014**, *30*, 376–382. [CrossRef]
43. Hillen, M.; van Tienhoven, G.; Bijker, N.; Laarhoven, H.; Vermeulen, D.; Smets, E. All eyes on the patient: The influence of oncologists' nonverbal communication on breast cancer patients' trust. *Breast Cancer Res. Treat.* **2015**, *153*, 161–171. [CrossRef]
44. Friemer, A. Digitale Technik droht? Bedroht? Wirklich nur? Kompetenzentwicklung in Veränderungsprojekten. In *Digitalisierung der Arbeit in der Langzeitpflege als Veränderungsprojekt*; Bleses, P., Busse, B., Friemer, A., Eds.; Springer: Berlin/Heidelberg, Germany, 2020; pp. 135–150. [CrossRef]

applied sciences

MDPI

Article

Prefetching Method for Low-Latency Web AR in the WMN Edge Server

Seyun Choi [1], Sukjun Hong [1], Hoijun Kim [2], Seunghyun Lee [3] and Soonchul Kwon [4,*]

1 Department of Smart System, Kwangwoon University, Seoul 01897, Republic of Korea
2 Department of Plasma Bio Display, Kwangwoon University, Seoul 01897, Republic of Korea
3 Department of Ingenium College Liberal Arts, Kwangwoon University, Seoul 01897, Republic of Korea
4 Graduate School of Smart Convergence, Kwangwoon University, Seoul 01897, Republic of Korea
* Correspondence: ksc0226@kw.ac.kr; Tel.: +82-2-940-8637

Abstract: Recently, low-latency services for large-capacity data have been studied given the development of edge servers and wireless mesh networks. The 3D data provided for augmented reality (AR) services have a larger capacity than general 2D data. In the conventional WebAR method, a variety of data such as HTML, JavaScript, and service data are downloaded when they are first connected. The method employed to fetch all AR data when the client connects for the first time causes initial latency. In this study, we proposed a prefetching method for low-latency AR services. Markov model-based prediction via the partial matching (PPM) algorithm was applied for the proposed method. Prefetched AR data were predicted during AR services. An experiment was conducted at the Nowon Career Center for Youth and Future in Seoul, Republic of Korea from 1 June 2022 to 31 August 2022, and a total of 350 access data points were collected over three months; the prefetching method reduced the average total latency of the client by 81.5% compared to the conventional method.

Keywords: wireless mesh network; edge server; augmented reality; prefetching

Citation: Choi, S.; Hong, S.; Kim, H.; Lee, S.; Kwon, S. Prefetching Method for Low-Latency Web AR in the WMN Edge Server. *Appl. Sci.* **2023**, *13*, 133. https://doi.org/10.3390/app13010133

Academic Editors: Radu Comes, Jing-Jing Fang, Dorin-Mircea Popovici and Calin Gheorghe Dan Neamtu

Received: 23 November 2022
Revised: 19 December 2022
Accepted: 20 December 2022
Published: 22 December 2022

1. Introduction

Studies have been conducted on augmented reality (AR) services in web browsers such as the WebXR Device API (Web eXtended Reality Device Application Programming Interface) [1], AR.js [2], and Three.js [3]. Users can access AR services through the web browser on their smartphone without installing a separate application; this helps improve user accessibility [4]. However, there are limitations in that users must always be connected to the services [5], and fetching causes delays when using an AR service [6].

The Institute of Electrical and Electronics Engineers (IEEE) has defined a standard called 802.11s, which is related to the mesh for a wireless mesh network (WMN). 802.11s conducts traffic forwarding via 802.11ac [7–10]. Internet wireless fidelity (Wi-Fi) can be provided without a shadow area throughout the service area that provides the AR service. Web data are saved on an edge server with a short physical distance hop. The client fetches the saved web data, which helps reduce latency. When downloading AR data, the edge server communicates with the client without a wide area network (WAN), and therefore, it is not affected by WAN latency [11,12]. Further, it reduces the latency required to access the server and operates at a stable and constant speed. The AR data can be downloaded relatively quickly [13]; however, if there is a considerable amount of high-capacity AR data, latency can still occur [14].

This study attempted to reduce user latency in AR services. To this end, we proposed a prefetching method that uses the Markov model. The Markov model enables predictions via the partial matching algorithm used for prefetching [15]. The proposed method considers the priority of each AR dataset to reduce latency, and it allows the prediction of the AR data that the user will request next. According to the proposed method, AR data are sequentially downloaded [16]. In this study, the following experiments were conducted: (1) The latency was measured according to the use of an edge server; (2) a comparative analysis of network traffic was performed; (3) the hit ratio and latency for each request, user, and data in the time order were measured; and (4) the waste ratio results for each user were calculated.

The remainder of this paper is organized as follows: Section 2 explains the background theory. Section 3 describes the proposed methods. Section 4 presents the experimental environment, evaluation method, and results. Finally, Section 5 presents the conclusions, limitations, and future research directions.

2. Background Theory

2.1. WebAR Service

AR allows the seamless integration of virtual data with the real world to provide users with sensory experiences that transcend reality [14,17]. AR is built and provided as a mobile application; AR data are pre-stored inside a client terminal and serviced [18–20]. The WebAR service starts downloading AR data when a webpage is accessed; therefore, this service does not require separate application installations compared to those required by native AR applications. Currently, the representative technologies include WebXR Device API, AR.js, and Three.js [21]. Several studies have focused on WebAR. For example, Qiao [14] conducted a study on a mechanism for the implementation of WebAR on mobile devices and presented various approaches to implement Web AR. Rodrigues [22] conducted a study using WebAR to use several types of media as AR objects.

2.2. Wireless Mesh Network

A WMN is a communication network that comprises a mesh router and mesh client; it provides broadband internet access, wireless local area network (LAN) coverage, and network connectivity to both mobile and stationary nodes. The WMN is the most efficient wireless technology compared to general networks such as ad hoc sensor networks [23]. Further, wireless 802.11 mesh networks have the advantages of low cost, easy and incremental deployment, and fault tolerance [24,25]. A WMN can be reconfigured dynamically. The nodes can automatically establish and maintain mesh connections internally, and it has advantages such as improved stability [26]. Thus far, various studies have been conducted on WMNs. For example, Benyamina [27] conducted a study to improve the performance of a WMN network design, and Akyildiz et al. [28] studied the protocol for a WMN. Figure 1 shows the wireless mesh network topology.

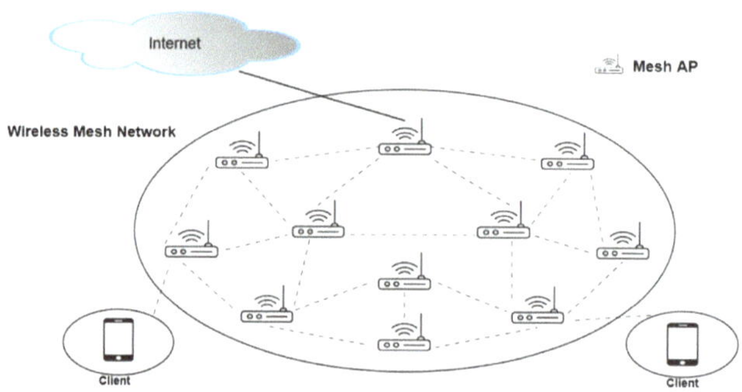

Figure 1. Wireless mesh network topology.

2.3. Edge Server

An edge server is a server on the edges of the network [29]; it is located where the corresponding function is required and distributed processing is performed [30]. The edge server performs compute offloading, data storage, caching, and processing. Further, it distributes request and delivery services from the cloud to the user [31].

Figure 2a shows the network distance between the client and cloud server, and Figure 2b shows the network distance between the client and edge server. The physical distance between the edge server and client is shorter than that between the cloud server and client. The edge server simplifies the network structure, and the time required to send and receive data is short [32]. The edge servers in the LAN layer can communicate data with clients in a stable manner. In the case of a cloud server, the data are transmitted from the client to the destination server via a metropolitan area network (MAN) and WAN. Latency such as bottlenecks and intermediate node systems can occur depending on the amount of data transmission [33]. Sukhman [34] conducted research on 5G, edge caching, and computing. Edge caching has been studied in the existing literature to minimize latency and load.

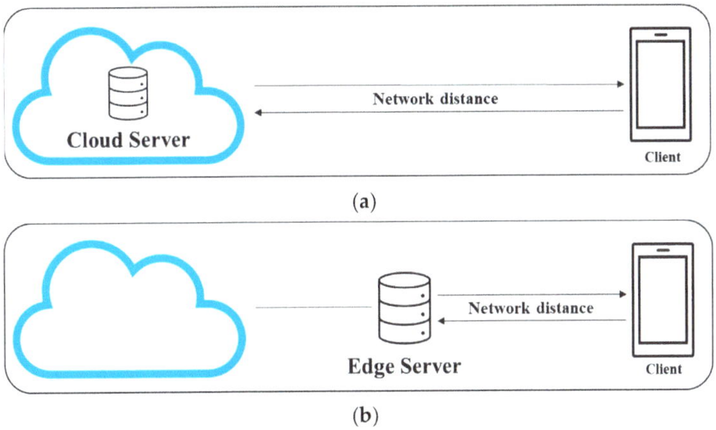

Figure 2. Network type and physical distance: (**a**) cloud server; (**b**) edge server.

2.4. Prefetching

Caching and prefetching methods have been proposed for the prediction of data usage patterns and to fetch data from a location close to the user in advance. The caching method sends cached data through a proxy server; this saves frequently requested data closer to the user, and it aims to reduce bandwidth consumption, network congestion, and traffic [15]. This caching method causes a bottleneck in the origin server with an increase in the number of users. This method becomes less efficient because of the limited system resources of the cache server. Prefetching was proposed to solve this caching problem [35]. The prefetching method solves bottlenecks and traffic jams, and it allows the faster transmission of data. A proxy can effectively handle more user requests than caching, and it can help reduce the load on the origin server. However, one disadvantage of the prefetching method is that prefetched data may not be requested by the user. To solve this problem, a high-accuracy prediction model needs to be used [36]. Domènech et al. [35] conducted a study on indices-related prediction, resource usage, and latency evaluation related to prefetching.

3. Proposed Method

3.1. AR Prefetching

We proposed a prefetching method which partitions data. Excessive traffic occurs during the first connection if a user downloads all the AR data simultaneously. Excessive traffic increases network traffic, and latency increases owing to limited network bandwidth [37]. The latency of other users increases because of the increase in traffic. Figure 3 shows the differences between prefetching and conventional methods. Figure 3a shows the conventional method in which a load event occurs once, and the entire AR content is prefetched simultaneously. Figure 3b shows the proposed method in which a load event occurs several times, and the predicted AR content is prefetched.

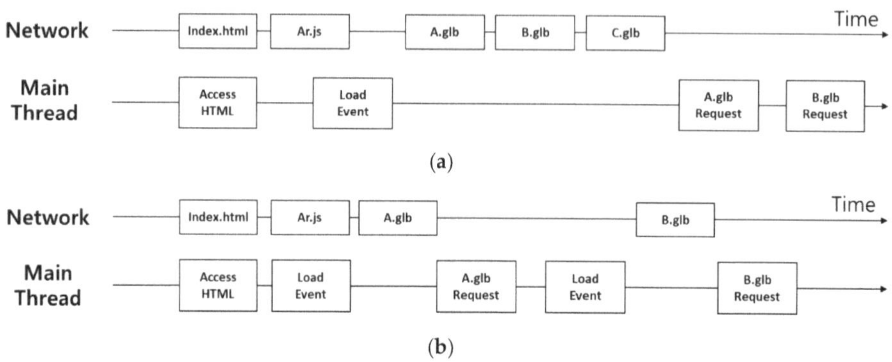

Figure 3. Resource loading sequence: (**a**) conventional method; (**b**) proposed method.

3.2. Client Server Architecture

Figure 4 shows the client and server architecture. This system consists of a client, web server, and database. The web server and database are located on edge servers.

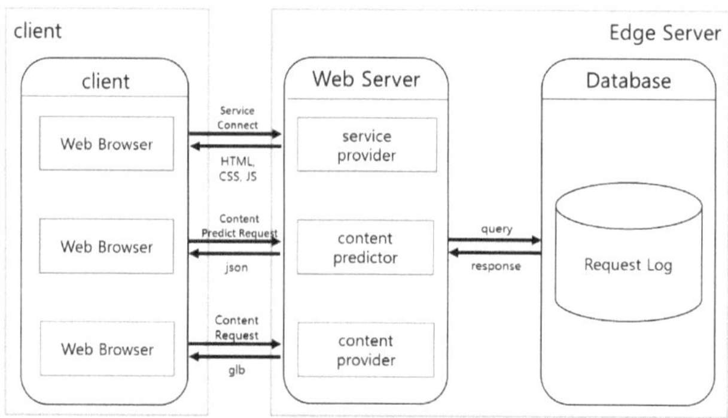

Figure 4. Client and server architecture.

3.2.1. Client

Figure 5 shows a flowchart of the client. The web browser sends a service access request to the web service provider and receives HTML, CSS, and JS to access AR services. When the AR is loaded, the client sends a request to the content predictor and initially receives the content information to be prefetched in JSON format. A list of content received from the content predictor is requested to the content provider and is prefetched. When the marker is recognized, a content output request is generated. If the content is prefetched, the content is provided immediately. However, if the content is not prefetched, the content is provided after prefetching the content. After providing the content, the list of content to be prefetched from the content predictor is received. If the list includes content that has not been prefetched, a request is sent to the content provider, and the content is prefetched.

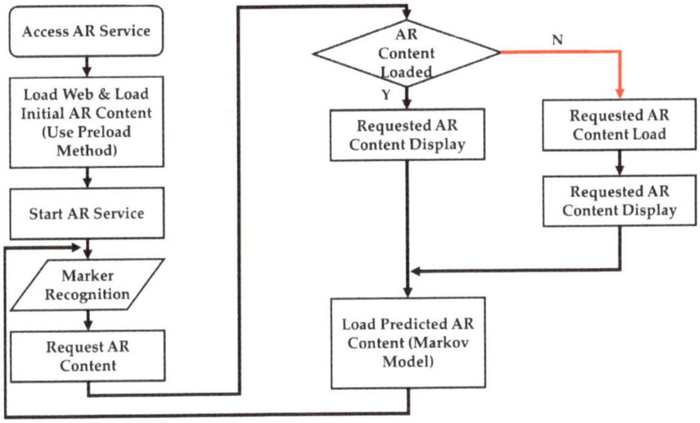

Figure 5. Client flowchart.

3.2.2. Edge Server

The edge server consists of a web server and database. The web server serves to transmit data to the client and consists of a service provider, content predictor, and content provider. The database stores request records.

The service provider provides a user interface to the client when the client accesses the AR service through a web browser. The information that the service provider provides to the client is in the form of HTML, CSS, and JS files, which compose the user interface.

The content predictor responds with a list of content to be prefetched in JSON format when a request for content prediction occurs in a web browser. Prefetching [34] based on the Markov model is used. The Markov model defines the transition probabilities between several states. The discrete-time Markov chain formula that predicts data is expressed as

$$\Pr(X_{n+1} = x|X_1, X2 = x_2, \ldots, X_n = x_n) = \Pr(X_{n+1} = x|X_n = x_n), \tag{1}$$

where n represents the order, and the state at n is defined as $x_1, x_2, \cdots, x_n$. Further, $X_1, X_2, \cdots, X_n$ represents the content. The formula for the calculation of statistical probability is

$$\check{P}(X(t+1) = x_c|X(n) = x_b) = \frac{n_{bc}}{\sum_{\alpha=a}^{0} n_{\alpha c}}, \tag{2}$$

where $X(t)$ denotes a random variable predicting AR content in time zone t; x_a, x_b, $\cdots$, x_o means $a \cdots o$ content; and $n_{\alpha c}$ represents the number of shifts from x_α to x_c content.

The content provider provides the corresponding 3D content as a glb file when a content prefetching request occurs in a web browser.

4. Experiments

4.1. Experimental Environment

For the experiment, an AR service was implemented in the "Nowon Career Center for Youth and Future" in Seoul, Republic of Korea, and the AR service data of users were collected. Figure 6 shows the mesh network access point (AP)/edge installation location and the AR image anchor location. In the experiment, 15 AR objects, each with a capacity of 10 MB to 10.5 MB, were used. The data were collected for three months from 1 June 2022 to 31 August 2022.

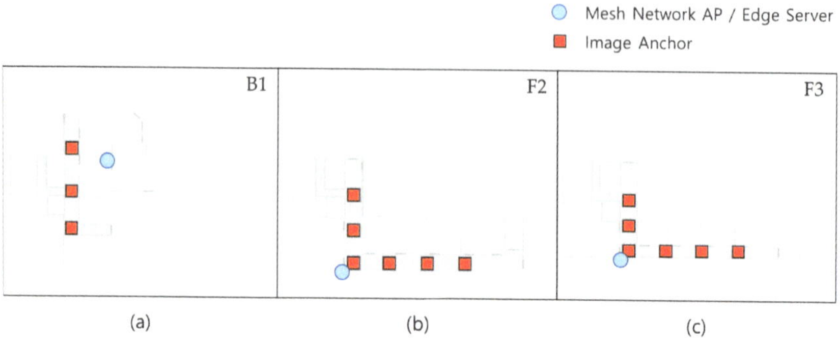

Figure 6. Test area drawings: (**a**) B1 drawing; (**b**) F2 drawing; (**c**) F3 drawing.

We placed mesh network AP, edge server, and anchor on building basement 1, floor 2, and floor 3. Figure 6 illustrates the test area drawings.

In the experiment, Samsung SM-T860 was used as the client device. The AP and edge server used VEEA's VHE10; it can communicate up to 300 Mbps using Wi-Fi-5-enabled devices. The AWS EC2 cloud server was used for an experimental comparison. AWS is the one of top cloud solution providers (CSPs), a pioneer, and the oldest cloud-service-providing company [38]. Table 1 lists the client information and Table 2 lists the server information used in this experiment.

Table 1. Client information used in the experiment.

	Client (Samsung Tab S6 SM-T860)
CPU	Qualcomm Snapdragon 855 SM8150 Platform
RAM	8 GB LPDDR4X SDRAM
OS	Android 11
Wi-Fi	Wi-Fi 1/2/3/4/5
Chrome	97.0.4692.98

Table 2. Server information used in the experiment.

	Edge Server (VEEA VHE10)	**Cloud Server (Amazon EC2)**
Type	-	t2.large
CPU	ARMv8 Quad Core processer, 1.5 GHz	2vCPU
RAM	8 GB DRAM	8 GB
Wi-Fi	Tri-band Wi-Fi5	-
NETWORK	1 Gbps	500 Mbps

In this experiment, we proposed a WMN edge server method for stably providing clients with low latency. The service area was expanded by installing an AP constituting each mesh with the IEEE 802.11 protocol. The WMN covered the entire AR service area using Wi-Fi. All APs were connected to each other in a mesh structure. The AP constituting the mesh amplified the WLAN signal and expanded the area; the edge server was configured in the same LAN layer as the client accessing the WMN. Further, it accessed the server only through communication with an internal network.

In the case of an edge server, network communication was performed using the internal network (LAN) without using the WAN and MAN; this reduced the effect of reducing network-related variables. Figure 7 shows the network configuration of the WMN and edge server.

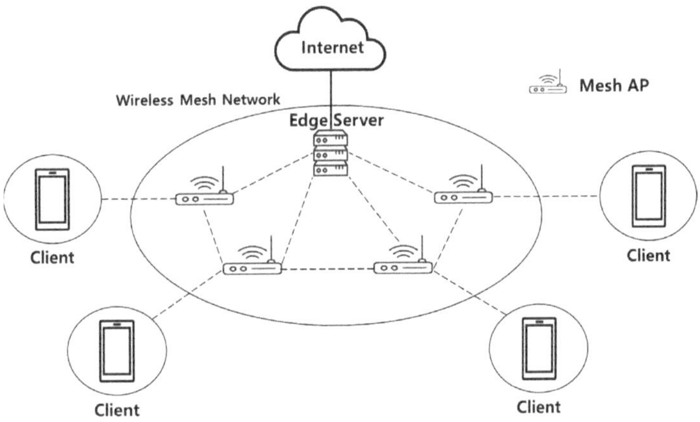

Figure 7. Wireless mesh network topology.

4.2. *Evaluation Method*

4.2.1. Hit Ratio

The hit ratio represents the ratio of the prefetch hits to the total number of objects requested by users. The formula for the *hit ratio* [39] of AR prefetching is expressed in Equation (3).

$$hit\ ratio\ (\%) = \left|\frac{\text{True}}{\text{True} + \text{False}}\right| \times 100 \tag{3}$$

where True represents the number of times a request occurs in the prefetching state, and False indicates the number of times the request has not been prefetched.

4.2.2. Waste Ratio

The waste ratio [40] refers to the ratio that has been prefetched; however, it is not used in the service. Equation (4) shows the *waste ratio* calculation formula.

$$waste\ ratio\ (\%) = \left|1 - \frac{\text{Prefetch Hits}}{\text{Prefetchs}}\right| \times 100, \tag{4}$$

where prefetch represents the number of data points prefetched by the client. The prefetch hits represent the number of prefetches used.

4.2.3. Latency

Latency [39] is an index that measures the delay that occurs in a client. It is used to measure the initial latency when connecting and the latency of the display output when requesting specific content. Equation (5) shows the *latency* calculation formula.

$$latency(\text{ms}) = |T_1 - T_2|, \tag{5}$$

where T_1 represents completed times, and T_2 represents start times.

4.2.4. Moving Average

The moving average [41] is an indicator of the hit ratio, waste ratio, and latency trends. Equation (6) shows the moving average calculation formula.

$$\overline{x}_k = \frac{x_{k-n+1} + x_{k-n+2} + \cdots + x_k}{n} = \frac{1}{n}(x_{k-n+1} + x_{k-n+2} + \cdots + x_k), \tag{6}$$

where $x_1, x_2, x_3 \cdots x_k$ represents the $1st, 2nd, 3rd \cdots k$ data, and k represents the total amount of data. Further, n represents the average number of data points.

4.3. Experimental Results

In this study, the average of next content usage intermediate time was divided by the average prefetching time to obtain the number of prefetching AR objects. The average of next content usage intermediate time of the collected data was 1592.23 ms, and the average prefetching time was 385.91 ms.

4.3.1. Comparison between the Edge and Cloud Servers

The first experiment compared a cloud server and an edge server with a traditional AR service. The AWS cloud servers located in Singapore, Virginia, and Seoul were used in this experiment. The experiment measured the AR content loading times of the cloud and edge servers. The experiment was performed ten times, and the mean and standard deviation were calculated.

Figure 8 shows the load time of the AR service for each server. The number of attempts denotes the number times each experiment was performed. Table 3 lists the average latency and standard deviation of the data in Figure 8. The AR content load time was 4329.50 ms when the edge server was used; it exhibited faster load times than that of cloud servers. Further, the standard deviation was stable at 170.31 ms. The edge server reduced delays and was 14.49% faster than the cloud server. Further, stability increased by 4.54% when using the edge server, and this showed that latency and stability were excellent because of the reduction in nodes when the physical distance between the server and client was reduced.

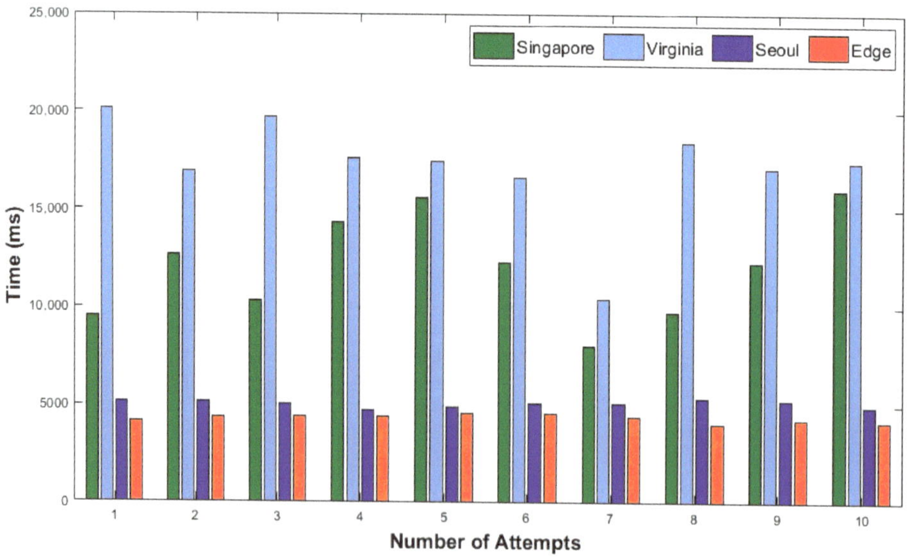

Figure 8. AR content load on the cloud server.

Table 3. Average and standard deviation of the AR content load on cloud servers.

	Average (ms)	Standard Deviation (ms)	Distance (km)
Singapore	12,070.50	2542.15	4688.87
Virginia	17,181.00	2506.36	11,137.60
Seoul	5062.90	178.41	11.34
Edge	4329.50	170.31	-

4.3.2. Comparative Analysis of the Network Traffic

Figure 9 shows the results of measuring traffic when users use AR content. Figures 9a and 8b show the traffic results of the conventional method and the traffic measurement results of the proposed method, respectively. In the conventional method, a relatively large amount of traffic was generated in the initial stage of accessing a web page. Compared with the conventional method, the proposed method was distributed and generated less initial traffic. In the proposed method, additional network traffic was generated by prefetching additional content during service use. The probability of content prefetching increased because of the increase in the number of requests. Therefore, additional traffic showed that the bytes per second decreased gradually with an increase in the request order.

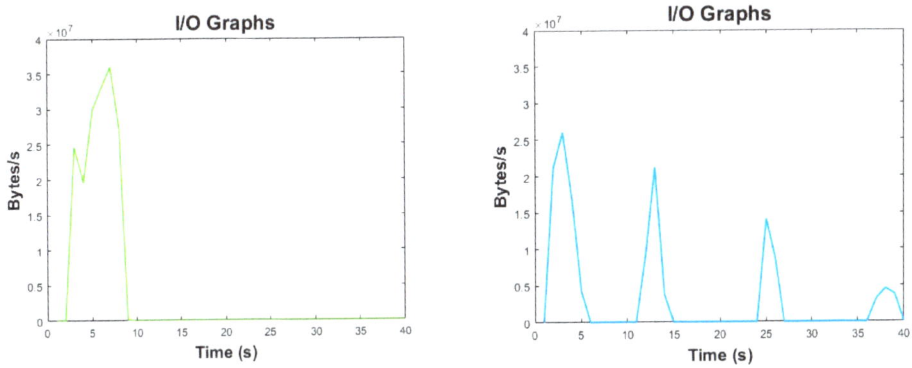

(a) (b)

Figure 9. Network traffic I/O graph: (**a**) conventional method; (**b**) proposed method.

Table 4 shows Mean and standard deviation of the AR content loading of the proposed method. The proposed method showed superior results in terms of initial latency and total latency compared with the conventional method. False prefetching indicates that the corresponding content is not prefetched when a content request occurs. High latency occurs because the content is provided after fetching. True prefetching indicates that the corresponding content is prefetched when the content is requested. The prefetched content is provided immediately.

Table 4. Mean and standard deviation of the AR content loading of the proposed method.

	Average (ms)	Standard Deviation (ms)
Initial time	295.60	34.99
Prefetching false	385.91	60.08
Prefetching true	17.98	8.68

4.3.3. Results per Request of the Proposed Method

Figure 10 shows the results of content requests over time. Figure 10a shows the hit ratio; the points represent real data, and in the case of a linear graph, the trend of the data is shown as a moving average, where the number of data points to be averaged is set to 30. The moving average of the hit ratio starts at 0% and increases as the user data collection progresses, which maintains it between 70% and 100%. Figure 10b shows the latency, which is inversely proportional to the hit ratio and shows a high delay time initially, which decreases to less than 100 ms.

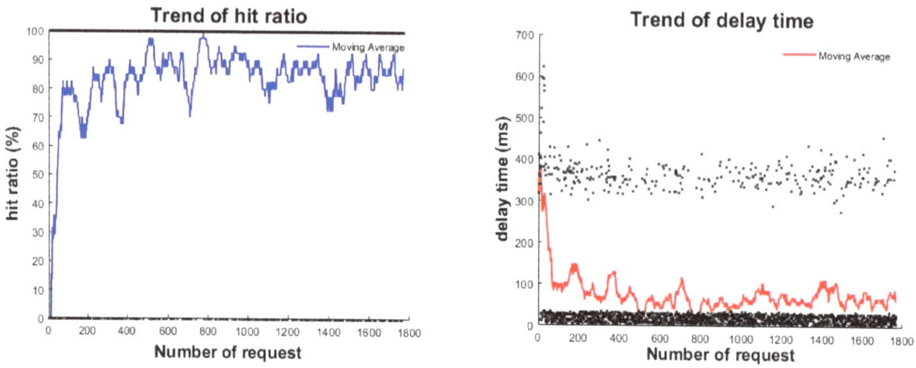

(a) (b)

Figure 10. Content request results in the chronological order of the proposed method: (**a**) hit ratio; (**b**) latency.

4.3.4. Average Result per User of the Proposed Method

Figure 11 shows the hit ratio and latency for each increase in user access. Figure 11a shows the average hit ratio for each user, and Figure 11b shows the total latency for each user. The total latency of a user was approximately 2000 ms. The total latency of a user also decreased to less than 400 ms with an increase in the hit ratio.

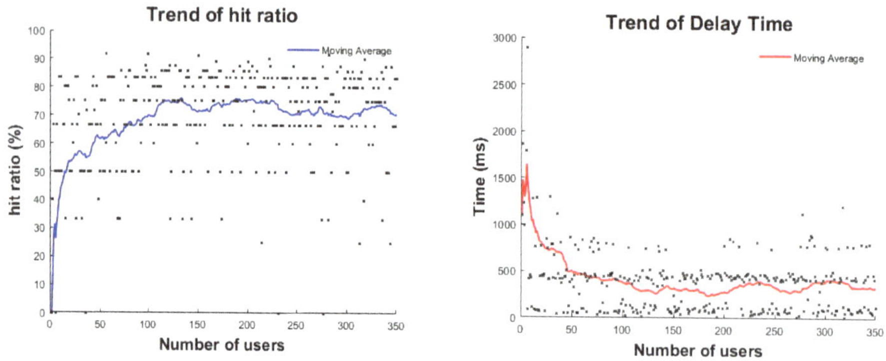

(a) (b)

Figure 11. Average content request results of the connected users of the proposed method: (**a**) hit ratio; (**b**) total latency.

As user data accumulated, the hit ratio increased.

4.3.5. Results Based on Content Request Order of the Proposed Method

Figure 12 shows the hit ratio and latency for each content request order. Figure 12a shows the hit ratio. The first request per user had a low hit ratio of 50% because the experiment was conducted in an environment where the starting location was not determined.

From the second request onward, the hit ratio increased to more than 80%. Subsequently, it gradually increased and reached a hit ratio of 100% from the eighth request. Figure 12b shows the latency. In the case of content requested for the first time by each user, it took more than 180 ms, and this was relatively time-consuming. After the eigth request, when the hit ratio became 100%, the output time was 20 ms or less. The AR content for which prefetching was completed also increased because the number of requests per user increased. Even if the prediction failed, there was a high probability that the prefetching was completed. Therefore, the hit ratio converged to 100%.

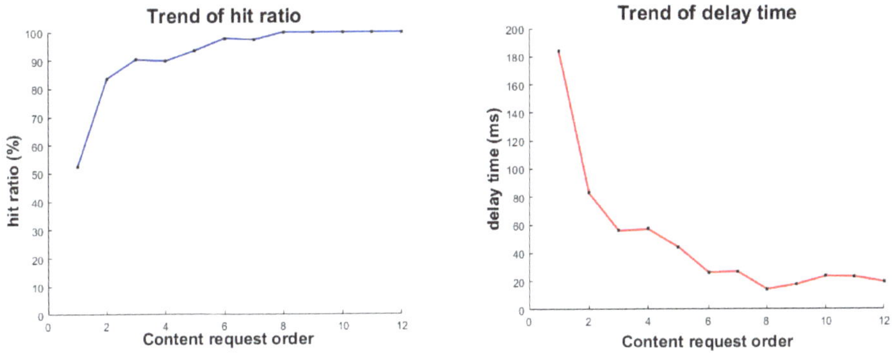

(**a**) (**b**)

Figure 12. Results of the content request order for the proposed method: (**a**) hit ratio; (**b**) latency.

4.3.6. Waste Ratio Results of the Proposed and Conventional Methods

Figure 13 shows the waste ratio that was prefetched but not used by the client. Figure 13a,b show the results of the conventional and proposed methods, respectively. The proposed method had an average waste ratio of 50.25%, and it was lower than that of the conventional method (66.28%). The proposed method initially exhibited a low waste ratio. Prefetching did not proceed because of the lack of user data and unpredictability. The amount of prefetching content increased as the user data accumulated, and this resulted in a waste ratio that increased to approximately 50% and was maintained.

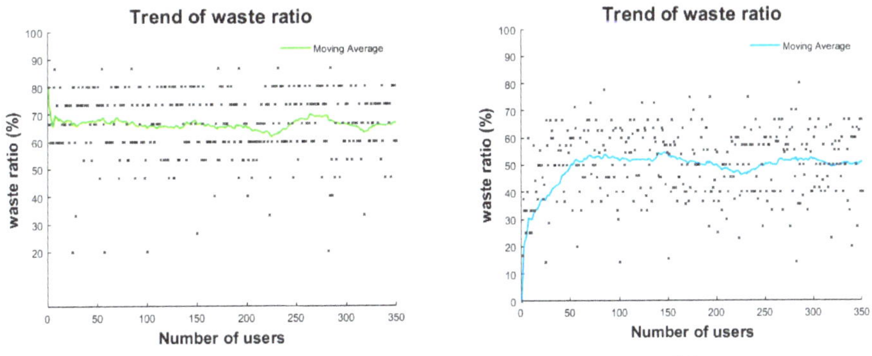

(**a**) (**b**)

Figure 13. Result of waste ratio: (**a**) conventional methods; (**b**) proposed method.

5. Conclusions

This study provides a method for faster and more efficient WebAR services. Large amounts of 3D data require latency from the users. A method was proposed that reduces latency in WebAR services by 81.5%. In the experiments, edge servers could physically reduce delays and were 14.49% faster than cloud servers. Further, the stability increased by 4.54%. The waste ratio related to unnecessary content prefetching was 16% lower than that of the conventional method. The Markov model was used to prefetch the predicted content rather than random prefetching to increase the hit ratio. The proposed method is more advantageous as it provides a large amount of AR content. Further, it is suitable for the realization of high-quality data in Web AR services. The results of this study have potential applications in areas such as AR games and AR docent services. A limitation of this study is that latency increased when prediction failed. Future research should increase the hit ratio by considering multiple parameters and advanced prediction algorithms. To this end, it is necessary to secure user data and apply machine learning.

Author Contributions: Conceptualization, S.C.; methodology, S.C.; software, S.C., S.H. and S.L.; investigation, S.H. and H.K.; writing—original draft preparation, S.C.; writing—review and editing, S.L. and S.K.; supervision, S.K.; project administration, S.K. All authors have read and agreed to the published version of the manuscript.

Funding: This research was supported by the Basic Science Research Program through the National Research Foundation of Korea (NRF) funded by the Ministry of Science and ICT (2020R1F1A1069079) and by Ministry of Culture, Sports and Tourism and Korea Creative Content Agency (Project Number: R2021040083).

Institutional Review Board Statement: Not applicable.

Informed Consent Statement: Not applicable.

Data Availability Statement: The data presented in this study are available upon request from the corresponding author. The data are not publicly available because of privacy concerns.

Conflicts of Interest: The authors declare no conflict of interest.

References

1. Web XR Device API. Available online: https://www.w3.org/TR/webxr/ (accessed on 1 May 2022).
2. Three.js. Available online: https://threejs.org/ (accessed on 1 May 2022).
3. AR.js. Augmented Reality on the Web. Available online: https://ar-js-org.github.io/AR.js-Docs/ (accessed on 1 May 2022).
4. Mai, S.; Liu, Y. Implementation of Web AR applications with fog radio access networks based on openairinterface platform. In Proceedings of the 2019 5th International Conference on Control, Automation and Robotics (ICCAR), Beijing, China, 19–22 April 2019; IEEE Publications: Beijing, China, 2019; pp. 639–643. [CrossRef]
5. Han, D.-I.; Tom Dieck, M.C.; Jung, T. User experience model for augmented reality applications in urban heritage tourism. *J. Herit. Tour.* **2018**, *13*, 46–61. [CrossRef]
6. Naka, R.; Hagiwara, N.; Ohta, M. Accelerating data loading for photo-based augmented reality on web browser. In Proceedings of the 2018 IEEE 7th Global Conference Consumer Electronics (GCCE), Nara, Japan, 9–12 October 2018; IEEE Publications: Nara, Japan, 2018; pp. 698–699. [CrossRef]
7. Banerji, S.; Chowdhury, R.S. On IEEE 802.11: Wireless LAN technology. *IJMNCT* **2013**, *3*, 45–64. [CrossRef]
8. IEEE. 802.11TM Wireless Local Area Networks. Available online: https://www.ieee802.org/11 (accessed on 5 May 2022).
9. IEEE. P802.11 Wireless LANs Draft Terms and Definitions for 802.11s. Available online: https://mentor.ieee.org/802.11/dcn/04/11-04-0730-01-000s-draft-core-terms-and-definitions-802-11s.doc (accessed on 5 May 2022).
10. IEEE. 802.11-s Tutorial Overview of the Amendment for Wireless Local Area Mesh Networking. Available online: https://www.ieee802.org/802_tutorials/06-November/802.11s_Tutorial_r5.pdf (accessed on 5 May 2022).
11. Lin, Y.; Kemme, B.; Patino-Martinez, M.; Jimenez-Peris, R. Enhancing edge computing with database replication. In Proceedings of the 2007 26th IEEE International Symposium on Reliable Distributed Systems (SRDS 2007), Beijing, China, 10–12 October 2007; IEEE Publications: Beijing, China, 2007; pp. 45–54. [CrossRef]
12. Seyun, C.; Woosung, S.; Sukjun, H.; Hoijun, K.; Seunghyun, L.; Soonchul, K. A Novle Method for Efficient Mobile AR Service in Edge Mesh Network. *Int. J. Internet Broadcast. Commun.* **2022**, *14*, 22–29.
13. Ren, J.; He, Y.; Huang, G.; Yu, G.; Cai, Y.; Zhang, Z. An edge-computing based architecture for mobile augmented reality. *IEEE Netw.* **2019**, *33*, 162–169. [CrossRef]
14. Xiuquan, Q.; Pei, R.; Schahram, D.; Ling, L.; Huadong, M.; Junliang, C.; Web, A.R. A promising future for mobile augmented reality—State of the art, challenges, and insights. *Proc. IEEE* **2019**, *107*, 651–666.
15. Ali, W.; Shamsuddin, S.M.; Ismail, A.S. A survey of web caching and prefetching. *Int. J. Adv. Soft Comput.* **2011**, *3*, 18–44.

16. Miyashita, T.; Meier, P.; Tachikawa, T.; Orlic, S.; Eble, T.; Scholz, V.; Gapel, A.; Gerl, O.; Arnaudov, S.; Lieberknecht, S. An augmented reality museum guide. In Proceedings of the 2008 7th IEEE/ACM International Symposium Mixed Augmented Reality, Cambridge, UK, 15–18 September 2008; IEEE Publications: Cambridge, UK, 2008; pp. 103–106. [CrossRef]
17. Lee, D.; Shim, W.; Lee, M.; Lee, S.; Jung, K.-D.; Kwon, S. Performance evaluation of ground AR anchor with WebXR device API. *Appl. Sci.* **2021**, *11*, 7877. [CrossRef]
18. Lee, G.A.; Dunser, A.; Kim, S.; Billinghurst, M. CityViewAR: A mobile outdoor AR application for city visualization. In Proceedings of the 2012 IEEE International Symposium Mixed Augmented Reality—Arts, Media, and Humanities (ISMAR-AMH), Atlanta, GA, USA, 5–8 November 2012; IEEE Publications: Atlanta, GA, USA, 2012; pp. 57–64.
19. Chung, N.; Han, H.; Joun, Y. Tourists' intention to visit a destination: The role of augmented reality (AR) application for a heritage site. *Comput. Hum. Behav.* **2015**, *50*, 588–599. [CrossRef]
20. He, J.; Ren, J.; Zhu, G.; Cai, S.; Chen, G. Mobile-based AR application helps to promote EFL children's vocabulary study. In Proceedings of the 2014 IEEE 14th International Conference on Advanced Learning Technologies, Athens, Greece, 7–10 July 2014; IEEE Publications: Athens, Greece, 2014; pp. 431–433. [CrossRef]
21. Nguyen, M.; Lai, M.P.; Le, H.; Yan, W.Q. A web-based augmented reality platform using pictorial QR code for educational purposes and beyond. In Proceedings of the 25th ACM Symposium on Virtual Reality Software Technology, Parramatta, Australia, 12–15 November 2019; ACM: Parramatta, NSW, Australia, 2019; pp. 1–2.
22. Barone Rodrigues, A.; Dias, D.R.C.; Martins, V.F.; Bressan, P.A.; de Paiva Guimarães, M. WebAR: A web-augmented reality-based authoring tool with experience API support for educational applications. In *International Conference on Universal Access in Human-Computer Interaction*; Springer International Publishing: Berlin/Heidelberg, Germany, 2017; pp. 118–128. [CrossRef]
23. Karthika, K.C. Wireless mesh network: A survey. In Proceedings of the 2016 International Conference on Wireless Communications, Signal Processing and Networking (WiSPNET), Chennai, India, 21–23 March 2016; IEEE Publications: Chennai, India, 2016; pp. 1966–1970. [CrossRef]
24. Passos, D.; Teixeira, D.V.; Muchaluat-Saade, D.C.; Magalhães, L.S.; Albuquerque, C. Mesh network performance measurements. In Proceedings of the International Information and Telecommunication Technologies Symposium (I2TS), Cuiabá, Brazil, 6–8 December 2006; pp. 48–55.
25. Navda, V.; Kashyap, A.; Das, S.R. Design and evaluation of IMesh: An infrastructure-mode wireless mesh network. In Proceedings of the Sixth IEEE International Symposium World of Wireless Mobile Multimedia Networks, Naxos, Italy, 13–16 June 2005; IEEE Publications: Taormina-Giardini Naxos, 2005; pp. 164–170. [CrossRef]
26. Paulon, J.V.M.; Olivieri de Souza, B.J.; Endler, M. Exploring data collection on Bluetooth mesh networks. *Ad Hoc Netw.* **2022**, *130*, 102809. [CrossRef]
27. Benyamina, D.; Hafid, A.; Gendreau, M. Wireless mesh networks design—A survey. *IEEE Commun. Surv. Tutor.* **2012**, *14*, 299–310. [CrossRef]
28. Akyildiz, I.F.; Xudong, W. A survey on wireless mesh networks. *IEEE Commun. Mag. Inst. Electr. Electron. Eng.* **2005**, *43*, S23–S30. [CrossRef]
29. Loven, L.; Lahderanta, T.; Ruha, L.; Leppanen, T.; Peltonen, E.; Riekki, J.; Sillanpaa, M.J. Scaling up an edge server deployment. In Proceedings of the 2020 IEEE International Conference on Pervasive Computing and Communications Workshops (PerCom Workshops), Austin, TX, USA, 13–17 March 2020; IEEE Publications: Austin, TX, USA, 2020; pp. 1–7. [CrossRef]
30. Wang, S.; Zhao, Y.; Xu, J.; Yuan, J.; Hsu, C.-H. Edge server placement in mobile edge computing. *J. Parallel Distrib. Comput.* **2019**, *127*, 160–168. [CrossRef]
31. Shi, W.; Cao, J.; Zhang, Q.; Li, Y.; Xu, L. Edge computing: Vision and challenges. *IEEE Internet Things J.* **2016**, *3*, 637–646. [CrossRef]
32. Premsankar, G.; Di Francesco, M.; Taleb, T. Edge computing for the internet of things: A case study. *IEEE Internet Things J.* **2018**, *5*, 1275–1284. [CrossRef]
33. Besson, E. Performance of TCP in a wide-area network: Influence of successive bottlenecks and exogenous traffic. In Proceedings of the Globecom'00—IEEE. Global Telecommunications Conference, Cat. No. 00CH37137, San Francisco, CA, USA, 27 November–1 December 2000; IEEE Publications: San Francisco, CA, USA, 2000; Volume 3, pp. 1798–1804.
34. Sukhmani, S.; Sadeghi, M.; Erol-Kantarci, M.; El Saddik, A. Edge caching and computing in 5G for mobile AR/VR and tactile internet. *IEEE Multimed.* **2019**, *26*, 21–30. [CrossRef]
35. Domènech, J.; Gil, J.A.; Sahuquillo, J.; Pont, A. Web prefetching performance metrics: A survey. *Perform. Eval.* **2006**, *63*, 988–1004. [CrossRef]
36. Pallis, G.; Vakali, A.; Pokorny, J. A clustering-based prefetching scheme on a Web cache environment. *Comput. Electr. Eng.* **2008**, *34*, 309–323. [CrossRef]
37. Robert, L.C.; Mark, E.C. Measuring bottleneck link speed in packet-switched networks. *Perform. Eval.* **1996**, *27–28*, 297–318.
38. Manish, S.; Tripathi, R.C. Cloud computing: Comparison and analysis of cloud service providers-AWs, Microsoft and Google. In Proceedings of the 9th International Conference System Modeling and Advancement in Research Trends (SMART), Moradabad, India, 4–5 December 2020; Volume 2020.
39. Christos, B.; Agisilaos, K.; Dionysios, K. Predictive Prefetching on the Web and Its Potential Impact in the Wide Area. *World Wide Web* **2004**, *7*, 143–179. [CrossRef]
40. Ibrahim, T.I.; Cheng-Zhong, X. Neural nets based predictive prefetching to tolerate WWW latency. In Proceedings of the 20th IEEE International Conference on Distributed Computing Systems, Taipei, Taiwan, 10–13 April 2000. [CrossRef]

41. Craig, A.E.; Simon, A.P. Is smarter better? A comparison of adaptive, and simple moving average trading strategies. *Res. Int. Bus. Financ.* **2005**, *19*, 399–411. [CrossRef]

virtual worlds

Concept Paper

Enhancing Nursing Simulation Education: A Case for Extended Reality Innovation

Shanna Fealy [1,2,*], Pauletta Irwin [1], Zeynep Tacgin [3], Zi Siang See [4] and Donovan Jones [1,2]

1 School of Nursing, Paramedicine and Healthcare Sciences, Faculty of Sciences and Health, Charles Sturt University, Port Macquarie, NSW 2444, Australia
2 School of Medicine and Public Health, College of Health and Wellbeing, University of Newcastle, Callaghan, NSW 2308, Australia
3 Social Science Vocational School, Marmara University, Istanbul 34865, Turkey
4 School of Education, College of Arts, Law and Education, University of Tasmania, Launceston, TAS 7250, Australia
* Correspondence: sfealy@csu.edu.au

Abstract: This concept paper explores the use of extended reality (XR) technology in nursing education, with a focus on three case studies developed at one regional university in Australia. Tertiary education institutions that deliver nursing curricula are facing challenges around the provision of simulated learning experiences that prepare students for the demands of real-world professional practice. To overcome these barriers, XR technology, which includes augmented, mixed, and virtual reality (AR, MR, VR), offers a diverse media platform for the creation of immersive, hands-on learning experiences, situated within virtual environments that can reflect some of the dynamic aspects of real-world healthcare environments. This document analysis explores the use of XR technology in nursing education, through the narrative and discussion of three applied-use cases. The collaboration and co-design between nursing educators and XR technology experts allows for the creation of synchronous and asynchronous learning experiences beyond traditional nursing simulation media, better preparing students for the demands of real-world professional practice.

Keywords: extended reality; nursing; educational technology; simulation education

Citation: Fealy, S.; Irwin, P.; Tacgin, Z.; See, Z.S.; Jones, D. Enhancing Nursing Simulation Education: A Case for Extended Reality Innovation. *Virtual Worlds* **2023**, 2, 218–230. https://doi.org/10.3390/virtualworlds2030013

Academic Editors: Radu Comes, Dorin-Mircea Popovici, Calin Gheorghe Dan Neamtu and Jing-Jing Fang

Received: 3 May 2023
Revised: 5 June 2023
Accepted: 3 July 2023
Published: 27 July 2023

1. Introduction

The provision of authentic learning experiences for undergraduate (pre-registration) nursing students is an ongoing challenge for tertiary education institutes globally [1]. Traditionally, real-world learning experiences were the sole approach to offer authentic learning experiences within nursing curricula, ensuring adequate and contextualised preparation for practice as a registered health professional [2,3]. Although workplace learning remains effective in preparing nursing students for the realities of professional practice [3,4], the shift from apprenticeship-style nursing education to university-based education and an increasingly competitive marketplace for industry-supported work experience, have led to a decrease in students being exposed to the contextual demands of real-world professional practice [2,5]. Moreover, workplace learning hours within nursing curricula vary substantially between countries. For example, the United Kingdom requires nursing students to achieve a minimum of 2300 h of workplace learning, and New Zealand requires a minimum of 1100 h, whereas Australian students are only required to achieve a minimum of 800 h of workplace learning prior to graduation. The variable hours and the competitive nature of gaining quality industry work placements for countries such as Australia, has contributed to an increasing reliance on educational institutions to provide authentic simulated learning experiences that adequately prepare nursing students for professional practice [2,5–7]. Paradoxically, the healthcare industry is increasingly demanding that new graduate nurses be "work ready", with the ability to autonomously apply skills learnt within their degree programs, within complex and continually changing healthcare environments [3,7–9].

1.1. Nursing Simulation Education

Simulated learning within nursing curricula generally encompasses learning experiences to assist students in attaining and practising skills within safe, physical environments that are designed to look like a hospital or other healthcare environment [10]. Often referred to as simulated learning environments (SLE), equipment such as low-to-high-fidelity (realism) task trainers and mannikins are typically used in combination with roleplay and simulated patient scenarios to facilitate incremental learning (i.e., novice to expert), without the risk of harming actual patients [3,7]. Extending beyond developing and rehearsing psychomotor skills, contemporary programs seek to create contextual asynchronous and synchronous experiences that also promote cognitive (facts, critical thinking, clinical reasoning), and affective skill (beliefs, emotional intelligence, empathy) development, while adhering to the principles of nursing education theory [5,8]. The experiential learning theory (ELT) conceptualised by Kolb [11] is most often used to underpin nursing simulation education, supporting the idea that the acquisition of knowledge is derived from learner experience (concrete or abstract) and relies upon reflection to form generalisations and a new understanding [11].

The value of simulated learning for practicing skills within a supportive environment prior to workplace learning, increasing self-efficacy, and increasing confidence and competence for workplace learning are well documented [3,10]. However, the effectiveness of simulated learning for preparing work-ready graduates is sparse [7,12,13]. Additionally, students have commented on a lack of perceived authenticity and realism in simulated learning, particularly when using mannikins within an SLE [7]. A systematic review and meta-synthesis of 27 studies by Handeland et al. [14] evaluating nursing students' experiences of using mannikins described the phenomena as "seeing the manikin as a doll or a patient". The manikin as a doll was drawn from students' perceptions that mannikins were akin to a plastic doll, devoid of human expression such as communication and emotion, which hindered the real learning of nursing practice through the application of affective skills such as empathy [14]. However, the unreal nature of the manikin allowed students to practice skills unhindered, without fear of hurting anyone (failsafe) [14]. Interestingly, a study investigating the realism and presence of utilising real-life human patients for nursing education within an SLE by MacLean et al. [15] found that nursing students commented on the need to increase the realism, to enhance learning. The students in this study noted a lack of authenticity, including a lack of background noise and distractions such as those from patient call buzzers, monitor alarms, and other nursing staff during the experience. A more recent study of nursing students' perceptions of simulated learning by Tan et al. [12] concluded that the authenticity of simulated learning experiences were important to nursing students, with real-world work perceived as more complex than what was portrayed within simulated learning [14]. Students specifically commented on the inability to simulate the management of multiple patients, time management skills, and resource management skills, as well as realistic interprofessional communication and opportunities for teamwork [12].

1.2. Making the Case for XR Innovation

Technology-enabled approaches, such as the use of extended reality (XR) media, including immersive virtual reality (IVR), augmented reality (AR), and mixed reality (MR) may be one way to afford nursing students more authentic simulated learning experiences that cannot be achieved with traditional simulation media [8,16–18]. The embedded media diversity of XR technology presents enormous potential for the development of simulated learning experiences that require active student engagement and participation, which are seen as crucial to improving learning outcomes [12,19]. One key advantage of XR technologies such as IVR is the ability to situate learners within virtual environments using head-mounted displays (HMDs), conveying the contextual (physical and mental) sensations of being present and immersed in the world around them, a virtual world [20,21]. Presence and embodiment are the main psychological concepts of building reality perception in IVR users, replacing the real world, and allowing for the feeling of being within an environment and interacting with the virtual environment [21]. Augmented reality (AR) is a technology that overlays digital information onto the real world, often using a mobile device or wearable technology, such as smart glasses [22,23]. AR can enhance a user's perception of reality, by adding digital objects or information to the live view of their environment, making it possible to interact with both the real and digital worlds simultaneously [22,23]. Mixed reality (MR) is a technology that blends elements of both AR and IVR to create a continuum of connection between digital objects and the real world [24]. MR creates a hybrid environment where users can interact with both digital and real-world objects (such as high-fidelity mannikins) in a seamless way.

Therefore, this concept paper explores the potential of XR technology in enhancing traditional nursing simulation within higher education institutions, through an exploration of three case studies developed within one large regional Australian university. Through this exploration, we aim to provide insights and practical guidance for nursing educators and instructional designers interested in using XR media to enhance simulated learning within higher education contexts.

2. Materials and Methods

The concept paper is guided by a document analysis methodology [25]. Document analysis can be particularly useful in evaluating the design features of XR software from a learning strategy perspective, enabling researchers to gain a better understanding of the software and its features, as well as the intended user experience and learning outcomes [26]. Therefore, this study employs a document analysis methodology to explore the design features of three XR applications developed to augment the simulated learning experience for undergraduate nursing students.

In 2018, a new educational design framework was initiated at one large regional Australian university, with a focus on promoting teaching innovation and expanding practical support and resources [27]. Within this context, a small group of nursing and midwifery educators proposed the development of three case studies using XR technology, to increase the realism and accessibility of simulated learning experiences for students within their nursing and midwifery programs. The case studies were developed as stand-alone research prototypes for initial testing among undergraduate nursing, midwifery, and medical student cohorts, rather than full curriculum and university system integration. Each case study was co-designed by nursing and midwifery educators and XR technology experts, with the prototype development funded by the institution's new educational design program.

The prototype development was guided by the scrum design framework [28]. Scrum is based on three principles: transparency, inspection, and adaptation, and is underpinned by the empirical process control theory, which emphasises that knowledge is gained from experience, and decision-making from what is known [28]. The transparency principle enables the team to collectively conceptualise and define the final product outcome and development endpoint [28]. The inspection and adaptation principles involve four key processes: the sprint planning, daily scrum, sprint review, and sprint retrospective. Sprints are considered the main aspect of the production phase, where the entire team plans a development sprint, whereby the deliverables or outcomes of each sprint are discussed, and the sprint duration is defined. Following a sprint, the team meets to reflect upon the progress and feasibility of the end outcome [28]. The prototypes presented were: (1) the Compromised Neonate (CN); (2) the Road to Birth (RtB); and (3) Conflict Resolution (Angry Stan). Each was conceptualised through regular team meetings over a three-month period, with each case study developed over twelve weeks, with sprints scheduled every two weeks, until each program was completed and ready for testing. The programs were designed using various hardware and instructional design components, for accessibility, and to target specific learning outcomes.

3. Results

3.1. The Compromised Neonate

The simultaneous application of psychomotor, cognitive, and affective skills required for neonatal resuscitation is an area in which the incorporation of XR technology, specifically IVR, has the potential to complement traditional simulated-learning media [16]. The compromised neonate program was designed in response to anecdotal student feedback of wanting more time to practise and/or refresh their neonatal resuscitation skills prior to workplace learning. Traditional simulation methods for practicing these skills outside of the curriculum-prescribed simulation learning were often inaccessible, or complicated by resource availability in terms of trained staff, equipment, and learning environment [29]. Nursing and midwifery educators therefore wanted to be able to make the practice of these lifesaving skills more accessible for their students from remote locations away from the educational institution, such as the students' residence.

The comprehensive design and initial testing of the program has been previously published [16]. The collective team aim was to be able to remotely immerse a student in a contemporary hospital-based birthing environment, where the student would be able to undertake self-directed learning of the procedural psychomotor skills of neonatal resuscitation, according to the Australian Resuscitation Council guidelines [16,30]. Approximately 10% of all neonates born in Australia will require some sort of resuscitation measure, with only 1% requiring advanced neonatal resuscitation skills [16,30]. As a result, all health-professional students working in maternity or neonatal care need to be well prepared for these events, ready to employ a range of resuscitation skills at any time, due to their unexpected and rare nature [8,16]. Given the focus of the brief, the program was produced for use by both immersive (IVR) and non-immersive (desktop VR) virtual reality media, with the final prototype accessible via desktop or laptop personal computer, tethered IVR (HTC VIVE and Samsung Oculus Rift) and untethered mobile IVR (Samsung Galaxy mobile phones and compatible Samsung – Oculus Gear VR headsets, sourced in Newcastle, Australia), accommodating for within-institution and remote student use [16].

Using IVR, and upon application of an immersive headset (with audio), students are presented with a 360-degree view of a virtual birthing room, where they are immersed within a scenario featuring a compromised neonate requiring resuscitation (Figure 1c). Students are then required to employ their theorical and practical knowledge of neonatal resuscitation by employing the procedural skills in their correct sequence, to resuscitate the neonate. The birthing environment, including equipment, was designed based on what was used within the Australian acute birthing care context, ensuring authenticity. To promote knowledge retention, and offer a scaffolded approach, two learning modes, a guided and unguided mode, were developed. The guided mode is based in behaviourist learning theory. Nursing has a long association with a behaviourist approach, wherein clinical skills have been honed using repetitious drills [31]. Within the guided mode, students are provided with a series of prompts required for successful resuscitation (Figure 1a), using handheld controllers for interaction with the environment (Figure 1b). Incorrect responses result in the student not being able to progress within the simulation, until the correct procedures have been identified [16].

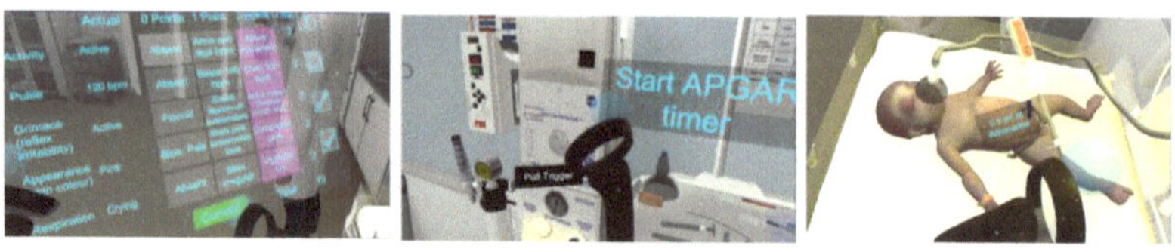

(a) (b) (c)

Figure 1. The Compromised Neonate virtual reality educational application. (**a**) Demonstration of conducting a neonatal resuscitation assessment. (**b**) Demonstration of interacting with the experience using a handheld controller. (**c**) Demonstration of the compromised neonate requiring medication.

A cognitivist approach is adopted throughout the program, which requires critical-thinking and problem-solving skills to be employed [32]. For example, students are challenged to distinguish the need for the escalation of care of the neonate, such as identifying the need for medical assistance, and interpreting the neonate's physical assessment score, as well as identifying the correct medications and dosages (Figure 1c) [16]. In addition, the application of affective skills is essential to successfully navigate the program. Students are required to interact with the baby's father, choosing appropriate family-centred communication, explaining what has happened to the baby, and identifying the need for post-resuscitation communication and education. More experienced students can perform these procedures using the unguided mode, which reflects how the student is required to autonomously practise during real-world workplace learning [16].

Following development, initial testing of the Compromised Neonate was undertaken within a small group ($n = 7$) of third year undergraduate midwifery students at the originating higher education institution [16]. During a usual neonatal resuscitation simulated learning experience that employed the use of high-fidelity simulation mannikins, students were additionally asked to test the Compromised Neonate program using mobile IVR (untethered Samsung-Oculus Gear VR headsets) and provide initial feedback on the Compromised Neonate program [16]. The feedback from anonymous post experience survey questions indicated that the simulation met the students' learning needs, allowed for interactive feedback and guidance, resembled a real-life situation, and was seen as an enjoyable experience that could likely improve their confidence in their neonatal resuscitation skills [16]. Due to the prototype nature of the program, empirical testing, such as a randomised controlled trial amongst a large cohort of students to evaluate its effectiveness compared to traditional simulation methods, was not possible, with testing mostly limited to ad hoc student use within the originating institution.

3.2. The Road to Birth

The use of XR technology is becoming increasingly popular, offering new ways to visualise and understand complex spatial concepts, such as human anatomical and physiological processes [20]. The initial concept for the RtB program evolved out of discussions among nursing and midwifery educators when brainstorming methods to enhance the teaching of complex spatial concepts, such as foetal positioning in utero in relation to maternal anatomy and physiology. Traditional learning approaches were typically static in nature (cadaveric specimens and plastic models), with access to these learning opportunities outside of education institutions often inaccessible for students, as described above [20]. Therefore, the primary design objective was to integrate XR technology, to provide nursing and midwifery students with an interactive and remote learning resource that could assist students in visualising the internal anatomical changes of pregnancy, and foetal positioning.

The collective team aim was to provide nursing and midwifery students with an internal view of pregnancy, allowing students to visualise the dynamic reproductive anatomical and physiological changes that occur over the 40+ weeks of human gestation [20,33]. The position and presentations of the foetus need to be clearly understood by all healthcare professionals working in maternity care. A number of these positions are favourable for a vaginal birth, whilst others may make a vaginal birth more difficult, and lead to complications in the birthing process, such as an operative birth by forceps, ventouse, or caesarean section [20]. The detailed development and testing of the RtB program have been previously published [20,33].

Allowing for within-institution and remote use, a multimodal approach was devised for interaction with the RtB environment [20,33]. The RtB was developed for use with IVR (SteamVR-compatible) mobile smartphone/tablet devices (both iOS and android), as well as being compatible for use on a personal computer (Figure 2a). In addition, the program was designed to run on the mixed reality Microsoft HoloLens headset (sourced in Newcastle, Australia), with gesture-controlled interactivity, as featured in (Figure 2b).

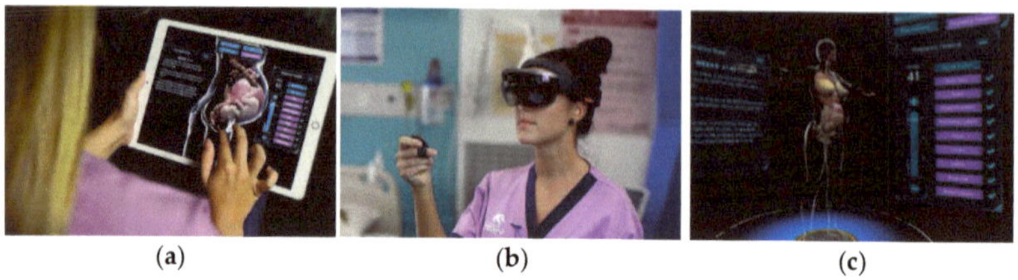

Figure 2. The Road to Birth multimodal XR learning program. (**a**) Demonstration of the RtB being used on a smart tablet. (**b**) Demonstration of a student using the RtB on the Microsoft HoloLens. (**c**) Demonstration of the RtB timeline interface.

Taking a constructivist educational perspective [34], the RtB program allows students to actively engage in their own learning, by exploring and manipulating the digital anatomy content, and thus building on their prior learning and experiences. The RtB program includes four main digital anatomy interfaces: (1) the base anatomy, (2) the pregnancy timeline (Figure 2c), (3) birth considerations, and (4) an adaptable quiz-mode function. As illustrated in Figure 2c, students can interact with the anatomy interfaces by manipulating the pregnancy animation, to view both the foetal and maternal anatomical changes that occur during each week of pregnancy. Students are also able to visualise and manipulate uncommon placental and foetal positions that may not be congruent with normal birth practices, requiring specialist consultation [20,33].

The active engagement with the program affords students the ability to construct their own understanding of the material, by relating it to their own experiences. From a behaviorist perspective, the program includes a quiz function that allows self-assessment and the reinforcement of knowledge, promoting the idea that behaviour is shaped by the reinforcement of correct knowledge acquisition [20,33]. Aligning with Kolb's ELT, the program also provides opportunities for learners to reflect on, and apply, their knowledge in real-world settings [11]. Due to its portability on phone/tablet devices, students can use the program during workplace learning, as a personal and consumer education tool, potentially enhancing health literacy amongst consumers, and promoting collaboration [20,33].

The initial testing of the RtB (in its smartphone/tablet and IVR forms) was undertaken amongst two cohorts of undergraduate midwifery students, one within the originating Australian university (n = 19) and one with a partner university in Belgium (n = 139) [20]. Amongst the Australian cohort, the results indicated that the program was a useful learning resource that assisted with visualising the internal anatomical changes of pregnancy, and understanding foetal positioning in utero [20]. The students in Belgium indicated that the program had an above-average usability, according to the System Usability Scale (SUS), and improved student understanding of female reproductive anatomy and foetal positioning. The students also found the program to be fun to use, and there were no perceived negative impacts on learning. The experience of both samples of students of using the program in the education context was positive. Further testing of the RtB program remains in progress. The RtB has been deployed for testing amongst a small cohort of medical students undertaking problem-based learning in one large Midwestern university in the United States of America (USA), a large cohort of Midwifery students for various education outcomes within the United Kingdom (UK) as part of a PhD project, and as a health practitioner and consumer engagement tool in one large Midwestern Hospital in the USA, with all study outcomes pending.

3.3. *Conflict Resolution—Angry Stan*

The Conflict Resolution program was designed as a proof of concept to provide a simulated learning experience wherein nursing students could be immersed in an intense conflict situation. It's an unfortunate reality that nursing, medical, and midwifery staff often find themselves in intense conversations with healthcare consumers, and these conversations require skills in conflict resolution [35]. In nursing, constructively managed conflict has been linked with improved patient safety and quality of nursing care. Alternatively, poorly managed conflict can adversely affect nurses' mental health, affecting the healthcare organisation overall, and lead to poor patient outcomes [35]. The teaching of these skills at the time of development was resource-intensive, requiring specialist trained staff and actors within a simulated learning environment, and was only featured during the students' second year of study. This meant that students could have been exposed to conflict situations while engaging in a work placement without having been exposed to, or equipped with, conflict resolution skills. Therefore, the collective brief was to be able to safely immerse undergraduate nursing students in an intense interaction with an emergency department patron, providing exposure to an intense interaction, while providing students with the opportunity to practice conflict resolution skills from the perspective of a registered healthcare professional.

The program was again designed for accessibility (i.e., within-institution and remote student use), including tethered and untethered IVR (Oculus Rift S and Lenovo Daydream headsets), and desktop VR. To increase the authenticity of the experience, the Conflict Resolution program was paired with an off-the-shelf heart rate wrist monitor, essentially using an elevated heart rate (above baseline) as a proxy measure for the stress response elicited by the simulated experience (Figure 3c). Upon application of the IVR headset (with audio), students are transported to an environment that replicates a contemporary Australian hospital emergency department (Figure 3a), where they meet Stan (Angry Stan, appearing in Figure 3b). Stan is trying to find out about the condition of his friend, who was involved in a car accident, and progressively becomes frustrated and angry during the interaction. In general, staying calm is a trait required by nurses in resolving conflict [36]. Based on this premise, the IVR headset was paired with the heart rate wrist monitor, measuring a student's heart rate (Figure 3c) as a proxy measure of biometric stress [37,38].

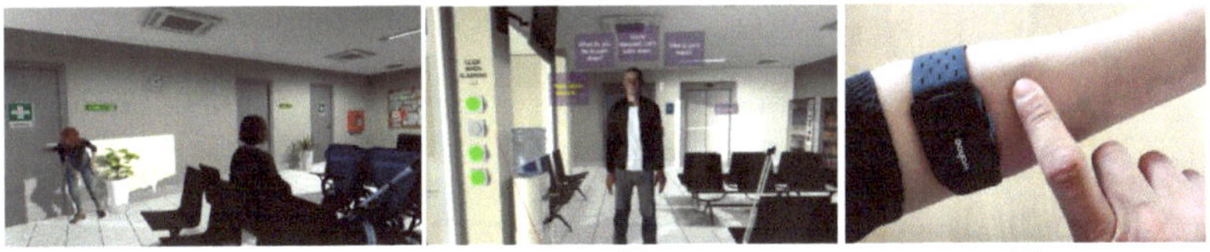

(a) **(b)** **(c)**

Figure 3. The Conflict Resolution (Angry Stan) program. (**a**) Demonstration of the emergency room environment. (**b**) Demonstration of Angry Stan & mini game. (**c**) Demonstration of heart rate writs monitor.

Students are required to interact with Stan by using the hand controllers to select appropriate responses that either assist in calming, or escalate Stan's emotions. The student's heart rate is detected by the IVR headset, and is used in combination with text-based prompts. Essentially, the higher a student's heart rate, the harder it is for a student to calm Stan. In addition, features were added to increase the cognitive load placed on the student, to reflect the challenging dynamics of real-world healthcare environments, beyond what is possible with traditional simulated-learning media [36–40]. These features included a mini game (Figure 3b) in which a flashing red light accompanied by an audio buzzer appears randomly throughout the experience, and needs to be switched off periodically, otherwise it will become increasingly louder and more distracting. Moreover, an intense background noise, including a crying baby, is also used, increasing the level of concentration and emotional intelligence required to successfully resolve Stan's grievances. Initial testing of the Conflict Resolution program is in progress, and is the focus of a PhD study at the originating institution. The program has been deployed in IVR amongst a large cohort (n = 400) of nursing students undertaking a nursing and mental health subject at the originating Australian university. The program is additionally being utilised amongst a cohort of business students within one large Midwestern university in the USA, for the initial testing of empathy traits, with all results pending.

4. Discussion

This article presents three novel XR simulated learning experiences that were co-created by university educators in the fields of nursing and midwifery, in collaboration with XR technology experts from a prominent regional university in Australia. The first case study describes the Compromised Neonate program, which was designed to enhance the development of the psychomotor, cognitive, and affective skills required when performing neonatal resuscitation in real-world contexts. The second case study, the RtB, was designed to provide students with an internal view of pregnancy over the course of human gestation, and to assist with the teaching of complex foetal–maternal anatomical spatial relationships. The third case study, Conflict Resolution, provides students the opportunity to be safely immerse in an intense interaction with an emergency department patron, with gamification features used to increase the realism and cognitive load, to reflect the dynamics of real-word professional practice environments. All case studies use multimodal XR media for within-institution and remote student use. Each experience showcases a unique design objective and development approach that reflects the nature of the XR content, to enhance simulated learning beyond traditional simulation media.

To date, the uptake of XR technology within nursing simulation education has been largely driven by small groups of technology and nursing content experts who are enthusiastic about using XR to optimise student learning. This is particularly true within the Australian higher education context [8,27]. Barriers to the broad upscaling of XR media within nursing curricula include a deficit in empirical efficacy studies, the sparse application of nursing learning theories underpinning design and development, difficulties in attracting funding, and difficulties in sustaining XR experiences beyond their development for curriculum and university system integration [8,27,41,42]. However, there is a growing recognition of the application of XR technology in nursing simulation education.

An umbrella review evaluating the use of metaverse technology in nursing education identified the application of virtual reality (VR) technology (desktop and IVR) as the primary technology medium being used to enhance simulated nursing education [43]. A systematic review by Shorey and Ng [44] evaluated the use of VR simulation among nursing students and registered nurses. Of the included studies, five utilised IVR technology, with most included studies using desktop VR, and high-fidelity simulation mannikins. Of the five studies that utilised IVR, all were used for psychomotor skill development, aiding in intravenous device insertion or venepuncture-type procedures [44]. Kim et al. [45] conducted a systematic review of XR-based paediatric nursing simulation programs, identifying fourteen studies for inclusion. Due to the varying definitions of VR and MR used within the article, only four included studies were identified that used IVR and AR for psychomotor skill development [45]. In this review, IVR and AR were used for teaching paediatric intensive care skills, such as basic infant care, feeding practices, the prevention of neonatal infection, paediatric airway management, injection practice, and wound care skills [45]. Lastly, a scoping review by Fealy et al. [8] evaluated the integration of IVR in nursing and midwifery education, identifying two studies. IVR was used in psychomotor skill development for cardiopulmonary resuscitation and urinary catheterisation [3]. These reviews suggest that the integration of XR technologies in nursing simulation education is emerging, with considerable scope for increasing the application of XR technology beyond IVR use for psychomotor skill development.

Incorporating learning theory into the design process is a crucial aspect of using these technologies in effective teaching and learning [42]. Learning theories serve as the foundation for understanding how students can acquire new knowledge, skills, and behaviours [7,46,47]. As a result, incorporating these theories into the design process ensures that educators are actively involved in creating XR experiences that are effective in promoting student learning [48–50]. Moreover, educators need to identify and select suitable technological equipment to support the learning outcomes [51]. Despite the proven advantages of IVR systems, simulated learning for skill acquisition using HMDs may not be the best method for every kind of student or teaching concept. As a result, educators, learning designers, and subject experts should follow scientific methods and/or frameworks during the instructional design process [51]. The utilisation of phases of design or design-based research methodologies, such as the scrum framework, can provide a practical approach to support XR content creators and educators. Figure 4 details a useful roadmap for conceptualising and organising the design of an XR learning environment. In particular, this roadmap can serve as a valuable guide to ensure the effective integration of learning theories and educational goals into the design process [51].

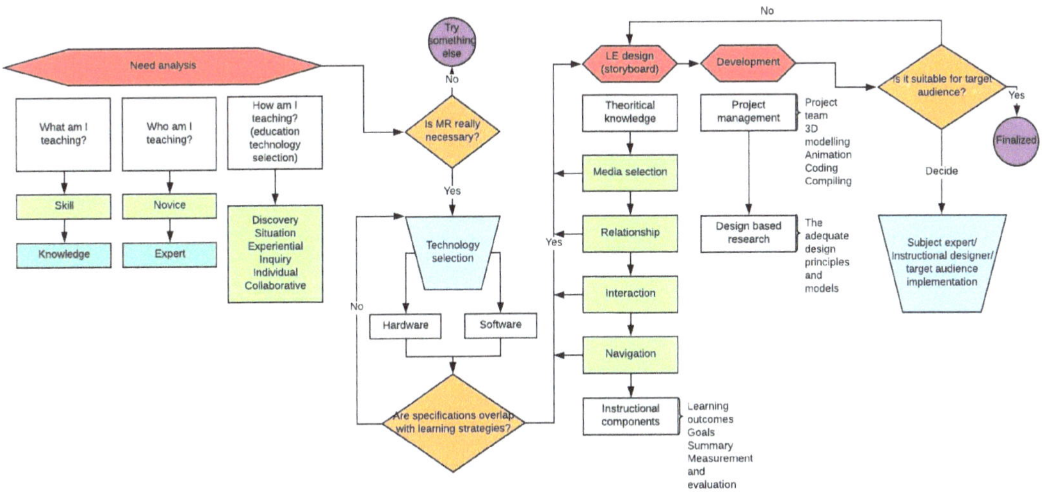

Figure 4. A pathway to assist with the educational interactive design process [51].

The Technological Pedagogical Content Knowledge (TPCK) framework, and the Substitution, Augmentation, Modification, Redefinition (SAMR) models are two widely used frameworks that can be additionally employed to assist nursing educators during the design process [52,53]. TPCK refers to the interplay between technological knowledge, pedagogical knowledge, and content knowledge, and asserts that for the effective integration of technology, all three types of knowledge are required, necessitating collaboration between experts [52,53]. The SAMR model categorises the different ways in which technology can be integrated into teaching and learning activities, ranging from simple substitution, to the creation of new and unique learning experiences, enabled by the application of various XR technology media [52,54]. The integration of learning theories into the design process, as highlighted in frameworks such as TPCK and SAMR, can serve as a guiding principle for the development of effective XR educational experiences.

An innovative policy-based co-creation model for the design of immersive health-related content has additionally been presented by Antoniou et al. [55]. The authors suggest an 8-step problem-solving framework when considering the application of XR technologies, as follows: (1) Defining the problem—XR technologies can be used to simulate many areas of healthcare. Involving the right people in the design process, and clearly identifying and defining the problem at hand can assist in providing a sense of direction and purpose to the project. (2) Assembling evidence—this involves gathering evidence to support the project, reviewing relevant information, such as what has been already done, and the current landscape, from various sources, providing valuable insights into the technology and content being created. (3) Constructing alternatives—based on the evidence gathered, this step involves developing a range of alternative courses of action or strategies to address the problem. This includes weighing up traditional development pipelines with alternative methods. (4) Selecting criteria—identifying criteria that can be used to measure and evaluate the effectiveness of the project, such as cost, technique, or pedagogical outcomes. (5) Projecting outcomes—making realistic projections of the outcomes or impacts of the project, considering how realistic or viable each outcome is, such as, *do we have the relevant personnel with technical skills?* (6) Confronting trade-offs—this involves weighing up the outcomes in relation to the selected evaluation criteria. (7) Decision-making—based on the previous steps, a final decision is made on the best strategy to address the problem. (8) Sharing the results of the process—this is the final stage, where the well-considered project process is shared in order to communicate the rationale behind the chosen problem, design, technology, outcomes, and evaluation methods [55].

The three case studies described in this paper broadly highlight how nursing educators can engage with the co-design of XR-enhanced simulated learning experiences for nursing student learning. By considering these examples, as well as applying theorical principles and frameworks, educators and XR content creators can ensure that their designs result in impactful and accessible learning experiences. It is important to acknowledge that learning is a multifaceted process. The effective integration of technology-enabled teaching approaches must be informed by an understanding of individual learner characteristics, and environmental factors that may impact learning outcomes [47,48,56]. The main limitation of all the presented case studies was that they were not developed or funded for broad curriculum or sustainable university system integration. Furthermore, empirical efficacy testing, in the form of randomised controlled trials of the three presented cases, has not been conducted, and this has been recognised as a barrier to XR adoption, based on the wider systematic review literature [42]. There is an urgent need to empirically examine the effectiveness of XR teaching methods for simulation nursing education, compared to traditional simulated media, in preparing work-ready graduates.

5. Conclusions

XR technologies may offer educational benefits beyond traditional simulated learning media, in the preparation of work-ready graduates. By providing learners with the opportunity to visualise abstract concepts in a 3D format, express their understanding of phenomena, observe the dynamic relationships between variables in a system, and experience events that may be inaccessible due to constraints such as distance, cost, time, safety, or scarcity, the integration of XR technology into nursing education offers a unique and innovative solution. The collaboration between nursing educators and XR technology specialists at one regional university in Australia has resulted in the development of three diverse and impactful case studies that demonstrate the potential of XR to enhance the simulated-learning experience for students. The embedded media diversity of XR technology provides students with the opportunity to actively engage in immersive and hands-on learning experiences, within virtual environments that can be designed to reflect the complexities of real-world healthcare situations, most importantly in psychomotor, affective, and cognitive skill acquisition.

Author Contributions: All listed authors made significant contributions to the manuscript. These are itemised as follows: S.F., conceptualisation, original draft preparation, writing and reviewing of the manuscript; D.J., conceptualisation, original draft preparation, reviewing and editing of the manuscript; P.I., original draft preparation, reviewing and editing of the manuscript; Z.T., original draft preparation, reviewing and editing of the manuscript; and Z.S.S., original draft preparation, reviewing and editing of the manuscript. All authors have read and agreed to the published version of the manuscript.

Funding: This research received no external funding. Internal institutional funding was gained to support the development of each XR program.

Institutional Review Board Statement: Not applicable.

Informed Consent Statement: Not applicable.

Data Availability Statement: Not applicable.

Acknowledgments: We would like to acknowledge Vandlella Pinto and the wider Newcastle University Innovation Team for the technical development of all three extended reality software programs. In addition, we would like to thank Sally Chan, Michael Hazelton, and Darrel Evans for funding and supporting the development of the programs.

Conflicts of Interest: The authors declare no conflict of interest.

References

1. Irwin, P.; Coutts, R.; Graham, I. Looking Good Sister! The Use of Virtual World to Develop Nursing Skills. In *Intersections in Simulation and Gaming*; Naweed, A., Bowditch, L., Sprickm, C., Eds.; Springer: Singapore, 2019; pp. 33–45.
2. Oliveira, S.N.d.; Prado, M.L.d.; Kempfer, S.S.; Martini, J.G.; Caravaca-Morera, J.A.; Bernardi, M.C. Experiential learning in nursing consultation education via clinical simulation with actors: Action research. *Nurse Educ. Today* **2015**, *35*, e50–e54. [CrossRef] [PubMed]
3. Thirsk, L.M.; Stahlke, S.; Bryan, V.; Dewart, G.; Corcoran, L. Lessons learned from clinical course design in the pandemic: Pedagogical implications from a qualitative analysis. *J. Adv. Nurs.* **2023**, *79*, 309–319. [CrossRef] [PubMed]
4. Hayden, J.K.; Smiley, R.A.; Alexander, M.; Kardong-Edgren, S.; Jeffries, P.R. The NCSBN National Simulation Study: A Longitudinal, Randomized, Controlled Study Replacing Clinical Hours with Simulation in Prelicensure Nursing Education. *J. Nurs. Regul.* **2014**, *5*, S3–S40. [CrossRef]
5. Edward, K.-l.; Ousey, K.; Playle, J.; Giandinoto, J.-A. Are new nurses work ready—The impact of preceptorship. An integrative systematic review. *J. Prof. Nurs.* **2017**, *33*, 326–333. [CrossRef] [PubMed]
6. Irwin, P.; Crepinsek, M.; Coutts, R. The use of avatars: Challenging longstanding approaches for experiential learning in nursing. *Interact. Learn. Environ.* **2022**, 1–10. [CrossRef]
7. Parker, B.A.; Grech, C. Authentic practice environments to support undergraduate nursing students' readiness for hospital placements. A new model of practice in an on campus simulated hospital and health service. *Nurse Educ. Pract.* **2018**, *33*, 47–54. [CrossRef]
8. Fealy, S.; Jones, D.; Hutton, A.; Graham, K.; McNeill, L.; Sweet, L.; Hazelton, M. The integration of immersive virtual reality in tertiary nursing and midwifery education: A scoping review. *Nurse Educ. Today* **2019**, *79*, 14–19. [CrossRef]
9. Hallaran, A.J.; Edge, D.S.; Almost, J.; Tregunno, D. New Nurses' Perceptions on Transition to Practice: A Thematic Analysis. *Can. J. Nurs. Res.* **2022**, *55*, 126–136. [CrossRef]
10. Cooper, S.; Cant, R.; Porter, J.; Bogossian, F.; McKenna, L.; Brady, S.; Fox-Young, S. Simulation based learning in midwifery education: A systematic review. *Women Birth* **2012**, *25*, 64–78. [CrossRef]
11. Kolb, D.A. *Experiential Learning: Experience as the Source of Learning And Development*; FT Press: Upper Saddle River, NJ, USA, 1984.
12. Tan, K.-A.Z.Y.; Seah, B.; Wong, L.F.; Lee, C.C.S.; Goh, H.S.; Liaw, S.Y. Simulation-Based Mastery Learning to Facilitate Transition to Nursing Practice. *Nurse Educ.* **2022**, *47*, 336–341. [CrossRef]
13. Cantrell, M.A.; Franklin, A.; Leighton, K.; Carlson, A. The evidence in simulation-based learning experiences in nursing education and practice: An umbrella review. *Clin. Simul. Nurs.* **2017**, *13*, 634–667. [CrossRef]
14. Handeland, J.A.; Prinz, A.; Ekra, E.M.R.; Fossum, M. The role of manikins in nursing students' learning: A systematic review and thematic metasynthesis. *Nurse Educ. Today* **2021**, *98*, 104661. [CrossRef]
15. MacLean, S.; Geddes, F.; Kelly, M.; Della, P. Realism and presence in simulation: Nursing student perceptions and learning outcomes. *J. Nurs. Educ.* **2019**, *58*, 330–338. [CrossRef]
16. Jones, D.; Evans, D.; Hazelton, M.; Siang See, Z.; Fealy, S. The development of the compromised neonate: A virtual reality neonatal resuscitation program. In *Interactive Learning Environments*, 1st ed.; Tacgin, Z., Hagan, A., Eds.; Cambridge Scholars Publishing: Newcastle upon Tyne, UK, 2022; pp. 46–54.
17. O'Connor, S.; Kennedy, S.; Wang, Y.; Ali, A.; Cooke, S.; Booth, R.G. Theories informing technology enhanced learning in nursing and midwifery education: A systematic review and typological classification. *Nurse Educ. Today* **2022**, *118*, 105518. [CrossRef]
18. Woon, A.P.N.; Mok, W.Q.; Chieng, Y.J.S.; Zhang, H.M.; Ramos, P.; Mustadi, H.B.; Lau, Y. Effectiveness of virtual reality training in improving knowledge among nursing students: A systematic review, meta-analysis and meta-regression. *Nurse Educ. Today* **2021**, *98*, 104655. [CrossRef]
19. Schuelke, S.; Krystal, D.; Barnason, S. Implementing Immersive Virtual Reality into a Nursing Curriculum. *Innov. Health Sci. Educ. J.* **2022**, *1*, 2. [CrossRef]
20. Jones, D.; Hazelton, M.; Evans, D.J.R.; Pento, V.; See, Z.S.; Leugenhaege, L.V.; Fealy, S. *Digital Anatomy, Applications of Virtual, Mixed and Augmented Reality*; Human–Computer Interaction Series; Springer: Berlin, Germany, 2021; pp. 325–342. [CrossRef]
21. Sherman, W.R.; Craig, A.B. *Understanding Virtual Reality: Interface, Application, and Design*; Morgan Kaufmann: Burlington, MA, USA, 2018.
22. Bansal, G.; Rajgopal, K.; Chamola, V.; Xiong, Z.; Niyato, D. Healthcare in Metaverse: A Survey on Current Metaverse Applications in Healthcare. *IEEE Access* **2022**, *10*, 119914–119946. [CrossRef]

23. Chengoden, R.; Victor, N.; Huynh-The, T.; Yenduri, G.; Jhaveri, R.H.; Alazab, M.; Bhattacharya, S.; Hegde, P.; Maddikunta, P.K.R.; Gadekallu, T.R. Metaverse for Healthcare: A Survey on Potential Applications, Challenges and Future Directions. *arXiv* **2022**, arXiv:2209.04160. [CrossRef]
24. Musamih, A.; Yaqoob, I.; Salah, K.; Jayaraman, R.; Al-Hammadi, Y.; Omar, M.; Ellahham, S. Metaverse in Healthcare Applications Challenges and Future Directions. *IEEE Consum. Electron. Mag.* **2023**, *12*, 33–46. [CrossRef]
25. Barab, S.A.; Hay, K.E.; Barnett, M.; Keating, T. Virtual solar system project: Building understanding through model building. *J. Res. Sci. Teach. Off. J. Natl. Assoc. Res. Sci. Teach.* **2000**, *37*, 719–756. [CrossRef]
26. Yin, X.; Wonka, P.; Razdan, A. Generating 3d building models from architectural drawings: A survey. *IEEE Comput. Graph. Appl.* **2008**, *29*, 20–30. [CrossRef] [PubMed]
27. Kluge, M.G.; Maltby, S.; Keynes, A.; Nalivaiko, E.; Evans, D.J.; Walker, F.R. Current state and general perceptions of the use of extended reality (XR) technology at the University of Newcastle: Interviews and surveys from staff and students. *SAGE Open* **2022**, *12*, 21582440221093348. [CrossRef]
28. Schwaber, K.; Sutherland, J. The Scrum Guide: The Definitive Guide to Scrum: The Rules of the Game. 2011. Available online: https://scrumguides.org/index.html (accessed on 3 February 2023).
29. Williams, J.; Jones, D.; Walker, R. Consideration of using virtual reality for teaching neonatal resuscitation to midwifery students. *Nurse Educ. Pract.* **2018**, *31*, 126–129. [CrossRef] [PubMed]
30. Australian and New Zealand Committee on Resuscitation [ANZCOR]. *ANZCOR Guideline 13.1 Introduction to Resuscitation of the Newborn Infant*; ANZCOR: Melbourne, Australia, 2018; pp. 1–10.
31. Lavoie, P.; Michaud, C.; Belisle, M.; Boyer, L.; Gosselin, E.; Grondin, M.; Larue, C.; Lavoie, S.; Pepin, J. Learning theories and tools for the assessment of core nursing competencies in simulation: A theoretical review. *J. Adv. Nurs.* **2018**, *74*, 239–250. [CrossRef]
32. Brown, A.L. The advancement of learning. *Educ. Res.* **1994**, *23*, 4–12. [CrossRef]
33. Jones, D.; See, Z.S.; Billinghurst, M.; Goodman, L.; Fealy, S. Extended Reality for Midwifery Learning: MR VR Demonstration. In Proceedings of the 17th International Conference on Virtual-Reality Continuum and Its Applications in Industry, Brisbane, Australia, 14–16 November 2019; pp. 1–2.
34. Knowles, M.S.; Holton, E.; Swanson, R.A. *The Adult Learner: The Definitive Classic in Adult Education and Human*; Taylor and Francis: Florence, Italy, 2015; Volume 265.
35. Labrague, L.J.; McEnroe–Petitte, D.M. An integrative review on conflict management styles among nursing students: Implications for nurse education. *Nurse Educ. Today* **2017**, *59*, 45–52. [CrossRef]
36. Başoğul, C.; Özgür, G. Role of Emotional Intelligence in Conflict Management Strategies of Nurses. *Asian Nurs. Res.* **2016**, *10*, 228–233. [CrossRef]
37. Gaggioli, A.; Pallavicini, F.; Morganti, L.; Serino, S.; Scaratti, C.; Briguglio, M.; Crifaci, G.; Vetrano, N.; Giulintano, A.; Bernava, G.; et al. Experiential Virtual Scenarios With Real-Time Monitoring (Interreality) for the Management of Psychological Stress: A Block Randomized Controlled Trial. *J. Med. Internet Res.* **2014**, *16*, e167. [CrossRef]
38. Nakayama, N.; Arakawa, N.; Ejiri, H.; Matsuda, R.; Makino, T. Heart rate variability can clarify students' level of stress during nursing simulation. *PLoS ONE* **2018**, *13*, e0195280. [CrossRef]
39. Lischke, A.; Jacksteit, R.; Mau-Moeller, A.; Pahnke, R.; Hamm, A.O.; Weippert, M. Heart rate variability is associated with psychosocial stress in distinct social domains. *J. Psychosom. Res.* **2018**, *106*, 56–61. [CrossRef]
40. Tokuno, J.; Carver, T.E.; Fried, G.M. Measurement and Management of Cognitive Load in Surgical Education: A Narrative Review. *J. Surg. Educ.* **2023**, *80*, 208–215. [CrossRef]
41. Idrees, A.; Morton, M.; Dabrowski, G. Advancing Extended Reality Teaching and Learning Opportunities Across the Disciplines in Higher Education. In Proceedings of the 2022 8th International Conference of the Immersive Learning Research Network (iLRN), Vienna, Austria, 30 May–4 June 2022; pp. 1–8.
42. Radianti, J.; Majchrzak, T.A.; Fromm, J.; Wohlgenannt, I. A systematic review of immersive virtual reality applications for higher education: Design elements, lessons learned, and research agenda. *Comput. Educ.* **2020**, *147*, 103778. [CrossRef]
43. De Gagne, J.C.; Randall, P.S.; Rushton, S.; Park, H.K.; Cho, E.; Yamane, S.S.; Jung, D. The Use of Metaverse in Nursing Education: An Umbrella Review. *Nurse Educ.* **2022**, *10*, 1097. [CrossRef]
44. Shorey, S.; Ng, E.D. The use of virtual reality simulation among nursing students and registered nurses: A systematic review. *Nurse Educ. Today* **2021**, *98*, 104662. [CrossRef]
45. Kim, E.J.; Lim, J.Y.; Kim, G.M. A systematic review and meta-analysis of studies on extended reality-based pediatric nursing simulation program development. *Child Health Nurs. Res.* **2023**, *29*, 24–36. [CrossRef]
46. Asad, M.M.; Naz, A.; Churi, P.; Tahanzadeh, M.M. Virtual Reality as Pedagogical Tool to Enhance Experiential Learning: A Systematic Literature Review. *Educ. Res. Int.* **2021**, *2021*, 7061623. [CrossRef]
47. Cant, R.P.; Cooper, S.J. Use of simulation-based learning in undergraduate nurse education: An umbrella systematic review. *Nurse Educ. Today* **2017**, *49*, 63–71. [CrossRef]
48. Bauce, K.; Kaylor, M.B.; Staysniak, G.; Etcher, L. Use of theory to guide integration of virtual reality technology in nursing education: A scoping study. *J. Prof. Nurs.* **2023**, *44*, 1–7. [CrossRef]
49. Hernon, O.; McSharry, E.; MacLaren, I.; Dunne, R.; Carr, P.J. The Use of Educational Technology in Undergraduate and Postgraduate Nursing and Midwifery Education: A Scoping Review. *CIN Comput. Inform. Nurs.* **2022**, *41*, 162–171. [CrossRef]

50. Morris, T.H. Experiential learning—A systematic review and revision of Kolb's model. *Interact. Learn. Environ.* **2020**, *28*, 1064–1077. [CrossRef]
51. Tacgin, Z. *Virtual and Augmented Reality: An Educational Handbook*; Cambridge Scholars Publishing: Newcastle upon Tyne, UK, 2020.
52. Bartolotti, L. From Traditional to Distance Learning: Chronicle of a Switch From Physical to Virtual—Using the Game Metaphor to Understand the Process. In *Handbook of Research on Teaching with Virtual Environments and AI*; Panconesi, G., Guida, M., Eds.; IGI Global: Hershey, PA, USA, 2021; pp. 119–139.
53. Koehler, M.J.; Mishra, P.; Cain, W. What is Technological Pedagogical Content Knowledge (TPACK)? *J. Educ.* **2013**, *193*, 13–19. [CrossRef]
54. Puentedura, R. SAMR and TPCK: Intro to Advanced Practice. 2010. Available online: http://hippasus.com/resources/sweden2010/SAMR_TPCK_IntroToAdvancedPractice.pdf (accessed on 3 February 2023).
55. Antoniou, P.E.; Pears, M.; Schiza, E.C.; Frangoudes, F.; Pattichis, C.S.; Wharrad, H.; Bamidis, P.D.; Konstantinidis, S.T. Eliciting Co-Creation Best Practices of Virtual Reality Reusable e-Resources. *Virtual Worlds* **2023**, *2*, 75–89. [CrossRef]
56. Hardie, P.; Darley, A.; Carroll, L.; Redmond, C.; Campbell, A.; Jarvis, S. Nursing & Midwifery students' experience of immersive virtual reality storytelling: An evaluative study. *BMC Nurs.* **2020**, *19*, 78. [CrossRef]

sensors

MDPI

Article

Extended Reality Telemedicine Collaboration System Using Patient Avatar Based on 3D Body Pose Estimation

Matko Šarić *,†, Mladen Russo †, Luka Kraljević and Davor Meter

Faculty of Electrical Engineering, Mechanical Engineering and Naval Architecture, University of Split, Ruđera Boškovića 32, 21000 Split, Croatia; mrusso@fesb.hr (M.R.); lkraljev@fesb.hr (L.K.); davor.meter.00@fesb.hr (D.M.)
* Correspondence: msaric@fesb.hr
† These authors contributed equally to this work.

Abstract: Recent advances in extended reality (XR) technology have opened the possibility of significantly improving telemedicine systems. This is primarily achieved by transferring 3D information about patient state, which is utilized to create more immersive experiences on VR/AR headsets. In this paper, we propose an XR-based telemedicine collaboration system in which the patient is represented as a 3D avatar in an XR space shared by local and remote clinicians. The proposed system consists of an AR client application running on Microsoft HoloLens 2 used by a local clinician, a VR client application running on the HTC vive Pro used by a remote clinician, and a backend part running on the server. The patient is captured by a camera on the AR side, and the 3D body pose estimation is performed on frames from this camera stream to form a 3D patient avatar. Additionally, the AR and VR sides can interact with the patient avatar via virtual hands, and annotations can be performed on a 3D model. The main contribution of our work is the use of 3D body pose estimation for the creation of a 3D patient avatar. In this way, 3D body reconstruction using depth cameras is avoided, which reduces system complexity and hardware and network resources. Another contribution is the novel architecture of the proposed system, where audio and video streaming are realized using WebRTC protocol. The performance evaluation showed that the proposed system ensures high frame rates for both AR and VR client applications, while the processing latency remains at an acceptable level.

Keywords: extended reality; telemedicine system; avatar; 3D body pose estimation

Citation: Šarić, M.; Russo, M.; Kraljević, L.; Meter, D. Extended Reality Telemedicine Collaboration System Using Patient Avatar Based on 3D Body Pose Estimation. *Sensors* **2024**, *24*, 27. https://doi.org/10.3390/s24010027

Academic Editors: Radu Comes, Dorin-Mircea Popovici, Calin Gheorghe Dan Neamtu and Jing-Jing Fang

Received: 21 November 2023
Revised: 15 December 2023
Accepted: 18 December 2023
Published: 20 December 2023

1. Introduction

Telemedicine systems are a well-known technology aimed at improving healthcare and reducing costs. The need for telemedicine was recognized during the COVID-19 pandemic, when physical interaction with patients was risky. Until recently, telemedicine relied on 2D modalities, that is, video conferencing, which substituted cell phone consultation. This includes audio and single-viewpoint video transmission. The drawback of the 2D approach is the limited availability of information about the patient's condition in comparison with a physical examination. With the recent advances in augmented reality (AR), virtual reality (VR), and mixed reality (MR), where all these technologies can be encompassed by the term extended reality (XR), it is feasible to transmit more information about patient states, primarily by including the third space dimension (3D). VR and AR technologies have practical advantages and disadvantages. While VR provides a highly immersive experience that is particularly suitable for educational purposes, users' field of view is blocked. On the other hand, AR adds computer-generated information to the user's field of view, but it lacks interaction with 3D objects. MR, and consequently XR solutions, overlay 3D objects onto a semi-transparent screen, preserving the user's view of the physical environment and making these technologies good candidates for telemedicine collaboration.

A 3D human avatar can be a valuable tool in telemedicine because it allows healthcare providers to remotely interact with patients in a more immersive and personalized way. Annotations of 3D models (human avatars) in extended reality (XR) can provide a valuable tool for telemedicine. In XR, healthcare professionals can use virtual annotations to highlight specific areas of a patient's anatomy or medical imaging, which can be viewed and manipulated in real-time. For example, a radiologist can use annotations to mark abnormalities in a CT scan or MRI, which can be viewed by other specialists at different locations. This approach can help with collaborative diagnosis and treatment planning and provide a more detailed understanding of the patient's condition. Additionally, annotations in XR can be used for patient education, allowing healthcare professionals to explain medical conditions and procedures to patients using a 3D avatar or model. This approach can be particularly useful for patients who may have difficulty understanding medical terminology or who have limited access to traditional education materials. Overall, annotations of 3D models in XR can enhance the telemedicine experience, providing healthcare professionals with a more detailed understanding of a patient's condition, facilitating collaboration and communication, and improving patient outcomes. Holographic communication is an emerging technology that extends traditional video conferencing with real-time 3D representations of participants. The typical steps in holographic communications include real-time 3D capture of an object or person, data processing for 3D model creation, its transmission through a network, presentation of the transmitted model on the receiving end, and real-time interaction with the 3D model. Although holographic communication has the potential to improve remote interaction in medicine and healthcare applications, it faces significant implementation challenges [1]. Three-dimensional data capture should be performed in real time; however, consequently, the precision of the acquired data is lower. For this purpose, time-of-flight (ToF) cameras or stereo cameras are used, but because of their narrow field of view, a multi-camera setup is often required. Three-dimensional reconstruction is performed on a large amount of the captured data, which implies longer processing time and, consequently, greater latency. The transmission of 3D data is related to three main challenges: ultra-high bandwidth, ultra-low latency, and network optimization. The use of 5G networks can only partially satisfy the transmission speed requirements of holographic communication systems. End-to-end transmission latency is influenced by all steps, from local site data capture to remote site rendering. Currently, holographic communication systems generate a latency of several hundred milliseconds [1], which is greater than the recommended value of 50–100 ms [2]. In this paper, we propose an XR-based telemedicine collaboration system that enables local doctors to consult with remote specialists where patients are represented as 3D human body avatars in a shared XR space. The local doctor, using the AR application running on an AR headset (Microsoft HoloLens 2), starts the remote session with a remote specialist who works with VR applications running on a VR headset (HTC Vive Pro). First, Web Real-Time Communication (WebRTC) is established between the AR side and VR side, where a remote specialist sees a real-time camera stream (captured by a HoloLens 2 camera or webcamera) of the patient. This stream is processed on the backend part of the system to obtain the data necessary for patient 3D avatar control. The data are subsequently sent to the AR and VR sides so that they can see the same 3D avatar matching the patient pose. In this way, both sides are present in the shared XR space, allowing interaction with the patient avatar in the form of virtual hands. For this purpose, hand pose data are exchanged between the AR and VR sides in real time. Since the 3D avatar of the patient is transmitted to the remote site, the proposed approach is an example of a holographic communication system. The main contribution of this paper is the use of 3D body pose estimation for the creation of a patient avatar. This approach is different from the approaches described in related work, where the patient is captured with depth camera(s) and reconstructed as a 3D model. In the proposed approach, 3D patient reconstruction is avoided, which eliminates the need for specialized equipment and reduces computational and network resources. In this way, we reduce processing time and the amount of data needed for 3D avatar creation, which are typical challenges met in holographic communication systems. Our system represents a simpler and more robust solution in comparison with other approaches from the literature. Another contribution is the novel system architecture exploiting the WebRTC protocol for audio and video streaming. This ensures lower latency, which is especially critical in video streaming applications. Additionally, in this way, direct peer-to-peer communication is established between the AR side and VR side, eliminating the need for additional servers. The paper is organized as follows. In Section 2, an overview of the related work is given. Section 3 provides a detailed description of the proposed system, and Section 4 presents the results obtained by system testing. Conclusions are given in Section 5.

2. Related Work

Regarding the usage of XR technology in telemedicine applications, we can mention the solution proposed in [3], where an MR teleconsultation system was realized. Azure Kinect DK is exploited on the patient side, while a doctor uses Microsoft HoloLens 2, which allows manipulation of 3D organ models and medical images. In this way, doctors can explain symptoms and educate patients through real-time video communication realized through Microsoft Teams. In [4], a platform for real-time remote medical consultations that combines VR and AR technologies was introduced. On the patient side, an RGB+D video is captured with a Microsoft Kinect device and sent, together with vital patient information, to the remote location where streamed data are visualized to the expert using a stereoscopic display. Augmented feedback is presented on the patient side using a projector previously calibrated with Kinect. Carbone et al. [5] developed an AR-based telemedicine platform using a see-through head mounted display (HMD) on the remote or local clinician side. In this way, both HMDs show the same image in which the hands of a remote specialist are overlaid on the actual scene to guide the local clinician. In [6], the authors described a 3D teleconsultation system intended for preclinical emergency scenarios. A depth camera captures the patient environment, and from this information, 3D reconstruction is performed on the remote expert side. Guidelines are transmitted to the patient side using a shared avatar representation of the expert, which is presented to the local clinician via an AR HMD. The system was compared to the 2D video teleconsultation approach on the task of electrocardiogram electrode placement, and it was shown that higher accuracy was obtained using the proposed 3D approach. In [7], an MR system for surgical telementoring was introduced. A remote expert utilizes a VR operating room, where gestures and annotations on a 3D patient model are sent to remote novice surgeons using the AR interface. The novice side is equipped with depth cameras capturing the operating room, with one attached to a surgical lamp to scan the patient's body. The novice surgeon uses the Microsoft HoloLens 2 device to run the AR interface, which has only passive elements to avoid distractions. The remote expert is equipped with a VR headset, HTC Vive Pro, and IMU-equipped gloves. Roth et al. [8] presented a mixed reality teleconsultation system intended for usage in intensive care units. It consists of three modules: a reconstruction module, a local expert module, and a remote expert module. The reconstruction module creates a local point cloud of the intensive care unit using frames obtained from six RGB-D cameras. The remote expert module uses a VR HMD to allow experts to join the reconstructed intensive care unit space. Remote experts are represented with avatars in the local expert module where the AR system is used. In [9], a mixed reality (MR) system for surgical telementoring was proposed. The patient is captured with a Kinect depth camera and reconstructed in a remote virtual environment where an expert surgeon can interact with the 3D patient model. The local surgeon is guided by 3D annotations projected in AR as well as the gestures of the avatar representing the expert surgeon that are shown using AR. Kalbas et al. [10] introduced an AR-based surgical telementoring system. Microsoft HoloLens 2 is used to share the operating surgeon's field of view, and accurate 3D annotations are provided with satisfactory accuracy. The application of a telemedicine system for remote patient monitoring is described in [11], where the use of a teleguided portable ultrasound with ultrasound image analysis was proposed for COVID-19 patients.

Using the proposed approach, individuals with limited medical backgrounds can achieve high accuracy in detecting COVID-19. Hill [12] demonstrated the use of the Microsoft HoloLens 2 device to improve outcomes in patients receiving negative pressure wound therapy. The bedside nurse used a HoloLens 2 to remotely consult wound care personnel, who could load previous wound images into the local nurse's field of view and perform 3D drawings to guide the procedure. The study group using AR technology had fewer complications than the control group. Borresen et al. [13] proposed an augmented reality telerehabilitation system for the remote examination of upper extremity strength and range of motion. The solution is based on two Kinect depth cameras that capture 3D videos of the patient's body and a Force Dimension Omega.3 Haptic Controller device for transmission of the patient's force. The results show that remote assessment performed remotely with the proposed system has promising agreement with in-person diagnoses.

3. Proposed Method

The purpose of the proposed solution is to enable patient examination by remote experts without the need for physical presence. The system consists of three components (Figure 1): a user application with an AR interface (AR client), used by a local doctor performing a physical examination of a patient; a user application with a VR interface (VR client), used by a remote expert; and an XR collaboration system (backend) running on a workstation/server. A local doctor using AR glasses (Microsoft HoloLens 2) starts a telemedicine session to receive guidelines from the remote expert. The webcamera view of the patient is streamed to the remote location where the expert uses VR glasses (HTC VIVE Pro). The camera stream is also processed on the server to obtain the data needed for controlling the 3D avatar of the patient. These data are subsequently sent to the VR and AR sides to match the pose of the avatar with the patient's pose. During collaboration, both sides share the common XR space and observe the same avatar. Additionally, in real time, the AR and VR sides exchange data related to the relative position of user/control modalities in the AR/VR interface. In this way, the transmission of the hands/controllers is enabled, and both users see virtual hands as a form of interaction with a 3D avatar. Both sides are able to annotate the 3D model. Microsoft HoloLens 2 is an augmented reality (AR) headset developed for mixed reality applications where the focus is on blending virtual elements with the real world. It is equipped with various sensors, including an RGB camera, a depth camera, head tracking cameras, eye-tracking cameras, and an IMU unit. It uses see-through waveguide lenses with 2048 × 1080 resolution and supports hand-tracking with various gesture readings. One feature that is exploited in the proposed system is holographic remoting, where the app interface is seen on a HoloLens 2 device, but it is actually running on a PC to utilize more powerful hardware to avoid a decrease in the frame rate. The HTC Vive is a VR headset featuring a dual AMOLED display with a resolution of 1080 × 1200 per eye. The refresh rate is 90 Hz with a 110-degree field of view. One of the important features of such systems is the use of a room-scale tracking system based on the base stations, which track the headset and handheld controllers used for interaction and navigation in the VR space.

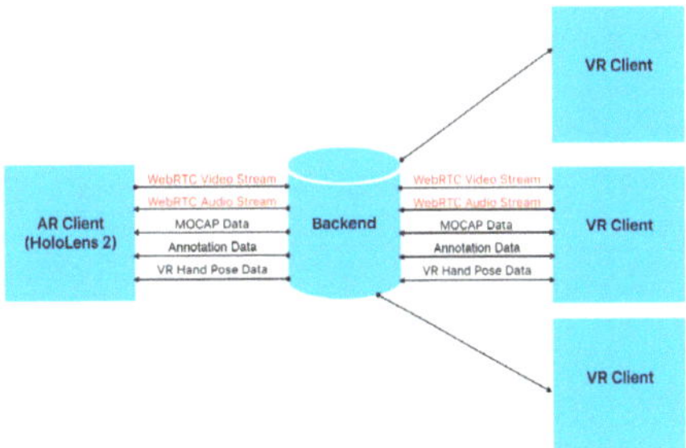

Figure 1. Architecture of the proposed system.

3.1. Avatar Control

By creating a 3D avatar of a patient, doctors can better visualize and understand the patient's physical condition, which can help with diagnosis and treatment planning. Additionally, patients can use 3D avatars to convey information about their symptoms and medical history to healthcare providers, even if they are not physically present in the same location. A human/patient avatar can help doctors better understand a patient's physical condition by providing a more detailed and visual representation of the patient's anatomy. By creating a 3D avatar of the patient, doctors can examine the avatar from different angles, zoom in on specific areas, and manipulate the avatar to better understand the patient's condition. This approach can be particularly useful when physical examination is limited, such as in telemedicine, or when the condition is complex and difficult to visualize. The avatar control workflow, shown in Figure 2, is an essential part of the proposed XR collaboration system. Several microservices are needed to establish real-time communication and process the camera stream.

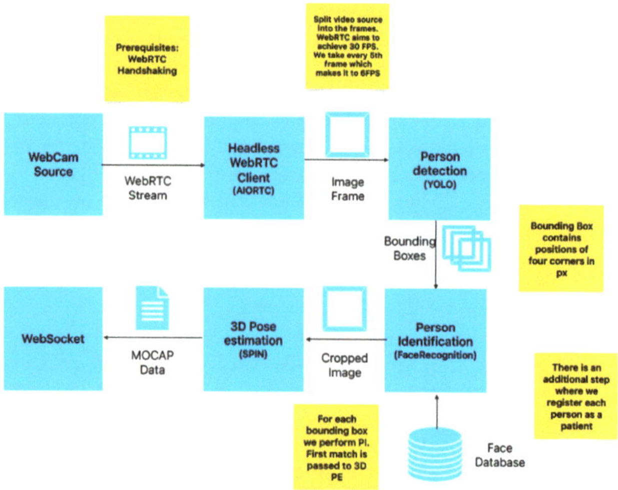

Figure 2. Avatar control workflow.

The REST service is employed for user authentication. The real-time communication (RTC) service used is based on the WebRTC protocol. WebRTC was chosen for this purpose because it offers several advantages:

- Low latency, which is especially important for real-time interaction in videoconferencing and telemedicine applications
- Peer-to-peer (P2P) communication, where video streams are sent directly between users, which eliminates the need for a server.
- High-quality supporting adaptive bitrates needed to handle varying network conditions.
- Open source and standardized: the developers' community ensures constant improvements.

In the proposed system, the RTC service is implemented as a headless WebRTC client that has two functions: the first one is audio and video communication between the AR and VR sides and the processing of the camera stream, and the second is the usage of different computer vision algorithms on the server side. The headless WebRTC client unpacks the video stream into individual frames, and every computer vision algorithm is represented as an individual microservice. The message exchange service, based on the WebSocket protocol, transfers the following JSON messages between the AR and VR sides:

- The WebRTC data (OFFER, ANSWER, ICECANDIDATES) needed for establishing a RTC connection.

- MOCAP data obtained by pose estimation, which are used for avatar control in the XR space (shared 3D space).
- Collaborative cross-platform hand pose data are 3D vectors that enable the visualization of the user's hands/controllers. In this way, the AR and VR sides are able to virtually collaborate on the patient's 3D model.
- Annotation data: the remote or local expert can annotate a point on an avatar and send its position and textual description.

The person detection service is realized using a real-time object detection algorithm from the MediaPipe library [14]. This object detector supports several models to balance the processing time and the detection accuracy. The recommended model is EfficientDet-Lite0 from the EfficientDet model family, which is introduced in [15]. It utilizes a weighted bi-directional feature pyramid network (BiFPN) for feature fusion and compound scaling of the resolution, depth and width for all backbone, feature network, and box/class prediction networks. The headless WebRTC client unpacks frames from the camera stream that are sent to the object detector, giving the person bounding box as output. The patient identification service exploits the Python library's face recognition [16], ensuring that the pose estimation data and annotation data are combined with the correct person representing the patient. This is especially important in cases where a connection is re-established or when there are several people present at the scene.

3.2. Pose Estimation

Three-dimensional pose estimation is the most important and most challenging step in the proposed system. Generally, pose estimation can be realized in several different ways. Two-dimensional pose estimation involves estimating the position of body joints in a two-dimensional image. It can be performed using methods such as single-person pose estimation or multi-person pose estimation. Three-dimensional pose estimation determines the position of body joints in three-dimensional space. It is usually realized using a combination of 2D image information and depth information. Kinematic pose estimation gives the full-articulated pose of a person by considering the kinematic relationships between body parts. Human pose estimation has many practical applications, such as in human–computer interactions, sports analysis, and medical diagnosis. It can also be used for tracking the movements of people in surveillance systems or for creating realistic virtual avatars. In the proposed system, a 3D pose estimation service is realized using the model proposed in [17]. This method involves the use of a 3D pose estimation system for the body, face, and hands using only monocular images. It outputs in the form of the SMPL-X model [18], which combines the skinned multi-person linear (SMPL) model [19], which represents the human body as a collection of interconnected joints, and the linear blend skinning model with the face and hands model. In this way, a low-dimensional representation of the human body, hands, and face is obtained. The SMPL-X model is able to model shape variations and body deformations with low-dimensional shape and pose parameters. The SMPL-X model extends the SMPL model to include articulated hands and an expressive face. The SMPL-X model, denoted by W, can be expressed as follows:

$$V_w = W(\phi_w, \theta_w, \beta_w, \psi_f) \quad (1)$$

where $\phi_w \in R^3$ is whole body global orientation, $\theta_w \in R^{(21+15+15)\times 3}$ refers to whole body pose parameters, $\beta \in R^{10}$ represents shape parameters, and $\psi_f \in R^{10}$ are facial expression parameters. Pose parameters θ are divided into 21 body parameters, 15 parameters for the left hand, and 15 parameters for the right hand. Pose parameters θ are defined with the angle-axis notation that defines relative rotation to the parent joint. The SMPL-X model has the mesh structure $V \in R^{10435\times 3}$. Three-dimensional body joint locations could be calculated using the regression function R on V_w:

$$J_w^{3D} = R_w(V_w) \quad (2)$$

where $J_w^{3D} \in R^{(22+15+15)\times 3}$. The hand model is defined using only hand parts from the SMPL-X model:

$$V_h = W(\phi_h, \theta_h, \beta_h) \tag{3}$$

where $\theta_h \in R^{3\times 15}$ represents hand pose parameters, β_h are hand shape parameters, and ϕ_h is the global orientation of the hand mesh. The output of the hand model is the hand mesh structure $V_h^{778\times 3}$, containing hand vertices extracted from the SMPL-X hand area. Three-dimensional hand joints can be calculated by regression:

$$J_h^{3D} = R_h(V_h) \tag{4}$$

where $J_h^{3D} \in R^{21\times 3}$ includes the wrist, 5 fingertips, and 15 finger joints. The 3D hand pose estimation model is built as an end-to-end deep neural network architecture, and is defined as follows:

$$[\phi_h, \theta_h, \beta_h, c_h] = M_H(I_H) \tag{5}$$

where I_h stands for the input RGB image cropped to show only the hand region and $c_h(t_h, s_h)$ represents the set of weak perspective camera parameters used for the projection of the obtained 3D model onto the input image. The 3D body pose estimation model is given by:

$$[\phi_b, \theta_b, \beta_b, c_b] = M_B(I_b) \tag{6}$$

where I_b represents the image cropped around the person's body. For this model, the method presented in [20] is exploited. Firstly, 2D joint localization is performed on input using a pretrained model, such as OpenPose. After that, the model utilizes a deep neural network to perform regression of the SMPL-X parameters. The regressed parameter values are further refined via an iterative optimization routine, where the model is aligned with the image based on 2D keypoints. This step minimizes the mismatch between the projected 3D joints in the SMPL-X model and the 2D joint positions in the image. The 3D face-estimation model presented in [21] is used to obtain the face poses θ_f and facial expressions ψ_f:

$$[\theta_f, \psi_f] = M_F(I_f) \tag{7}$$

The final output of the described model is formed by combining outputs from the face, hands, and body modules into the SMPL-X representation.

The output of the model contains the positions of the body joints, and these data are used for kinematic graph calculations according to the SMPL-X model, where each joint movement is expressed as a function of the other joints' movements. A kinematic graph gives rotation data for 24 joints that represent MOCAP data, which are sent using a message exchange service to the AR and VR sides and mapped to the avatar. The Z-anatomy 3D model is exploited to visualize different systems of the human body (cardiovascular, skeletal, nervous, etc.). This model is modified in Blender to obtain the skin mesh, which is connected with the skeletal system of the SMPL-X. Regarding the accuracy of the 3D pose estimation model [17] exploited in our system, an evaluation by the authors shows that the mean vertex-to-vertex distance (V2V) in millimeters is 63.5 mm, where the vertex refers to the SMPL-X model.

4. Results

To better illustrate the usage of the proposed system, examples of the AR client view and VR client view are shown in Figures 3 and 4, respectively. The VR client shows the 3D patient avatar presented to the remote specialist wearing the HTC VIVE Pro VR headset. This view also includes WebRTC preview of the camera from the AR side. The AR client view, presented to the local doctor using Microsoft HoloLens 2, overlays the 3D patient avatar with the physical environment view. The AR client enables avatar translation, rotation, and scaling to better match the patient's body in a real environment. Figure 3 shows an example of annotation on the 3D avatar as well as a virtual hand that guides the local doctor. Figure 4 illustrates that the system is robust to varying patient poses, with the avatar matching the patient in the sitting position. Since 3D body pose estimation is used instead of 3D reconstruction, the matching accuracy is not sufficient for tasks requiring high precision, such as surgical procedures. Interaction with a patient avatar is achieved with a virtual hand, which represents the hand of a remote specialist. Different human body systems can be chosen for visualization according to the doctor's preferences.

Since the time delay of avatar movement is critical for system usability, data streaming experiments were performed to determine the times needed for each step in the avatar control workflow. The execution times for different services are shown in Table 1. Frame grabbing, person detection, person identification, and 3D pose estimation services were run on the following server configurations: AMD CPU Ryzen 9 5900X, RAM 3200 Mhz 4 × 16 GB, GPU NVIDIA RTX A5000 24 GB, and SAMSUNG SSD 980 PRO 1TB M.2. Peer-to-peer delay (WebRTC) and MOCAP data message exchange delay are measured on the LAN network. The unity 3D model transformation on the VR side was run on a laptop with the following configurations: CPU Intel(R) Core(TM) i5-9300H CPU @ 2.40GHz, GPU NVIDIA GeForce GTX 1650, SSD NVMe Micron_2200 _MTFD _16GB, and RAM DDR4 16 GB 3.2 GHz. The VIVE Pro headset was connected to a laptop to present the 3D model to a remote specialist. HoloLens 2, used on the AR side, can run applications using onboard hardware or a PC in holographic remoting mode. It can be seen that running the client application on the laptop, which is the only available option on the VR side, is significantly faster compared to the running time when the client application runs on HoloLens 2 hardware. It should be noted that, in the holographic remoting mode, the HoloLens camera is not accessible from the code, and therefore an external webcamera is used for patient capture. As expected, WebRTC communication significantly contributes to the overall delay, which has values ranging from 340 to 560 ms. The individual computer vision service requires time ranging from 15 to 60 ms. Compared to approaches using 3D reconstruction for avatar creation, the usage of 3D body pose estimation in the proposed system reduces the amount of transferred data and requires less processing time, which is comparable to the time needed for other computer vision algorithms in avatar control workflow. Although direct comparison of latency with other systems from the literature is not possible due to the specific features of each architecture, the obtained values are comparable to the latency of other holographic communication systems, which have values of several hundred milliseconds [1]. The mixed reality telemedicine system proposed in [8] has similar latency values (300–400 ms). It uses depth cameras and 3D reconstruction of the intensive care unit, but the reconstruction module, network transmission, and streaming processing are implemented in C++/CUDA to reduce processing time. In the proposed approach, Python implementations of computer vision services for avatar control are used to determine the possibility of further reducing the time delay by C++ implementation of some tasks.

The frame rate obtained in client applications on the VR and AR sides is a critical factor for system usability; therefore, the frame rate (Table 2) is measured in two lightning scenarios (light and no light) and the human body system (Z-anatomy model) chosen for visualization. A constant frame rate is obtained for the AR client application (60 fps) running on a laptop (AR-remote) and for the VR client application (120 fps) also running on the same laptop (VR-build). It can be seen that, for the AR client running on the HoloLens 2 hardware, the frame rate is variable and depends on the type of body system chosen for visualization. The main difference between the proposed method and the existing approaches is the construction of the patient avatar using 3D body pose estimation from 2D images. A similar system was proposed in [8]; however, instead of a patient, remote experts are represented as avatars in the 3D-reconstructed intensive care unit. The body poses of remote clinicians are obtained with trackers attached to the ankles, wrists, and hip, while in the proposed approach, additional sensors are not needed to construct a patient avatar. In [7], a 3D reconstruction of the patient body is performed using depth images captured by a Microsoft Azure Kinect camera. Since the Kinect camera is attached to a surgical lamp, this setup is suitable for patients in a lying position. The proposed solution does not require a depth camera and could also be used for other patient poses (Figure 4). Limitations of the proposed system include the accuracy of 3D body pose estimations, which affect the alignment of the 3D avatar with the patient's body. Because of that, the proposed system is not suitable for surgical applications, but it could be exploited for remote patient evaluation, such as remote triage, nonsurgical remote medical interventions, and educational purposes.

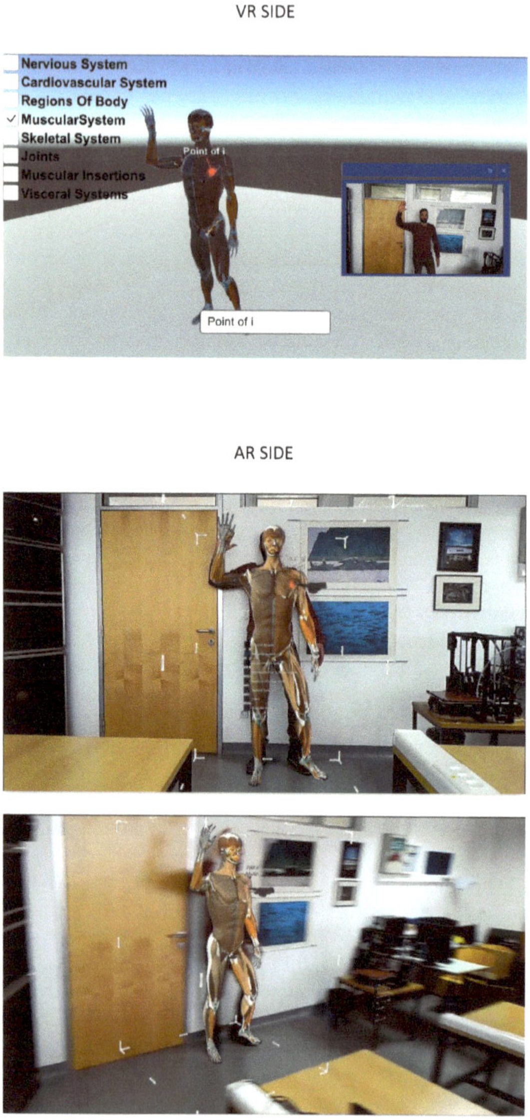

Figure 3. VR and AR client views. The red point on the avatar represents point of interest, and the virtual hand (in gray color) represents the remote specialist hand.

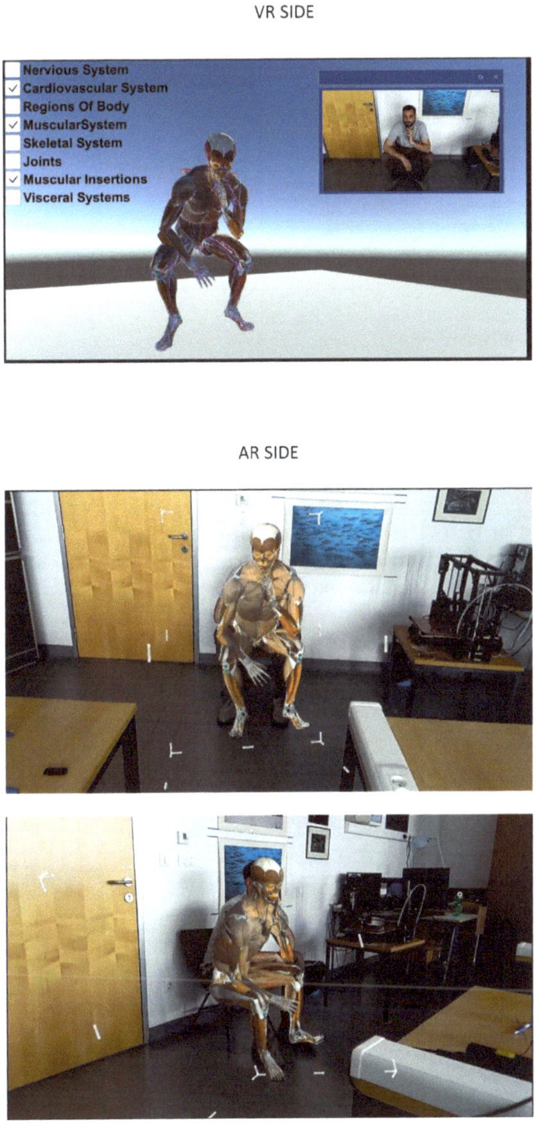

Figure 4. VR and AR client view for patient in a sitting pose.

Table 1. Time delay of avatar movement.

Service	Time Delay (ms)
WebRTC P2P	200–300
Grab frame	3–8
Person detection	25–60
Person identification	30–60
3D pose estimation	15–50
WebSocket MOCAP	50
Unity 3D model transformation (running on laptop)	5–15
Unity 3D model transformation (running on HoloLens 2)	10–25

Table 2. Performance of the AR and VR client applications.

Body System	AR Build		AR Remote		VR Build	
	No Light (FPS)	Light (FPS)	No Light (FPS)	Light (FPS)	No Light (FPS)	Light (FPS)
Visceral system	26	25	60	60	120	120
Muscural system	13	12	60	60	120	120
Cardiovascular system	8	8	60	60	120	120
Nervous system and sence organs	13	13	60	60	120	120
Regions of human body/skin	54	51	60	60	120	120
Skeletal system	28	28	60	60	120	120
Joints	38	36	60	60	120	120
Muscular insertion	26	26	60	60	120	120
Lymphoid organs	50	46	60	60	120	120

5. Conclusions

In this paper, we introduce an XR-based telemedicine collaboration system based on the 3D avatar modality for patient body representation. Instead of relying on 3D reconstructions of the patient's body using depth cameras, 3D body pose estimation from 2D images is utilized for this purpose. In this way, there is no need for an array of depth cameras that are preinstalled and calibrated in a controlled environment, which reduces the cost and system complexity. Additionally, the processing time and amount of transferred data are reduced compared to those of approaches utilizing depth cameras and 3D reconstruction. The remote expert (VR side) and local doctor (AR side) exchange information by interacting with the same patient avatar in a shared XR space. This process is performed with virtual hands and textual annotations on the patient avatar. Use cases of the proposed system include remote education of the patient or doctor as well as remote consultations where remote experts could guide local clinicians. A limitation of the proposed system is that it is not intended for use in high-precision tasks such as surgical procedures because of the limited accuracy of matching the avatar and patient body. Future work will include test cases in which clinicians perform real medical procedures. Further evaluation will be performed to obtain the system usability score for different tasks and investigate the agreement between the in-person assessment and the remote examination performed by the proposed system. Latency improvement will also be addressed by the C++ implementation of steps critical for processing speeds.

Author Contributions: Conceptualization, M.Š. and M.R.; methodology, M.R., M.Š. and L.K.; software, L.K. and D.M.; validation, M.Š., L.K. and D.M.; formal analysis, M.Š.; investigation, M.R.; resources, L.K.; data curation, L.K. and D.M.; writing—original draft preparation, M.Š.; writing—review and editing, M.Š., L.K. and M.R.; visualization, L.K. and M.Š.; supervision, M.R.; project administration, M.R.; funding acquisition, M.R. All authors have read and agreed to the published version of the manuscript.

Funding: This research was funded by the Virtual Telemedicine Assistance (VITA), a project co-financed by the Croatian Government and the European Union through the European Regional Development Fund: the Competitiveness and Cohesion Operational Programme (KK.01.1.1.01).

Institutional Review Board Statement: Not applicable.

Informed Consent Statement: Not applicable.

Data Availability Statement: Data are contained within the article.

Conflicts of Interest: The authors declare no conflict of interest.

References

1. Petkova, R.; Poulkov, V.; Manolova, A.; Tonchev, K. Challenges in Implementing Low-Latency Holographic-Type Communication Systems. *Sensors* **2022**, *22*, 9617. [CrossRef] [PubMed]
2. Qualcomm Technologies, Inc. *VR and AR Pushing Connectivity Limits*; Qualcomm Technologies, Inc.: San Diego, CA, USA, 2018.

3. Lin, P.J.; Tsai, B.C.; Tsai, Y.W. Telemedicine System Based on Mixed Reality and Cognitive Speech Service Technologies. In Proceedings of the 2022 IEEE 4th Eurasia Conference on Biomedical Engineering, Healthcare and Sustainability (ECBIOS), Tainan, Taiwan, 27–29 May 2022; pp. 241–244.
4. Anton, D.; Kurillo, G.; Yang, A.Y.; Bajcsy, R. Augmented telemedicine platform for real-time remote medical consultation. In Proceedings of the MultiMedia Modeling: 23rd International Conference, MMM 2017, Reykjavik, Iceland, 4–6 January 2017; Proceedings, Part I 23; Springer: Cham, Switzerland, 2017; pp. 77–89.
5. Carbone, M.; Freschi, C.; Mascioli, S.; Ferrari, V.; Ferrari, M. A wearable augmented reality platform for telemedicine. In Proceedings of the Augmented Reality, Virtual Reality, and Computer Graphics: Third International Conference, AVR 2016, Lecce, Italy, 15–18 June 2016; Proceedings, Part II 3; Springer: Cham, Switzerland, 2016; pp. 92–100.
6. Strak, R.; Yu, K.; Pankratz, F.; Lazarovici, M.; Sandmeyer, B.; Reichling, J.; Weidert, S.; Kraetsch, C.; Roegele, B.; Navab, N.; et al. Comparison between video-mediated and asymmetric 3d teleconsultation during a preclinical scenario. In Proceedings of the Mensch und Computer 2021, Ingolstadt, Germany, 5–8 September 2021; pp. 227–235.
7. Gasques, D.; Johnson, J.G.; Sharkey, T.; Feng, Y.; Wang, R.; Xu, Z.R.; Zavala, E.; Zhang, Y.; Xie, W.; Zhang, X.; et al. ARTEMIS: A collaborative mixed-reality system for immersive surgical telementoring. In Proceedings of the 2021 CHI Conference on Human Factors in Computing Systems, Yokohama, Japan, 8–13 May 2021; pp. 1–14.
8. Roth, D.; Yu, K.; Pankratz, F.; Gorbachev, G.; Keller, A.; Lazarovici, M.; Wilhelm, D.; Weidert, S.; Navab, N.; Eck, U. Real-time mixed reality teleconsultation for intensive care units in pandemic situations. In Proceedings of the 2021 IEEE Conference on Virtual Reality and 3D User Interfaces Abstracts and Workshops (VRW), Lisbon, Portugal, 27 March–1 April 2021; pp. 693–694.
9. Weibel, N.; Gasques, D.; Johnson, J.; Sharkey, T.; Xu, Z.R.; Zhang, X.; Zavala, E.; Yip, M.; Davis, K. Artemis: Mixed-reality environment for immersive surgical telementoring. In Proceedings of the Extended Abstracts of the 2020 CHI Conference on Human Factors in Computing Systems, Honolulu, HI, USA, 25–30 April 2020; pp. 1–4.
10. Kalbas, Y.; Jung, H.; Ricklin, J.; Jin, G.; Li, M.; Rauer, T.; Dehghani, S.; Navab, N.; Kim, J.; Pape, H.C.; et al. Remote Interactive Surgery Platform (RISP): Proof of Concept for an Augmented-Reality-Based Platform for Surgical Telementoring. *J. Imaging* **2023**, *9*, 56. [CrossRef] [PubMed]
11. Sultan, L.R.; Haertter, A.; Al-Hasani, M.; Demiris, G.; Cary, T.W.; Tung-Chen, Y.; Sehgal, C.M. Can Artificial Intelligence Aid Diagnosis by Teleguided Point-of-Care Ultrasound? A Pilot Study for Evaluating a Novel Computer Algorithm for COVID-19 Diagnosis Using Lung Ultrasound. *AI* **2023**, *4*, 875–887. [CrossRef] [PubMed]
12. Hill, R. Using augmented reality to improve patient outcomes with negative pressure wound therapy. *Wounds* **2022**, *33*, 47–50. [CrossRef] [PubMed]
13. Borresen, A.; Chakka, K.; Wu, R.; Lin, C.K.; Wolfe, C.; Prabhakaran, B.; Annaswamy, T.M. Comparison of in-person and synchronous remote musculoskeletal exam using augmented reality and haptics: A pilot study. *PM&R* **2023**, *15*, 891–898.
14. Mediapipe Object Detection. 2023. Available online: https://developers.google.com/mediapipe/solutions/vision/object_detector (accessed on 13 October 2023).
15. Tan, M.; Pang, R.; Le, Q.V. Efficientdet: Scalable and efficient object detection. In Proceedings of the IEEE/CVF Conference on Computer Vision and Pattern Recognition, Seattle, WA, USA, 13–19 June 2020; pp. 10781–10790.
16. Python Package Face-Recogntion. 2023. Available online: https://pypi.org/project/face-recognition/ (accessed on 13 October 2023).
17. Rong, Y.; Shiratori, T.; Joo, H. Frankmocap: A monocular 3d whole-body pose estimation system via regression and integration. In Proceedings of the IEEE/CVF International Conference on Computer Vision, Montreal, BC, Canada, 11–17 October 2021; pp. 1749–1759.
18. Pavlakos, G.; Choutas, V.; Ghorbani, N.; Bolkart, T.; Osman, A.A.; Tzionas, D.; Black, M.J. Expressive body capture: 3d hands, face, and body from a single image. In Proceedings of the IEEE/CVF Conference on Computer Vision and Pattern Recognition, Long Beach, CA, USA, 15–20 June 2019; pp. 10975–10985.
19. Loper, M.; Mahmood, N.; Romero, J.; Pons-Moll, G.; Black, M.J. SMPL: A skinned multi-person linear model. In *Seminal Graphics Papers: Pushing the Boundaries, Volume 2*; Association for Computing Machinery: New York, NY, USA, 2023; pp. 851–866.
20. Kolotouros, N.; Pavlakos, G.; Black, M.J.; Daniilidis, K. Learning to reconstruct 3D human pose and shape via model-fitting in the loop. In Proceedings of the IEEE/CVF International Conference on Computer Vision, Seoul, Republic of Korea, 27 October–2 November 2019; pp. 2252–2261.
21. Sanyal, S.; Bolkart, T.; Feng, H.; Black, M.J. Learning to regress 3D face shape and expression from an image without 3D supervision. In Proceedings of the IEEE/CVF Conference on Computer Vision and Pattern Recognition, Long Beach, CA, USA, 15–20 June 2019; pp. 7763–7772.

computers

MDPI

Article

The Readiness of Lasem Batik Small and Medium Enterprises to Join the Metaverse

Theresia Dwi Hastuti [1,*], Ridwan Sanjaya [2] and Freddy Koeswoyo [1]

1 Accounting Department, Faculty of Economics and Business, Soegijapranata Catholic University, Semarang 50234, Indonesia
2 Information Systems Department, Faculty of Computer Science, Soegijapranata Catholic University, Semarang 50234, Indonesia
* Correspondence: theresia@unika.ac.id

Abstract: Today's business competitiveness necessitates the capacity of all company players, particularly small and medium enterprises (SMEs), to enter a broader market through information technology. However, the Lasem Batik SMEs have endured a great deal of turmoil during the COVID-19 pandemic. Marketing has been conducted through physical and internet channels, but the results have not been maximized. The purpose of this research was to consider the possibilities of Lasem Batik SMEs adopting metaverse technology as a marketing medium to enhance sales. The investigation was conducted on 40 Lasem Batik SMEs who met the requirements of using online media to sell their products, having a medium-sized firm, and displaying marketing that has reached the provincial level. The findings of this study are as follows: (1) The majority of participants stated that the metaverse is a virtual 3D space. This understanding is deepened by discussions about virtual 3D spaces that combine VR and AR, which today is often referred to as the metaverse. (2) Batik business owners hope that by using the metaverse, they will be able to obtain many benefits, especially related to market expansion. (3) Lasem Batik SMEs show great interest in expanding their marketing channels to a wider area; Lasem Batik entrepreneurs also accept the challenge of studying the metaverse with new knowledge and techniques they have never considered. (4) Overall, 75% of participants were ready to use the metaverse, and 25% still required guidance. (5) Local communities, universities, and large corporations provide great support for the use of the metaverse. (6) The commercial success of Lasem Batik SMEs is defined by product quality; ongoing online and offline advertising; originality and innovation; and the capacity to capitalize on possibilities, retain local wisdom, and preserve strong customer connections. The main conclusion is that the readiness of batik entrepreneurs to use the metaverse is highly dependent on the support of various parties. A strong desire to progress and develop one's business is the main factor determining one's intention to use the metaverse. As a result of the research, a prototype of a metaverse platform for Lasem Batik exhibitions has been developed. SMEs can use the room template provided by the platform and join other SMEs to hold a metaverse exhibition to attract global customers. These results can be connected to create a metaverse exhibition to attract global customers.

Keywords: augmented reality; marketing; metaverse; readiness; SMEs; virtual reality

Citation: Hastuti, T.D.; Sanjaya, R.; Koeswoyo, F. The Readiness of Lasem Batik Small and Medium Enterprises to Join the Metaverse. *Computers* **2023**, *12*, 5. https://doi.org/10.3390/computers12010005

Academic Editors: Radu Comes, Dorin-Mircea Popovici, Calin Gheorghe Dan Neamtu and Jing-Jing Fang

Received: 6 November 2022
Revised: 21 December 2022
Accepted: 21 December 2022
Published: 26 December 2022

1. Research Background

Over the last thirty years, immersive virtual reality (VR) and augmented reality (AR) technologies have continued to advance. Over the same period, network speeds have increased, culminating in the deployment of 5G mobile networks. Combined, these advances have greatly increased the prospects for the worldwide adoption of VR and AR. Facebook launched the metaverse and was followed by other platform providers with different names [1]. Facebook spent more than USD 10 billion in 2021 in developing metaverse technologies, and it is predicted that its investment will increase in the coming years [2]. The metaverse is generally considered a network of 3D virtual worlds wherein people can interact, conduct business, and establish social relations through their virtual "avatars". It can be regarded as the virtual reality version of today's internet [3].

Over the past 18 months, public interest in the metaverse has soared, along with significant increases within companies [1]. The effects of the pandemic, especially in terms of restrictions on physical gatherings and travel, have spurred companies to seek new methods of working that can accommodate more authentic, cohesive, and interactive processes of remote and hybrid interaction and communication. The metaverse can address this need in four main ways: (1) new forms of immersive team collaboration; (2) the emergence of new digital partners that support artificial intelligence; (3) accelerated learning and skill acquisition through virtualization and gamified technology; (4) improving the economy through economic activities with metaverse media.

Widayani et al. [4] stated that today's business competition requires the capability of all businesses, especially SMEs, to penetrate a wider market and develop themselves by directing their business processes through technology and information advancements. The addition of online sales channels is an inevitable choice. The use of e-marketplaces is one of the easiest ways to get involved in online sales globally [5]. There are various factors influencing the readiness of SMEs to implement information technology, including the optimism, knowledge, and skills of SME actors, while the inhibiting factors include perceptions of discomfort and reluctance to change. Research conducted by Firmansyah et al. [6] found that the perception of the use of information technology (IT) depends on the factors of optimism and innovation. They also concluded that (1) insecurity is a limiting factor, (2) the perception of the use of IT is a factor determining the intention to use IT, and (3) SME actors need to maintain a positive attitude in understanding IT.

Research conducted by Kurniati and Prajanti [7] states that the role of batik entrepreneur owners is very large in innovation, which includes product innovation, marketing innovation, and business alliances. The role of entrepreneurship in marketing innovation has the highest elasticity concerning the production and sales of batik, followed by the roles of product innovation and business alliances. In a competitive industrial environment, batik industry entrepreneurs have an important role in improving the economy of the company and its industry. Innovation is not limited to large-scale enterprises, which generally have a research and development (R & D) division, but also includes small businesses such as batik SMEs, which also require innovation activities [4,6–10]. SMEs benefit from organizational flexibility in responding to environmental changes, but most SMEs have drawbacks in access and innovation capacity due to limited resources and economies of use [11].

Rosenberg [1] stated that over the past thirty years, virtual reality (VR) and augmented reality (AR), as immersive technologies, have continued to evolve as sophisticated forms of technology, enabling users to develop various business processes using VR and AR. During the same period, the demand for network speed has continued to increase progressively. These advances increase the prospects for the worldwide adoption of VR and AR. The metaverse, as a platform provider that can combine VR and AR, has begun to be widely used in the business world and the world of education to develop networks and promote their products. The increase in the use of the metaverse has had a huge impact on society. It is very important to consider the risks and prepare appropriate regulations so that the negative aspects of using information technology can be minimized.

This study was designed based on the practice gap between small and medium enterprises (SMEs) facing problems related to data volumes that are too large, a lack of information, and a lack of knowledge. In fact, to be able to develop better, SMEs must be able to make timely decisions. On the other hand, the metaverse is associated with high-level technologies that take advantage of VR and AR together, which brings many advantages and benefits to businesses. The technology gap is very clear in this regard, and the capabilities of SMEs must be developed in such a way as to allow a technological pursuit of the metaverse [12].

Lasem is a small area in the form of a sub-district in Rembang Regency, Central Java, which is associated with the classical style of coastal batik craft. Lasem Batik is rich in motifs and colors due to the accumulation of local culture (Javanese) influenced by immigrant culture, mainly derived from Champa (Vietnam), India, China, and the Netherlands. The main characteristics of Lasem's hand-drawn batik lie in the color display in the form of a combination of bright colors, such as red (bang-bangan), blue, yellow, and green, which is different from other forms of coastal batik [13]. Lasem Batik will continue to prosper, in addition to marketing and tourism development. Lasem, known as Little China, also has the potential to develop its tourism sector.

Lasem Batik's marketing has experienced a great deal of turmoil and is greatly affected by the economic conditions. Efforts to conduct marketing through offline and online channels have been made. Marketing with an online model is achieved, among other things, by performing live streaming through Instagram. The pandemic conditions and changes in transportation routes between cities and between provinces, which were moved to toll roads, no longer passing through Lasem, greatly affected the marketing of Lasem Batik products. Efforts made by Lasem Batik include more aggressive marketing through Facebook, WhatsApp, and Instagram. The originality of this research is the investigation of the possibility of Lasem Batik SMEs conducting marketing through the metaverse.

2. Literature Review

2.1. Metaverse

"Metaverse" has different definitions depending on the context in which it is described. Generally, the metaverse is related to virtual reality (VR) and augmented reality (AR). The metaverse is a persistent and immersive world of simulation experienced in the first person, as well as in a large group of users simultaneously present in a large space that becomes a completely virtual environment (virtual world), or it can exist as layers of virtual content overlaid in the real world with convincing registration [1]. Virtual reality (VR) is an immersive and interactive simulation environment experienced in the first person and offers the user a strong sense of presence. Mystakidis [14] defined the metaverse as a post-reality universe, a perpetual and persistent multiuser environment merging physical reality with digital virtuality. It is based on the convergence of technologies that enable multisensory interactions with virtual environments, digital objects, and people, such as virtual reality (VR) and augmented reality (AR). Laeeq [3] described the concept of a fully immersive virtual world where people gather to socialize, play, and work. It is a simulated digital environment that combines augmented reality (AR), virtual reality (VR), blockchain, and social media principles to create areas for rich user interaction that imitate the real world. Based on the above definitions, it can be concluded that the metaverse is a persistent simulated world that combines augmented reality (AR), virtual reality (VR), blockchain, and social media principles to create an area for interaction between platform users and allows users to simulate the real world.

2.2. Trade in the Metaverse

Trading in the metaverse is relatively new and yields quite promising results when businesses make use of its advantages and obtain good outcomes. For example, virtual real estate company Gucci, a fashion brand, is collaborating with game developer Roblox to sell products in the metaverse. Balenciaga partnered with Epic Games, the creators of Fortnite, to provide a virtual boutique. RTFKT, a well-known metaverse brand with a collection of shoes, was purchased by Nike to expand its sales. An 18-year-old designer sold more than USD 3 million in virtual shoes in less than seven minutes. Nike is looking to hire virtual apparel designers and trademark apps [3].

The whole world is experiencing a significant shift from the actual economy to the digital economy. Work and life are increasingly dependent on the internet because various activities depend on information obtained from online systems. The internet is often the main gateway for millions of people to interact and socialize with each other, sell products, and transact through a virtual environment; long distances are not an obstacle. Technology is key to the maintenance of many jobs. The demand for virtual reality is growing along with the industry that utilizes the metaverse [15]. In the metaverse, a virtual world that transcends reality, artificial intelligence, and blockchain technology are combined. With new technologies related to the development of computers, graphics, and hardware, cyberspace has become a reality. More and more digital asset transfers will occur on the blockchain via avatars. It is expected that the digital value paradigm will form a new economic model.

Soepeno [16] states that the metaverse is a 3D virtual augmented reality where anyone can experience anything in a virtual environment and connect. The use of the application in an extended and tactical virtual environment, meeting people in virtual reality, engaging in physical activities in a virtual holographic metaverse, and many more opportunities and activity options are offered.

2.3. Technology Acceptance Model

The Technology Acceptance Model (TAM) was developed by Davis [17]. It explains how the acceptance of technology by users will affect the use of the technology itself. This theory was adapted from several models built to analyze and understand the factors that influence the acceptance of using new technologies. The Technology Acceptance Model is part of the Theory of Reasoned Action, which is most widely used by researchers to explain the reasons for using information technology [15,16,18]. TAM is a theory designed to explain how users apply and understand information technology. TAM aims to explain and predict the acceptance of information relations with technology-based users. In addition, TAM is also used to explain the behavior of end users with variations, and the number of user populations is increasing. TAM has three key variables: perceived usefulness (PU), perceived ease of use (PEU), and behavioral intention to use (BIU). Perceived usefulness and ease of use of IT are the most significant factors influencing the desire to adopt information technology.

Since its introduction by Davis [17], TAM has been widely used by researchers to explain the user acceptance of technology. The model explains that if a technology is deemed useful, the technology will be adopted, which seems to be supported by the PEOU. There is a positive and strong correlation between the acceptance and use of technology variables and user satisfaction. The results of this study are useful not only for managers but also for manufacturers, technical support, online support, and after-sales services because they are advised to develop strategies for user satisfaction [19].

Davis [17] developed and validated a new scale for two specific variables, perceived usefulness and perceived ease of use (see Figure 1), which were hypothesized to be fundamental determinants of user acceptance. Davis' main goals were as follows: first, the theory presented should be able to enhance our understanding of the user acceptance process, providing new theoretical insights into the design and implementation of successful information systems; second, TAM must provide a theoretical basis for the testing of acceptance among users of the system.

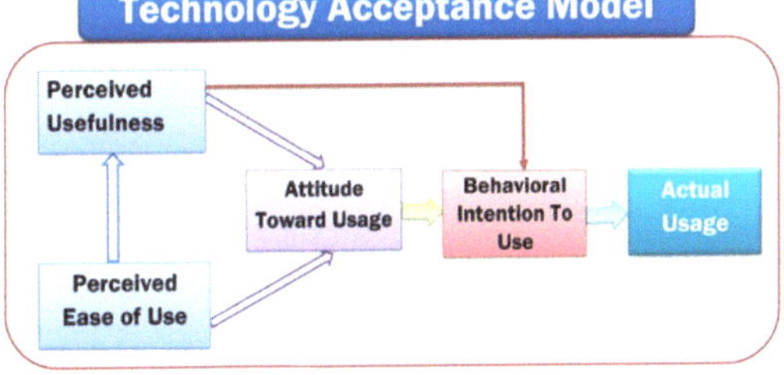

Figure 1. TAM. Source: Davis (1989).

Davis [17] found that usability has a much greater correlation with user behavior than ease of use. Perceived ease of use may, in fact, be a causal antecedent for perceived usefulness; that is, PEOU affects technology acceptance (TA) indirectly through PU. In the last decade, TAM has received much attention and empirical support (see Gefen and Straub [20]; Venkatesh [21]). It is estimated that around 100 studies were published in journals, proceedings, or technical reports related to TAM between 1989 and 2001.

2.4. Theory of Planned Behavior

The Theory of Planned Behavior was developed by [22] and is often used to explain individual behavior associated with the use of information technology. Many studies have proven this and provide empirical evidence for researchers. Intention to behave with different types of technology can be predicted with high accuracy from attitudes towards behavior, subjective norms, and perceived behavioral control. Nita considers this in conjunction with perceived behavioral control, explaining the considerable variation in actual behavior. Huang and Chen [23] stated that the Theory of Planned Behavior developed by [22] has become the main theory used to explain actual intentions and behavior in various fields. The Theory of Planned Behavior considers attitudes, subjective norms, and perceived behavioral control (PBC) as three useful factors in predicting actual intentions and behavior.

3. Research Methods

The sample of this research consists of the owners of Lasem Batik SMEs in the middle-to-upper business category whose sales have reached the provincial, national, and international levels. The criteria for selecting this sample referred to the Indonesian Government's Law No. 20 of 2018 [24] regarding the following criteria for SMEs: (1) a minimum net worth of IDR 500 million, and (2) a sales turnover in one year of at least IDR 2.5 billion. Based on these criteria, the selection of SMEs was conducted through the Lasem Batik entrepreneur cooperative. There are 79 batik entrepreneurs who are members of the batik entrepreneur cooperative. The selection was carried out on 79 batik entrepreneurs, and 40 batik business owners who met these criteria were obtained.

This study uses an interpretive phenomenological analysis (IPA) approach, which provides the researcher with the best opportunity to understand in depth the research participants' experiences of the metaverse. As a 'participant-oriented' approach, the interpretive phenomenological analysis approach allows the research participants to express themselves and provide their recollections of their experiences as they see fit, without distortion and/or prosecution. The primary aim of the IPA approach is to explore the 'hands-on experience' of the research participants and to enable them to generate research findings through their experiences [25]. Qualitative research methods impart an added advantage to exploratory abilities. Qualitative methodologies enable researchers to advance and apply their interpersonal skills and subjectivity to their exploratory research process. In a study with an interpretive phenomenological analysis (IPA) approach, IPA provides the best opportunity for researchers to understand the details of the 'life experiences' of research participants in depth.

The research process was conducted as a focus group discussion, which started with an explanation of the metaverse and the various functions of the metaverse. The process of applying the metaverse for marketing in Lasem Batik was also conducted, with the assistance of various workshops on materials related to creating a metaverse space, photography, branding, and promotion through a metaverse. The focus group discussion focused on understanding the metaverse, the readiness of the owners of Lasem Batik to consider the metaverse, the obstacles and challenges that will occur, and the prospects for marketing through the metaverse.

4. Results and Discussion

4.1. The Understanding of the Metaverse

A focus group discussion was conducted to discuss the possibility of using the metaverse to increase the marketing of Lasem Batik. The initial question in this research was regarding the participants' understanding of the metaverse. In the focus group discussion, the researcher explained in detail what the metaverse is, with the various functions and uses of the metaverse. Participants were asked to respond to questions about their understanding of the metaverse and the likelihood that they would use the metaverse to expand their marketing channels. The results of the focus group discussion are depicted in Figure 2.

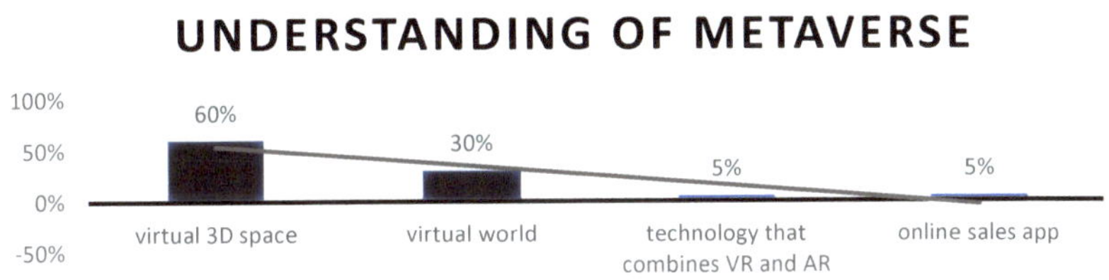

Figure 2. The understanding of the metaverse. Source: processed primary data, 2022.

Based on Figure 2, the majority of participants stated that the metaverse is a virtual 3D space. This understanding was deepened by discussions about virtual 3D spaces that combine VR and AR, which today is often referred to as the metaverse. The metaverse can be used by various institutions and associations to conduct online meetings and can even be used to market products, such as through model exhibitions. In the acceptance model theory, this stage involves explaining how technology is accepted by users. The acceptance of technology begins with an understanding of the technology itself [3,22,23].

The introduction of the metaverse technology was conducted by providing examples of various batik exhibitions conducted with AR and VR technologies. The control of metaverse technology towards Lasem Batik entrepreneurs can be seen in Figure 3. This exhibition was designed to include various activities that were photographed and videotaped in the metaverse space. Exhibitors could observe various models of batik, and, if interested, they could perform transactions with batik owners.

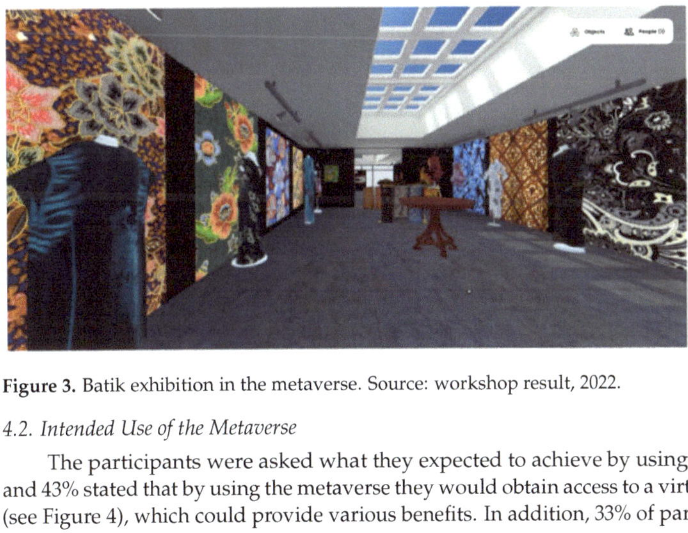

Figure 3. Batik exhibition in the metaverse. Source: workshop result, 2022.

4.2. Intended Use of the Metaverse

The participants were asked what they expected to achieve by using the metaverse, and 43% stated that by using the metaverse they would obtain access to a virtual community (see Figure 4), which could provide various benefits. In addition, 33% of participants stated that using the metaverse would create a growing trade, and 25% of participants stated that they would obtain familiarity with a different world. We can conclude that batik business owners hope that by using the metaverse, they will be able to achieve many benefits, especially related to market expansion, which is quite different from the brand's past experiences.

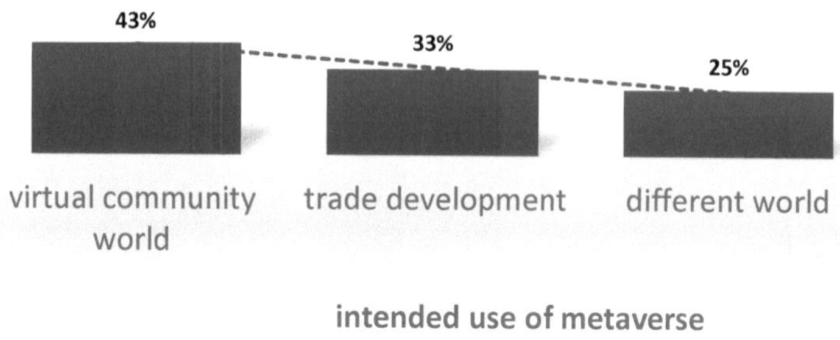

Figure 4. Intended use of the metaverse. Source: processed primary data, 2022.

Based on the responses of the batik entrepreneurs who were invited to discuss their attitudes towards using the metaverse, they showed great interest in expanding their marketing channels to a wider area. Lasem Batik entrepreneurs also accept the challenge of studying the metaverse with new knowledge and techniques never considered before. Great interest in using the metaverse is one of the keys to successfully using this type of information technology. It has been explained that TAM has three main variables: perceived usefulness (PU), perceived ease of use (PEU), and behavioral intention to use (BIU) [15–18]. Interest in using the metaverse is a determining factor in whether or not this information technology platform is used. This is also supported by the behavioral control conducted by the researchers by providing examples of the use of the metaverse and descriptions of development opportunities that can be explored. Such conditions align with the conditions described in the Theory of Planned Behavior [15–18].

In its development, the process of implementing the metaverse to expand the marketing channels for Lasem Batik was well-received by the local community. This is shown by the large number of mass media interested in becoming involved, particularly by publicizing training activities and workshops related to the metaverse conducted by researchers at Lasem [26–29]. Marketing activities constitute an interaction between the environment and the companies, which are self-centered during their operations. Such activities have included functional, transactional, competitive, mixed, integral, and relational aspects, among others [30].

4.3. Constraints of Using the Metaverse

Aware of the current condition, whereby batik business owners are not fully familiar with the metaverse or the various tools needed, we asked whether any obstacles were expected to greatly affect the use of the metaverse platform as a marketing tool for Lasem Batik. Participants' responses were as follows: 48% of Lasem Batik owners stated that they lacked knowledge about the metaverse (see Figure 5), and 8% of participants stated that they would refuse to use the metaverse because their industry adheres to traditional practices. Meanwhile, 10% of participants stated that the main obstacle faced was that the infrastructure required to use the metaverse did not yet exist. In addition, 15% of participants stated that they had to improve their human resources and were willing to perform marketing through the metaverse. Finally, 20% of participants stated that they required high creativity in marketing their products through the metaverse platform, while their current business processes were focused on the patterns and development of batik motifs.

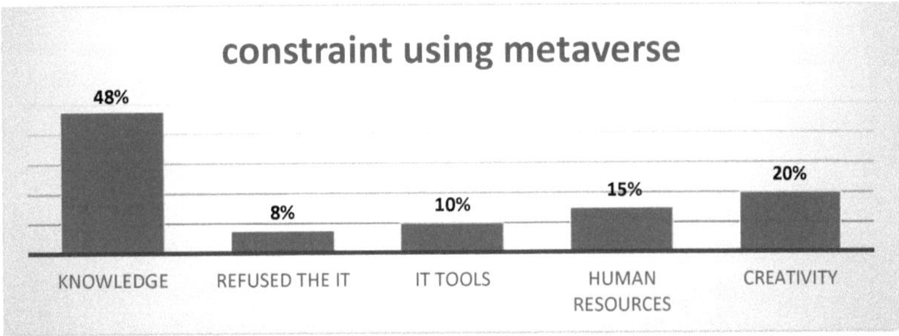

Figure 5. Constraints of using the metaverse. Source: processed primary data, 2022.

The obstacles faced by Lasem Batik entrepreneurs in using the metaverse are not fully considered to be inhibiting factors in developing their knowledge and marketing channels. Although they are still unfamiliar with the metaverse and the tools used to access the metaverse, the high willingness to learn among these batik entrepreneurs could help them to overcome the obstacles that they face. As revealed by [29], Lasem Batik entrepreneurs have established a cooperative formed to develop their businesses with various activities, including savings and loans, workshops, and discussions on batik development. In this cooperative, many problems have been resolved, including the problem of expanding the batik marketing channel.

4.4. The Possibility of Using the Metaverse Platform as a Marketing Tool

In general, the enthusiasm to participate in various metaverse-use preparation programs is extremely high. Based on the analysis of the responses of batik entrepreneurs when asked about the possibility of using the metaverse to market their batik, the answers were as follows: 13% of participants said they would not use the metaverse platform, their main reason being there is no evidence that the metaverse can increase sales; 48% of participants stated that they would use the metaverse platform; another 40% were still hesitant to use the metaverse platform for marketing their products.

The considerations were the same as those of the participants who answered "no"—namely, there is no convincing evidence that marketing with the metaverse can be achieved and can increase sales. The condition of batik entrepreneurs who are still unsure is in accordance with the research results of Hastuti et al. [31], which states that Lasem Batik entrepreneurs have not used information technology as a tool in managing the business. This is illustrated in Figure 6. These results support what is stated in the Technology Acceptance Model. There is a positive and strong correlation between the acceptance and use of technology and user satisfaction. The results of this study are useful not only for managers but also for manufacturers, technical support, online support, and after-sales services, as they are important in the development of user satisfaction strategies [23].

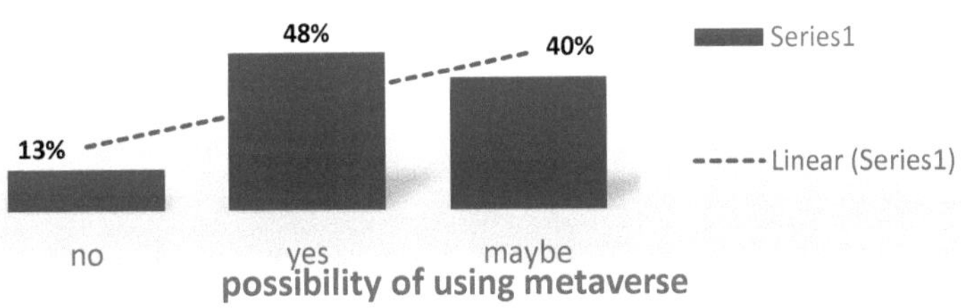

Figure 6. The possibility of using the metaverse platform. Source: processed primary data, 2022.

The involvement of Lasem Batik entrepreneurs in activities designed to prepare them for using the metaverse platform is quite high. Preparations include creating a metaverse platform, preparing a space for exhibitions, and creating metaverse assets. To expedite the process of placing batik assets in the metaverse, a photography workshop was held. This workshop was intended to document Lasem Batik's work in the metaverse. In addition, a workshop was also held on exploring batik branding and promotion on the metaverse platform. With these workshops, it was hoped that the Lasem Batik entrepreneur could increase his understanding of the metaverse to overcome his concerns about using it. In addition, a metaverse platform prototype was also developed for the Lasem Batik exhibition. Several ready-made metaverse room templates were provided for Lasem Batik SMEs to make it easier for them to utilize the technology for their business. SMEs can use the room templates provided by the platform and collaborate with other SMEs to hold metaverse exhibitions to attract global customers. This is consistent with what is stated in the Theory of Planned Behavior. The Theory of Planned Behavior was developed by [17] and is often used to explain individual behaviors related to the use of information technology.

4.5. The Hope after Knowing the Metaverse

It was hoped that the workshop provided as part of the preparatory process for using this platform could provide deeper and more detailed insights for Lasem Batik business owners. During the workshop process, in addition to providing knowledge and skills enrichment materials about the metaverse, an activity evaluation and analysis of increasing interest was also conducted using the metaverse platform. Based on the evaluation results, it was found that 75% of participants would continue to use the metaverse platform as an alternative to the Lasem Batik marketing platform and 25% of participants stated that their use of the metaverse platform required assistance in its operation (see Figure 7). Based on this evaluation, it can be concluded that 100% of participants would use the metaverse platform as an alternative method of marketing batik products. Based on the results, it can also be concluded that the metaverse workshop and its supporting tools, provided by the researchers, encourage batik entrepreneurs to use the metaverse platform. Participants who are hesitant at first are encouraged to become involved in using the metaverse, even if they require assistance initially.

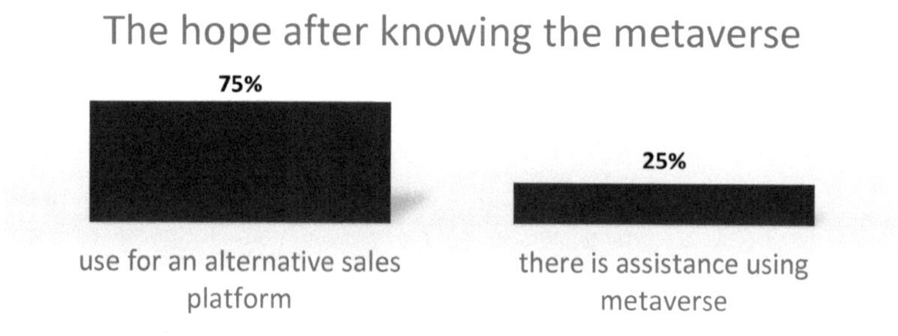

Figure 7. The hope of using the metaverse. Source: processed primary data, 2022.

4.6. Environmental Support

The batik business can develop well if there is support from various parties, such as family members, the surrounding community, and the government. Government support in the form of exhibitions and events will increase product marketing and encourage the emergence of batik product innovation. This is possible because the exhibitors could visit each other and discuss the uniqueness of each of their products. Government support can also be provided in the form of skills development and training for batik craftsmen [32]. Batik has been recognized as one of the products developing rapidly in the creative economy in Indonesia. The batik trade has grown and developed in Indonesia as a form of preserving regional cultural wealth, which has been developed as a form of local wisdom [33].

Recently, the central government, through the village development program, has formed a tourist village in an effort to develop regional potential and provide a place to foster community creativity. Tourism villages can also increase the incomes of local entrepreneurs. The community's strong support for the creativity of its citizens—for example, the creativity in producing batik and other food businesses—is achieved by purchasing these products. This will increase the turnover of the village economy. In addition, batik entrepreneurs can also encourage their employees to take part in the training provided so that they can jointly develop their own abilities and support the batik business in which they work. Small and medium enterprises (SMEs) face unique challenges in the business environment. SMEs must be able to keep up with change if they are to survive and grow and meet the expectations of creating investment and job opportunities. SMEs are expected to successfully adapt to technological changes and advances, customer expectations, supplier requirements, the regulatory environment, and increasing competition [34–36].

The government must ensure stable macroeconomic conditions, especially regarding exchange rates, interest rates, and inflation. Policies for SMEs must be able to protect and support their businesses in times of low economic growth. Governments can increase the promotional channels for new business development through intensive mentoring and removing known barriers. SMEs are introduced to an integrated multi-sector SME strategy. They are provided with partnership facilitation, entrepreneurship promotion and support, ease of access to financing, a focus on export promotion, and competitiveness development [22,23].

In this study, the community's support for batik businesses' efforts to expand their marketing through the metaverse platform was perceived by batik business owners. This support is depicted in Figure 8 as follows: 65% of participants stated that they received full support from the community, 13% of participants stated that they encountered obstacles, and 23% of participants wished to learn more about the metaverse. This indicates a society open to new developments that will advance the region.

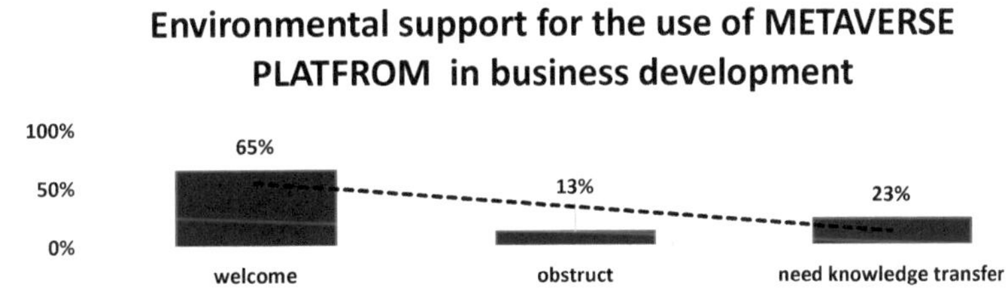

Figure 8. Environmental support for the use of the metaverse platform in business development.

4.7. *Continuity of Business Planning*

Continuous business plans and strategies provide effective solutions for multi-cloud and microservice approaches. A business continuity plan can help to provide a backup and measures for disaster recovery. In the business plan, actions have been raised to ensure sustainable business processes during disasters and emergencies. Business continuity planning methods include risk assessment, impact analysis, and a full business continuity strategy [37].

The talent for making Batik that has been owned by the people of Lasem and combined with the cultural heritage program by the government has made Lasem Batik continues to grow to this day. Cultural and Batik observers from universities and non-governmental organizations also coloured the development of Lasem Batik [38].

The ups and downs of Lasem Batik occur because the main thing is the willingness of the Lasem people themselves to keep the cultural heritage growing in Lasem or not.

Many Lasem Batik businesses have gone out of business because there is no successor to their business. The heirs are more likely to work in other sectors and outside Lasem. This growing awareness of the importance of the Lasem Batik business being maintained and developed is a crucial factor that the Batik community and the Rembang district government as well as cultural observers realize so that until now Lasem Batik is getting better and better [39].

Based on the focus group discussions with batik business owners (results can be seen in Figure 9), we obtained the factors that influence the growth of Lasem Batik. Focus group discussion participants stated that the factors that determined the sustainability of Lasem Batik were as follows: 28% of participants stated that they maintained the quality of their products, 23% of participants stated that they conducted continuous promotions both online and offline, and 18% of participants stated that the continuity of the batik business was due to the creativity and innovation of batik owners, who continued to grow. Moreover, 3% of participants stated that to develop their business they had to add employees, while 9% of participants stated that they had to use the opportunity to develop as much as possible. Meanwhile, 3% of participants stated that they had to maintain the traditional nature of Lasem Batik, and 15% of participants stated that they had to always maintain good relations with customers and expand their relationships.

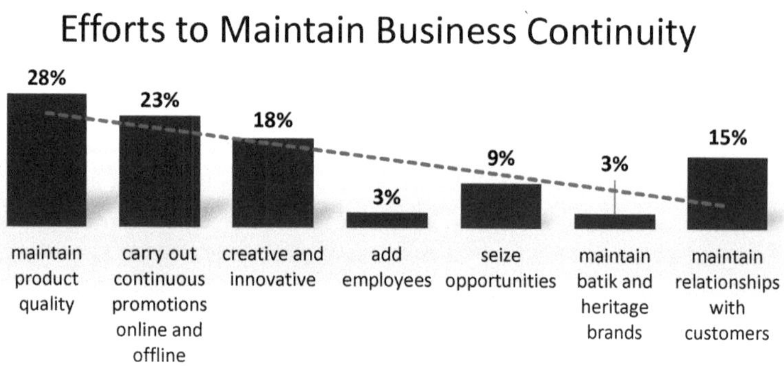

Figure 9. Efforts to maintain business continuity.

Lasem Batik has developed over time and has experienced some turmoil. The cultural value in Lasem continues to be developed by the local community and government [40]. The Lasem community's talent for batik, combined with the government's cultural heritage program, has allowed Lasem Batik to continue to grow to this day. Observers of culture and batik from universities and non-governmental organizations have also promoted the development of Lasem Batik [41,42].

The turmoil and success experienced byLasem Batik has occurred because of the willingness of the Lasem people themselves to maintain the cultural heritage that has developed in Lasem. This is the main requirement. Many Lasem Batik businesses have become bankrupt because there are no successors. Successors are more likely to work in other sectors and move outside Lasem. The growing awareness of the importance of the Lasem Batik business to be maintained and developed is a crucial factor that the batik-making community should be aware of. This can be strengthened by the support of the Rembang District government, as well as culturalists around Lembang, or even by national culturalists paying more attention to the development of Lasem Batik so that Lasem Batik can continue to grow and expand.

5. Conclusions

Studies on the readiness of SMEs in Lasem Batik for using the metaverse as a marketing channel have not been conducted widely. The originality of this research is its focus on metaverse applications in SMEs. Thus far, the metaverse has been used in large institutions, both in the world of business and the world of education. This study describes the readiness of Lasem Batik SMEs to utilize the metaverse by adopting an interpretive phenomenological analysis (IPA) approach. The phenomenological analysis provides researchers with an opportunity to understand, in-depth, the research participants' experiences of the metaverse. The study results show that the readiness of batik entrepreneurs to use the metaverse is highly dependent on the support of various parties. A strong desire to progress and develop one's business is the main factor determining one's intention to use the metaverse. Support from other parties, especially those who provide assistance regarding new technologies that businesses have never used before, is urgently needed by batik SMEs. The results of this study prove that information technology assistance can eliminate doubts about using the metaverse and promote strong beliefs to encourage involvement and the exploitation of opportunities to develop the business. The involvement of the mass media and non-governmental organizations is also a factor that can provide support for the intention of SMEs to use the metaverse. With mass media publications, it will be possible to increase the news about batik itself; this will raise the prestige of batik in the eyes of buyers and prospective buyers. Lasem Batik will also be increasingly recognized by many people. From mass media publications, we may also attract the government's attention to assist in the development of batik SMEs.

Implementing the metaverse for batik marketing includes creating a metaverse platform, preparing a space for exhibitions, and creating metaverse assets. To expedite the process of placing batik assets in the metaverse, a photography workshop was held. A workshop was also held exploring batik branding and promotion on the metaverse platform. With these workshops, it was hoped that the Lasem Batik entrepreneur would increase their understanding of the metaverse so that they could overcome their concerns about using the metaverse.

The main obstacle faced by Lasem Batik entrepreneurs in using the metaverse is their fear of not being able to use the tools to access the metaverse. In addition, the sustainability of using the metaverse depends on the ability of batik entrepreneurs to obtain the optimal benefits from the metaverse. Another challenge facing batik entrepreneurs is that SMEs must be able to keep up with change if they are to survive and grow and meet expectations by creating investment and job opportunities. SMEs are expected to successfully adapt to technological changes and advances, customer expectations, supplier requirements, the regulatory environment, and increasing competition.

Based on the results of this study, researchers can implement the use of the metaverse among Lasem Batik entrepreneurs and cooperate with the local government based on the Lasem Batik SMEs' characteristics. As a result of the research, a prototype of a metaverse platform for a Lasem Batik exhibition has been developed. Several ready-to-use metaverse room templates have been provided for the Lasem Batik SMEs to ease the process of utilizing the technology for their business. The SMEs can use the room template provided by the platform and join other SMEs to hold a metaverse exhibition to attract global customers. These rooms will be connected to create a metaverse exhibition to attract global customers. Although the platform can not only be viewed using a metaverse headset but also can be accessed by laptop users or smartphone users, the most immersive experience can be achieved by the use of a metaverse headset. Batik cloth and batik outfits that are displayed in 3 dimensions in the immersive room and can be seen in detail will create a new experience for the customers who see those clothes. The new experiences that customers feel can increase better interest in batik cloth and batik outfits. The development of exhibition spaces within the metaverse can be an alternative to displaying Lasem Batik products virtually and regularly in various countries that the SMEs have never visited before. From the results presented, future research could analyze the impact of the metaverse on the marketing of Lasem Batik by measuring the increase in sales, both in terms of the quantity and quality of its customers.

6. Recommendations

Recommendations are provided for Lasem Batik entrepreneurs. They can use the results of this study, which show that strong intentions accompanied by support and assistance will help to strengthen the use of information technology as one of the channels that will expand the range of sales of Lasem Batik products. Lasem Batik entrepreneurs can use this research as a reference to ensure that their knowledge is up to date, especially so that the batik that they produce can reach a global level. The batik business can thus grow rapidly because it can keep up with the latest marketing developments but can also anticipate the risks that will occur. Innovation and creativity continue to be developed as one of the keys to business success. The main recommendation for the government is that they must continue to support Lasem Batik SMEs so that the cultural heritage can be well maintained and develop into a national asset that is known internationally. Recommendations for future research are that research can be conducted using quantitative methods that examine the impact of using the metaverse to improve financial performance, increase Lasem Batik branding, and expand its marketing.

Author Contributions: Conceptualization, T.D.H. and R.S.; methodology, T.D.H.; validation, R.S.; formal analysis, T.D.H.; investigation, T.D.H.; resources, T.D.H.; data curation, F.K.; writing—original draft preparation, T.D.H.; writing—review and editing, R.S.; visualization, F.K.; supervision, R.S.; project administration, T.D.H. and F.K.; funding acquisition, T.D.H., R.S. and F.K. All authors have read and agreed to the published version of the manuscript.

Funding: This research and APC was funded by the Indonesian Ministry of Education, Culture, Research, and Technology.

Data Availability Statement: All data has been present in main text.

Acknowledgments: This article was a part of a research project supported by the Indonesian Ministry of Education, Culture, Research, and Technology under the scheme of the Matching Fund Kedaireka in 2022, titled Metaverse-Based Batik Event Organizing Platform for Increasing and Expanding Lasem Batik Sales Channels.

Conflicts of Interest: The authors declare no conflict of interest.

References

1. Rosenberg, L. Regulation of the Metaverse: A Roadmap the Risks and Regulatory Solutions for Largescale Consumer Platforms. In Proceedings of the 6th International Conference on Virtual and Augmented Reality Simulations, Brisbane, Australia, 25–27 March 2022; pp. 21–26.
2. Culliford, E.; Balu, N. Facebook Invests Billions in Metaverse Efforts as Ad Business Slows. Available online: https://www.reuters.com/technology/facebook-revenue-misses-estimates-apples-privacy-rules-bite-2021-10-25/ (accessed on 21 December 2022).
3. Laeeq, K. Metaverse: Why, How and What. Available online: https://www.researchgate.net/profile/Kashif-Laeeq/publication/358505001_Metaverse_Why_How_and_What/links/62053bb0afa8884cabd70210/Metaverse-Why-How-and-What.pdf (accessed on 21 December 2022).
4. Widayani, A.; Astuti, E.S.; Saifi, M. Competence and readiness of small and medium industries against of industrial revolution 4.0. In *IOP Conference Series: Earth and Environmental Science*; IOP Publishing: Bristol, UK, 2020; Volume 485.
5. Sanjaya, R.; Hastuti, T.D.; Koeswoyo, G.F. Accounting-based Digital Payment Systems for SMEs. In Proceedings of the International Conference on Computer and Information Sciences (ICCOINS), Kuching, Malaysia, 13–15 July 2021; pp. 226–229.
6. Firmansyah, A.; Yani, N.A.; Pontoh, G.T.; Arifuddin, A. Readiness of Micro, Small and Medium Enterprises Using Information Technology (Study in Selayar District). *AFEBI Acc. Rev.* **2022**, *6*, 100. [CrossRef]
7. Kurniati, E.D.; Prajanti, S.D.W. Batik SMEs Efficiency and Entrepreneurship Role in Innovation. *Jejak* **2018**, *11*, 375–389. [CrossRef]
8. Ganzer, P.P.; Chais, C.; Olea, P.M. Product, process, marketing and organizational innovation in industries of the flat knitting sector. *RAI Rev. Adm. Inovação* **2017**, *14*, 321–332. [CrossRef]
9. Charoenrat, T.; Harvie, C. Technical Efficiency of Thai Manufacturing SMEs: A Stochastic Frontier Analysis. *Australas Account. Bus. Financ. J.* **2013**, *16*, 99–121. [CrossRef]
10. Karabulut, A.T. Effects of Innovation Types on Performance of Manufacturing Firms in Turkey. *Proc. Soc. Behav. Sci.* **2015**, *195*, 1355–1364. [CrossRef]
11. Acs, Z.J.; Desai, S.; Hessels, J. Entrepreneurship, Economic Development and Institutions. *Small Bus. Econ.* **2008**, *31*, 219–234. [CrossRef]
12. Papachristodoulou, E.; Koutsaki, M.; Kirkos, E. Journal of Intelligence Studies in Business. *J. Intell. Stud. Bus.* **2017**, *7*, 70–78.

13. Aryani, R.; Widodo, W. The determinant of organizational culture and its impact on organization: A conceptual framework. *Int. J. High. Educ.* **2020**, *9*, 64–70. [CrossRef]
14. Mystakidis, S. Metaverse. *Encyclopedia* **2022**, *2*, 486–497. [CrossRef]
15. Fernando, M.; George, A.S. Metaverse: The Next Stage of Human Culture and the Internet. *Int. J. Adv. Res. Trends Eng. Technol.* **2021**, *8*, 1–10.
16. Soepeno, R. Metaverse: A Potential Threat to Humanity and Ethics. Bachelor's Thesis, Sampoerna University, Jakarta, Indonesia, 2021.
17. Davis, F.D. Perceived Usefulness, Perceived Ease of Use, and User Acceptance of Information Technology. *MIS Q. Manag. Inf. Syst.* **1989**, *13*, 319–339. [CrossRef]
18. Mukerjee, H.S.; Deshmukh, G.K.; Prasad, U.D. Technology Readiness and Likelihood to Use Self-Checkout Services Using Smartphone in Retail Grocery Stores: Empirical Evidences from Hyderabad, India. *Bus. Perspect. Res.* **2019**, *17*, 1–15. [CrossRef]
19. Bayraktaroglu, S. Application of Expanded Technology Acceptance Model for Enhancing the HRIS Usage in SMEs. *Int. J. Appl.* **2019**, *18*, 48–66.
20. Gefen, D.; Straub, D. The Relative Importance of Perceived Ease of Use in IS Adoption: A Study of E-Commerce Adoption. *J. Assoc. Inf. Syst.* **2000**, *1*, 1–30. [CrossRef]
21. Venkatesh, V. A Theoretical Extension of the Technology Acceptance Model: Four Longitudinal Field Studies. *Manag. Sci.* **2002**, *46*, 186–204. [CrossRef]
22. Ajzen, I. The Theory of Planned Behavior. *Organ. Behav. Hum. Decis. Process.* **1991**, *50*, 179–211. [CrossRef]
23. Huang, C.; Chen, T. Moral Norm and the Two-Component Theory of Planned Behavior Model in Predicting Knowledge Sharing Intention: A Role of Mediator Desire. *Psychology* **2015**, *6*, 1685–1699. [CrossRef]
24. Law of the Republic of Indonesia Number 20 of 2008. Available online: https://eng.kppu.go.id/wp-content/uploads/LAW-OF-THE-REPUBLIC-OF-INDONESIA-20-OF-2008.pdf (accessed on 21 December 2022).
25. Alase, A. The Interpretative Phenomenological Analysis (IPA): A Guide to a Good Qualitative Research Approach. *Int. J. Educ. Lit. Stud.* **2017**, *5*, 9. [CrossRef]
26. Agus. Increasing Batik Lasem Sales, Unika Develops Metaverse. Available online: https://www.krjogja.com/berita-lokal/read/471284/tingkatkan-penjualan-batik-lasem-unika-kembangkan-metaverse (accessed on 2 November 2022). (In Indonesian).
27. Holy. Increasing Sales of Rembang Lasem Batik, Unika Soegijapranata Develops Metaverse. Available online: https://kuasakata.com/read/berita/58662-tingkatkan-penjualan-batik-lasem-rembang-unika-soegijapranata-kembangkan-metaverse (accessed on 2 November 2022). (In Indonesian).
28. Luhur, P.A. Exhibit Lasem Batik through Metaverse, Collaboration between Unika Soegijapranata Academics and the Business World. Available online: https://lenterajateng.com/pamerkan-batik-lasem-lewat-metaverse/ (accessed on 2 November 2022). (In Indonesian).
29. Rizqyana, A. Increasing Batik Lasem Sales, Unika Develops Metaverse. Available online: https://jateng.tribunnews.com/2022/09/04/tingkatkan-penjualan-batik-lasem-unika-kembangkan-metaverse (accessed on 2 November 2022). (In Indonesian).
30. Acosta, F.J. The Community in Business: Strategic Relationship between Companies and Environment and Marketing. *Int. J. Psychol. Res.* **2014**, *7*, 8–11. [CrossRef]
31. Hastuti, T.D.; Sanjaya, R.; Koeswoyo, F. The Investment Opportunity, Information Technology and Financial Performance of SMEs. In Proceedings of the International Conference on Computer and Information Sciences (ICCOINS), Kuching, Malaysia, 13–15 July 2021; pp. 247–251.
32. Siregar, D.A.; Nizma, C. Batik Industry Development Strategy in Medan Batik Village. In *Multi-Disciplinary National Seminar on Science*; Abulyatama University: Aceh, Indonesia, 2019; pp. 901–917.
33. Hamidin, A.S.; Pranowo, L.P.A. *Original Indonesian Cultural Heritage Batik*; Narasi: Yogyakarta, Indonesia, 2010. (In Indonesian)
34. Ganyaupfu, E.M. Entrepreneurand Firm Characteristics Affecting Success of Small and Medium Enterprises (SMEs) in Gauteng Province. *Int. J. Innov. Res. Manag.* **2013**, *9*, 1–8.
35. Friedman, A.L.; Miles, S. SMEs and the environment: Evaluating dissemination routes and handholding levels. *Bus. Strateg. Environ.* **2002**, *11*, 324–341. [CrossRef]
36. Banham, H.C. External Environmental Analysis for Small and Medium Enterprises (SMEs). *J. Bus. Econ. Res.* **2010**, *8*, 19–26. [CrossRef]
37. Kumar, A. Business Continuity Plan. *South Asian J. Eng. Technol.* **2020**, *10*, 1–4. [CrossRef]
38. Steelyana, E. Batik, a Beautiful Cultural Heritage that Preserve Culture and Supporteconomic Development in Indonesia. *Binus Bus. Rev.* **2012**, *3*, 116. [CrossRef]
39. Rahayu, M.D. The Development of Chinese Lasem Batik Motifs Descendants of the Year 1900–1960. *Avatara* **2014**, *2*, 36–49. (In Indonesian)
40. Dwikurniarini, D. Acculturation of Traditional Javanese Batik with Chinese. *Informasi* **2013**, *39*, 1–14. (In Indonesian)

41. De Jorge, J.; Suárez, C. Influence of R&D subsidies on efficiency: The case of Spanish manufacturing firms. *Cuad. Econ. Dir. Empres.* **2011**, *14*, 185–193.
42. Esmaeel, R.I.; Zakuan, N.; Jamal, N.M.; Taherdoost, H. Fit manufacturing; Integrated Model of Manufacturing Strategies. *Procedia Manuf.* **2018**, *22*, 975–981. [CrossRef]

applied sciences

MDPI

Article

Creating an Interactive Urban Traffic System for the Simulation of Different Traffic Scenarios

Marco Weißmann *, Dennis Edler, Julian Keil and Frank Dickmann

Geomatics Group, Institute of Geography, Ruhr-University Bochum (RUB), 44801 Bochum, Germany; dennis.edler@rub.de (D.E.); julian.keil@rub.de (J.K.); frank.dickmann@rub.de (F.D.)

* Correspondence: marco.weissmann@rub.de

Abstract: The social and political efforts to fight climate change have contributed to a re-thinking of traffic systems, especially in urban areas under constant transformation. To simulate and visualize planning scenarios of urban traffic systems in a realistic way, the possibilities of virtual 3D environments have regularly been used. The modern potentials of (immersive) virtual reality, however, still require exploration, evaluation, and further development. Using the game engine Unity, an immersive virtual environment was developed to visualize and experience dynamic traffic conditions of a highly dense urban area. The case study is based on the characteristic model of a Central European city (not a representation of a real city), which brings together the specific considerations of urban traffic, such as mirroring the complex interplay of pedestrians as well as individual and public transport. This contribution has an applied methodological focus and considers possibilities as well as difficulties in the design of a reliably running (open-end) traffic system. The applied tool for the creation of a modular and customizable traffic system in Unity resulted in a traffic system that is capable of reacting to the individual behavior of the user (including the individualized motion of the avatar), without leading to accidents or uncorrectable traffic jams. Therefore, the tool used could be a valuable option for any developer of immersive virtual environments in Unity to equip these immersive virtual environments with a traffic system, without the use of additional third-party software.

Keywords: virtual reality; smart mobility; transport geography; human–computer interaction; game engine

Citation: Weißmann, M.; Edler, D.; Keil, J.; Dickmann, F. Creating an Interactive Urban Traffic System for the Simulation of Different Traffic Scenarios. *Appl. Sci.* **2023**, *13*, 6020. https://doi.org/10.3390/app13106020

Academic Editors: Radu Comes, Dorin-Mircea Popovici, Calin Gheorghe Dan Neamtu and Jing-Jing Fang

Received: 12 April 2023
Revised: 10 May 2023
Accepted: 12 May 2023
Published: 13 May 2023

1. Introduction

The ongoing worldwide debates on the consequences of climate change, digitization, and urban migration have led to new political and planning concepts for governing and redesigning cities and their urban systems. An important field of action is inner-city traffic, whose emissions (pollutant emissions and noise) and dynamics have a major impact on the lives of citizens [1–3]. New approaches to transport systems in the future that pursue smart and climate-neutral goals are leading to significant changes in the urban landscape; for example, the replacement of combustion engines with electric motors, the increase in public transport with a decrease in cars at the same time, the increase in bicycle traffic with more bicycle paths, new approaches in unmanned parcel delivery, more charging stations for electric mobility, more greenery at the roadside, etc.

In order to simulate and plan this complex interaction of new approaches in the urban traffic system, modern approaches to visualization in virtual reality (VR) are suitable. VR-based visualizations enable different actors in the planning process to experience the entire construct in an immersive approach. In addition, by assigning rules of motion and behavior to each relevant traffic object, a system can be created (and changed in terms of individual parameters) that simulates the multisensory impact of inner-city traffic.

This article aims to present an example of a transferable VR-based traffic system in the model (typical traffic situation at an intersection) of a Central European city. After a summary of VR-based approaches to urban traffic simulation (Section 2), the core steps and characteristics of a new approach (Section 3) are presented, and the limitations of the approach (Section 4) are discussed. In terms of methodology, the approach presented in this article is based on the current possibilities of the game engine Unity.

2. Virtual Reality in Urban Traffic Simulations

The idea of simulating urban traffic systems, in the sense of "traffic as a simulation of object" [4], has a long tradition and has made regular advances with new technology and methods (see also [5]). Several research efforts have been made to apply technological and methodological innovations to simulate traffic situations, such as CAD and GIS [6–8], parallel computing [9], and 3D modelling [10,11]. With increasing computing power, the number of objects has also increased within virtual traffic models cf. [12–14]. Approaches to the use of virtual reality began to play an increasingly important role in the 2010s (e.g., [15]).

Today, VR technologies are known in geoinformation sciences for the development of immersive environments and have so far only been used sporadically for traffic simulation. To bring together traffic planning and the design of sustainable urban spaces, bike simulators that facilitate immersive VR have recently been developed [16–18]. With respect to inner-city automobile traffic, few studies are available to date that address specific components of VR-based simulations.

Edler et al. [19] discussed approaches to the dynamic visualization of 3D sound for VR-based road traffic simulations. Beyond the visualization of urban soundscape ecology, Wu et al. [20] used 3D sound in immersive VR to study pedestrian decisions in intersection situations. Using deep learning approaches, Kalatian and Farooq [21] attempted to analyze pedestrian and vehicle interactions in immersive VR. Currently, research on the technical development of interacting transportation systems in immersive VR is scarce. This study follows up on this by presenting an approach to an interacting traffic system in immersive VR.

When it comes to traffic simulations within the game engine Unity, which became free to use in 2015 for personal users, there is a lack of publications dealing with the creation of transport systems from a non-expert developer perspective. Rundel and De Amicis [22] created a workflow based on a combination of different proprietary and freely available stand-alone software to implement a traffic system into the game engine Unity. The use of proprietary software in this workflow might be a hurdle for developers who want to benefit from freely available software such as Unity and also implement a traffic system without the use of additional third-party software. Liao et al. [23] used the freely available traffic simulation software SUMO to implement traffic into Unity, but focused on the analysis than the implementation and visualization of the traffic system. Chen and De Luca [24] used a visual programming language to simulate random traffic and autonomous driving.

Thus, in this paper, the proposed method provides a cost-effective solution to allow developers of immersive virtual environments without a technical background in traffic simulation to quickly add traffic to their immersive virtual environments in Unity, without the need to learn and use additional third-party (proprietary) software.

3. New Approach to Urban Traffic Simulation in (Immersive) VR

For the development and creation of a 3D environment in the form of an exemplary inner-city intersection situation, the game engine Unity was used in this study. The future purpose of this 3D environment is to use it in geography classes to familiarize students with possible sustainable urban development concepts. The creation of additional 3D objects was realized using the Blender software. Unity provides developers with the ability to contribute their own 3D models and compatible software to the game engine using the Unity Asset Store. The development and implementation of an urban traffic system were performed using the "Simple Traffic System" asset, available in the Unity Asset Store by the developer TurnTheGameOn. This asset offers the possibility to build a modular traffic system with the help of a dedicated editor.

Locomotion in the virtual environment took place through a keyboard and mouse controllable first-person avatar. The application was released as Web Graphics Library (WebGL), which creates the possibility to run and use the application in a web browser. The 3D environment was additionally developed to be experienced with a head-mounted display and controller using teleportation as the type of locomotion. The implementation was performed using SteamVR, and the virtual reality application was released as a Windows standalone.

The initial point for the development of an urban traffic situation inside an immersive virtual environment was the idea of an intersection situation that can be found within the traffic network of a Central European city. The representation of the city in the virtual environment itself is not built on any real existing urban environment. It is considered a representative model. The intersection situation consists of a main road with four motorized traffic lanes and one lane for a tram. In addition, there are two side streets for motorized traffic (Figure 1). Around the streets, the environment is modelled with buildings (perimeter block development). The focus of transportation planning for the road network is on motorized traffic.

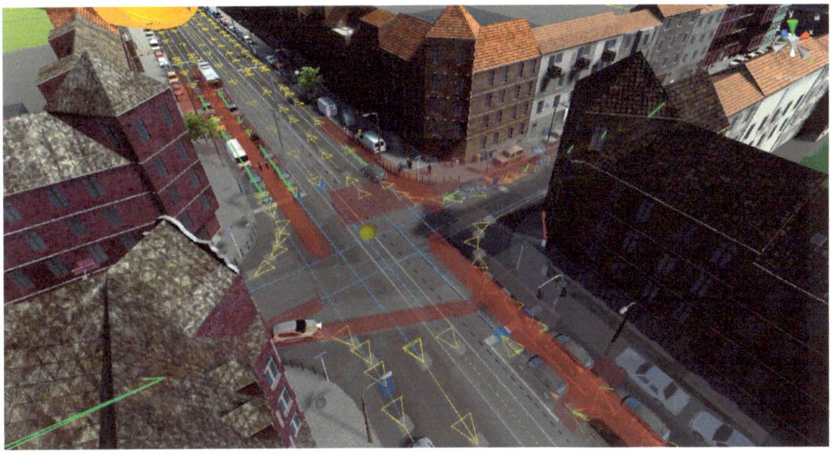

Figure 1. The inner-city intersection situation. The yellow arrows represent the driving direction of the waypoint routes, while the green lines represent the next waypoint of a vehicle on a route that will be approached.

3.1. *Requirements for Object Interaction in the Traffic System*

The preconditions of the possible interactions to be applied in the transport system should be defined in advance of development. The implementation of the simulated virtual motorized traffic was performed after the virtual environment was created. The traffic system consists of vehicles, traffic lights, the traffic network (represented by interconnected waypoint routes), and an avatar that interacts with each other. The interaction between the vehicles should take place in such a way that no accidents occur. This means that vehicles should recognize other vehicles and also initiate the braking process when the vehicle in front of them brakes. In addition, the vehicles should be able to interact with the traffic light system. The traffic light system component is expected to ensure that vehicles react in accordance with the current traffic light circuit. Since the virtual environment can be experienced through a first-person avatar and, accordingly, the road can be walked on, the vehicles should interact with the avatar in such a way that the avatar is not run over by vehicles. This requires that the traffic system is able to react to individual user motion represented by the avatar. For example, the vehicles must be able to recognize an avatar when it is too close to them in order to stop and avoid accidents. After the actions take place based on the avatar's position, the traffic has to continue without producing uncorrectable traffic problems (accidents, traffic jams at the intersection, and obstruction of the traffic routes of trams or cyclists). The traffic system in its entirety should run in a loop without interruptions (open-end). Therefore, it was defined that the traffic lights have a fixed continuous running circuit, which cannot be altered by the actions of the avatar.

The walkability of the virtual environment by the avatar is limited to the area of the intersection situation. Moving further is restricted by an invisible wall with a collider attached to it. When the avatar is navigated into the inaccessible area, the limit of the freely explorable environment becomes visible through an impenetrable red transparent wall, and an acoustic signal is then played. The walkable virtual environment is shown in Figure 2. The figure indicates that the road network goes beyond the walkable area for the avatar. The interaction features for the educational learning tasks, which are connected to interactable 3D objects, can be found in the area accessible to the avatar. Vehicles are loaded from areas that are not accessible and visible to the avatar. When the player is looking towards the areas that are not accessible, the impression is simulated that the environment is larger than it really is. For example, a train runs along the end of the main street. This is to give the impression that the virtual environment and the traffic is not limited to the intersection.

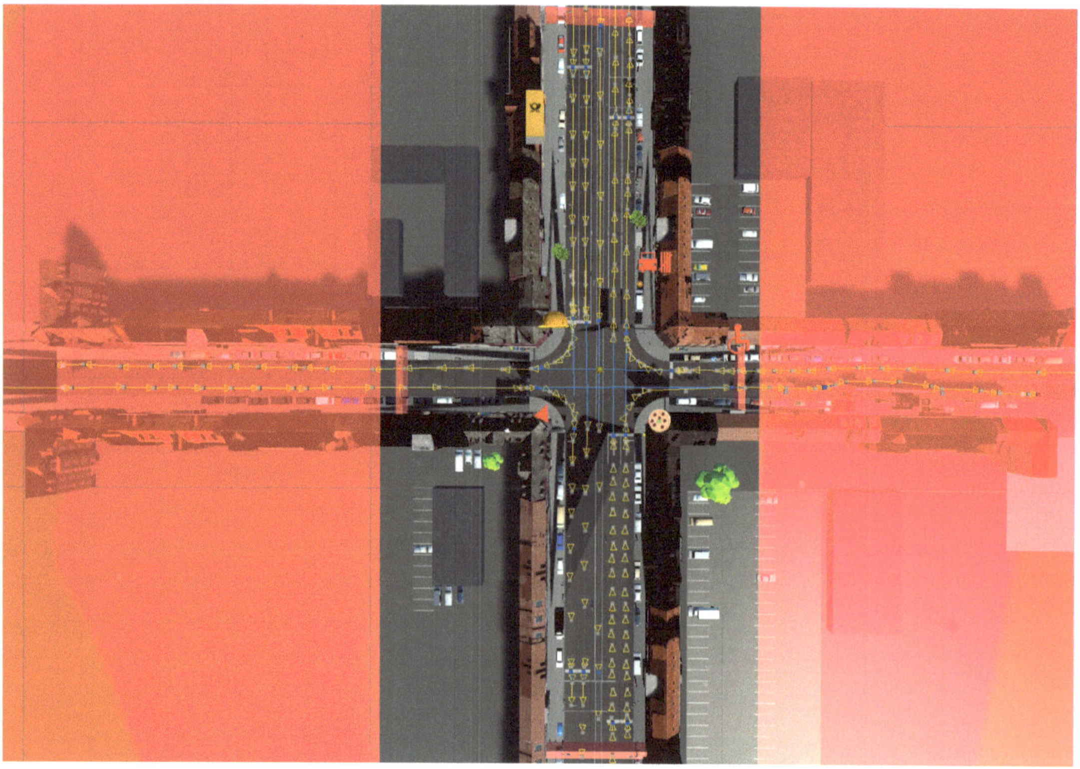

Figure 2. Limits of the explorable area of the crossing situation indicated in the development environment.

3.2. Creating a Road Network, Road Waypoints, and a Waypoint Route

As the basis of the road network, it is necessary to equip the 3D-modelled roads of the virtual environment with waypoints. These waypoints represent the traffic network on which the vehicles should drive. For the creation of waypoint routes, the asset offers a dedicated editor. First, an AITrafficController is loaded into the unity scene using the editor button. This AITrafficController controls the other components of the traffic system. Then, using the AITrafficWaypointRoute button of the user interface, a waypoint route is loaded into the unity scene. Each waypoint route consists of at least two connected waypoints. The waypoints are manually inserted into the environment. The first waypoint is the start point and the last waypoint is the endpoint of a road in the traffic system, as shown in red in Figure 3. In order to connect different waypoint routes, the asset provides a configuration mode that allows connecting the endpoints of one waypoint route to the starting point of another.

Figure 3. An individual waypoint route consisting of multiple waypoints can be implemented in virtual environments, which serve as the basic construct of the traffic system. (The yellow arrows indicate the direction of travel).

On every waypoint, the speed of the vehicles driving on the route from that waypoint to the next waypoint can be set via the script settings in Unity. To create a waypoint in the virtual environment, a so-called AITrafficController is loaded into the Unity scene via the tool window, which controls the movement of the cars along the created routes. After that, an AITrafficWaypointRoute has to be loaded via the tool window. It contains an array of waypoints that can be created by holding down the shift key and clicking the left mouse button. It is possible to create individual waypoints for waypoint routes manually.

Since the vehicles are to be loaded onto the waypoint routes outside the visibility range of the avatar, multiple connected waypoint routes were created for this purpose. Since the accessibility of the virtual environment by the avatar was limited to the intersection, the traffic system was not interconnected by several connected waypoint routes. Vehicles were loaded into the traffic system through those waypoint routes that were pointing towards the intersection. When the vehicles reached the end of the waypoint routes, they were loaded back to their starting waypoint route and drove the route using the predefined path.

3.3. Traffic Lights

As a next step, the traffic lights are integrated into the virtual environment in the waypoint network that has been created so far (Figure 4). Once a waypoint route is implemented into the unity scene, it is possible to connect traffic lights to them via the dedicated editor window. For this purpose, an AITrafficLightManager is loaded into the scene that consists of a Unity Game Object called AITrafficLight. The Game Object AITrafficLight contains three separate objects that represent the traffic light colors red, yellow, and green as a mesh. Using the edit function of the tool window, the AITrafficLight is connected to the endpoints of a waypoint route. These endpoints serve as stopping points at which the vehicles stop when the traffic light phase displays red or yellow. In the settings of the AITrafficManager, the time in seconds for the red, yellow, and green phases can be set for each created AITrafficLight. In addition, traffic light cycles can be set according to the sequence in which the respective pairs of traffic lights execute their traffic light phase. Once the traffic light circuit and the sequential order of the traffic lights have been set, the traffic lights run open-end when the application is started.

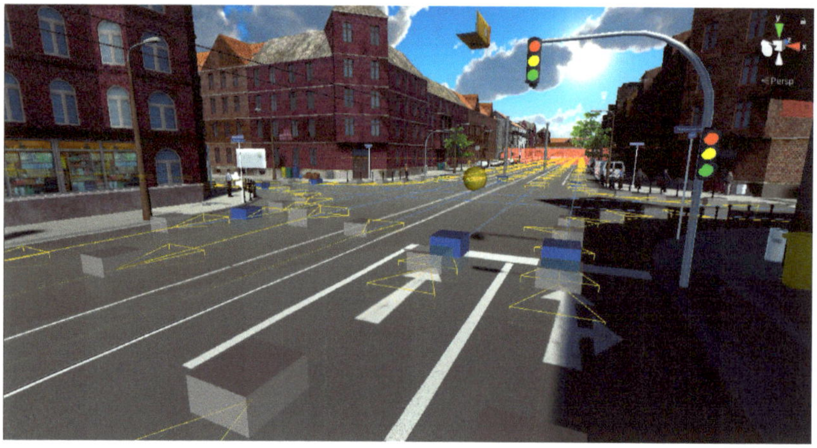

Figure 4. Traffic light meshes attached to a 3D model of a traffic light VR intersection situation.

3.4. Vehicles

After the waypoints have been connected to the traffic lights, the vehicles are loaded into the waypoint routes where the vehicles are to appear and travel accordingly along the predefined route. Vehicles are the components in the traffic system that move along the predefined waypoints of the waypoint routes, waypoint by waypoint, and are reloaded to their original waypoint route when the vehicles reach the last waypoint. Thus, the vehicles consist of a modelled body and tires, which are equipped with Unity's own wheel colliders. In order to detect obstacles (vehicles or avatars) when driving along the waypoints of the interconnected waypoint routes and to stop accordingly after detecting them, the vehicles are equipped with three colliders. Two are located on the left and right sides of the vehicle and one is in front of the vehicle.

To integrate the vehicles into the already built traffic system, the 3D models of the vehicles are connected to a waypoint route for this purpose. In order to implement them, the waypoint routes have an array of Unity Game Objects attached to them, into which the vehicle models can be loaded via drag and drop.

4. Discussion: Technical Limitations and Solutions

Theoretically, the implementation and connection of the individual components of the asset should result in a functional urban traffic system that runs open-end without errors. However, issues have occurred in the development process of the traffic system that occasionally brought it to a complete breakdown, as shown for example in Figure 5. In this particular case, traffic accidents occurred in the areas of the starting waypoint routes used to load vehicles. This error occurred when two vehicles took different routes on turning points but reached the endpoints of the different waypoint routes at the same time, which also caused them to be loaded to their starting waypoint route at the same time. The cause of this error was that the vehicles were loaded to their starting waypoint routes at the same time. This caused these vehicles to collide with each other, fall over and become unable to drive, leading to a blockage of the road, which prevented other vehicles from continuing their route, since these crashed vehicles were recognized as obstacles. This highly relevant issue counteracting the idea of an open-end loop could not be handled by the opportunities of the asset itself. It required the customized implementation of an adjustment.

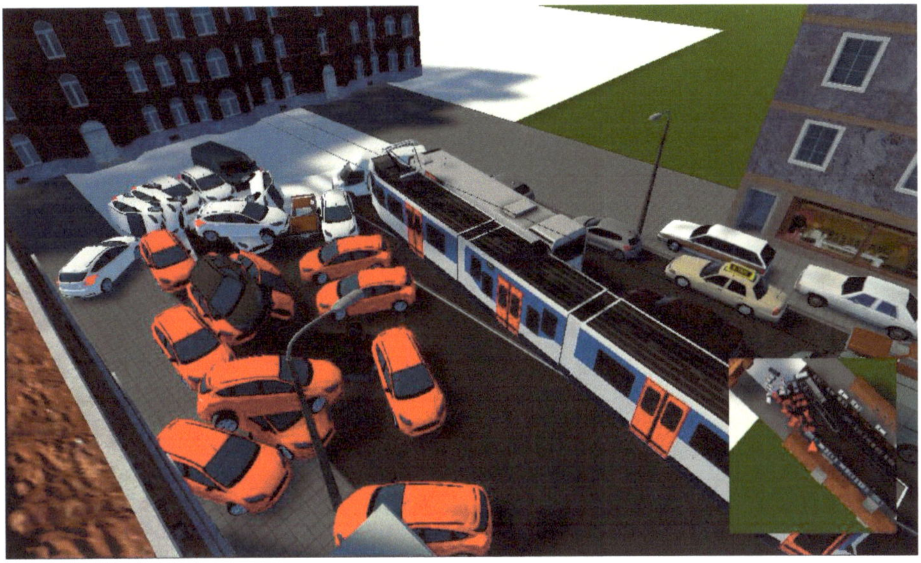

Figure 5. Traffic accident triggered by simultaneous loading of vehicles onto the waypoint route.

To solve this issue, a collider was placed in the location of the waypoint routes used to load the vehicles. Additionally, blockades were placed at the ends of the waypoints. The collider at the loading waypoint routes is used to check whether there are currently any vehicles in the waypoint route area. If this is the case, the deployed collider at the end waypoint routes is activated and prevents vehicles from reaching the endpoint and being loaded to the starting point of their waypoint route. Other solutions to this error, such as disabling the vehicle colliders while on the starting waypoint route, are imaginable.

Another issue is that by actively moving the avatar into the interaction through the user, a gridlock of the traffic system can be triggered because the avatar is set to be recognized by the vehicles as an obstacle and ensures that the vehicles stop. If the avatar is placed within the intersection in such a way that the vehicles stop and block each other, since the avatar is detected as an obstacle, this leads to a traffic gridlock situation as shown in Figure 6. Such a traffic gridlock would not resolve itself and would persist until the application is restarted.

To resolve such gridlocks caused by irrational user behavior, vehicles that have not moved for a fixed time period are loaded back to their starting waypoint routes and disappear from their current position in the environment. The waiting time has been set longer than the stop time of the traffic light phase so that the vehicles waiting at the traffic lights are not mistakenly loaded to their starting waypoint routes. Considering that the vehicles disappear from the environment after the waiting time has expired, it could lead to a negative impact on the user's immersion if the disappearance is perceived.

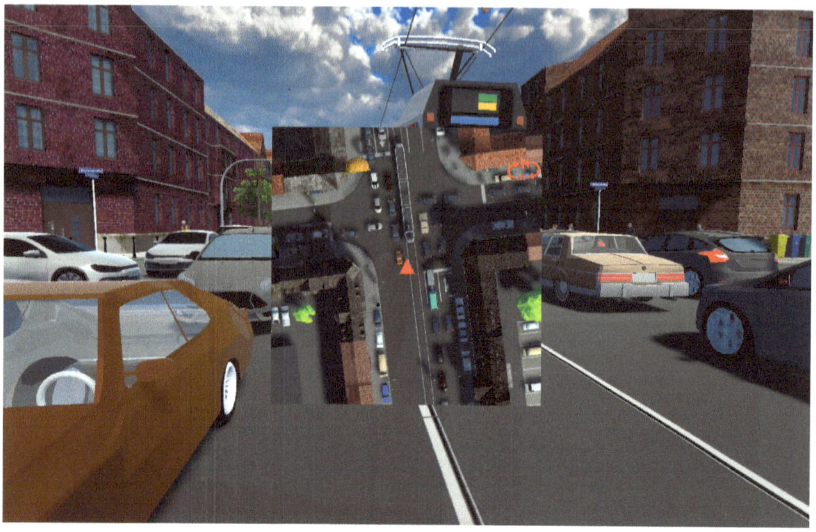

Figure 6. Traffic gridlock triggered by the user through the avatar displayed on the mini-map as a red arrow.

There could be other difficulties in implementing a transportation system that is not encountered in the application example presented here. The traffic system implemented here did not consist of a closed system of waypoint routes, since the area of the virtual environment was limited to the intersection. Especially in the case of a further developed, more complex, and closed traffic network with more traffic volume, further sources of error and difficulties would be imaginable. Further developments in traffic systems should deal with the irrational behavior of users in order to avoid errors triggered by irrational behavior. In addition, studies are needed to identify the key factors of accidents and errors in traffic simulations as has been carried out by Liu et al. [25], who elaborated on the key factors of the severity of traffic accidents between automobiles and two-wheelers.

Despite the errors and the described limitations of the traffic system, the implementation into the already existing virtual environment in Unity is user-friendly due to the modular structure of the individual components and the user interface. Developers who value and prefer a fast and user-friendly implementation of a traffic system with a focus on traffic visualization could benefit from this tool without relying on other additional software. Due to the availability of the source code, adaptations by developers who want to go beyond the sole purpose of traffic visualization and extend the tool for analytical application purposes are conceivable.

5. Summary

The simulation of traffic systems in virtual environments has been a topic attracting a multidisciplinary research community for decades [4,18]. With new political and planning concepts for urban transformation, as well as with the increasing computational power and software solutions, [13,14], the complexity and applications of traffic simulations have increased.

The current opportunities for developing realistic, immersive, and intelligent VR-based traffic systems in Game Engines provide a new dimension of interaction. Individual motion paths of the user's 'virtual ego' (avatar) require a permanent interaction and reaction of other animated objects within the system. This leads to an individual chain of follow-up reactions. To avoid a collapse of the permanent loop of the traffic system, rules must be defined in the development phase that guarantee a running system and do not restrict the freedom of user motion and the perception of a realistic scenario. The present study uses the opportunities of the asset "Simple Traffic System" and added individual solutions to guarantee such criteria.

With the presented asset, it was possible to equip the virtual environment created in Unity with a traffic system consisting of a waypoint network, traffic light circuits, and the associated vehicles. The interface simplicity of the tool makes it convenient to extend existing static virtual environments with traffic. However, it should be noted that currently, it is only possible to manually create the traffic network with its routes based on waypoints.

The automated creation of the waypoints based on an existing modelled road network or its representation in the form of geospatial data is, therefore, not possible. This circumstance could complicate the implementation of complex city models that have already been created. For example, for 3D city models that were automatically created in Unity based on OpenStreetMap (OSM) and CityGML data [26], developing an automated implementation of the traffic network based on the OSM data could be equipped with the components of the presented asset and could animate the static urban environment with traffic.

It should also be noted that the tool in its current state can only be used to simulate traffic. Virtual tools for analyzing specific traffic parameters, such as volume, pollutant emissions, and noise, have not yet been implemented. Due to the availability of the source code, it is conceivable to develop the asset further and to use it for other tasks that are not only limited to the simulation of traffic.

6. Outlook: The Application in Geography School Education

A highly relevant field for VR applications is education cf. [27–30]. The presented application has the potential to be implemented in geography education. Together with geography teachers and researchers in the field of didactics, the running traffic system is currently being developed to share knowledge about urban development and smart cities. The traffic system will have different traffic components in the future state of modern cities, which will allow a comparison with the present state. This builds a foundation for geographical discussion in the educational context of secondary schools. The first testing and evaluation of the application was conducted (Figure 7) and organized by the Ministry of Education, North Rhine-Westphalia, Germany. The traffic model also has the potential to be used as a standardized urban scene for laboratory studies focused on the impact of urban traffic transformation on the physiological responses of citizens [31].

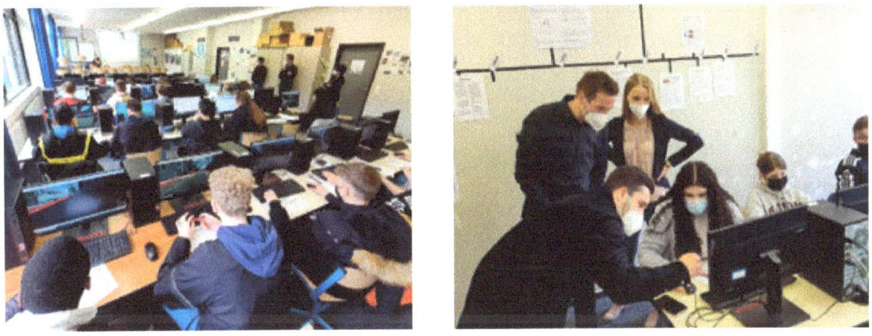

Figure 7. Evaluating the VR traffic simulation at school: learning smart mobility scenarios in geography classes.

Author Contributions: Conceptualization, M.W., D.E. and F.D.; methodology, M.W., D.E., F.D. and J.K.; software, M.W.; validation, M.W., D.E., J.K. and F.D.; formal analysis, M.W., D.E., J.K. and F.D.; investigation, M.W., D.E., J.K. and F.D.; resources, M.W., D.E., J.K. and F.D.; data curation, M.W., D.E., J.K. and F.D.; writing—original draft preparation, M.W. and D.E.; writing—review and editing, M.W. and D.E.; visualization, M.W.; supervision, F.D. and D.E.; project administration, M.W.; funding acquisition, D.E. and F.D. All authors have read and agreed to the published version of the manuscript.

Funding: This research was funded by Ministry of Education North Rhine-Westfalia: Az 412-5.01.02.03-154677.

Institutional Review Board Statement: Not applicable.

Informed Consent Statement: Not applicable.

Data Availability Statement: Not applicable.

Acknowledgments: This contribution is part of the project "On a virtual exploration in the smart city: development of VR-based, model-based urban development scenarios for interaction in geography school education" (2021–2024). The project is funded by the Ministry of Education, North Rhine-Westphalia (Az 412-5.01.02.03-154677). Based on the solar power plant installed in the Cartography Lab at the Ruhr-University Bochum (RUB), this research was conducted using solar power. The authors have no competing interests to declare that are relevant to the content of this article.

Conflicts of Interest: The authors declare no conflict of interest.

References

1. Beben, D.; Maleska, T.; Bobra, P.; Duda, J.; Anigacz, W. Influence of traffic-induced vibrations on humans and residential building—A case study. *Int. J. Environ. Res. Public Health* **2022**, *19*, 5441. [CrossRef]
2. Jacyna, M.; Wasiak, M.; Lewczuk, K.; Karoń, G. Noise and environmental pollution from transport: Decisive problems in developing ecologically efficient transport systems. *J. Vibroeng.* **2017**, *19*, 5639–5655. [CrossRef]
3. Morillas, J.M.B.; Gozalo, G.R.; González, D.M.; Moraga, P.A.; Vílchez-Gómez, R. Noise pollution and urban planning. *Curr. Pollut. Rep.* **2018**, *4*, 208–219. [CrossRef]
4. Pursula, M. Simulation of traffic systems—An overview. *J. Geogr. Inf. Decis. Anal.* **1999**, *3*, 1–8. Available online: https://publish.uwo.ca/~jmalczew/gida_5/Pursula/Pursula.html (accessed on 11 April 2023).
5. Qiao, F.; Liu, T.; Sun, H.; Guo, L.; Chen, Y. Modelling and simulation of urban traffic systems: Present and future. *Int. J. Cybern. CyberPhysical Syst.* **2021**, *1*, 1–32. [CrossRef]
6. Despine, G.; Baillard, C. Realistic road modelling for driving simulators using GIS data. In *Advances in Cartography and GIScience. Volume 2*; Ruas, A., Ed.; Lecture Notes in Geoinformation and Cartography; Springer: Berlin/Heidelberg, Germany, 2011; Volume 6, pp. 431–448. ISBN 978-3-642-19213-5.
7. Etches, A.; Claramunt, C.; Bargiela, A.; Kosonen, I. An integrated temporal GIS for model traffic systems. *GIS Res. UK VI Natl. Conf.* **1998**, 1–12. Available online: https://www.researchgate.net/publication/266527833_An_Integrated_Temporal_GIS_Model_for_Traffic_Systems (accessed on 11 April 2023).
8. Thériault, M.; Vandersmissen, M.H.; Lee-Gosselin, M.; Leroux, D. Modeling commuter trip length and duration within GIS: Application to an O-D survey. *J. Geogr. Inf. Decis. Anal.* **1999**, *3*, 41–55. Available online: https://www.researchgate.net/publication/228944562_Modelling_commuter_trip_length_and_duration_within_GIS_Application_to_an_OD_survey (accessed on 11 April 2023).
9. Nagel, K.; Schleicher, A. Microscopic traffic modeling on parallel high performance computers. *Parallel Comput.* **1994**, *20*, 125–146. [CrossRef]
10. Ambroz, M.; Krasna, S.; Prebil, I. 3D road traffic situation simulation system. *Adv. Eng. Softw.* **2005**, *36*, 77–86. [CrossRef]
11. Deng, Y.; Cheng, J.C.P.; Anumba, C. A framework for 3D traffic noise mapping using data from BIM and GIS integration. *Struct. Infrastruct. Eng.* **2016**, *12*, 1267–1280. [CrossRef]
12. Wang, C.; Chen, G.; Liu, Y.; Horne, M. Virtual-reality based integrated traffic simulation for urban planning. In Proceedings of the 2008 International Conference on Computer Science and Software Engineering, Wuhan, China, 12–14 December 2008; IEEE: New York, NY, USA, 2008; pp. 1137–1140. [CrossRef]
13. Chao, Q.; Deng, Z.; Ren, J.; Ye, Q.; Jin, X. Realistic data-driven traffic flow animation using texture synthesis. *IEEE Trans. Visual. Comput. Graph.* **2018**, *24*, 1167–1178. [CrossRef]
14. Yang, X.; Su, W.; Deng, J.; Jin, X.; Tan, G.; Pan, Z. Real-virtual fusion model for traffic animation: Real-virtual fusion model for traffic animation. *Comput. Anim. Virtual Worlds* **2017**, *28*, e1740. [CrossRef]
15. Yu, Y.; El Kamel, A.; Gong, G.; Li, F. Multi-agent based modeling and simulation of microscopic traffic in virtual reality system. *Simul. Model. Pract. Theory* **2014**, *45*, 62–79. [CrossRef]
16. Matviienko, A.; Müller, F.; Zickler, M.; Gasche, L.A.; Abels, J.; Steinert, T.; Mühlhäuser, M. Reducing virtual reality sickness for cyclists in VR bicycle simulators. In Proceedings of the CHI Conference on Human Factors in Computing Systems, New Orleans, LA, USA, 29 April–5 May 2022; ACM: New York, NY, USA, 2022; pp. 1–14. [CrossRef]
17. Ullmann, D.; Kreimeier, J.; Götzelmann, T.; Kipke, H. BikeVR: A virtual reality bicycle simulator towards sustainable urban space and traffic planning. In Proceedings of the Mensch und Computer 2020, Magdeburg, Germany, 6–9 September 2020; Tagungsband. Alt, F., Schneegass, S., Hornecker, E., Eds.; ACM: New York, NY, USA, 2020; pp. 511–514.

18. Zeuwts, L.H.R.H.; Vanhuele, R.; Vansteenkiste, P.; Deconinck, F.J.A.; Lenoir, M. Using an immersive virtual reality bicycle simulator to evaluate hazard detection and anticipation of overt and covert traffic situations in young bicyclists. *Virtual Real.* **2023**, 1–21. [CrossRef]
19. Edler, D.; Kühne, O.; Keil, J.; Dickmann, F. Audiovisual cartography: Established and new multimedia approaches to represent soundscapes. *KN J. Cartogr. Geogr. Inf.* **2019**, *69*, 5–17. [CrossRef]
20. Wu, H.; Ashmead, D.H.; Adams, H.; Bodenheimer, B. Using virtual reality to assess the street crossing behavior of pedes-trians with simulated macular degeneration at a roundabout. *Front. ICT* **2018**, *5*, 27. [CrossRef]
21. Kalatian, A.; Farooq, B. Decoding pedestrian and automated vehicle interactions using immersive virtual reality and interpretable deep learning. *Transp. Res. Part C Emerg. Technol.* **2021**, *124*, 102962. [CrossRef]
22. Rundel, S.; De Amicis, R. Leveraging digital twin and game-engine for traffic simulations and visualizations. *Front. Virtual Real.* **2023**, *4*, 1048753. [CrossRef]
23. Liao, X.; Zhao, X.; Wang, Z.; Han, K.; Tiwari, P.; Barth, M.J.; Wu, G. Game theory-based ramp merging for mixed traffic with unity-SUMO co-simulation. *IEEE Trans. Syst. Man Cybern. Syst.* **2022**, *52*, 5746–5757. [CrossRef]
24. Chen, Y.; De Luca, G. Traffic simulation and autonomous driving experiment in VIPLE. In Proceedings of the 5th International Symposium for Intelligent Transportation and Smart City (ITASC), Virtual, 20–21 May 2022; Zeng, X., Xie, X., Sun, J., Ma, L., Chen, Y., Eds.; Lecture Notes in Electrical Engineering. Springer Nature: Singapore, 2023; Volume 1042, pp. 1–13, ISBN 978-981-9922-51-2.
25. Liu, L.; Ye, X.; Wang, T.; Yan, X.; Chen, J.; Ran, B. Key factors analysis of severity of automobile to two-wheeler traffic accidents based on Bayesian network. *Int. J. Environ. Res. Public Health* **2022**, *19*, 6013. [CrossRef]
26. Keil, J.; Edler, D.; Schmitt, T.; Dickmann, F. Creating immersive virtual environments based on open geospatial data and game engines. *KN J. Cartogr. Geogr. Inf.* **2021**, *71*, 53–65. [CrossRef]
27. Edler, D.; Keil, J.; Wiedenlübbert, T.; Sossna, M.; Kühne, O.; Dickmann, F. Immersive VR experience of redeveloped post-industrial sites: The example of "Zeche Holland" in Bochum-Wattenscheid. *KN J. Cartogr. Geogr. Inf.* **2019**, *69*, 267–284. [CrossRef]
28. Klippel, A.; Zhao, J.; Jackson, K.L.; La Femina, P.; Stubbs, C.; Wetzel, R.; Blair, J.; Wallgrün, J.O.; Oprean, D. Transforming earth science education through immersive experiences: Delivering on a long held promise. *J. Educ. Comput. Res.* **2019**, *57*, 1745–1771. [CrossRef]
29. Lindner, C.; Ortwein, A.; Staar, K.; Rienow, A. Different levels of complexity for integrating textured extra-terrestrial elevation data in game engines for educational augmented and virtual reality applications. *KN J. Cartogr. Geogr. Inf.* **2021**, *71*, 253–267. [CrossRef]
30. Prisille, C.; Ellerbrake, M. Virtual Reality (VR) and geography education: Potentials of 360° 'experiences' in secondary schools. In *Modern Approaches to the Visualization of Landscapes*; Edler, D., Jenal, C., Kühne, O., Eds.; RaumFragen: Stadt–Region–Landschaft; Springer Fachmedien Wiesbaden: Wiesbaden, Germany, 2020; pp. 321–332, ISBN 978-3-658-30955-8.
31. Keil, J.; Weißmann, M.; Korte, A.; Edler, D.; Dickmann, F. Measuring physiological responses to visualizations of urban planning scenarios in immersive virtual reality. *KN J. Cartogr. Geogr. Inf.* **2023**, 1–10. [CrossRef]

sensors

MDPI

Article

A Physical Fatigue Evaluation Method for Automotive Manual Assembly: An Experiment of Cerebral Oxygenation with ARE Platform

Wanting Mao [1], Xiaonan Yang [2,3,4,*], Chaoran Wang [2], Yaoguang Hu [2] and Tianxin Gao [5]

1 Department of Civil and Environmental Engineering, Imperial College London, London SW7 2AZ, UK; w.mao23@imperial.ac.uk
2 School of Mechanical Engineering, Beijing Institute of Technology, Beijing 100081, China; chaoranwang@bit.edu.cn (C.W.); hyg@bit.edu.cn (Y.H.)
3 Key Laboratory of Industry Knowledge & Data Fusion Technology and Application, Ministry of Industry and Information Technology, Beijing Institute of Technology, Beijing 100081, China
4 Yangtze Delta Region Academy, Beijing Institute of Technology, Jiaxing 314019, China
5 School of Life Science, Beijing Institute of Technology, Beijing 100081, China; gtx@bit.edu.cn
* Correspondence: yangxn@bit.edu.cn

Abstract: Due to the complexity of the automobile manufacturing process, some flexible and delicate assembly work relies on manual operations. However, high-frequency and high-load repetitive operations make assembly workers prone to physical fatigue. This study proposes a method for evaluating human physical fatigue for the manual assembly of automobiles with methods: NIOSH (National Institute for Occupational Safety and Health), OWAS (Ovako Working Posture Analysis System) and RULA (Rapid Upper Limb Assessment). The cerebral oxygenation signal is selected as an objective physiological index reflecting the human fatigue level to verify the proposed physical fatigue evaluation method. Taking auto seat assembly and automobile manual assembly as an example, 18 group experiments were carried out with the ARE platform (Augmented Reality-based Ergonomic Platform). Furthermore, predictions of metabolic energy expenditure were performed for experiments in Tecnomatix Jack. Finally, it is concluded that the proposed physical fatigue evaluation method can reflect the human physical fatigue level and is more accurate than the evaluation of metabolic energy consumption in Tecnomatix Jack because of the immersion that comes with the AR devices and the precision that comes with motion capture devices.

Keywords: physical fatigue; automotive manual assembly; cerebral oxygenation; metabolic energy consumption

Citation: Mao, W.; Yang, X.; Wang, C.; Hu, Y.; Gao, T. A Physical Fatigue Evaluation Method for Automotive Manual Assembly: An Experiment of Cerebral Oxygenation with ARE Platform. *Sensors* **2023**, *23*, 9410. https://doi.org/10.3390/s23239410

Academic Editor: Stefano Berretti

Received: 16 September 2023
Revised: 27 October 2023
Accepted: 22 November 2023
Published: 26 November 2023

1. Introduction

Assembly and manufacturing processes usually involve a mass of flexible and elaborate manual operations performed by human operators working in the workshop. Especially in the automotive assembly industry, there is much assembly work that is done manually by workers, and these assembly tasks, including lifting, handling, and installation, are usually characterized by high frequency and high load [1]. Long hours of high workload can easily lead to worker fatigue, physical strength decline, and even cause injury and disease [2]. Workers in a fatigued state easily have low efficiency and more operational errors, which would have a negative impact on both company revenue and workers' physical health [3]. These problems can only be avoided if ergonomics are properly applied so that workers are able to perform assembly work within their physical capabilities. Therefore, accuracy in evaluating workers' fatigue is very crucial [4].

Energy expenditure is an important factor in physical fatigue because muscle contraction during exercise uses up stored energy in the body [5,6]. When people are in a state of fatigue, the internal catabolism and anabolism of the body are difficult to maintain in balance, causing muscle contractions to become weak, inhibiting the central nervous system, and finally exhausting the whole body [7]. By decomposing assembly movements, acquiring movement parameters, and calculating human fatigue assessment based on energy consumption, the fatigue level of workers performing assembly work can be assessed [8]. Tecnomatix Jack 8.0 is a human modeling and simulation software developed by Siemens Digital Industries Software (The company is headquartered in Plano, TX, USA), that is a powerful tool for human-centric design and ergonomic analysis. It aids in creating work environments that are not only efficient and productive, but also considerate of human factors to enhance safety and well-being. However, the traditional energy-based physical fatigue assessment, such as Tecnomatix Jack, has disadvantages, such as the influence of individual differences and the influence of external environmental factors, so it cannot assess human fatigue more accurately [9]. Especially for the prediction of energy expenditure in Tecnomatix Jack, its prediction accuracy cannot reach a high level due to limitations in model accuracy, assumptions about static environments, insufficient individual differences, and inaccurate modeling of complex actions, [10,11].

The brain is a highly energy-consuming organ, consuming 20% of the body's energy at about 2% of the body's weight, and can be irreversibly damaged by brief periods of hypoxic conditions [12]. The rapid consumption of energy by the brain during exercise can lead to changes in cerebral oxygen saturation, thus cerebral oxygen saturation can be used to evaluate physical fatigue [13,14]. Cerebral oxygen saturation is usually measured by near-infrared spectroscopy (NIRS). NIRS cerebral oxygen saturation monitoring quantifies the relative concentrations of oxyhemoglobin and deoxyhemoglobin within a target tissue by relying on the transmission and absorption of near-infrared light through the tissue, allowing for an estimate of the balance between cerebral oxygen supply and demand [13]. Matsuura et al. studied changes in brain and muscle oxygenation in humans during static and dynamic knee extension to voluntary fatigue, and used cerebral oxygen during exercise to assess the level of cerebral reoxygenation and thus the degree of fatigue [15]. Monroe et al. explored the changes in fatigue level and cerebral oxygenation produced by exercise at different intensities, and used cerebral oxygenation to explain the changes in fatigue and energy during exercise recovery [16]. Hiura et al. analyzed cerebral oxygenation in rowing athletes, which varied at different exercise intensities and fatigue levels, thus assessing the level of fatigue [17].

This paper conducted a field investigation and in-depth research on a well-known Chinese auto manufacturer. In order to improve the accuracy of physical fatigue evaluation, considering the different action characteristics in the manual assembly process, the process in the automobile manual assembly line is divided into three stages: the lifting stage (Figure 1a,b), the carrying stage (Figure 1c), and the static stage (Figure 1d). The lifting stage mainly refers to the workers lifting the car doors, tires, seats, and other auto parts from the designated area; then workers carry these pre-assembled parts to the front of the auto body; finally, in this stage, workers need to bend over to operate, their torsos are static and only hands are performing fine operations, so this stage is called the static stage.

The main goal of this paper is to study a physical fatigue evaluation method for automobile manual assembly. This method combines the action characteristics of different stages in manual assembly, objective experimental data, and the characteristics of fatigue accumulation over time. It pays more attention to the dynamic behavior of workers and makes a more comprehensive and accurate physical fatigue evaluation of procedural behavior. To achieve this, we address the following issues:

- Can brain oxygen saturation represent the degree of fatigue in the human body?
- Do different carrying weights and attitude holding heights affect the degree of fatigue?
- Which of the fatigue evaluation methods proposed in this paper and energy expenditure in Tecnomatix Jack can better reflect fatigue?

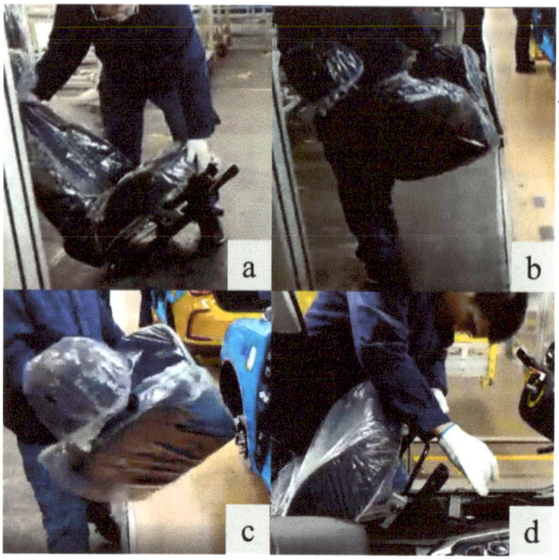

Figure 1. Car seat assembly process in a famous Chinese auto manufacturer: (**a**) Lifting start; (**b**) Lifting end; (**c**) Carrying stage; (**d**) Static stage.

2. Methods

2.1. Fatigue Evaluation Method

The process of automobile manual assembly is divided into three stages: the lifting stage, the carrying stage, and the static stage. Therefore, the appropriate ergonomic methods should be selected for these stages. The NIOSH 1991 (National Institute for Occupational Safety and Health) equation is selected for the lifting stage and the lifting index (LI) is used to represent the value of NIOSH 1991 [18,19]; Ovako Working Posture Analysis System (OWAS) is selected for the carrying stage, in order to reflect the effect of the quality of the object being handled on physical fatigue, a single digit was added to describe the weight to the three-digit version of OWAS proposed by Karhu et al. in 1977. The four digits are used for upper limb states, lower limb states, back states, and weight-bearing, respectively [20,21]; the Rapid Upper Limb Assessment (RULA) is selected for the static stage, which mainly involves the assembly details of the worker's upper limbs [22,23]. These three methods are commonly used in the assessment of the risk of musculoskeletal injuries, whereas incorrect posture and repetitive high-load work resulting in energy depletion and rapid physical fatigue are the key factors leading to musculoskeletal injuries, and therefore these three methods can be used to assess the physical fatigue.

To establish a quantitative method of physical fatigue for automobile manual assembly, it is first necessary to determine the weights of NIOSH, OWAS, and RULA. The entropy weight method is used to calculate the weight of the above three methods. The entropy weight method calculates weights based on objective data changes [24], which can avoid the limitations and constraints of subjective conditions brought about by the weights given by methods, such as the analytic hierarchy process, based on personal experience and subjective judgment of evaluation experts [25,26]. For the index x_i, the greater the difference between the values x_{ij} of the experimental data under the index, the greater the role of the index in the comprehensive evaluation [27]. Thus, the weights corresponding to NIOSH, OWAS, and RULA are, respectively w_1, w_2 and w_3.

Then, the values of NIOSH, OWAS, and RULA are normalized and the changes of these values are fixed at [0, 1] without changing the original distribution of the data. The formula is as follows,

$$r_{ij} = \frac{r'_{ij} - Min\left(r'_{ij}\right)}{Max\left(r'_{ij}\right) - Min\left(r'_{ij}\right)}, \quad (1)$$

Among them, r'_{ij} is the actual score during the experiment of NIOSH, OWAS, and RULA, and r_{ij} is the normalized result of this value.

On this basis, because fatigue is a dynamic and cumulative process over time, the time-weighted method is used to weigh the actual duration of the lifting stage, the carrying stage, and the static stage, so that the final quantitative value of fatigue is

$$e_j = \frac{\sum_{i=1}^{3} r_{ij} w_i t_i}{\sum_{i=1}^{3} t_i} \quad (2)$$

Among them, e_j is the fatigue quantification value corresponding to group j experiments. w_i (i = 1, 2, 3) is the weight values of three indexes: NIOSH, OWAS, and RULA, respectively, and t_i (i = 1, 2, 3) is the actual duration of the three stages in each group of experiments: lifting, carrying, and static stage. Therefore, the construction of the physical fatigue evaluation method for automobile manual assembly is completed.

2.2. Experimental Design

2.2.1. Experimental Hypothesis

The independent variables in this experiment are the seat weight and the height of the car body from the ground. The seat weights were, respectively 8 kg, 14 kg and 20 kg. The heights of the car bottom from the ground were selected as 15 cm and 45 cm. The dependent variable of the experiment was the level of physical fatigue of the manual assemblers. The level of physical fatigue is represented by three indicators, which are the difference of cerebral oxygen saturation, the value of physical fatigue evaluation method and metabolic energy expenditure. On this basis, the hypothesis of the experiment is that different seat weights and the height of the vehicle bottom from the ground have an effect on the level of physical fatigue.

2.2.2. Experimental Manual Assembly Task

All experiments were carried out in the morning to ensure the consistency of the participants' physical condition to a large extent, and each experiment was only performed once a day for each participant. The experimental site was in an ergonomic laboratory with good sound insulation to reduce the interference of external noise to participants. The laboratory was spacious and ventilated, with good lighting conditions and a suitable temperature to ensure the comfort and stability of the experimental environment. This experiment took the car seat assembly in the vehicle manual assembly as an example. The car seats were objects of equal quality, and the vehicle body was a virtual model displayed through the ARE platform. The distance between the seat and the vehicle body was kept consistent with the actual industrial site distance of 3 m. This experiment was an intra-group experiment, which was divided into 6 group experiments, with 3 participants in each group. First, participants needed to lift an object with the same weight as the seat at the starting point; then, the participants carried the object 3 m to the virtual vehicle body model; finally, they bent over to assemble the object into the correct position on the vehicle body, during which time their bodies remain static and only their hands can perform detailed operations for 10 s. The duration of each experiment was 30 min.

2.3. Apparatus and Platform

2.3.1. Cerebral Oximeter

The near-infrared tissue blood oxygen nondestructive monitor used in this experiment is wearable wireless oxygen saturation monitoring on the head (WORTH) (Figure 2a). The device is a wireless monitoring device independently developed by the Brain Network Group Research Center of the Institute of Automation, Chinese Academy of Sciences, which is founded in Beijing in 2017. A highly integrated central block is embedded in the device body, which includes an optical module, a microprocessor unit, a wireless communication module, and a power management module. Moreover, WORTH has the accuracy of recording cerebral oxygen saturation with an accuracy comparable to that of current clinically used cerebral oxygen monitors and has proved that it is effective during exercise tasks [28].

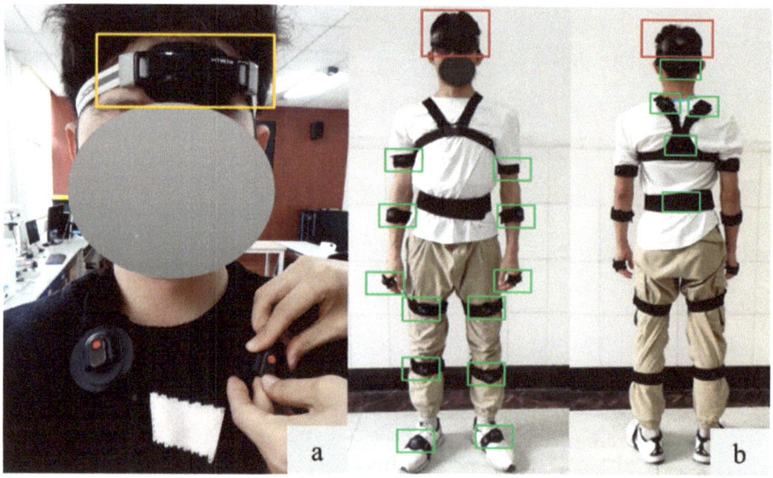

Figure 2. (**a**) Cerebral oximeter (yellow box); (**b**) Augmented reality devices (red box) and motion capture systems (green boxes).

2.3.2. Experiment Platform

The construction of the experimental environment and the calculation of ergonomic indexes (NIOSH, OWAS, RULA) were completed by the Augmented Reality (AR)-based Ergonomic Platform (ARE Platform) [29]. The ARE platform can put virtual manufacturing models in the physical environment based on the AR device, providing the participants with a semi-immersive working experience and retaining the constraints of the physical environment, thus completing the environment for fatigue experiments. Moreover, the ARE platform uses the motion capture system to collect a set of ergonomics indexes (NIOSH, OWAS, RULA), accessibility, and visibility verification data, which meets the real-time data required (NIOSH, OWAS, RULA) for the fatigue evaluation method. In addition, the accuracy of the ergonomics indexes provided by the ARE platform has been verified.

1. A commercial AR device Microsoft Hololens2 (Hololens2) (Figure 2b) is used for this platform. The total weight of Hololens2 is 566 g. The setup is equipped with four visible light cameras, two infrared cameras, a 1-MP time-of-flight depth sensor, and an inertial sensor. HoloLens2 can provide users with hand tracking, eye tracking, voice commands, spatial mapping, mixed reality capture, 6 degrees of freedom tracking, and other functions;
2. The motion capture system used in this platform is the Noitom Perception Neuron 3 (PN3) (Figure 2b), which can collect and process human posture data in real-time. PN3 includes 17 inertial sensors and the size of each inertial sensor is

27.9 × 16.2 × 11.6 mm, and the weight is 4.1 g, which makes users feel lighter and more flexible. It provides a data output frame rate of up to 60 Hz, and the static attitude accuracy is Roll/Pitch 1°, Yaw 2°. Moreover, PN3 connects the sensor data with computers through the Type-C interface, and the transmission delay is within 20 ms.

2.4. Participants

Three adult male participants were recruited to participate in this laboratory study (the seat assembly workers in the actual work site are men, so men were selected as subjects), and all participants were healthy without muscle strain. Participation was voluntary, with written consent, and anonymous. The ages of the participants ranged from 23 to 24 years (mean = 23.67 years), with average height and weight of 176.3 cm and 68.28 kg. Before the experiment, the participants were required to ensure adequate sleep, avoid any food and drugs that stimulate or inhibit the central nervous system, including coffee, alcohol, and tea, and avoid strenuous exercise. Before the start of the experiment, each participant was required to fully understand the entire experimental procedure, requirements, and testing methods, and to be proficient in the required work.

2.5. Outcome Measures

2.5.1. Cerebral Oxygen Saturation

Cerebral oxygen saturation was chosen to represent fatigue in the experiment because changes in cerebral blood oxygen saturation are closely related to the cerebral circulation. Disease or physical activity can affect cerebral circulation, thereby altering cerebral blood oxygen saturation [30]. During intense exercise, hyperventilation reduces the carbon dioxide tension in the arteries and slows blood flow to the brain, which can lead to insufficient oxygen delivery to the brain, leading to the development of fatigue [31]. And the lack of oxygen in the brain causes a decrease in the cerebral oxygen saturation. This experiment uses rSO_2 to represent fatigue, which is the weighted average of cerebral arterial, capillary, and venous oxygen saturation [32,33]. In actual monitoring, rSO_2 is generally defined as the percentage of oxygen carried by hemoglobin at the target monitoring point, and its formula is

$$rSO_2 = \frac{C_{HbO_2}}{C_{HbO_2} + C_{HbR}} \times 100\% \quad (3)$$

Among them, C_{HbO_2} is the concentration of oxyhemoglobin; C_{HbR} is the concentration of reduced hemoglobin, which refers to the content of the corresponding type of hemoglobin in the unit volume of blood.

The fluctuations of the cerebral oxygen saturation of the three participants in a calm state were detected many times, and the fluctuations of the cerebral oxygen saturation within 40 min were all between −0.5% and 0.5%. Therefore, it is assumed that the cerebral oxygen saturation did not change within 40 min of the three participants in a calm state.

2.5.2. Physical Fatigue Evaluation Method

Using PN3, 17 inertial sensors were placed at specific joints of the body (Figure 2b). After the human body pose was calibrated, the kinematics data were collected and transmitted to the ARE platform for processing. After participants began lifting objects, the NIOSH score and lifting time were recorded; in the carrying stage, the OWAS score and carrying time were recorded; in the static stage, the RULA score was recorded and the default duration was 10 s. After the experiment, the NIOSH, OWAS, and RULA scores recorded were processed with the entropy weight method to obtain their respective weights. Next, the NIOSH, OWAS, and RULA scores were normalized according to Formula (1). Finally, according to the actual experimental duration of the three stages, Formula (2) was used to get the final quantitative value of the physical fatigue in each experiment.

2.5.3. Jack MEE

The limitation of energy supply is the classic hypothesis of muscle fatigue, whereby energy deficit is an important factor in fatigue [34]. Tecnomatix Jack software, a module from the Siemens PLM digital factory portfolio, is a tool in the field of human factors reliability [35]. Tecnomatix Jack provides some advanced analysis tools for ergonomic analysis. Metabolic Energy Expenditure (MEE) is based on the defined human virtual model and divides typical tasks into 25 task behaviors such as lifting, carrying, sitting, standing, walking, and bending. On this basis, index parameters such as the working cycle time of the current task, specific working posture, and task load are set to predict the metabolic energy consumption of the current task.

Firstly, virtual human models were established in Tecnomatix Jack based on the height and weight of participants. On this basis, the proportion of each working posture was calculated according to the duration of different working postures in the experiment. The duration of each experiment was 30 min. According to the total number of times the participants performed under the conditions of different vehicle body heights and seat weights, the cycle time for completing a task can be calculated. According to the actual seat assembly workflow and the settings of this experiment, the lifting stage corresponds to the lifting task type in the MEE tool, the lifting stage corresponds to the handling task type in the MEE tool, and the static stage corresponds to the low position task type in the MEE tool. The energy consumption formulas of the working posture are as follows,

$$E_{pos} = K_{pos} \times T_{pos} \times W \tag{4}$$

$$E_T = \sum_{i=1,\ldots,n} E_i + E_{standing} + E_{sitting} + E_{benting} \tag{5}$$

Among them, K_{pos} represents the energy consumption coefficient of different working postures, T_{pos} represents the duration of the current posture, and W is the weight of the current operator. E_i is the energy consumption of each action, where i represents the specific number of the action sequence, and E_T represents the total energy consumption for completing the entire task.

2.6. Experimental Procedures

This experiment strictly followed the experimental ethics code, requiring participants to participate voluntarily after knowing the purpose of the experimental data. Firstly, participants practiced until they became familiar with the seat assembly process, with an average practice time of about 5 min. Then, they needed to wear the WORTH correctly for about 10 min and be in a calm state during this period, avoiding intense exercise or intense emotions to ensure the stability and accuracy of cerebral oxygen saturation data.

After taking off WORTH, participants needed to wear the PN3 motion capture system. They chose to use a strap of appropriate length to choose the position with the least amount of muscle to wear, and inserted PN3 sensors into the base of the strap to ensure that they would not fall off due to activities. Due to the variability of wearers and the inconsistency of each wearing part, it was necessary to calibrate participants' posture data. Then, participants put the HoloLens2 on the head and adjusted the knob on the back of the device to adjust the tightness to ensure that it was comfortable to wear and did not shake with the head movement. After wearing HoloLens2 participants could see the virtual vehicle body model placed 3 m away. First, participants lifted the seat equivalent of a specific weight (8 kg, 14 kg, 20 kg); secondly, they carried the equivalent and walked 3 m to the virtual vehicle body model; finally, they placed the object on a specific vehicle body height (15 cm, 45 cm), and simulated 10 s of static assembly operation, and repeated the above operation until the 30 min mark (Figure 3). The MEE tool in Tecnomatix Jack performs simulations that do not involve detailed operations of the upper limbs, therefore boxes with the same quality as the three weights of seats were chosen for the experiment, thus comparing the method proposed in this paper with the results of MEE tool in Tecnomatix Jack performs simulations.

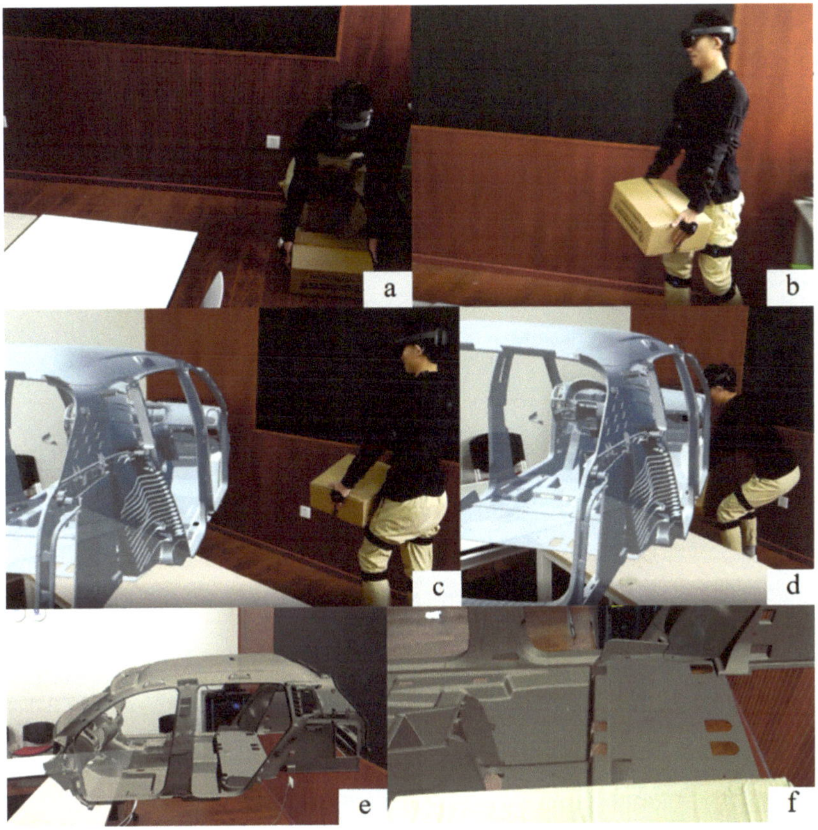

Figure 3. (**a**) Lifting start; (**b**) Lifting end; (**c**) Carrying stage; (**d**) Static stage; (**e**) First view of lifting end; (**f**) First view of static stage.

After the experiment was completed, participants took off the HoloLens2 and wore the WORTH again for about 10 min, and remained in a calm state within ten minutes, avoiding intense exercise or intense emotions. Then, they removed the WORTH and PN3 motion capture system.

2.7. Statistical Data Analysis

The dependent variable is the human physical fatigue level, which is represented by three indicators, which are the experimental results of the physical fatigue evaluation method and the difference of cerebral oxygen saturation. On this basis, the MEE simulation in Tecnomatix Jack was carried out for each group. Before the statistical analysis, the normality of the experimental results of physical fatigue evaluation method, the difference of cerebral oxygen saturation, and the simulation results of Jack MEE were tested by Shapiro–Wilk, and they all conformed to the normality. Then, the experimental results of the physical fatigue evaluation method, the difference of cerebral oxygen saturation, and the simulation results of Jack MEE were analyzed by two-way analysis of variance (ANOVA). The independent variables are (1) Seat weight: 8 kg, 14 kg, 20 kg, and (2) Vehicle body height: 15 cm, 45 cm. The statistical significance of ANOVA was $p \leq 0.05$, and if statistical significance was found, a Pearson correlation analysis was performed to further clarify the differences between techniques.

3. Results

3.1. Cerebral Oxygen Saturation

The rSO_2 of each participant was measured for 10 min by the WORTH before and after the experiment, and selected the stabilized data from the monitored values as the baseline data for the subjects. According to the rSO_2 difference after and before the experiment in 18 groups, the results are shown in Table 1 below.

Table 1. The change value of rSO_2 before and after the experiment.

Vehicle Body Height (cm) \ Seat Weight (kg)	8	14	20
15	−4.26% ± 0.5% −4.12% ± 0.5% −4.02% ± 0.5%	−9.92% ± 0.5% −9.92% ± 0.5% −9.9% ± 0.5%	−15.11% ± 0.5% −16.25% ± 0.5% −18.46% ± 0.5%
45	−2.57% ± 0.5% −2.34% ± 0.5% −2.63% ± 0.5%	−6.33% ± 0.5% −6.42% ± 0.5% −7.62% ± 0.5%	−12.89% ± 0.5% −13.04% ± 0.5% −15.58% ± 0.5%

According to the experimental hypothesis, the hypothesis made on the height of the vehicle body from the ground and the seat weight are as follows,

$\mathbf{H_{0A}}$: *Different vehicle body heights (15 cm, 45 cm) have no significant effect on the rSO_2 difference;*

$\mathbf{H_{1A}}$: *Different vehicle body heights (15 cm, 45 cm) have a significant impact on the rSO_2 difference.*

$\mathbf{H_{0B}}$: *Different seat weights (8 kg, 14 kg, 20 kg) have no significant effect on the rSO_2 difference;*

$\mathbf{H_{1B}}$: *Different seat weights (8 kg, 14 kg, 20 kg) have a significant impact on the rSO_2 difference.*

Therefore, the two-way ANOVA was performed on the data in Table 1, and the following are the analysis results. A two-way ANOVA demonstrated that the effect of vehicle body height was significant for rSO_2 difference, $F(1, 2) = 29.623$, $p < 0.001$. And the effect of seat weight was significant for rSO_2 difference, $F(2, 2) = 224.652$, $p < 0.001$.

3.2. Physical Fatigue Evaluation Method

Firstly, the entropy weight method was used to process the 18 groups of NIOSH, OWAS, and RULA scores collected during the experiment (as Table 2), to obtain the respective weights, as shown in Table 3 below.

Table 2. The value of NIOSH, OWAS, and RULA.

Experiment No.	Value of NIOSH	Value of OWAS	Value of RULA
1	0.46	1	6
2	0.59	1	6
3	0.43	1	6
4	1.1	3	6
5	1.28	3	6
6	0.93	3	7
7	1.88	3	5
8	2.01	3	6
9	2.51	4	7
10	0.59	1	3
11	0.42	1	4
12	0.51	1	4
13	0.9	2	4
14	0.95	3	4
15	0.87	3	4
16	1.83	3	4
17	1.94	3	4
18	2.18	3	5

Table 3. Weights of NIOSH, OWAS, and RULA.

Evaluation Method	Information Entropy Value e	Information Utility Value d	Weights (%)
NIOSH	0.854	0.146	40.616
OWAS	0.852	0.148	41.194
RULA	0.935	0.065	18.19

Then, the NIOSH, OWAS, and RULA values were normalized according to Formula (1). Finally, based on the specific duration data of the experiment and the Formula (2), the results obtained by the physical fatigue evaluation method are shown in Table 4. In order to ensure the accuracy of the subsequent comparison with the calculation results of the MEE tool, the calculation results of the physical fatigue evaluation method are not rounded.

Table 4. The results obtained by the physical fatigue evaluation method.

Seat Weight (kg) / Vehicle Body Height (cm)	8	14	20
15	0.010766997 0.011034003 0.01072171	0.019983377 0.020297028 0.020373405	0.020962028 0.022100687 0.027797152
45	0.008193415 0.008682337 0.008965525	0.014098114 0.01775242 0.017608327	0.020047302 0.020818436 0.020569058

According to the experimental hypothesis, the data in Table 3 were subjected to two-way ANOVA, and the results are as follows. A two-way ANOVA demonstrated that the effect of vehicle body height was significant for physical fatigue evaluation method results, F (1, 2) = 15.309, $p = 0.002$. And the effect of seat weight was significant for physical fatigue evaluation method results, F (2, 2) = 88.684, $p < 0.001$.

After that, a Pearson correlation analysis was used to analyze the correlation between the rSO_2 difference and the physical fatigue evaluation method results, and the correlation coefficient is obtained as shown in Table 5.

Table 5. Correlation analysis results of rSO_2 difference and physical fatigue evaluation method.

Variable	rSO_2 Difference	Physical Fatigue Evaluation Method Results
rSO_2 Difference	1 (<0.001)	−0.938 (<0.001)
Physical Fatigue Evaluation Method Results	−0.938 (<0.001)	1 (<0.001)

According to Table 4, we found a strong correlation between rSO_2 difference and physical fatigue evaluation method, r = −0.938, $p < 0.001$.

3.3. Jack MEE

After filling in the parameters such as task type and load in the MEE interface according to the experimental data, 18 sets of metabolic energy consumption (kcal) consumed by the experiment are shown in Table 6.

Table 6. The metabolic energy expenditure (kcal) in Tecnomatix Jack.

Seat Weight (kg) / Vehicle Body Height (cm)	8	14	20
15	1267.80 1295.80 1349.33	1575.37 1573.48 1747.11	1886.35 1870.81 1814.05
45	1215.47 1235.22 1190.07	1519.52 1537.95 1535.00	1867.15 1901.10 1691.50

According to the experimental hypothesis, the data in Table 5 were subjected to two-way ANOVA, and the results are as follows. A two-way ANOVA demonstrated that the effect of vehicle body height was significant for metabolic energy expenditure, F (1, 2) = 6.525, $p = 0.023 < 0.05$. And the effect of seat weight was significant for metabolic energy expenditure, F (2, 2) = 125.845, $p < 0.001$.

After that, a Pearson correlation analysis was used to analyze the correlation between the rSO_2 difference and metabolic energy expenditure, and the correlation coefficient is shown in Table 7.

Table 7. Correlation analysis results of rSO_2 difference and metabolic energy expenditure.

Variable	rSO_2 Difference	Jack MEE Results
rSO_2 Difference	1 (<0.001)	−0.924 (<0.001)
Jack MEE results	−0.924 (<0.001)	1 (<0.001)

According to Table 7, we found a strong correlation between rSO_2 difference and metabolic energy expenditure, r = −0.924, $p < 0.001$.

4. Discussion

This paper systematically studied the effects of different seat weights and vehicle heights from the ground on physical fatigue during the manual seat assembly. The main research results showed that when the vehicle height was 15 cm and the seat weight was 20 kg, the physical fatigue level was the highest. On the contrary, when the vehicle height was 45 cm and the seat weight was 8 kg, the physical fatigue level was the lowest. The cerebral oxygen saturation was used as the objective physiological signal for fatigue detection in the experiment, and the correlation between the proposed physical fatigue evaluation method and the rSO_2 difference was slightly higher than that between the metabolic energy expenditure in Jack and the rSO_2 difference, which means the proposed physical fatigue evaluation method is more accurate than the evaluation of metabolic energy consumption in Tecnomatix Jack (Figure 4). The horizontal axis presents the numbers of the eighteen sets of experiments, and the vertical coordinates are the normalized values of the three fatigue evaluation methods.

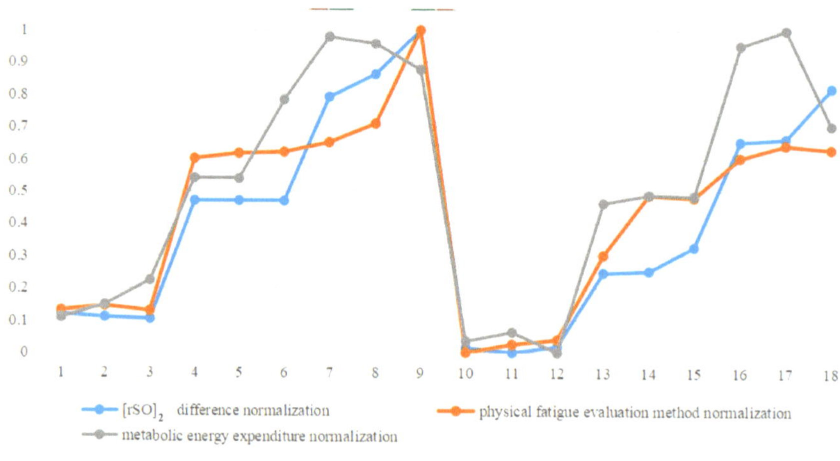

Figure 4. Normalization of rSO_2 difference, normalization of physical fatigue evaluation method, and that of metabolic energy expenditure in 18 groups of experimental trends comparison.

4.1. Cerebral Oxygen Saturation

According to Table 1, when the seat weight was 8 kg and 14 kg, the impact of the vehicle height on the rSO_2 difference was more obvious than when the seat weight was 20 kg. When the vehicle height was constant, the influence of different seat weights on the rSO_2 difference was obvious. In Table 2, the results of ANOVA between vehicle height and seat weight on rSO_2 difference can show that these two independent variables both have a significant impact on rSO_2 difference.

4.2. Physical Fatigue Evaluation Method

According to the weights of NIOSH, OWAS, and RULA in Table 3, the degree of variation in the scores of NIOSH and OWAS among the experiments was greater than that of RULA. It showed that the influence of the vehicle height on the results of the physical fatigue evaluation method was less significant than that of the seat weight. In the two-way ANOVA results in Table 5, the vehicle body height and seat weight were significant to the results of the physical fatigue evaluation method. However, the significance of vehicle height to the results of physical fatigue evaluation method was weaker than its significance to rSO_2 difference. It showed that the physical fatigue evaluation method was slightly less sensitive to the vehicle body height. In Table 6, the correlation coefficient between rSO_2 difference and the results of the physical fatigue evaluation method was −0.938, and the p value was less than 0.05, indicating that there was a strong correlation between rSO_2 difference and the physical fatigue evaluation method. Because rSO_2 difference can represent the level of human physical fatigue, the physical fatigue evaluation method can reflect human physical fatigue level to a large extent.

4.3. Jack MEE

The p value of the vehicle body height to the metabolic energy expenditure from Jack MEE was 0.023. The p value was less than 0.05, the vehicle body height had a significant impact on the Jack MEE simulation results, but compared with the rSO_2 difference and physical fatigue evaluation method, the significant impact was smaller. Obviously, the sensitivity of the Jack MEE simulation to the vehicle body height was lower than that of the cerebral oxygen saturation signal and the physical fatigue evaluation method. According to the Pearson correlation analysis results, it can be concluded that there was a strong correlation between the Jack MEE simulation results and the rSO_2 difference, while the correlation coefficient was −0.924. However, the correlation coefficient between the results of the physical fatigue evaluation method and the rSO_2 difference was −0.938, which was closer to −1 than the difference between metabolic energy expenditure and rSO_2. Therefore, the physical fatigue evaluation method, to a certain extent, can more accurately reflect the level of human physical fatigue than the metabolic energy expenditure prediction in Tecnomatix Jack, and was more sensitive in maintaining the height of posture in the static stage.

5. Conclusions

This paper conducts an in-depth study on the evaluation method of human physical fatigue, oriented by the practical problems in the manual assembly of automobiles. This paper divides the automobile manual assembly process into three stages: the lifting stage, the carrying stage, and the static stage, and uses NIOSH, OWAS, and RULA to analyze these stages, respectively. Moreover, the ARE platform provides an AR environment and the calculation of ergonomic indexes (NIOSH, OWAS, and RULA) for the experiment. On this basis, the entropy weight method and time weighting are used to process the experimental data to complete the physical fatigue evaluation method. And using the MEE tool in Tecnomatix Jack to simulate and predict the metabolic energy expenditure in the experiment. In this paper, the vehicle seat assembly in the auto manual assembly is taken as an example to carry out experiments. The independent variables are seat weight and vehicle body height from the ground, and the dependent variable is the human physical fatigue level. Eighteen groups of effective experiments have been completed. Finally, this paper conducts a Pearson correlation analysis on the physical fatigue evaluation method and the difference between cerebral oxygen saturation and metabolic energy expenditure in Tecnomatix Jack. The results prove that compared to the metabolic energy expenditure tool in Tecnomatix Jack, the physical fatigue evaluation method refines and summarizes the entire dynamic manual assembly process of automobiles to obtain a more accurate physical fatigue evaluation level, which is exactly the innovation of this article. This provides a new ergonomic solution for intelligent manufacturing and provides a reference and support for the future development direction of human fatigue evaluation. In recent years, more and more researchers have made new explorations in the direction of physical fatigue evaluation. Just as the method used in this paper, there are many cases of using wearable devices for fatigue evaluation, and most of them have also achieved good results [36–38]. The use of wearable devices has the advantages of high precision, high flexibility and high adaptability. In the future it may become the primary means of accurately assessing physical fatigue.

However, some aspects of the current research content of this paper still need to be further studied. In the current physical fatigue evaluation method, the worker's posture is approximated as a static action during the last stage of assembly. But in fact, the workers' fingers still perform assembly movements. Therefore, in future research, the upper limbs should be decomposed and analyzed in more detail to improve the accuracy of the fatigue evaluation method. Because the number of experiments in this study is limited, it is necessary to increase the number of experiments, further explore the characteristics of experimental data, and improve the accuracy of the fatigue evaluation method in future research, while enabling the Physical Fatigue Evaluation Method to give a specific fatigue level. Moreover, this paper does not discuss the impact of the load brought by AR to the experiment in the physical fatigue evaluation, so it can be studied in future research on fatigue evaluation in the AR environment.

Author Contributions: Conceptualization, W.M.; methodology, W.M.; investigation, Y.H.; resources, X.Y. and T.G.; data curation, X.Y., Y.H. and T.G.; writing—original draft preparation, W.M. and C.W.; writing—review and editing, W.M. and C.W. All authors have read and agreed to the published version of the manuscript.

Funding: This research was funded by the National Natural Science Foundation, grant number 52205513 and 52175451.

Institutional Review Board Statement: Ethical review and approval were waived for this study due to the non-invasive nature of the experiments in this study.

Informed Consent Statement: Informed consent was obtained from all subjects involved in the study.

Data Availability Statement: In the informed consent form filled out by the subjects before the start of the experiment, it was written "Only the research team will have access to the data". In order to protect the privacy of the subjects, we decided not to disclose the experimental data.

Acknowledgments: We express our sincere gratitude to National Key Laboratory of Special Vehicle Design and Manufacturing Integration Technology, item (GZ2022KF012).

Conflicts of Interest: The authors declare no conflict of interest.

References

1. Graham, R.B.; Agnew, M.J.; Stevenson, J.M. Effectiveness of an on-Body Lifting Aid at Reducing Low Back Physical Demands during an Automotive Assembly Task: Assessment of EMG Response and User Accetability. *Appl. Ergon.* **2009**, *40*, 936–942. [CrossRef]
2. Landau, K.; Rademacher, H.; Meschke, H.; Winter, G.; Schaub, K.; Grasmueck, M.; Moelbert, I.; Sommer, M.; Schulze, J. Musculoskeletal disorders in assembly jobs in the automotive industry with special reference to age management aspects. *Int. J. Ind. Ergon.* **2008**, *38*, 561–576. [CrossRef]
3. Russo, A.; Vojković, L.; Bojic, F.; Mulić, R. The Conditional Probability for Human Error Caused by Fatigue, Stress and Anxiety in Seafaring. *J. Mar. Sci. Eng.* **2022**, *10*, 1576. [CrossRef]

4. Abdous, M.-A.; Delorme, X.; Battini, D.; Sgarbossa, F.; Berger-Douce, S. Assembly Line Balancing Problem with Ergonomics: A New Fatigue and Recovery Model. *Int. J. Prod. Res.* **2023**, *61*, 693–706. [CrossRef]
5. Ament, W.; Verkerke, G.J. Exercise and fatigue. *Sports Med.* **2009**, *39*, 389–422. [CrossRef] [PubMed]
6. Andrea, M.; Lucia, V.; Gianluca, M.; Antonella, C.; Gabriele, M.; Elena, A.; Franca, D. Energy Expenditure and Oxygen Consumption During Activities of Daily Living in People with Multiple Sclerosis and Healthy Subjects: An Ecological Approach to Estimate Real-Life Fatigue and Fatigability. *Arch. Phys. Med. Rehabil.* **2021**, *102*, 1482–1489.
7. Felipe, D.; Filipe, M.C.; Israel, T. The effect of physical fatigue on the performance of soccer players: A systematic review. *PLoS ONE* **2022**, *17*, e0270099.
8. Garg, A.; Chaffin, D.B.; Herrin, G.D. Prediction of metabolic rates for manual materials handling jobs. *Am. Ind. Hyg. Assoc. J.* **1978**, *39*, 661–674. [CrossRef] [PubMed]
9. Sun, J.; Sun, R. Development of a biomathematical model for human alertness and fatigue risk assessment based on the concept of energy. *Ergonomics* **2022**, 1–16. [CrossRef]
10. Demirel, H.O.; Duffy, V.G. Applications of Digital Human Modeling in Industry. *Lect. Notes Comput. Sci.* **2007**, *4561*, 824–832.
11. Hovanec, M. Digital factory as a prerequisite for successful application in the area of ergonomics and human factor. *Theor. Issues Ergon. Sci.* **2017**, *18*, 35–45. [CrossRef]
12. Benjamin, D.H.; Edward, J.T.; Gregory, R.B. Functional Transcranial Doppler Ultrasound for Monitoring Cerebral Blood Flow. *J. Vis. Exp. JoVE* **2021**, *2021*, e62048.
13. Gumulak, R.; Lucanova, L.C.; Zibolen, M. Use of near-infrared spectroscopy (NIRS) in cerebral tissue oxygenation monitoring in neonates. *Biomed. Pap. Med. Fac. Univ. Palacky Olomouc. Czech Repub.* **2017**, *161*, 128–133. [CrossRef] [PubMed]
14. Lucas-Cuevas, A.G.; Quesada, J.I.P.; Pérezsoriano, P.; Llana-Belloch, S. Effects of the exercise in the cerebral blood flow and metabolism. A review (Article). *J. Hum. Sport Exerc.* **2015**, *10*, 150–160. [CrossRef]
15. Matsuura, C.; Gomes, P.S.C.; Haykowsky, M.; Bhambhani, Y. Cerebral and muscle oxygenation changes during static and dynamic knee extensions to voluntary fatigue in healthy men and women: A near infrared spectroscopy study. *Clin. Physiol. Funct. Imaging* **2011**, *31*, 114–123. [CrossRef] [PubMed]
16. Monroe, D.C.; Gist, N.H.; Freese, E.C.; O'Connor, P.J.; Mccully, K.K.; Dishman, R.K. Effects of sprint interval cycling on fatigue, energy, and cerebral oxygenation (Article). *Med. Sci. Sports Exerc.* **2016**, *48*, 615–624. [CrossRef]
17. Mikio, H.; Yusuke, S.; Hirohide, S.; Akio, F.; Katsumi, T.; Yoichi, K. Estimation of Cerebral Hemodynamics and Oxygenation During Various Intensities of Rowing Exercise: An NIRS Study. *Front. Physiol.* **2022**, *13*, 828357.
18. Waters, T.R.; Putz-Anderson, V.; Garg, A.; Fine, L.J. Revised NIOSH equation for the design and evaluation of manual lifting tasks. *Ergonomics* **1993**, *36*, 749–776. [CrossRef]
19. Chung, M.K.; Kee, D. Evaluation of lifting tasks frequently performed during fire brick manufacturing processes using NIOSH lifting equations. *Int. J. Ind. Ergon.* **2000**, *25*, 423–433. [CrossRef]
20. Karhu, O.; Kansi, P.; Kuorinka, I. Correcting working postures in industry: A practical method for analysis. *Appl. Ergon.* **1977**, *8*, 199–201. [CrossRef]
21. Lins, C.; Fudickar, S.; Hein, A. OWAS inter-rater reliability. *Appl. Ergon.* **2021**, *93*, 103357. [CrossRef]
22. McAtamney, L.; Corlett, E.N. RULA: A survey method for the investigation of work-related upper limb disorders. *Appl. Ergon.* **1993**, *24*, 91–99. [CrossRef] [PubMed]
23. Joshi, M.; Deshpande, V. Identification of indifferent posture zones in RULA by sensitivity analysis. *Int. J. Ind. Ergon.* **2021**, *83*, 103123. [CrossRef]
24. Teixeira, S.J.; Ferreira, J.J.; Wanke, P.; Moreira Antunes, J.J. Evaluation model of competitive and innovative tourism practices based on information entropy and alternative criteria weight. *Tour. Econ.* **2021**, *27*, 23–44. [CrossRef]
25. Kumar, R.; Bilga, P.S.; Singh, S. Multi objective optimization using different methods of assigning weights to energy consumption responses, surface roughness and material removal rate during rough turning operation (Article). *J. Clean. Prod.* **2017**, *164*, 45–57. [CrossRef]
26. Zhu, Y.; Tian, D.; Yan, F. Effectiveness of Entropy Weight Method in Decision-Making. *Math. Probl. Eng.* **2020**, *2020*, 1–5. [CrossRef]
27. Mukhametzyanov, I.Z. Specific character of objective methods for determining weights of criteria in mcdm problems: Entropy, critic, sd. *Oncol. Res.* **2021**, *28*, 76–105. [CrossRef]
28. Si, J.; Zhang, X.; Li, M.; Yu, J.; Zhang, Z.; He, Q.; Chen, S.; Zhu, L. Wearable wireless real-time cerebral oximeter for measuring regional cerebral oxygen saturation. *Sci. China Inf. Sci.* **2021**, *64*, 1–10. [CrossRef]
29. Mao, W.; Hu, Y.; Yang, X.; Ren, W.; Fang, H. ARE-Platform: An Augmented Reality-Based Ergonomic Evaluation Solution for Smart Manufacturing. *Int. J. Hum.-Comput. Interact.* **2023**, 1–16. [CrossRef]
30. Zhong, W.; Ji, Z.; Sun, C. A Review of Monitoring Methods for Cerebral Blood Oxygen Saturation. *Healthcare* **2021**, *9*, 1104. [CrossRef]
31. Nybo, L.; Rasmussen, P. Inadequate cerebral oxygen delivery and central fatigue during strenuous exercise. *Exerc. Sport Sci. Rev.* **2007**, *35*, 110–118. [CrossRef]
32. Wabnitz, H.; Hornberger, C. Approaches for calibration and validation of near-infrared optical methods for oxygenation monitoring. *Biomed. Tech.* **2018**, *63*, 537–546.

33. Cour, A.l.; Greisen, G.; Hyttel-Sorensen, S. In vivo validation of cerebral near-infrared spectroscopy: A review. *Neurophotonics* **2018**, *5*, 040901.
34. Sahlin, K.; Tonkonogi, M.; Söderlund, K. Energy supply and muscle fatigue in humans. *Acta Physiol. Scand.* **1998**, *162*, 261–266. [CrossRef]
35. Hovanec, M.; Korba, P.; Solc, M. Tecnomatix for successful application in the area of simulation manufacturing and ergonomics. *Proc. Int. Multidiscip. Sci. GeoConf. SGEM* **2015**, *4*, 347–352.
36. Marotta, L.; Scheltinga, B.L.; van Middelaar, R.; Bramer, W.M.; van Beijnum, B.J.F.; Reenalda, J.; Buurke, J.H. Accelerometer-Based Identification of Fatigue in the Lower Limbs during Cyclical Physical Exercise: A Systematic Review. *Sensors* **2022**, *22*, 3008. [CrossRef]
37. Tahir, A.; Bai, S.; Shen, M. A Wearable Multi-Modal Digital Upper Limb Assessment System for Automatic Musculoskeletal Risk Evaluation. *Sensors* **2023**, *23*, 4863. [CrossRef]
38. Toro, S.F.D.; Santos-Cuadros, S.; Olmeda, E.; Álvarez-Caldas, C.; Díaz, V.; San Román, J.L. Is the use of a low-cost sEMG sensor valid to measure muscle fatigue? *Sensors* **2019**, *19*, 3204. [CrossRef]

sensors

Article

A Concept of a Plug-In Simulator for Increasing the Effectiveness of Rescue Operators When Using Hydrostatically Driven Manipulators

Rafał Typiak

Faculty of Mechanical Engineering, Military University of Technology, 2 Gen. S. Kaliskiego Str., 00-908 Warsaw, Poland; rafal.typiak@wat.edu.pl

Abstract: The introduction of Unmanned Ground Vehicles (UGVs) into the field of rescue operations is an ongoing process. New tools, such as UGV platforms and dedicated manipulators, provide new opportunities but also come with a steep learning curve. The best way to familiarize operators with new solutions are hands-on courses but their deployment is limited, mostly due to high costs and limited equipment numbers. An alternative way is to use simulators, which from the software side, resemble video games. With the recent expansion of the video game engine industry, currently developed software becomes easier to produce and maintain. This paper tries to answer the question of whether it is possible to develop a highly accurate simulator of a rescue and IED manipulator using a commercially available game engine solution. Firstly, the paper describes different types of simulators for robots currently available. Next, it provides an in-depth description of a plug-in simulator concept. Afterward, an example of a hydrostatic manipulator arm and its virtual representation is described alongside validation and evaluation methodologies. Additionally, the paper provides a set of metrics for an example rescue scenario. Finally, the paper describes research conducted in order to validate the representation accuracy of the developed simulator.

Keywords: teleoperation; simulators; sensors

Citation: Typiak, R. A Concept of a Plug-In Simulator for Increasing the Effectiveness of Rescue Operators When Using Hydrostatically Driven Manipulators. *Sensors* **2024**, *24*, 1084. https://doi.org/10.3390/s24041084

Academic Editors: Calin Gheorghe Dan Neamtu, Radu Comes, Jing-Jing Fang and Dorin-Mircea Popovici

Received: 31 October 2023
Revised: 22 January 2024
Accepted: 22 January 2024
Published: 7 February 2024

1. Introduction

Unmanned Ground Vehicles (UGVs) are being more and more frequently used in demining and rescue scenarios. This is due to both the fact that these activities are often carried out in environments that are dangerous to humans, and the fact that the tools used in these cases are not adapted to be man-portable and man-operated [1–4]. This is a trend which will continue as we move closer and closer into machine-only autonomous rescue and demining operations. However, because of the complexity and the dynamic nature of such missions, we can still see a wide range of unmanned machines being deployed and operated remotely. This creates a need to train IED/EOD and rescue operators in order to increase the operational safety and effectiveness of unmanned units [5]. One of the methods to increase the number of possible training instances and reduce costs at the same time is the use of simulators [6,7]. Useful for training in a wide range of tasks, ranging from maintenance to manipulation, these solutions must use highly accurate virtual models in order to be effective [8,9]. The high level of model detail should cover both the robot's or UGV's base platform's structure and its kinematics, and the functionality of its tools/manipulators, with a wide range of control options like speed and torque control [10–12].

As teleoperation is the most commonly used mode for controlling UGVs in demining and rescue operations, these types of simulators should not only provide sensor data commonly found in real-world products, like torque or vision sensors, i.e., RGB and RGB-D cameras, but also additional information which may be beneficial from a training standpoint [13]. Less common, but more relevant from that perspective, especially as computation capabilities increase, is the possibility of having deformable environmental objects and terrain [14]. Conducted analyses have shown that there are several simulators which offer extensive use case possibilities [15–18]. A solution commonly used in research is the MuJoCo [19]. A demonstrated use case was the ability to use a gripper-hand manipulation to solve a Rubik's cube using a 24DOF robotic hand driven using tendons [20]. A different example could be the MuJoCo simulator which researchers have used to build and simulate robotic manipulators in order to check initial concepts [21] to then transition them into real-world systems [15,22–24]. The described simulator supports most of the functions required in mobile robots with the exception of inverse kinematics and path planning. For research related to the analysis of object collisions, Pybullet [25] is being widely used, especially in the dynamics of gripping [24], and for manipulation of deformable objects (e.g., fabric) [26]. Another possible solution would be Gazebo [25], which is mostly being used for research on manipulation robots [27,28]. While none of these studies rely on Gazebo to perform skillful manipulations, one study clearly extended the simulation to external algorithms to deal with non-rigid bodies. Gazebo provides a simulation environment with the necessary actuators and sensors to enable manipulation. It also provides the Robotic Operating System (ROS) support which provides forward and reverse kinematics packages as well as path and motion planning. Another possible solution is the CoppeliaSim. It is a robotics simulator with a range of user-centric features, including sensor and actuator models, as well as motion planning, and support for simple and inverse kinematics. PyRep was recently introduced as a Python toolkit for teaching robots. It has been used to manipulate, pick up, and place cubes with the Kinova robot arm [29]. While the above-mentioned simulators focus on manipulation tasks which are in the scope of this article, they mainly focus on the machine–environment interactions. It should be stated however, that it is not the only requirement for robot/UGV training simulators, and the focus should be placed mainly on the need to train operators with the Human Machine Interfaces (HMIs) they will inevitably have to use in order to carry out a rescue operation. Most of the previously mentioned solutions rely on consumer-grade controllers for operator input. While sometimes found in real-world solutions of certain robots, they lack the interaction levels a controller has with its control station, as it is being replaced by an interaction with an operation system of a PC.

The main aim of this work was to develop a simulator capable of accepting commands coming from a control station typically used when operating UGVs or robots for IED and rescue missions [2]. Additionally, emphasis has been placed on achieving a high level of accuracy when recreating a real-world robotic arm for IED missions. In order to do so, the robotic arm has been equipped with a sensor suite for special tracking. Alongside a proposed data mapping method, data recorded from those sensors have been used to recreate real-world behaviors of the robotic arm in the simulated environment and were also later used for accuracy validation of said model.

2. Materials and Methods

Studies have shown [30–33] that the increase of an operator's immersion yields better learning results when using simulators. In order to take advantage of this fact, this paper proposes a solution which would allow for a plug-in simulator operation with the ability to assess mission critical parameters by an outside observer as well as to log test data for future analysis and the operator's effectiveness tracking (Figure 1). The plug-in operation refers to the ability to connect an existing control station of a UGV to the simulator and to be able to send data between them just like it would happen during normal operation. Because of this, the system introduces a hardware/software component called a gateway. This device is meant to work bidirectionally and translate data between the communication protocol of the UGV and the simulator. To not disclose said protocols, the simulator offers an open communication protocol with the need for implementation of the gateway shifted to UGV manufacturers.

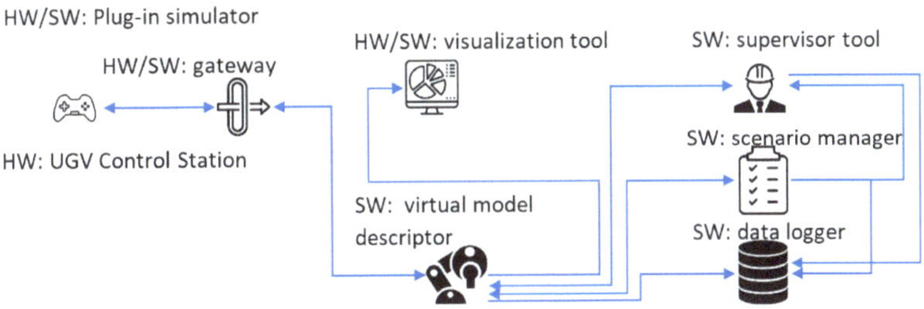

Figure 1. System structure of a plug-in simulator for rescue operations.

Within the simulator, data sent from the gateway is being processed by a software component called the virtual model descriptor. It is meant to house all the code used to model the simulated device and use it along with control signals to calculate its output state during simulation. That state is then sent to another software component called the scenario manager which houses all the virtual descriptions of objects taking part in the simulation. Its aim is to determine the ways in which the virtual model interacts with the environment on a scenario level. For example, if the scenario includes a person search and rescue operations, the object defined in the scenario manager may be a human model. Possible modifications to the model may include limb or body deformations, which the search and rescue operator should be able to detect prior to manipulations. A given set of parameters describing objects in the scene is then forwarded to another piece of software called the supervisor tool. The aim of this component is to provide the person supervising the training with sufficient data to enable performance assessment of the operator in real-time, and to help and guide him/her during testing, if needed. To do so, the supervisor tool is also able to access information from the virtual model descriptor. This allows to also measure the operator's level of familiarity with the controlled device. The next component included in the plug-in simulator is the visualization tool. It is meant to be used by the trainee to control the virtual model in order to interact with the environment. The main requirement for this module is that it needs to represent the virtual device's surroundings as accurately as possible. This covers both the hardware as well as the software side of things. The last piece of code running on the simulator is the data logger. Its aim is to record selected data for more in-depth analysis and post-mission assessment. That is why this component is receiving inputs from the virtual model descriptor, the scenario manager, and the supervisor tool.

2.1. Model Descriptor's and Supervisor Tool's Building Methodology

Testing methodology for the plug-in simulator consists of two main parts: the model's building methodology and the experiment's methodology. The first one describes the way the virtual model needs to be prepared to be able to be tested and the second one describes the way the model is going to be tested and how to process recorded data. The plug-in simulator assumes that the virtual representation and the real-world solution, which it is based upon, should resemble each other as closely as possible. This covers such aspects as kinematic description, manipulation functionalities, mechanical structure, physical dimensions, control scheme, and dynamic description. Because current robot development heavily relies on computer-based designs, developing all but the last two aspects is relatively easy. It is possible to export meshes of the robot's components to external formats and reimport them into the game engine. Then, using built-in functionalities, stitch them together the same way it is being performed in real-life. The more work-intensive part is related to the last two aspects: control scheme and dynamic description. The first one requires a process of mapping the gateway protocol with the model, while the second one requires the development of a component called Dynamic Model Description (DMD). The creation of a DMD is a 3-stage process. The first stage is the parameter identification phase, carried out on the real-world unit. Its goal is to acquire time domain-based reference position data in the time domain from the controlled device based on a set of discrete control signals for each of the device's functionality. An example of such an approach could be an IED/EOD manipulator arm (Figure 2). The data set should have twice the resolution of the control signal used to create the virtual model. The reason for it is that the unused datasets (every second datapoint in the dataset) will be used in the second (validation) stage. With the gathered data, an initial DMD can be developed ensuring that each joint can achieve the same movement speeds at the same positions in the time domain as its real-world counterpart. This creates a layered model for different control signal values. Its accuracy can be later increased by using approximation functions on each of the control signal speed and position datasets. For the purpose of this article, general polynomials have been assumed. By minimizing the approximation function using the sum of squared differences criterion, it is possible to obtain a continuous function of speed at certain rotational angles. To increase the DMD's accuracy, it is possible to run this scenario in both directions, going from the starting angle to maximum and back for each of the joints (Figure 2).

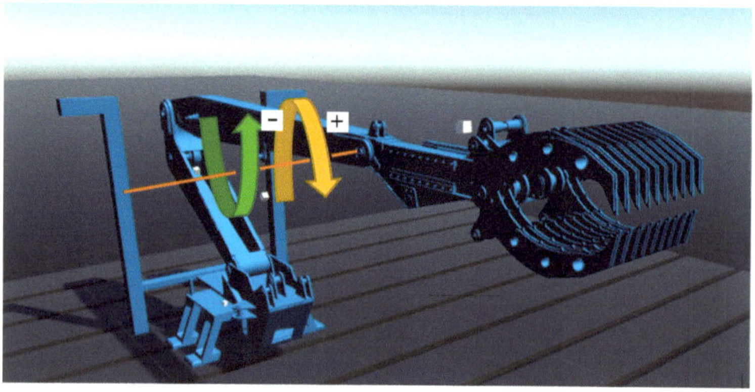

Figure 2. Testing angle directions used during the development of the DMD.

The above-described tasks should produce a layered DMD such as the one in Figure 3. While continuous for a set control signal, the DMD is still discrete in the control signal domain. In order to mitigate this problem, it has been assumed that a linear function would be calculated from two sets of known angular speeds for corresponding control signal values above and below the value currently generated by the operator. The output value is then proportional to the position of control signal value with relation to edge cases.

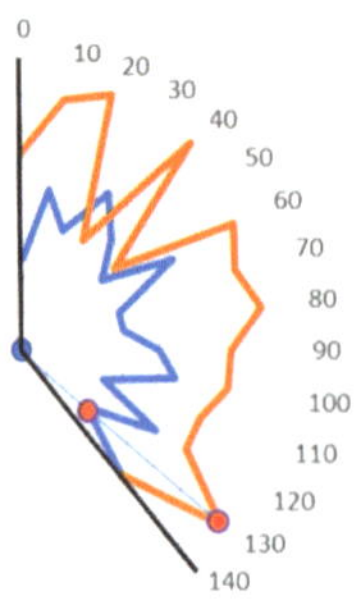

Figure 3. Visualization of the method for calculating angular joint speeds which are not covered by measured data. Colored lines represent speed values for consecutive, discrete control values. In order to calculate in between values, a line equation is being calculated based on two points from the known speed values, marked as red circles on the figure. The blue line symbolizes that line.

To generate data for the supervisor tool, the model needs to be configured in a way which enables data propagation between components. Table 1 lists the parameter types enabled for recording.

Table 1. Manipulator's parameter list.

ID	Name	Parameter Name	Type	Visualized	Recorded
1	Joint angle	jax_y	Float	No	Yes
2	Joint speed	jsx_y	Float	No	Yes
3	Joint collision	jcx_y	Bool	Possible	Yes
4	Object name per joint collision	onx_y_z	String	No	Yes
5	Joint movement start	tjmx_y_start	Bool	No	Yes
6	Joint movement stop	tjmx_y_stop	Bool	No	Yes
7	Joint maximum position overload	tjox_y_max	Bool	No	Yes
8	Joint minimum position overload	tjox_y_min	Bool	No	Yes
9	Time start	tstart	Long	Yes	Yes
10	Time end	tstop	Long	Yes	Yes

The same concept applies to the supervisor's tool. Table 2 shows the data made available by this component. The list differentiates between a body and an object.

Table 2. Environmental object parameter list.

ID	Name	Parameter Name	Type	Visualized	Recorded
1	Human body collision	h_{cx}	Bool	Possible	Yes
2	Human body maximum force in collision point	h_{cxf}	Float	No	Yes
3	Object collision	o_{cx}	bool	No	Yes
4	Object maximum force in collision point	o_{cxf}	Float	No	Yes
5	Maximum force on body without manipulator contact	h_{cxf_nm}	Float	No	Yes
6	Maximum force on object without manipulator contact	o_{cxf_nm}	Float	No	Yes

The testing phase covers not only the objective aspects of the rescue operation like precision of movement, equipment handling, and object handling, but also subjective ones. The reason for it is to measure the operator's response to the training process and determine if he is becoming more familiar with the scenario. This knowledge is then used to determine two basic factors: environmental familiarity and scenario fatigue.

Transferring the operator's control from a real-world solution to a simulated one introduces new stimuli for the operator. While a lot of care has been given toward a precise representation of the controlled object, the visual feedback the operator receives differs from what he will have to interact with. As such, there is a learning phase that needs to be carried out before the operator familiarizes himself with the simulator (environmental familiarity) and can start to learn behavioral responses which he will then be able to transfer over to the real world. The second aspect is scenario fatigue—it is a state where the operator knows all the specifics of a scenario and is becoming bored with it, which may introduce errors not present in real-world scenarios. In this case, a new scenario needs to be introduced to provide a new challenge and reintroduce uncertainty. For the above-mentioned purposes, two parameters were introduced that can be recorded: subjective accuracy and subjective situational awareness. The first one represents the operator's assessment on how good he was doing during the test. The second one allows to determine how well the operator thought he knew about what was going on around the controlled object during the test. This assessment needs to be carried out after the operator has finished the test and should be recorded alongside the objective parameters.

2.2. Data Evaluation

Data evaluation is a process that is being conducted both in real time and after the tests. Its aim is to compute an overall effectiveness score for the tested operator. This includes objective, measurable factors as well as subjective aspects of an operator's state and his or her perception of the completed task. The simulator uses a performance factor value to introduce a unified scoring system that has been described in detail in the author's thesis [34] as a performance indicator (PI) methodology for teleoperated unmanned ground systems. The main requirement of this method is having a reference dataset. The original implementation has used manned operated units for that purpose. With the plug-in simulator, there is a referencing initial stage for each of the tested operators. It needs to be stated that not all of the previously listed object and manipulator parameters are being used in the PI. The remaining ones are either used for post-test assessments or for additional processing. Calculation of the PI is described using the following Expression (1):

$$PI_x = \frac{t_{x\_ref}}{t_{x\_y}}(no_{col} + nb_{col} + no_{max} + no_{min} + s_a + s_{sa})k \tag{1}$$

where:

PI_x—performance indicator index;
t_{x_y} —test duration;
t_{x_ref}—reference test duration;
no_{col}—number of object collisions when the force exceeded max value;
nb_{col}—number of body collisions when the force exceeded max value;
no_{max}—number of overloads in the max direction;
no_{min}—number of overloads in the min direction;
s_a—subjective accuracy;
s_{sa}— subjective situational awareness;
k—completion indicator.

Test duration (t_{x_y}) is the timespan calculated from $\mathrm{t_{start}}$ and $\mathrm{t_{stop}}$. Reference test duration (t_{x_ref}) is calculated in a similar fashion but for the reference test phase. The completion indicator (k) is a 0 or 1 value given out per test by the supervisor via the supervisor tool. All the other components of the PI have certain weights attached to them. This was conducted in order to allow for higher testing flexibility if the operator is intended to focus more on a certain operational parameter. Setting these weight values is conducted freely, however, it needs to be recorded alongside the dataset. By default, the weight values per objective parameters equal 20 and per subjective 10. An example of this implementation is shown in (2).

$$no_{col} = 20 - 5\sum_{y=1}^{n} \mathrm{j_{cx\_y}} \tag{2}$$

It has been assumed that, for the purpose of this simulator, the maximum number of mistakes an operator can make equals 4. If he exceeds that number, the calculated component's value should not be calculated as being below 0, but instead, such state should result in an automatic test termination with a k factor equaling 0, unless the supervisor states otherwise.

2.3. Hydrostatic Arm Model

The plug-in simulator was created using the Unity game engine. The main reason for it was that it supports a robust physics engine, which is being used to calculate world interactions in real time [7]. Additionally, thanks to its target audience, it is relatively easy to develop HMIs for both the operator as well as the supervisor.

In order to create a virtual representation of a hydrostatically driven manipulator arm, 3D construction models were used for mesh implementation. Next, a set of joints were created. They are a configurable physical constraint which forces a certain type of relation between connected objects. For the purpose of the manipulator's definitions, joints were used both in a relation between the manipulator's segments (i.e., an arm, boom, or a gripper) as well as between an actuator and a segment (Figure 4). Due to their configurable nature, it is possible to change their settings during simulation, which allows for the development of complex relations.

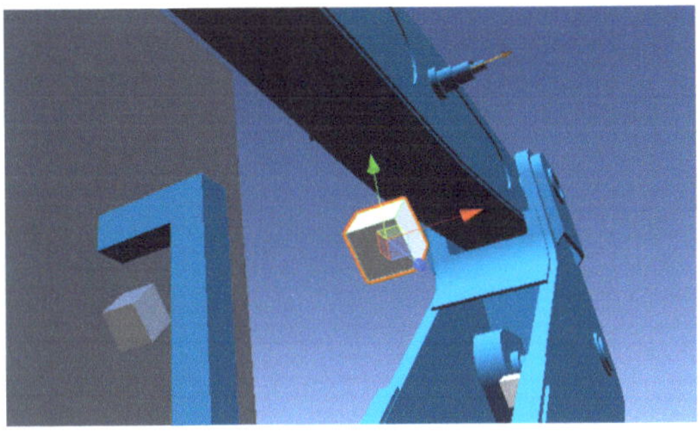

Figure 4. Hydraulic actuator's representation in the virtual model with an anchor point on the arm.

In order to enable world interactions, Unity uses constructs called colliders. They are a geometric representation used in physics calculations. It is separate from a mesh representation of an object because most of the time, the latter are too complex to allow for real-time computations. This does not mean that the manipulator's model has rudimentary collision detections. Figure 5 shows the number of basic colliders being used for the lower jaw of the recreated hydrostatic IED/EOD manipulator.

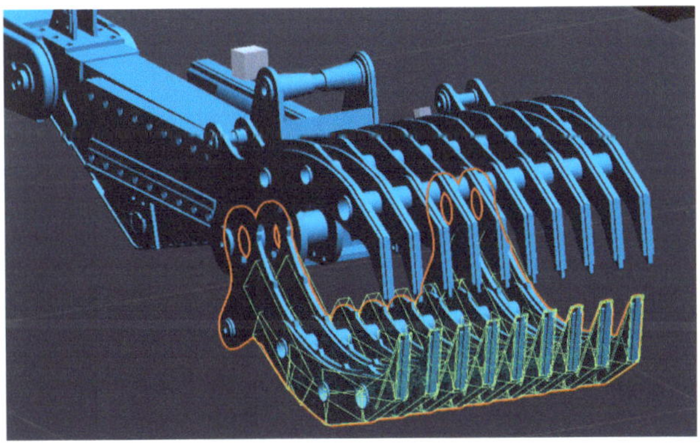

Figure 5. Structure of colliders on the manipulator's lower jaw.

The dataset for the simulator was gathered using absolute sensors (Figure 6a) connected to an input card. Gathered data (Figure 6b) were then processed to be used in the virtual model. Each manipulator segment's speed was registered for varying control signal levels from −250 to 250, with a 10-unit step. This value span is compliant with the J1939

CAN standard, which is normally used with digitally driven hydraulic valves, like the PVED-CC series spool valves from Danfoss. The simulator was created using 40-unit step increments, with the same signal-level range. This means that real-world angular speeds of each of the manipulator's segments were measured with valve control signals being: 0, 40, 80, 120, 160, 200, 250 and 0, −40, −80, −120, −160, −200, −250. In order to solve the problem of missing speed data for control signals in between consecutive control points (which correspond to the manipulator's arm speed), the linear approximation method described earlier in this article was used.

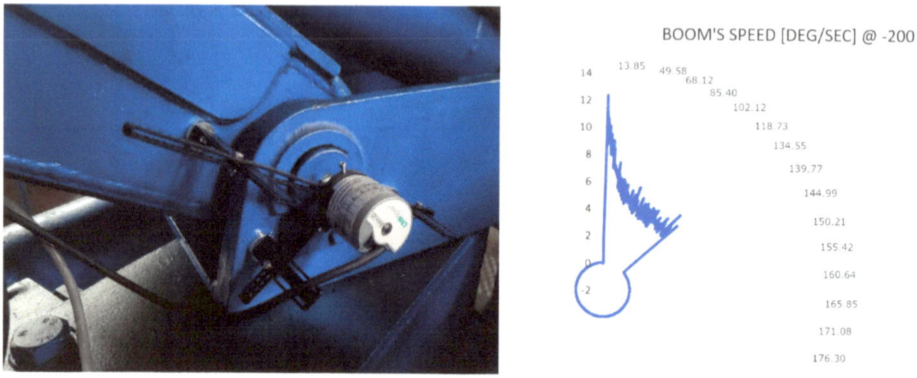

(**a**) (**b**)

Figure 6. Boom's speed identification: (**a**) Sensor setup and (**b**) Dataset for a control signal of "−200".

2.4. Simulator's Functionality

The main aspect of the developed simulator is its ability to interface with standard control stations. In Figure 7b, the solution presented is a CAN-bus-based UGV control panel, which is connected to the simulator PC using a specially developed CAN gateway. This solution acts as a translator between the proprietary control protocol and Windows API for HMI devices (used by the simulator).

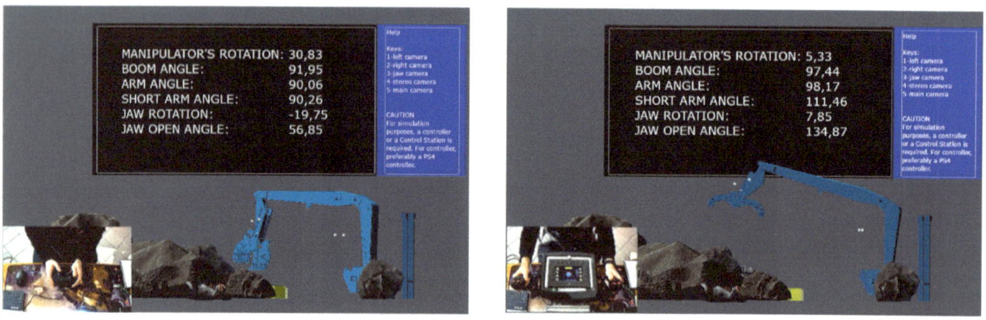

(**a**) (**b**)

Figure 7. Simulator view of an operator using a standard controller (**a**) and a plug-in control station (**b**).

The Unity-based simulator has the ability to utilize a wide range of objects to create complex scenarios. Figure 8 shows an example of a scene created for person retrieval tests.

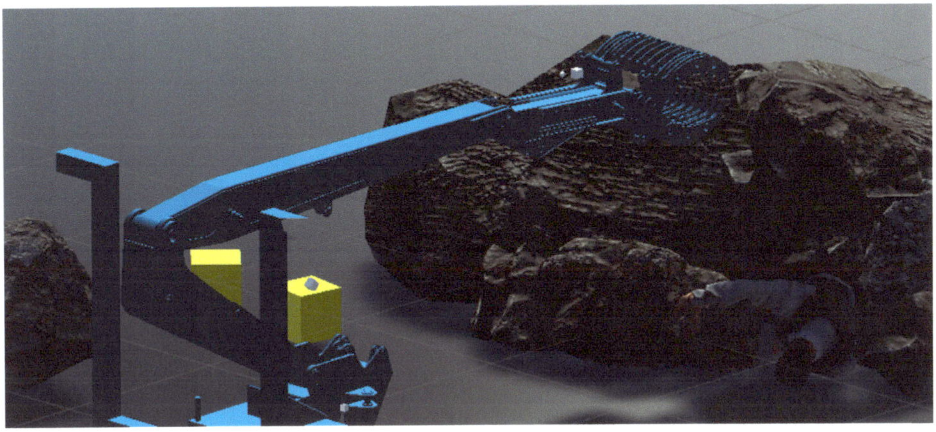

Figure 8. A rescue operation scenario created using the developed simulator.

As was the case with the manipulator, objects in the environment also possess physical traits, such as mass and dimensions. This is especially critical for interactions and assessing the operator's effectiveness. While it is possible to use mesh colliders for environmental objects, using it on humans is not efficient due to how the skeletal structure is being managed in Unity. Because of this, the use of multiple simple colliders was required (Figure 9).

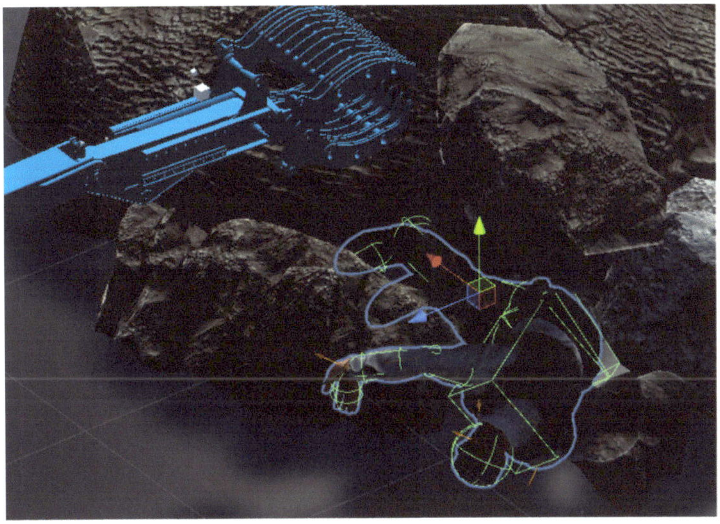

Figure 9. Collider structure of a male body model used for collisions during a rescue operation (green boxes and spheres).

The simulator's output is a timestamped file with all of the previously mentioned parameters logged for evaluation purposes. In order to automate the process of assessing and scoring the operators, a VBA script was developed which reads all the parameters, classifies them, and implements the evaluation methodology to produce an output Excel file with the final PI score as well as a score breakdown with regards to subjective and objective parameters. Additionally, a suggestion regarding the next aspect of the rescue scenario, where the operator needs to put more focus on, was generated.

3. Results

In order to determine the level of precision at which the virtual model represents the real-life solution, the following metrics were used: Mean Squared Error (MSE), Root Mean Squared Error (RMSE), and Mean Absolute Error (MAE).

The method of evaluating the developed simulator assumed additional real-world speed measurements were taken for each of the intermediate steps, with a constant increment of the control signal. This means that speed measurements for the following control signal groups were registered:

- 0, 20, 60, 100, 140, 180, 220.
- 0, −20, −60, −100, −140, −180, −220.

Afterward, each segment of the simulator was driven with the same control signal values and its angular speeds were measured. Later, both of these signal groups were compared using the previously mentioned metrics.

Table 3 presents the average values from each of the approximated levels for each of the manipulator's segments. Of note is the fact that the highest levels of average differences in speeds are observed for the simulator's boom segment and this trend persists for each consecutive segment. Several factors may be responsible for such an occurrence: approximation errors, simulator joint configuration, and weight differences between the model and the real-world unit. The last reason was considered the most probable because of the observed trend in MAE values. If it were the approximation errors, these values should not form a trend like that. It would be expected that they would remain somewhat constant between each segment. Joint configuration also does not provide a clear explanation as to why this trend is observed, but weight estimation errors could provide a reasonable explanation in that the simulation model stacks all the stack segments of a kinematic chain starting from the one being controlled. As such, if there would be a weight calculation error (said calculations were conducted using CAD designs and selected material information), that weight difference would affect each segment independently but would be summed when trying to move a stack of segments, rather than just one (i.e., jaws).

Table 3. Error table for each of the manipulator's segments.

Manipulator Segment	MAE	MSE	RMSE
Boom	0.0589	0.0006	0.0244
Arm	0.0530	0.0004	0.0220
Long arm	0.0424	0.0003	0.0154
Short arm	0.0381	0.0003	0.0123
Jaws	0.0343	0.0002	0.0111

The maximum average residual variance levels of angular speeds of 0.0589 deg/s allow to determine that the simulator is not generating speeds which would produce unexpected results for the operator controlling it. It should be noted that the maximum speed errors obtained were for the Boom segment, with the highest control signal levels of 220 and equated to less than 0.1 deg/s (Table 4). This signal has produced an error of approx. 1.9% with the average Boom speed for that control signal being 5.048 deg/s.

Table 4. MAE values per control signal value for the Boom segment of the simulator.

Control signal	20	60	100	140	180
MAE	0.0445	0.0424	0.0554	0.0665	0.0795
Control signal	−20	−60	−100	−140	−180
MAE	0.0401	0.0386	0.0406	0.0611	0.0694

The deviation levels, when compared to registered results, can be considered low, with a maximum value of 0.0244. This provides a stable foundation for a thesis, that the proposed method of transcribing real-world speed values onto a virtual model can be used without the model behaving "alien" or somehow "off" to the operator.

4. Conclusions

The plug-in simulator presented in this paper is a complete solution for the evaluating and training of rescue personnel in unmanned machine operation. By using existing control stations, it is possible for the operators to familiarize themselves with the HMI layout and control behaviors. The machine's model implemented in the simulator strives to provide an accurate representation of its real-world counterpart through the use of functional identity, dynamic response levels, mechanical constraints, and environmental interactions. Additionally, an ever-growing repository of external objects allows for building complex scenarios with multiple factors and conditions being introduced. This is largely due to the usage of a commercially available Unity game engine. The research presented in this paper show that it is possible to create a fully functional plug-in simulator solution, which aims at faithfully representing the mechanical and dynamic aspects of the real-world unit.

Funding: This research was funded by Military University of Technology, grant number UGB 708/2024.

Institutional Review Board Statement: Not applicable.

Informed Consent Statement: Not applicable.

Data Availability Statement: The data presented in this study are available on request from the author. Certain data may have share restrictions due to parts of the software being used in actions with restricted access.

Conflicts of Interest: The author declares no conflicts of interest.

References

1. Amit, D.; Neel, S.; Pranali, A.; Sayali, K. Fire Fighter Robot with Deep Learning and Machine Vision. *Neural Comput. Appl.* **2021**, *34*, 2831–2839.
2. Bishop, R. A survey of intelligent vehicle applications worldwide. In Proceedings of the IEEE Intelligent Vehicles Symposium 2000 (Cat. No. 00TH8511), Dearborn, MI, USA, 5 October 2000; IEEE: Piscataway, NJ, USA, 2000; pp. 25–30.
3. Giuseppe, Q.; Paride, C. Rese_Q: UGV for Rescue Tasks Functional Design. In Proceedings of the ASME 2018 International Mechanical Engineering Congress and Exposition, Pittsburgh, PA, USA, 9–15 November 2018. Volume 4A: Dynamics, Vibration, and Control.
4. Halder, S.; Afsari, K. Robots in Inspection and Monitoring of Buildings and Infrastructure: A Systematic Review. *Appl. Sci.* **2023**, *13*, 2304. [CrossRef]
5. Mao, Z.; Yan, Y.; Wu, J.; Hajjar, J.F.; Padlr, T. Towards Automated Post-Disaster Damage Assessment of Critical Infrastructure with Small Unmanned Aircraft Systems. In Proceedings of the 2018 IEEE International Symposium on Technologies for Homeland Security (HST), Woburn, MA, USA, 23–24 October 2018.
6. Martirosov, S.; Hořejší, P.; Kopeček, P.; Bureš, M.; Šimon, M. The Effect of Training in Virtual Reality on the Precision of Hand Movements. *Appl. Sci.* **2021**, *11*, 8064. [CrossRef]
7. Shi, X.; Yang, S.; Ye, Z. Development of a Unity–VISSIM Co-Simulation Platform to Study Interactive Driving Behavior. *Systems* **2023**, *11*, 269. [CrossRef]
8. De Luca, A.; Siciliano, B. Closed-form dynamic model of planar multilink lightweight robots. *IEEE Trans. Syst. Man Cybern.* **1991**, *21*, 826–839. [CrossRef]
9. Giorgio, I.; Del Vescovo, D. Energy-based trajectory tracking and vibration control for multi-link highly flexible manipulators. *Math. Mech. Complex Syst.* **2019**, *7*, 159–174. [CrossRef]
10. Kim, P.; Park, J.; Cho, Y.K.; Kang, J. UAV-Assisted Autonomous Mobile Robot Navigation for as-Is 3D Data Collection and Registration in Cluttered Environments. *Autom. Constr.* **2019**, *106*, 102918. [CrossRef]
11. Stampa, M.; Jahn, U.; Fruhner, D.; Streckert, T.; Röhrig, C. Scenario and system concept for a firefighting UAV-UGV team. In Proceedings of the 2022 Sixth IEEE International Conference on Robotic Computing (IRC), Naples, Italy, 5–7 December 2022.
12. Szrek, J.; Jakubiak, J.; Zimroz, R. A Mobile Robot-Based System for Automatic Inspection of Belt Conveyors in Mining Industry. *Energies* **2022**, *15*, 327. [CrossRef]
13. Zhu, S.; Xiong, G.; Chen, H.; Gong, J. Guidance Point Generation-Based Cooperative UGV Teleoperation in Unstructured Environment. *Sensors* **2021**, *21*, 2323. [CrossRef] [PubMed]

14. Va, H.; Choi, M.-H.; Hong, M. Efficient Simulation of Volumetric Deformable Objects in Unity3D: GPU-Accelerated Position-Based Dynamics. *Electronics* **2023**, *12*, 2229. [CrossRef]
15. Mahler, J.; Goldberg, K. Learning deep policies for robot bin picking by simulating robust grasping sequences. *Proc. Mach. Learn. Res.* **2017**, *78*, 515–524. Available online: http://proceedings.mlr.press/v78/mahler17a.html (accessed on 21 January 2024).
16. Mora-Soto, M.E.; Maldonado-Romo, J.; Rodríguez-Molina, A.; Aldape-Pérez, M. Building a Realistic Virtual Simulator for Unmanned Aerial Vehicle Teleoperation. *Appl. Sci.* **2021**, *11*, 12018. [CrossRef]
17. Nuaimi, A.; Ali, F.; Zeddoug, J.; Nasreddine, B.A. Real-time Control of UGV Robot in Gazebo Simulator using P300-based Brain-Computer Interface. In Proceedings of the 2022 IEEE International Conference on Bioinformatics and Biomedicine (BIBM), Las Vegas, NV, USA, 6–8 December 2022.
18. Sánchez, M.; Morales, J.; Martínez, J.L. Reinforcement and Curriculum Learning for Off-Road Navigation of an UGV with a 3D LiDAR. *Sensors* **2023**, *23*, 3239. [CrossRef] [PubMed]
19. Todorov, E.; Erez, T.; Tassa, Y. MuJoCo: A physics engine for model-based control. In Proceedings of the 2012 IEEE/RSJ International Conference on Intelligent Robots and Systems, Vilamoura-Algarve, Portugal, 7–12 October 2012; pp. 5026–5033.
20. Akkaya, I.; Andrychowicz, M.; Chociej, M.; Litwin, M.; McGrew, B.; Petron, A.; Paino, A.; Plappert, M.; Powell, G.; Ribas, R.; et al. Solving Rubik's cube with a robot hand. *arXiv* **2019**, arXiv:1910.07113. Available online: http://arxiv.org/abs/1910.07113 (accessed on 21 January 2024).
21. Pathak, D.; Gandhi, D.; Gupta, A. Self-supervised exploration via disagreement. *Proc. Mach. Learn. Res.* **2019**, *97*, 5062–5071. Available online: http://proceedings.mlr.press/v97/pathak19a.html (accessed on 21 January 2024).
22. Christiano, P.; Shah, Z.; Mordatch, I.; Schneider, J.; Blackwell, T.; Tobin, J.; Abbeel, P.; Zaremba, W. Transfer from simulation to real-world through learning deep inverse dynamics. *arXiv* **2016**, arXiv:1610.03518. Available online: http://arxiv.org/abs/1610.03518 (accessed on 21 January 2024).
23. Rusu, A.A.; Večerík, M.; Rothörl, T.; Heess, N.; Pascanu, R.; Hadsell, R. Sim-to-real robot learning from pixels with progressive nets. *Proc. Mach. Learn. Res.* **2017**, *78*, 262–270. Available online: http://proceedings.mlr.press/v78/rusu17a.html (accessed on 21 January 2024).
24. Tobin, J.; Fong, R.; Ray, A.; Schneider, J.; Zaremba, W.; Abbeel, P. Domain randomization for transferring deep neural networks from simulation to the realworld. In Proceedings of the 2017 IEEE/RSJ International Conference on Intelligent Robots and Systems (IROS), Vancouver, BC, Canada, 24–28 September 2017; pp. 23–30.
25. Koenig, N.; Howard, A. Design and use paradigms for Gazebo, an opensource multi-robot simulator. *IEEE/RSJ Int. Conf. Intell. Robot. Syst.* **2004**, *3*, 2149–2154. Available online: http://ieeexplore.ieee.org/document/1389727 (accessed on 21 January 2024).
26. Matas, J.; James, S.; Davison, A.J. Sim-to-real reinforcement learning for deformable object manipulation. *arXiv* **2018**, arXiv:1806.07851. Available online: http://arxiv.org/abs/1806.07851 (accessed on 21 January 2024).
27. Jin, H.; Chen, Q.; Chen, Z.; Hu, Y.; Zhang, J. Multi-LeapMotion sensor based demonstration for robotic refine tabletop object manipulation task. *CAAI Trans. Intell. Technol.* **2016**, *1*, 104–113. Available online: http://www.sciencedirect.com/science/article/pii/S2468232216000111 (accessed on 21 January 2024). [CrossRef]
28. Kunze, L.; Beetz, M. Envisioning the qualitative effects of robot manipulation actions using simulation-based projections. *Artif. Intell.* **2017**, *247*, 352–380. Available online: http://www.sciencedirect.com/science/article/pii/S0004370214001544 (accessed on 21 January 2024). [CrossRef]
29. James, S.; Davison, A.J.; Johns, E. Transferring end-to-end visuomotor control from simulation to real-world for a multi-stage task. *Proc. Mach. Learn. Res.* **2017**, *78*, 334–343. Available online: http://proceedings.mlr.press/v78/james17a.html (accessed on 21 January 2024).
30. Alexander, A.L.; Brunyé, T.; Sidman, J.; Weil, S.A. *From Gaming to Training: A Review of Studies on Fidelity, Immersion, Presence, and Buy-in and Their Effects on Transfer in Pc-Based Simulations and Games, DARWARS Training Impact Group*; Aptima Inc.: Woburn, MA, USA, 2005; Volume 5, pp. 1–14.
31. Aline, M.; Torchelsen, R.; Nedel, L. The effects of VR in training simulators: Exploring perception and knowledge gain. *Comput. Graph.* **2022**, *102*, 402–412.
32. Coulter, R.; Saland, L.; Caudell, T.; Goldsmith, T.E.; Alverson, D. The effect of degree of immersion upon learning performance in virtual reality simulations for medical education. In *Medicine Meets Virtual Reality*; IOS Press: Amsterdam, The Netherlands, 2007; Volume 15, p. 155.
33. Salman, N.; Colombo, S.; Manca, D. Testing and analyzing different training methods for industrial operators: An experimental approach. *Comput. Aided Chem. Eng.* **2013**, *32*, 667–672. Available online: https://www.sciencedirect.com/science/article/pii/B9780444632340501123 (accessed on 21 January 2024).
34. Typiak, R. Wpływ Konfiguracji Układu Akwizycji Obrazu na Sterowanie Bezzałogową Platformą Lądową. Ph.D. Thesis, Wojskowa Akademia Techniczna, Warsaw, Poland, 2017.

MDPI AG
Grosspeteranlage 5
4052 Basel
Switzerland
Tel.: +41 61 683 77 34

MDPI Books Editorial Office
E-mail: books@mdpi.com
www.mdpi.com/books

www.ingramcontent.com/pod-product-compliance
Lightning Source LLC
Chambersburg PA
CBHW041430210926
51850CB00013B/3397

* 9 7 8 3 7 2 5 8 4 1 3 9 4 *